Lecture Notes in Compute

Edited by G. Goos, J. Hartmanis and

Springer
Berlin
Heidelberg
New York
Barcelona
Hong Kong
London
Milan
Paris
Tokyo

Mário Figueiredo   Josiane Zerubia
Anil K. Jain (Eds.)

Energy Minimization Methods
in Computer Vision
and Pattern Recognition

Third International Workshop, EMMCVPR 2001
Sophia Antipolis, France, September 3-5, 2001
Proceedings

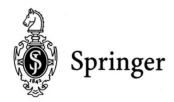

Springer

Series Editors

Gerhard Goos, Karlsruhe University, Germany
Juris Hartmanis, Cornell University, NY, USA
Jan van Leeuwen, Utrecht University, The Netherlands

Volume Editors

Mário Figueiredo
Instituto de Telecomunicacoes and Instituto Superior Tecnico
1049-001 Lisboa, Portugal
E-mail: mtf@lx.it.pt

Josiane Zerubia
INRIA, 2004 Route des Lucioles
06902 Sophia-Antipolis cedex, France
E-mail: Josiane.Zerubia@sophia.inria.fr

Anil K. Jain
Michigan State University, Department of Computer Science and Engineering
East Lansing, MI 48824, USA
E-mail: jain@cse.msu.edu

Cataloging-in-Publication Data applied for

Die Deutsche Bibliothek - CIP-Einheitsaufnahme

Energy minimization methods in computer vision and pattern recognition :
third international workshop ; proceedings / EMMCVPR 2001, Sophia Antipolis,
France, September 3 - 5, 2001 / Mário Figueiredo ... (ed.). - Berlin ; Heidelberg ;
New York ; Barcelona ; Hong Kong ; London ; Milan ; Paris ; Tokyo : Springer, 2001
  (Lecture notes in computer science ; Vol. 2134)
  ISBN 3-540-42523-3

CR Subject Classification (1998): I.4, I.5, I.2.10, I.3.5, F.2.2, F.1.1

ISSN 0302-9743
ISBN 3-540-42523-3 Springer-Verlag Berlin Heidelberg New York

Springer-Verlag Berlin Heidelberg New York
a member of BertelsmannSpringer Science+Business Media GmbH

http://www.springer.de

© Springer-Verlag Berlin Heidelberg 2001
Printed in Germany

Typesetting: Camera-ready by author, data conversion by Olgun Computergrafik
Printed on acid-free paper   SPIN 10840101   06/3142   5 4 3 2 1 0

Preface

This volume consists of the 42 papers presented at the International Workshop on Energy Minimization Methods in Computer Vision and Pattern Recognition (EMMCVPR 2001), which was held at INRIA (*Institut National de Recherche en Informatique et en Automatique*) in Sophia Antipolis, France, from September 3 through September 5, 2001. This workshop is the third of a series, which was started with EMMCVPR'97, held in Venice in May 1997, and continued with EMMCVR'99, which took place in York, in July 1999.

Minimization problems and optimization methods permeate computer vision (CV), pattern recognition (PR), and many other fields of machine intelligence. The aim of the EMMCVPR workshops is to bring together people with research interests in this interdisciplinary topic. Although the subject is traditionally well represented at major international conferences on CV and PR, the EMMCVPR workshops provide a forum where researchers can report their recent work and engage in more informal discussions.

We received 70 submissions from 23 countries, which were reviewed by the members of the program committee. Based on the reviews, 24 papers were accepted for oral presentation and 18 for poster presentation. In this volume, no distinction is made between papers that were presented orally or as posters. The book is organized into five sections, whose topics coincide with the five sessions of the workshop: "Probabilistic Models and Estimation", "Image Modelling and Synthesis", "Clustering, Grouping, and Segmentation", "Optimization and Graphs", and "Shapes, Curves, Surfaces, and Templates".

In addition to the contributed presentations, EMMCVPR 2001 had the privilege of including keynote talks by three distinguished scientists in the field: Donald Geman, Geoffrey Hinton, and David Mumford. These invited speakers have played seminal roles in the development of modern computer vision and pattern recognition, and continue to be involved in cutting-edge research.

We would like to thank a number of people who have helped us in making EMMCVPR 2001 a successful workshop. We thank Marcello Pelillo and Edwin Hancock for allowing us to take care of the EMMCVPR series, which they started, and for the important advice that made our organizational tasks easier. We also want to acknowledge all the program committee members for carefully reviewing papers for EMMCVPR.

Finally, we thank the various organizations that have provided support for EMMCVPR: the International Association for Pattern Recognition, who sponsored the workshop and provided publicity, the INRIA Sophia Antipolis, who hosted the workshop and provided financial support.

June 2001   Mário Figueiredo, Josiane Zerubia, and Anil K. Jain

Organization

Program Co-Chairs

Mário Figueiredo   Instituto Superior Técnico, Lisboa, Portugal
Josiane Zerubia   INRIA Sophia Antipolis, France
Anil K. Jain   Michigan State University, East Lansing, MI, USA

Program Commitee

Yali Amit   University of Chicago, USA
Joachim Buhmann   University of Bonn, Germany
Roland Chin   University of Science and Technology, Hong Kong
Byron Dom   IBM Almaden Research Center, USA
Marie Pierre Dubuisson-Jolly   Siemens Corp. Research, USA
Davi Geiger   New York University, USA
Christine Graffigne   Université René Descartes, France
Edwin Hancock   University of York, UK
Tin Ho   Bell Laboratories, USA
Kanti Mardia   University of Leeds, UK
Marcello Pelillo   University of Venice, Italy
Eugene Pechersky   Institute of Information Transmission Problems, Russia
Anand Rangarajan   Yale University, USA
Kaleem Siddiqi   McGill University, Canada
Richard Szeliski   Microsoft Research, USA
Alan Yuille   Smith-Kettlewell Eye Research Institute, USA
Ramin Zabih   Cornell University, USA
Song-Chun Zhu   Ohio State University, USA

Sponsoring Institutions

INRIA Sophia Antipolis
International Association for Pattern Recognition
Conseil General des Alpes-Maritimes

Table of Contents

III   Clustering, Grouping, and Segmentation

IV   Optimization and Graphs

V   Shapes, Curves, Surfaces, and Templates

Part I

Probabilistic Models and Estimation

A Double-Loop Algorithm
to Minimize the Bethe Free Energy

Alan Yuille

Smith Kettlewell Eye Research Institute, San Francisco CA 94965, USA
`yuille@ski.org`

Abstract. Recent work (Yedidia, Freeman, Weiss [22]) has shown that stable points of belief propagation (BP) algorithms [12] for graphs with loops correspond to extrema of the Bethe free energy [3]. These BP algorithms have been used to obtain good solutions to problems for which alternative algorithms fail to work [4], [5], [10] [11]. In this paper we introduce a discrete iterative algorithm which we prove is guaranteed to converge to a minimum of the Bethe free energy. We call this the double-loop algorithm because it contains an inner and an outer loop. The algorithm is developed by decomposing the free energy into a convex part and a concave part, see [25], and extends a class of mean field theory algorithms developed by [7],[8] and, in particular, [13]. Moreover, the double-loop algorithm is formally very similar to BP which may help understand when BP converges. In related work [24] we extend this work to the more general Kikuchi approximation [3] which includes the Bethe free energy as a special case. It is anticipated that these double-loop algorithms will be useful for solving optimization problems in computer vision and other applications.

1 Introduction

Local belief propagation (BP) algorithms [12] have long been known to converge to the correct marginal probabilities for tree-like graphical models. Recently, several researchers have empirically demonstrated that BP algorithms often perform surprisingly well for graphs with loops [4], [5], [10] [11] and, in particular, for practical applications such as learning low level vision [4] and turbo decoding [10]. (See [11], however, for examples where BP algorithms fail). It is important to understand when and why BP, and related algorithms, perform well on graphs with loops.

More recently Yedidia, Freeman and Weiss [22] proved that the stable fixed points of BP algorithms correspond to extrema of the Bethe free energy [3]. Therefore if a BP algorithm converges it must go to an extremum (i.e. maximum, minimum, or saddle point) of the Bethe free energy (and empirically this extremum seems always to a minimum [22]). Yedidia *et al* describe how these results can be generalized to Kikuchi approximations [3] which include the Bethe free energy as a special case. Overall, Yedidia *et al*'s work gives an exciting link between belief propagation and inference algorithms based on statistical physics.

M.A.T. Figueiredo, J. Zerubia, A.K. Jain (Eds.): EMMCVPR 2001, LNCS 2134, pp. 3–18, 2001.

This paper develops the connections between BP and the Bethe free energy (see [24] for extensions to Kikuchi free energy). The main result is a novel discrete iterative algorithm, called the *double-loop algorithm* which is guaranteed to converge to a minimum of the Bethe free energy. The double-loop algorithm is similar to BP because it also proceeds by passing "messages" between nodes of the graph (and there are interesting formal similarities between the two algorithms).

The double-loop algorithm is developed by decomposing the free energy into the sum of a convex term and a concave term. This is a general principle which can be applied to develop discrete iterative algorithms for a range of optimization problems, see [25]. In particular, it can be applied to mean field theory algorithms for solving optimization problems [7],[8],[13]. (Physicist readers should note that the "mean" is with respect to the Gibbs distribution but we do *not*, unlike most physics applications, assume that the "mean field" is spatially constant).

In Section (6), we place this work in context of mean field theory approaches to optimization (see [7],[8],[13] and chapters by Peterson and Yuille in [2]). This material is essentially a review (and some readers might prefer to read it before the rest of the paper).

Section (2) describes the Bethe free energy and BP algorithms. Section (3) gives the two basic design principles of our double-loop algorithm: (i) showing how to construct discrete iterative algorithms to minimize energy functions which are sums of a concave and a convex term, (ii) designing an iterative update algorithm guaranteed to enforce linear constraints. In Section (4) we apply these principles to the Bethe free energy and show that the specific nature of the constraints means that the iterative algorithm to solve the constraints takes a particularly simple form. Section (5) summarizes the double-loop algorithm and discusses formal similarities to BP. We conclude in Section (6) by briefly discussing how the scheme in this paper can be extended to obtain different statistical estimators, how temperature annealing can be done, and how the approach relates directly to mean field theory algorithms.

2 The Bethe Free Energy and the BP Algorithms

This section introduces the Bethe Free Energy and the BP algorithm following the formulation of Yedidia *et al* [22].

Consider a graph with nodes $i = 1, ..., N$. The state of a node is denoted by x_i (each x_i has M possible states). Each unobserved node is connected to an observed node y_i. The joint probability function is given by:

$$P(x_1, ..., x_N | y) = \frac{1}{Z} \prod_{i,j:i>j} \psi_{ij}(x_i, x_j) \prod_i \psi_i(x_i, y_i), \qquad (1)$$

where $\psi_i(x_i, y_i)$ is the local "evidence" for node i, Z is a normalization constant, and $\psi_{ij}(x_i, x_j)$ is the (symmetric) compatibility matrix between nodes i and j. We use the convention $i > j$ to avoid double counting. To simplify notation, we write $\psi_i(x_i)$ as shorthand for $\psi_i(x_i, y_i)$. If nodes i, j are *not* connected then we set $\psi_{ij}(x_i, x_j) = 1$.

The goal is to determine estimate $\{b_i(x_i)\}$ of the marginal distributions $\{P(x_i|y)\}$. It is convenient also to make estimates $\{b_{ij}(x_i, x_j)\}$ of the joint distributions $\{P(x_i, x_j|y)\}$ of nodes i, j which are connected in the graph. (Again we use the convention $i > j$ to avoid double counting). The $\{b_i(x_i)\}$ can then be used to calculate approximations to the minimum variance (MV) estimators for the variables $\{x_i\}$, see Section (6.1).

The BP algorithm introduces variables $m_{ij}(x_j)$ which correspond to "messages" that node i sends to node j (in the next subsection we will see how these messages arise as Lagrange multipliers). The BP algorithm is given by:

$$m_{ij}(x_j; t+1) = c_{ij} \sum_{x_i} \psi_{ij}(x_i, x_j)\psi_i(x_i) \prod_{k \neq j} m_{ki}(x_i; t), \qquad (2)$$

where c_{ij} is a normalization constant (i.e. it is independent of x_j). We use the convention that $m_{ki}(x_i, t) = 1$ if nodes i, k are *not* connected. Nodes are not connected to themselves (i.e $m_{ii}(x_i, t) = 1, \forall i$).

The messages determine additional variables $b_i(x_i), b_{ij}(x_i, x_j)$ corresponding to the approximate marginal probabilities at node i and the approximate joint probabilities at nodes i, j (with convention $i > j$). These are given in terms of the messages by:

$$b_i(x_i; t) = \hat{c}_i \psi_i(x_i) \prod_k m_{ki}(x_i; t), \qquad (3)$$

$$b_{ij}(x_i, x_j; t) = \bar{c}_{ij} \phi_{ij}(x_i, x_j) \prod_{k \neq j} m_{ki}(x_i; t) \prod_{l \neq i} m_{lj}(x_j; t), \qquad (4)$$

where $\phi_{ij}(x_i, x_j) = \psi_{ij}(x_i, x_j)\psi_i(x_i)\psi_j(x_j)$ and $\hat{c}_i, \bar{c}_{ij}$ are normalization constants.

For a tree, the BP algorithm of equation (2) is guaranteed to converge and the resulting $\{b_i(x_i)\}$ will correspond to the posterior marginals [12].

The Bethe free energy of this system is written as [22]:

$$F_\beta(\{b_{ij}, b_i\}) = \sum_{i,j:i>j} \sum_{x_i, x_j} b_{ij}(x_i, x_j) \log \frac{b_{ij}(x_i, x_j)}{\phi_{ij}(x_i, x_j)}$$

$$- \sum_i (n_i - 1) \sum_{x_i} b_i(x_i) \log \frac{b_i(x_i)}{\psi_i(x_i)}, \qquad (5)$$

where n_i is the number of neighbours of node i.

Because the $\{b_i\}$ and $\{b_{ij}\}$ correspond to marginal and joint probability distributions they must satisfy *linear* consistency constraints:

$$\sum_{x_i, x_j} b_{ij}(x_i, x_j) = 1, \forall i, j : i > j \quad \sum_{x_i} b_i(x_i) = 1, \forall i,$$

$$\sum_{x_i} b_{ij}(x_i, x_j) = b_j(x_j), \forall j, x_j, \quad \sum_{x_j} b_{ij}(x_i, x_j) = b_i(x_i), \forall i, x_i. \qquad (6)$$

The Bethe free energy consist of two terms. The first is of the form of a Kullback-Leibler (K-L) divergence between $\{b_{ij}\}$ and $\{\phi_{ij}\}$ (but it is not actually a K-L divergence because $\{\phi_{ij}\}$ is not a normalized distribution). The second is *minus* the form of the Kullback-Leibler divergence between $\{b_i\}$ and $\{\psi_i\}$ (again $\{\psi_i\}$ is not a normalized probability distribution). It follows that the first term is *convex* in $\{b_{ij}\}$ and the second term is *concave* in $\{b_i\}$. This will be of importance for the derivation of our algorithm in Section (3).

Yedidia *et al* [22] proved that the fixed points of the BP algorithm correspond to extrema of the Bethe free energy (with the linear constraints of equation (6)).

Yedidia *et al*'s work can be interpreted in terms of the dynamics of the dual energy function [24] where we extremize the Bethe Free Energy to express the $\{b_i\}, \{b_{ij}\}$ in terms of the Lagrange multiplers $\{\lambda_{ij}\}, \{\gamma_{ij}\}$. It can be shown that the messages $\{m_{ij}\}$ can be expressed as simple functions of the Lagrange parmeters. In this formulation Yedidia *et al*'s proof of convergence follows directly.

3   Convexity and Concavity

We now develop an algorithm that is guaranteed to converge to a minimum of the Bethe free energy. This section describes how we can exploit the fact that the Bethe free energy is the sum of a convex and a concave term, see Section (2).

Our main results are given by Theorem's 1,2,3 and show that we can obtain discrete iterative algorithms to minimize energy functions which are the sum of a convex and a concave term. (A similar result can be obtained using the Legendre transform, see [25]). We first consider the case where there are no constraints for the optimization. Then we generalize to the case where linear constraints are present.

Theorem 1. *Consider an energy function $E(z)$ (bounded below) of form $E(z) = E_{vex}(z) + E_{cave}(z)$ where $E_{vex}(z), E_{cave}(z)$ are convex and concave functions of z respectively. Then the discrete iterative algorithm $z^t \mapsto z^{t+1}$ given by:*

$$\nabla E_{vex}(z^{t+1}) = -\nabla E_{cave}(z^t), \tag{7}$$

is guaranteed to monotonically decrease the energy $E()$ as a function of time and hence to converge to a minimum of $E(z)$.

Proof. *The convexity and concavity of $E_{vex}(.)$ and $E_{cave}(.)$ means that:*

$$E_{vex}(z_2) \geq E_{vex}(z_1) + (z_2 - z_1) \cdot \nabla E_{vex}(z_1)$$
$$E_{cave}(z_4) \leq E_{cave}(z_3) + (z_4 - z_3) \cdot \nabla E_{cave}(z_3), \tag{8}$$

for all z_1, z_2, z_3, z_4. Now set $z_1 = z^{t+1}, z_2 = z^t, z_3 = z^t, z_4 = z^{t+1}$. Using equation (8) and the algorithm definition (i.e. $\nabla E_{vex}(z^{t+1}) = -\nabla E_{cave}(z^t)$) we find that:

$$E_{vex}(z^{t+1}) + E_{cave}(z^{t+1}) \leq E_{vex}(z^t) + E_{cave}(z^t), \tag{9}$$

which proves the claim.

Theorem 1 generalizes previous results by Marcus, Waugh and Westervelt [9],[19] on the convergence of discrete iterated neural networks. (They discussed the case where one function was convex and the second function was linear).

We can extend this result to allow for linear constraints on the variables z. This can be given a geometrical intuition. Firstly, properties such as concavity and concaveness are preserved when linear constraints are imposed. Secondly, because the constraints are linear they determine a hyperplane on which the constraints are satisfied. Theorem 1 can then be applied to the variables on this hyperplane.

Theorem 2. *Consider a function $E(z) = E_{vex}(z) + E_{cave}(z)$ subject to k linear constraints $\phi^\mu \cdot z = c^\mu$ where $\{c^\mu : \mu = 1, ..., k\}$ are constants. Then the algorithm $z^t \mapsto z^{t+1}$ given by:*

$$\nabla E_{vex}(z^{t+1}) = -\nabla E_{cave}(z^t) - \sum_{\mu=1}^{k} \alpha^\mu \phi^\mu, \tag{10}$$

where the parameters $\{\alpha^\mu\}$ are chosen to ensure that $z^{t+1} \cdot \phi^\mu = c^\mu$ for $\mu = 1, ..., k$, is guaranteed to monotonically decrease the energy $E(z^t)$ and hence to converge to a minimum of $E(z)$.

Proof. *Intuitively the update rule has to balance the gradients of E_{vex}, E_{cave} in the unconstrained directions of z and the term $\sum_{\mu=1}^{k} \alpha^\mu \phi^\mu$ is required to deal with the differences in the directions of the constraints. More formally, we define orthogonal unit vectors $\{\psi^\nu : \nu = 1, ..., n-k\}$ which span the space orthogonal to the constraints $\{\phi^\mu : \mu = 1, ..., k\}$. Let $y(z) = \sum_{\nu=1}^{n-k} \psi^\nu(z \cdot \psi^\nu)$ be the projection of z onto this space. Define functions $\hat{E}_{cave}(y), \hat{E}_{vex}(y)$ by:*

$$\hat{E}_{cave}(y(z)) = E_{cave}(z), \quad \hat{E}_{vex}(y(z)) = E_{vex}(z). \tag{11}$$

Then we can use the algorithm of Theorem 1 on the unconstrained variables $y = (y_1, ..., y_{n-k})$. By definition of $y(z)$ we have $\partial z / \partial y_\nu = \psi^\nu$. Therefore the algorithm reduces to:

$$\psi^\nu \cdot \nabla_z E_{vex}(z^{t+1}) = -\psi^\nu \cdot \nabla_z E_{cave}(z^t), \quad \nu = 1, ..., n-k. \tag{12}$$

This gives the result (recalling that $\phi^\mu \cdot \psi^\nu = 0$ for all μ, ν).

It follows from Theorem 2 that we only need to impose the constraints on $E_{vex}(z^{t+1})$ and not on $E_{cave}(z^t)$. In other words, we set

$$\bar{E}_{vex}(z^{t+1}) = E_{vex}(z^{t+1}) + \sum_\mu \alpha^\mu \phi^\mu \cdot z^{t+1}, \tag{13}$$

and use update equations:

$$\frac{\partial \bar{E}_{vex}}{\partial z}(z^{t+1}) = -\frac{\partial E_{cave}}{\partial z}(z^t), \tag{14}$$

where the coefficients $\{\alpha^\mu\}$ must be chosen to ensure that the constraints $\phi^\mu \cdot z^{t+1} = c^\mu \ \forall \mu$ are satisfied.

We now restrict ourselves to the specific case where $E_{vex}(z) = \sum_i z_i \log \frac{z_i}{\zeta_i}$. (This form of $E_{vex}(z)$ will arise when we apply Theorem 2 to the Bethe free energy, see Section (4)). We let $h(z) = \nabla E_{cave}(z)$. Then the update rules of Theorem 2, see equation (10), *can be expressed as selecting z^{t+1} to minimize a convex cost function $E^{t+1}(z^{t+1})$ which, by duality, implies that the constraint coefficients $\{\alpha^\mu\}$ can be found by maximizing a dual energy function.* More formally, we have the following result:

Theorem 3. *Let $E_{vex}(z) = \sum_i z_i \log \frac{z_i}{\zeta_i}$, then the update equation of Theorem 2 can be expressed as minimizing the convex energy function:*

$$E^{t+1}(z^{t+1}) = z^{t+1} \cdot h + \sum_i z_i^{t+1} \log \frac{z_i^{t+1}}{\zeta_i} + \sum_\mu \alpha^\mu \{\phi^\mu \cdot z^{t+1} - c^\mu\}, \qquad (15)$$

where $h = \nabla E_{cave}(z^t)$. By duality the solution corresponds to

$$z_i^{t+1} = \zeta_i e^{-h_i} e^{-1} e^{-\sum_\mu \alpha^\mu \phi_i^\mu}, \qquad (16)$$

where the Lagrange multipliers $\{\alpha^\mu\}$ are constrained to maximize the (concave) dual energy:

$$\hat{E}^{t+1}(\alpha) = -\sum_i \zeta_i e^{-h_i} e^{-1} e^{-\sum_\nu \phi_i^\nu \alpha^\nu} - \sum_\mu \alpha^\mu c^\mu. \qquad (17)$$

Moreover, maximizing $\hat{E}^{t+1}(\alpha)$ with respect to a specific α^μ enables us to satisfy the corresponding constraint exactly.

Proof. *This is given by straightforward calculations. Differentiating E^{t+1} with respect to z_i^{t+1} gives:*

$$1 + \log \frac{z_i}{\zeta_i} = -h_i - \sum_\mu \alpha^\mu \phi_i^\mu, \qquad (18)$$

which corresponds to the update equation (10) of Theorem 2. Since $E^{t+1}(z)$ is convex, duality ensures that the dual $\hat{E}^{t+1}(\alpha)$ is concave [18], and hence has a unique maximum which corresponds to the constraints being solved. Setting $\frac{\partial \hat{E}^{t+1}}{\partial \alpha^\mu} = 0$ ensures that $z^{t+1} \cdot \phi^\mu = c^\mu$, and hence satisfies the μth constraint.

By using Theorem 3, we see that solving for the constraint coefficients in Theorem 2 can be reduced to maximizing a concave energy function in the $\{\alpha^\nu\}$.

Moreover, for the specific constraints used in the Bethe free energy we will be able to determine an efficient discrete iterative algorithms for solving for the constraints. This is by generalizing work by Kosowsky and Yuille [7],[8] who used a result similar to Theorem 3 to obtain an algorithm for solving the linear assignment problem. (Kosowsky and Yuille [7],[8] also showed that this result could be used to derive an energy function for the classic Sinkhorn algorithm [17] which converts positive matrices into doubly stochastic ones.) Rangarajan *et al* [13] applied this result to obtain double loop algorithms for a range of optimization problems subject to linear constraints.

In the next section we apply Theorems 2 and 3 to the Bethe free energy. In particular, we will show that the nature of the linear constraints for the Bethe free energy mean that solving for the constraints in Theorem 3 can be done efficiently.

4   Constraints for the Bethe Free Energy

In this section we return to the Bethe free energy and describe how we can implement an algorithm of the form given by Theorems 1,2 and 3. This *double-loop* algorithm is designed by splitting the Bethe free energy into convex and concave parts. An inner loop is used to impose the linear constraints. (This design was influenced by the work of Rangarajan *et al* [13]).

First we split the Bethe free energy in two parts:

$$E_{vex} = \sum_{i,j:i>j} \sum_{x_i,x_j} b_{ij}(x_i,x_j) \log \frac{b_{ij}(x_i,x_j)}{\phi_{ij}(x_i,x_j)} + \sum_i \sum_{x_i} b_i(x_i) \log \frac{b_i(x_i)}{\psi_i(x_i)},$$

$$E_{cave} = -\sum_i n_i \sum_{x_i} b_i(x_i) \log \frac{b_i(x_i)}{\psi_i(x_i)}. \tag{19}$$

This split enables us to get non-zero derivatives of E_{vex} with respect to both $\{b_{ij}\}$ and $\{b_i\}$. (Other choices of split are possible).

We now need to express the linear constraints, see equation (6), in the form used in Theorems 2 and 3. To do this, we set $z = (b_{ij}(x_i,x_j), b_i(x_i))$ so that the first $\frac{N(N-1)}{2}M^2$ components of z correspond to the $\{b_{ij}\}$ and the later NM components to the $\{b_i\}$ (recall that there are N nodes of the graph each with M states). The dot product of z with a vector $\phi = (T_{ij}(x_i,x_j), U_i(x_i))$ is given by $\sum_{i,j:i>j} \sum_{x_i,x_j} b_{ij}(x_i,x_j)T_{ij}(x_i,x_j) + \sum_i \sum_{x_i} b_i(x_i)U_i(x_i)$.

There are two types of constraints: (i) normalization $- \sum_{x_p,x_q} b_{pq}(x_p,x_q) = 1 \ \forall \ p,q : p > q$, and (ii) consistency $- \sum_{x_p} b_{pq}(x_p,x_q) = b_q(x_q) \ \forall p,q,x_q : p > q$ and $\sum_{x_q} b_{pq}(x_p,x_q) = b_p(x_p) \ \forall q,p,x_p : p > q$.

We index the normalization constraints by pq (with $p > q$). Then we can express the constraint vectors $\{\phi^{pq}\}$, the constraint coefficients $\{\alpha^{pq}\}$, and the constraint values $\{c^{pq}\}$ by:

$$\phi^{pq} = (\delta_{pi}\delta_{qj}, 0), \quad \alpha^{pq} = \gamma_{pq}, \quad c^{pq} = 1, \ \forall p,q. \tag{20}$$

The consistency constraints are indexed by pqx_q (with $p > q$) and qpx_p (with $p > q$). The constraint vectors, the constraint coefficients, and the constraint values are given by:

$$\phi^{pqx_q} = (\delta_{ip}\delta_{jq}\delta_{x_j,x_q}, -\delta_{iq}\delta_{x_i,x_q}), \quad \alpha^{pqx_q} = \lambda_{pq}(x_q), \quad c^{pqx_q} = 0, \ \forall p,q,x_q$$

$$\phi^{qpx_p} = (\delta_{ip}\delta_{jq}\delta_{x_ix_p}, -\delta_{ip}\delta_{x_i,x_p}), \quad \alpha^{qpx_p} = \lambda_{qp}(x_p), \quad c^{qpx_p} = 0, \ \forall q,p,x_p. \tag{21}$$

We now apply Theorem 2 to the Bethe free energy and obtain:

Theorem 4. *The following update rule is guaranteed to reduce the Bethe free energy provided the constraint coefficients $\{\gamma_{pq}\}, \{\lambda_{pq}\}, \{\lambda_{qp}\}$ can be chosen to ensure that $\{b_{ij}(t+1)\}, \{b_i(t+1)\}$ satisfy the linear constraints of equation (6):*

$$b_{ij}(x_i, x_j; t+1) = \phi_{ij}(x_i, x_j)e^{-1}e^{-\lambda_{ij}(x_j)}e^{-\lambda_{ji}(x_i)}e^{-\gamma_{ij}},$$

$$b_i(x_i; t+1) = \psi_i(x_i)e^{-1}e^{n_i}\left(\frac{b_i(x_i;t)}{\psi_i(x_i)}\right)^{n_i}e^{\sum_k \lambda_{ki}(x_i)}. \tag{22}$$

Proof. *Substitute equation (19) into equation (10) and use equations (20,21) for the constraints. The constraint terms $\sum_\mu \alpha^\mu \phi^\mu$ simplify owing to the form of the constraints (e.g. $\sum_{p,q:p>q} \gamma_{pq}\delta_{ip}\delta_{jq} = \gamma_{ij}$).*

Finally, we use Theorem 3 to obtain an algorithm which ensures that the constraints are satisfied. Recall that finding the constraint coefficients is equivalent to maximizing the dual energy $\hat{E}^{t+1}(\alpha)$ and that performing the maximization with respect to the μth coefficient α^μ corresponds to solving the μth constraint equation. For the Bethe free energy it is possible to solve the μth constraint equation to *obtain an analytic expression for the μth coefficient* in terms of the remaining coefficients. Therefore we can maximize the dual energy $\hat{E}^{t+1}(\alpha)$ with respect to any coefficient α^μ analytically. Hence we have an algorithm that is guaranteed to converge to the maximum of $\hat{E}^{t+1}(\alpha)$: *select a constraint μ, solve for the equation $\frac{\partial \hat{E}^{t+1}}{\partial \alpha^\mu}$ for α^μ analytically, and repeat.*

More formally:

Theorem 5. *The constraint coefficients $\{\gamma_{pq}\}, \{\lambda_{pq}\}, \{\lambda_{qp}\}$ of Theorem 4 can be solved for by a discrete iterative algorithm, indexed by τ, guaranteed to converge to the unique solution. At each step we select coefficients $\gamma_{pq}, \lambda_{pq}(x_q)$ or $\lambda_{qp}(x_p)$ and update them by:*

$$e^{\gamma_{pq}(\tau+1)} = \sum_{x_p, x_q} \phi_{pq}(x_p, x_q)e^{-1}e^{-\lambda_{pq}(x_q, \tau)}e^{-\lambda_{qp}(x_p;\tau)},$$

$$e^{2\lambda_{pq}(x_q;\tau+1)} = \frac{\sum_{x_p} \phi_{pq}(x_p, x_q)e^{-\lambda_{qp}(x_p;\tau)}e^{-\gamma_{pq}(\tau)}}{\psi_q(x_q)e^{n_q}\left(\frac{b_q(x_q;t)}{\psi_q(x_q;t)}\right)^{n_q}e^{\sum_{j\neq p}\lambda_{jq}(x_q;\tau)}},$$

$$e^{2\lambda_{qp}(x_p;\tau+1)} = \frac{\sum_{x_q} \phi_{pq}(x_p, x_q)e^{-\lambda_{pq}(x_q;\tau)}e^{-\gamma_{pq}(\tau)}}{\psi_p(x_p)e^{n_p}\left(\frac{b_p(x_p;t)}{\psi_p(x_p;t)}\right)^{n_p}e^{\sum_{j\neq q}\lambda_{jp}(x_p;\tau)}} \tag{23}$$

Proof. *We use the update rule given by Theorem 4 and calculate the constraint equations, $\mathbf{z} \cdot \phi^\mu = c^\mu, \forall \mu$. For the Bethe free energy we obtain equations (23) where the upper equation corresponds to the normalization constraints and the lower equations to the consistency constraints. We observe that we can solve each equation analytically for the corresponding constraint coefficients $\gamma_{pq}, \lambda_{pq}(x_q), \lambda_{qp}(x_p)$. By Theorem 3, this is equivalent to maximizing the dual energy, see equation (17), with respect to each coefficient. Since the dual energy is concave solving for each coefficient $\gamma_{pq}, \lambda_{pq}(x_q), \lambda_{qp}(x_p)$ (with the others fixed) is* *guaranteed to increase the dual energy. Hence we can maximize the dual energy, and hence ensure the constraints are satisfied, by repeatedly selecting coefficients and solving the equations (23).*

Observe that we can update all the coefficients $\{\gamma_{pq}\}$ simultaneously because their update rule (i.e. the right hand side of the top equation of 23) depends only on the $\{\lambda_{pq}\}$. Similarly, we can update many of the $\{\lambda_{pq}\}$ simultaneously because their update rules (i.e. the right hand sides of the middle and bottom equation of 23) only depend on a subset of the $\{\lambda_{pq}\}$. (For example, when updating $\lambda_{pq}(x_q)$ we can simultaneously update any $\lambda_{ij}(x_j)$ provided $i \neq p \neq j$ and $i \neq q \neq j$.)

5   The Double-Loop Algorithm and BP

In this section we summarize the double-loop algorithm and then show that it has some interesting similarities to the belief propagation algorithm as formulated by Yedidia *et al* [22].

The double-loop algorithm consists of an outer loop which implements equation (22) plus an inner loop, given by equations (23) which imposes the constraints. The double loop design of the algorithm was influenced by the work of Rangarajan *et al* [13].

A convergence proof and theoretical analysis of Rangarajan *et al*'s algorithm was given in [14]. It is not clear how many iterations of the internal loop are needed to ensure the constraints are satisfied (though techniques developed by [7],[8] and [14] might be used to bound the number of iterations). In practice, the convergence of these inner loops seems to go quickly [7],[8] [13].

The algorithm consists of an inner and an outer loop. The outer loop has (discrete) time parameter t and is given by:

$$b_{ij}(x_i, x_j; t+1) = \phi_{ij}(x_i, x_j)e^{-1}e^{-\lambda_{ij}(x_j)}e^{-\lambda_{ji}(x_i)}e^{-\gamma_{ij}}, \tag{24}$$

$$b_i(x_i; t+1) = \psi_i(x_i)e^{-1}e^{n_i}\left(\frac{b_i(x_i; t)}{\psi_i(x_i)}\right)^{n_i}e^{\sum_k \lambda_{ki}(x_i)}, \tag{25}$$

and the inner loop to determine the $\{\gamma_{pq}\}, \{\lambda_{pq}\}, \{\lambda_{qp}\}$ has time parameter τ and is given by:

$$e^{\gamma_{pq}(\tau+1)} = \sum_{x_p, x_q} \phi_{pq}(x_p, x_q)e^{-1}e^{-\lambda_{pq}(x_q; \tau)}e^{-\lambda_{qp}(x_p; \tau)},$$

$$e^{2\lambda_{pq}(x_q; \tau+1)} = \frac{\sum_{x_p} \phi_{pq}(x_p, x_q)e^{-\lambda_{qp}(x_p; \tau)}e^{-\gamma_{pq}(\tau)}}{\psi_q(x_q)e^{n_q}\left(\frac{b_q(x_q; t)}{\psi_q(x_q; t)}\right)^{n_q}e^{\sum_{j \neq p} \lambda_{jq}(x_q; \tau)}}$$

$$e^{2\lambda_{qp}(x_p; \tau+1)} = \frac{\sum_{x_q} \phi_{pq}(x_p, x_q)e^{-\lambda_{pq}(x_q; \tau)}e^{-\gamma_{pq}(\tau)}}{\psi_p(x_p)e^{n_p}\left(\frac{b_p(x_p; t)}{\psi_p(x_p; t)}\right)^{n_p}e^{\sum_{j \neq q} \lambda_{jp}(x_p; \tau)}}. \tag{26}$$

Recall that the inner loop is required to impose linear constraints on the $\{b_{ij}\}, \{b_i\}$. For example, the update rule for $\lambda_{pq}(x_q)$ imposes the constraint $\sum_{x_p} b_{pq}(x_p, x_q) = b_q(x_q)$.

We now show that there are formal similarities between this algorithm and belief propagation as specified by equations (2,3, 4).

We can relate the messages $\{m_{ij}\}$ of BP to lagrange multipliers $\{\lambda_{ij}\}$ by $m_{ji}(x_i) = e^{\lambda_{ji}(x_i)}e^{-\frac{1}{n_i-1}\sum_k \lambda_{ki}(x_i)}$ and the inverse $e^{-\lambda_{ij}(x_j)} = \prod_{k \neq i} m_{kj}(x_j)$ $\forall i, j, x_i, x_j$ (see [22],[24]). Using these relations, and comparing equations (4,24), we see that the update equations for the $\{b_{ij}\}$ are identical for the double-loop algorithm and for BP. (In fact, the $\{b_{ij}\}$ variables play no role in the dynamics of either algorithm and need not be evaluated at all until the algorithm has converged).

The main difference between the two algorithms is that the double-loop algorithm has an outer loop to update the $\{b_i\}$ (equation (25)) and an inner loop (equation (26)) to update the $\{\lambda_{ij}, \gamma_{ij}\}$. By contrast, in the BP algorithm all the dynamics (equation (2)) can be expressed in terms of the messages $\{m_{ij}\}$, or the lagrange parameters $\{\lambda_{ij}\}$ (which directly determine the $\{b_i\}$ by equation (3)).

To go further, we express the BP update rules, equations (2,3), in terms of the lagrange multipliers. This gives:

$$e^{\lambda_{ij}(x_j;t+1)}\, e^{-\frac{1}{n_j-1}\sum_k \lambda_{kj}(x_j;t+1)} = c\sum_{x_i} \psi_{ij}(x_i, x_j)\psi_i(x_i)e^{-\lambda_{ji}(x_i;t)}, \quad (27)$$

$$b_i(x_i;t)\ = \hat{c}\psi_i(x_i)e^{-\frac{1}{n_i-1}\sum_l \lambda_{li}(x_i;t)}, \quad (28)$$

which we can compare to the equations for the double-loop algorithm:

$$e^{2\lambda_{pq}(x_q;\tau+1)} = \frac{\sum_{x_p} \psi_{pq}(x_p, x_q)\psi_p(x_p)e^{-\lambda_{qp}(x_p;\tau)}e^{-\gamma_{pq}}}{e^{n_q}\{\frac{b_q(x_q)}{\psi_q(x_q)}\}^{n_q}e^{\sum_{j \neq p} \lambda_{jq}(x_q;\tau)}}, \quad (29)$$

$$b_i(x_i;t+1) = \psi_i(x_i)e^{-1}e^{n_i}\{\frac{b_i(x_i;t)}{\psi_i(x_i)}\}^{n_i}e^{\sum_k \lambda_{ki}(x_i)}, \quad (30)$$

where (as before) we use the variables τ and t for the time steps in the inner and outer loops respectively. We also use the relationship $\phi_{pq}(x_p, x_q) = \psi_{pq}(x_p, x_q)\psi_p(x_p)\psi_q(x_q)$. (We ignore the "normalization dynamics" – updating the $\{\gamma_{pq}\}$ – because it is straightforward and can be taken for granted. With this understanding we have dropped the dependence of the $\{\gamma_{pq}\}$ on τ).

Now suppose we try to approximate the double-loop algorithm by setting $b_i(x_i;t) = \hat{c}\psi_i(x_i)e^{-\frac{1}{n_i-1}\sum_l \lambda_{li}(x_i;t)}$ from equation (28). This "collapses" the outer loop of the double-loop algorithm and so only the inner loop remains. This reduces equation (29) to:

$$e^{2\lambda_{pq}(x_q;\tau+1)} \times \{e^{-\lambda_{pq}(x_q;\tau)}e^{-\frac{1}{n_q-1}\sum_j \lambda_{jq}(x_q;\tau)}\}$$
$$= \sum_{x_p} \psi_{pq}(x_p, x_q)\psi_p(x_p)e^{-\lambda_{qp}(x_p;\tau)}e^{-\gamma_{pq}}, \quad (31)$$

which is almost exactly the same as the BP algorithm, equation (27). (Use the identity $\{e^{-\frac{1}{n_q-1}\sum_l \lambda_{lq}(x_q)}\}^{n_q}e^{\sum_{j \neq p} \lambda_{jq}(x_q)} = e^{-\frac{1}{n_q-1}\sum_j \lambda_{jq}(x_q)}e^{-\lambda_{pq}(x_q)}$). The only difference is the factor $\{e^{-\lambda_{pq}(x_p;\tau)}e^{-\frac{1}{n_q-1}\sum_j \lambda_{jq}(x_q;\tau)}\}$ is evaluated at time τ from equation (31) and at time $t+1$ for equation (27).

It is also straightforward to check that equation (30) for updating the outer loop has $b_i(x_i) = \hat{c}\psi_i(x_i)e^{-\frac{1}{n_i-1}\sum_l \lambda_{li}(x_i)}$ as a fixed point. More precisely, if we converge to a state where $\lambda_{ij}(x_j;\tau+1) = \lambda_{ij}(x_j;\tau) \; \forall \; i,j,x_j$ then substituting $b_i(x_i;t) = \hat{c}\psi_i(x_i)e^{-\frac{1}{n_i-1}\sum_l \lambda_{li}(x_i;t)}$ into equation (30) gives $b_i(x_i;t+1) = b_i(x_i;t) \; \forall \; i,x_i$.

To conclude, the BP algorithm can be thought of as an approximation to the double-loop algorithm. The approximation is done by assuming a fixed functional form for the $\{b_i\}$ in terms of the $\{\lambda_{ij}\}$, thereby collapsing the outer loop of the algorithm, and modifying the update equations for the inner loop (by evaluating certain terms at $\tau+1$ instead of at τ).

6 Discussion

This section covers three additional topics which are essentially review material (i.e. no novel results are presented here). Firstly, we discuss the relationship of the Bethe approximation to MAP/MV estimation and how a temperature parameter can be introduced to obtain deterministic annealing. Secondly, we describe how the Bethe and mean field free energies can be obtained from an information geometry viewpoint [1] using Kullback-Leibler divergences. Relations of the double-loop algorithm to mean field theory are described in [25].

6.1 MV and MAP Estimation and Deterministic Annealing

We now briefly discuss the use of the Bethe approximations for estimation and how they can be modified to allow for temperature annealing [6]. For simplicity we concentrate only on the Bethe Free Energy.

The input to a double-loop algorithm is a probability distribution function $P(x_1,...,x_N|y)$, see equation (1). The output of the algorithm is an estimate of the marginal and joint probability distributions.

In many optimization problems it is desired to estimate the variables $\{x_i\}$ from $P(x_1,...,x_N|y)$. Two common estimators are the the Minimal Variance (MV) Estimator and the Maximum a Posteriori (MAP). From the estimates of the marginal probability distributions $\{b_i(x_i)\}$, provided by minimizing the Bethe free energy, it is possible to directly obtain an approximation to the MV estimate by computing $\bar{x}_i = \sum_{x_i} x_i b_i(x_i)$.

The MAP estimate can be obtained by introducing a temperature parameter T. We replace the probability distribution $P(x_1,...,x_N|y)$ by $\{P(x_1,...,x_N|y)\}^{1/T}$ which implies, by equation (1), replacing $\{\psi_i\},\{\psi_{ij}\},\{\phi_{ij}\}$ by $\{\psi_i^{1/T}\},\{\psi_{ij}^{1/T}\}$, $\{\phi_{ij}^{1/T}\}$ and scaling by a factor T. This gives a family of Bethe free energies:

$$F_\beta^T(\{b_{ij}, b_i\}) = T \sum_{i,j:i>j} \sum_{x_i,x_j} b_{ij}(x_i, x_j) \log b_{ij}(x_i, x_j)$$

$$- \sum_{i,j:i>j} \sum_{x_i,x_j} b_{ij}(x_i,x_j) \log \phi_{ij}(x_i,x_j)$$

$$-T \sum_i (n_i - 1) \sum_{x_i} b_i(x_i) \log b_i(x_i)$$

$$+ \sum_i (n_i - 1) \sum_{x_i} b_i(x_i) \log \psi_i(x_i), \qquad (32)$$

where the original Bethe Free Energy, see equation (5), is be obtained by setting $T = 1$. We see that equation (32) is equivalent to having energy terms $-\sum_{i,j:i>j} \sum_{x_i,x_j} b_{ij}(x_i,x_j) \log \phi_{ij}(x_i,x_j) + \sum_i (n_i - 1) \sum_{x_i} b_i(x_i) \log \psi_i(x_i)$ (independent of temperature T) and temperature dependent entropy terms given by $T \sum_{i,j:i>j} \sum_{x_i,x_j} b_{ij}(x_i,x_j) \log b_{ij}(x_i,x_j) - T \sum_i (n_i - 1) \sum_{x_i} b_i(x_i) \log b_i(x_i)$. This is the same form for mean field annealing, see for example [7], [13].

Minimizing F_β^T gives a family of marginal distributions $\{b_i^T(x_i)\}$. As $T \mapsto 0$ the marginals $\{b_i^T(x_i)\}$ will become sharply peaked about the most probable values $x_i^{*,T} = \arg\max_{x_i} b_i^T(x_i)$. Therefore the estimates $\{x_i^{*,T}\}$ will become approximations to the MAP estimates $\{x_i^*\} = \arg\max_{\{x_i\}} P(x_1, ..., x_N | y)$. (Provided some technical conditions apply, see [23] for a theoretical analysis of what conditions are needed for the mean field theory approximation).

In addition, for many optimization problems it may be desirable to have some form of temperature annealing to help avoid local minima. This can be achieved by calculating the estimates of the marginals $\{b_i^T(x_i)\}$, and the joint distribution $\{b_{ij}^T(x_i,x_j)\}$, at high values of the temperature T and using these as initializations for the estimates for smaller values of the T. See [23], [13] for examples of this approach and for further references.

6.2   Kullback-Leibler Approximations and Information Geometry

Amari's theory of information geometry [1] gives a framework for obtaining approximations to probability distributions (where the approximations are restricted to have specific functional forms). This gives some insight into the Bethe approximations. The material on the mean field theory approximation is related to Saul $et\ al$ [16] and the Bethe free energy is similar to the derivation by Yedidia $et\ al$ [22].

Let the target distribution be $P(x_1, ..., x_N) = \frac{1}{Z} \prod_{i,j:i>j} \psi_{ij}(x_i,x_j) \prod_i \psi_i$ (x_i, y_i) (see equation (1)). Suppose we want to approximate it by a factorizable distribution $P_F(x_1, ..., x_N) = \prod_{i=1}^N b_i(x_i)$ (with $\sum_{x_i} b_i(x_i) = 1 \ \forall \ i$). One measure of similarity, suggested by information geometry, is to seek the distribution $P_F(x_1, ..., x_N)$ which minimizes the Kullback-Leibler divergence to $P(x_1, ..., x_N)$:

$$D(P_F||P) = \sum_{x_1,...,x_N} P_F(x_1, ..., x_N) \log \frac{P_F(x_1, ..., x_N)}{P(x_1, ..., x_N)}. \qquad (33)$$

We can re-express this as:

$$D(P_F||P) = - \sum_i \sum_{x_i} b_i(x_i) \log \psi_i(x_i) - \sum_{i,j} \sum_{x_i,x_j} b_i(x_i)b_j(x_j) \log \psi_{ij}(x_i,x_j)$$

$$+ \sum_i \sum_{x_i} b_i(x_i) \log b_i(x_i) + \log Z. \qquad (34)$$

Minimizing $D(P_F||P)$ with respect to the $\{b_i\}$ (with the constraints that $\sum_i b_i(x_i) = 1 \ \forall i$) gives the mean field free energy used for many optimization applications, see for example [23], [13]. (The notation is different in those papers. For example to obtain the formulation used in [23] we relate the variables x_i, x_j to a, b and identify the variables $\{b_i(x_i)\}$ with the matching variables $\{S_{ia}\}$ and the terms $-\log \psi_i(x_i)$ and $-\log \psi_{ij}(x_i, x_j)$ with terms $-A_{ia}$ and T_{ijab}. The variables are constrained so that $\sum_a S_{ia} = 1, \ \forall \ i$.)

The Bethe free energy can be obtained in a similar way (although, as we will discuss, an additional approximation is needed if the graph has closed loops). We seek to approximate the distribution $P(x_1, ..., x_N)$ by a distribution $P_\beta(x_1, ..., x_N)$ which has marginals $\{b_i(x_i)\}$ and joint distributions $\{b_{ij}(x_i, x_j)\}$. Once again, we attempt to find the approximation $P_\beta(x_1, ..., x_N)$ which minimizes the Kullback-Leibler divergence:

$$\begin{aligned} D(P_\beta||P) &= \sum_{x_1,...,x_N} P_\beta(x_1, ..., x_N) \log \frac{P_\beta(x_1, ..., x_N)}{P(x_1, ..., x_N)} \\ &= \sum_{x_1,...,x_N} P_\beta(x_1, ..., x_N) \log P_\beta(x_1, ..., x_N) \\ &\quad - \sum_{x_1,...,x_N} P_\beta(x_1, ..., x_N) \log P(x_1, ..., x_N). \end{aligned} \qquad (35)$$

The second term of the Kullback-Leibler, see equation (35), can be expressed as $-\sum_i \sum_{x_i} b_i(x_i) \log \psi_i(x_i) - \sum_{i,j} \sum_{x_i, x_j} b_{ij}(x_i, x_j) \log \psi_{ij}(x_i, x_j) + \log Z$.

The first term is the entropy of the approximating distribution $P_\beta(x_1, ..., x_N)$. The Bethe approximation consists of assuming that we can express this as:

$$\begin{aligned} &\sum_{x_1,...,x_N} P_\beta(x_1, ..., x_N) \log P_\beta(x_1, ..., x_N) \\ &\approx \sum_{i,j} \sum_{x_i, x_j} b_{ij}(x_i, x_j) \log b_{ij}(x_i, x_j) - \sum_i (n_i - 1) \sum_{x_i} b_i(x_i) \log b_i(x_i). \end{aligned} \qquad (36)$$

It can be shown that this approximation is exact *if the graph has no loops*. (Recall that we only define joint distribution $b_{ij}(x_i, x_j)$ for nodes i, j which are directly joined in the graph. Also n_i is the number of neighbours). If the graph has no loops then the marginal and joint distributions (combined with the maximum entropy principle) determine a unique probability distribution (see, for example, [15]):

$$P_\beta(x_1, ..., x_N) = \frac{\prod_{i,j} b_{ij}(x_i, x_j)}{\prod_i \{b_i(x_i)\}^{n_i - 1}}. \qquad (37)$$

In this case, the entropy can be computed directly to give equation (36). But *if the graph has loops then $P_\beta(x_1, ..., x_N)$ given by equation (37) is not a* *normalized distribution.* The Bethe approximation assumes that the entropy can be written as equation (36) even when the graph has closed loops.

Using equation (36) for the entropy gives the result:

$$
D(P_\beta || P) \approx - \sum_i \sum_{x_i} b_i(x_i) \log \psi_i(x_i) - \sum_{i,j} \sum_{x_i,x_j} b_{ij}(x_i, x_j) \log \psi_{ij}(x_i, x_j)
$$
$$
+ \sum_{i,j} \sum_{x_i,x_j} b_{ij}(x_i, x_j) \log b_{ij}(x_i, x_j)
$$
$$
- \sum_i (n_i - 1) \sum_{x_i} b_i(x_i) \log b_i(x_i), \tag{38}
$$

which is exact for graphs with no loops and an approximation otherwise.

It can be quickly verified that the right hand side of equation (38) is the Bethe free energy (which involves using the relations $\phi_{ij}(x_i, x_j) = \psi_{ij}(x_i, x_j)\psi_i(x_i)$ $\psi_j(x_j)$ and the identity $\sum_{i,j} \sum_{x_i,x_j} b_{ij}(x_i, x_j) \log \psi_i(x_i) = \sum_i n_i \sum_{x_i} b_i(x_i)$ $\log \psi_i(x_i)$).

In summary, the mean field and the Bethe free energies can be obtained replacing the true distribution $P(x_1, ..., x_n)$ by approximations with probability distributions with specified marginal distributions (mean field) or specified marginal and joint distributions (Bethe). The Bethe free energy requires an additional approximation, about the entropy, if the graph has closed loops. The Kikuchi approximation can be obtained in a similar way. Essentially all these approaches (mean field, Bethe, Kikuchi) seek to approximate the true distributions $P(x_1, ..., x_N)$ by distributions which are easier to compute with.

7   Conclusion

The aims of this paper were to analyze the BP algorithm of Yedidia *et al* [22] and to design a double-loop algorithm which can be proven to converge to a minimum of the Bethe free energy. It may also be helpful to determine when BP, and related algorithms, converge to the correct result – see [20].

More constructively, we derived a double-loop algorithm based on separating the Bethe free energy into concave and convex parts and then using a discrete iterative algorithm to solve for the constraints. We showed that the BP algorithm is formally similar to the double-loop algorithm (and might be an effective approximation in some cases).

In other work, see [24]. we generalized our results to the Kikuchi free energy. This yielded both a dual formulation of the free energy and a double-loop algorithm that can be proven to converge to a minimum of the Kikuchi free energy.

Finally, we described how previous mean field theory work could be interpreted within this framework. It seems that the differences between mean field theory and the Bethe methods is merely the degree of the approximation used (i.e. do we try to approximate the target distribution by a factorizable distribution – the mean field approach – or do we look for a higher order Bethe approximation). Mean field theory algorithms can be very effective on difficult optimization problems (e.g., see [13]) provided the factorization assumptions is good enough but they also fail on other difficult problems such as the non-Euclidean Traveling Salesman Problem (Rangarajan – personal communication).

Current work is also to implement the double-loop algorithm on computer vision problems and compare its performance to alternatives such as mean field theory algorithms. It has already been demonstrated [21] that the BP algorithms give good results in situations where mean field algorithms break down.

Acknowledgements

I would like to acknowledge helpful conversations with James Coughlan and Huiying Shen. Yair Weiss pointed out a conceptual bug in the original dual formulation. Anand Rangarajan pointed out the connections to Legendre transforms. Sabino Ferreira read the manuscript carefully, made many useful comments, and gave excellent feedback. Jonathan Yedidia pointed out a faulty assumptions about the $\{c_r\}$. This work was supported by the National Institute of Health (NEI) with grant number RO1-EY 12691-01.

References

1. S. Amari. "Differential Geometry of curved exponential families – Curvature and information loss. Annals of Statistics, vol. 10, no. 2, pp 357-385. 1982.
2. M. Arbib (Ed.) **The Handbook of Brain Theory and Neural Networks**. A Bradford Book. The MIT Press. 1995.
3. C. Domb and M.S. Green (Eds). **Phase Transitions and Critical Phenomena**. Vol. 2. Academic Press. London. 1972.
4. W.T. Freeman and E.C. Pasztor. "Learning low level vision". In *Proc. International Conference of Computer Vision*. ICCV'99. pp 1182-1189. 1999.
5. B. Frey. **Graphical Models for Pattern Classification, Data Compression and Channel Coding**. MIT Press. 1998.
6. S. Kirkpatrick, C. Gelatt (Jr.), and M. Vecchi. "Optimization by Simulated Annealing". *Science*, 220:671-680. 1983.
7. J. Kosowsky and A.L. Yuille. "The Invisible Hand Algorithm: Solving the Assignment Problem with Statistical Physics". *Neural Networks.*, Vol. 7, No. 3, pp 477-490. 1994.
8. J. Kosowsky. **Flows Suspending Iterative Algorithms**. PhD Thesis. Division of Applied Sciences. Harvard University. Cambridge, Massachusetts. 1995.
9. C.M. Marcus and R.M. Westervelt. "Dynamics of iterated- map neural networks". *Physical Review A*, 40, pp 501-504. 1989.
10. R.J. McEliece, D.J.C. Mackay, and J.F. Cheng. "Turbo decoding as an instance of Pearl's belief propagation algorithm". *IEEE Journal on Selected Areas in Communication.* 16(2), pp 140-152. 1998.
11. K.P. Murphy, Y. Weiss, and M.I. Jordan. "Loopy belief propagation for approximate inference: an empirical study". In *Proceedings of Uncertainty in AI*. 1999.
12. J. Pearl. **Probabilistic Reasoning in Intelligent Systems**. Morgan Kaufmann. 1988.

13. A. Rangarajan, S. Gold, and E. Mjolsness. "A Novel Optimizing Network Architecture with Applications". *Neural Computation*, 8(5), pp 1041-1060. 1996.
14. A. Rangarajan, A.L. Yuille, S. Gold. and E. Mjolsness."A Convergence Proof for the Softassign Quadratic assignment Problem". In *Proceedings of NIPS'96*. Snowmass. Colorado. 1996.
15. B.D. Ripley. "Pattern Recognition and Neural Networks". Cambridge University Press. 1996.
16. L. K. Saul, T. Jaakkola, and M. I. Jordan. "Mean Field Theory for Sigmoid Belief Networks". *Journal of Artificial Intelligence Research*, 4, 61-76, 1996.
17. R. Sinkhorn. "A Relationship Between Arbitrary Positive Matrices and Doubly Stochastic Matrices". *Ann. Math. Statist.*. 35, pp 876-879. 1964.
18. G. Strang. **Introduction to Applied Mathematics**. Wellesley-Cambridge Press. Wellesley, Massachusetts. 1986.
19. F.R. Waugh and R.M. Westervelt. "Analog neural networks with local competition: I. Dynamics and stability". *Physical Review E*, 47(6), pp 4524-4536. 1993.
20. Y. Weiss. "Correctness of local probability propagation in graphical models with loops". *Neural Computation* 12 (1-41) 2000.
21. Y. Weiss. "Comparing the mean field method and belief propagation for approximate inference in MRFs". To appear in **Advanced Mean Field Methods**. Saad and Opper (Eds). MIT Press. 2001.
22. J.S. Yedidia, W.T. Freeman, Y. Weiss. "Bethe free energy, Kikuchi approximations and belief propagation algorithms". To appear in NIPS'2000. 2000.
23. A.L. Yuille and J.J. Kosowsky. "Statistical Physics Algorithms that Converge." Neural Computation. **6**, pp 341-356. 1994.
24. A.L. Yuille. "A Double-Loop Algorithm to Minimize the Bethe and Kikuchi Free Energies". Submitted to *Neural Computation*. 2001.
25. A.L. Yuille and A. Rangarajan. "The Concave-Convex Procedure (CCCP)". Submitted to *Neural Computation*. 2001.

A Variational Approach to Maximum
a *Posteriori* Estimation for Image Denoising*

A. Ben Hamza and Hamid Krim

Department of Electrical and Computer Engineering
North Carolina State University, Raleigh, NC 27695-7914, USA
{abhamza,ahk}@eos.ncsu.edu

Abstract. Using first principles, we establish in this paper a connection between the maximum *a posteriori* (MAP) estimator and the variational formulation of optimizing a given functional subject to some noise constraints. A MAP estimator which uses a Markov or a maximum entropy random field model for a prior distribution can be viewed as a minimizer of a variational problem. Using notions from robust statistics, a variational filter called *Huber gradient descent flow* is proposed. It yields the solution to a Huber type functional subject to some noise constraints, and the resulting filter behaves like a total variation anisotropic diffusion for large gradient magnitudes and like an isotropic diffusion for small gradient magnitudes. Using some of the gained insight, we are also able to propose an information-theoretic gradient descent flow whose functional turns out to be a compromise between a neg-entropy variational integral and a total variation. Illustrating examples demonstrate a much improved performance of the proposed filters in the presence of Gaussian and heavy tailed noise.

1   Introduction

Linear filtering techniques abound in many image processing applications and their popularity mainly stems from their mathematical simplicity and their efficiency in the presence of additive Gaussian noise. A mean filter for example is the optimal filter for Gaussian noise in the sense of mean square error. Linear filters, however, tend to blur sharp edges, destroy lines and other fine image details, fail to effectively remove heavy tailed noise, and perform poorly in the presence of signal-dependent noise. This led to a search for nonlinear filtering alternatives. The research effort on nonlinear median-based filtering has resulted in remarkable results, and has highlighted some new promising research avenues [1]. On account of its simplicity, its edge preservation property and its robustness to impulsive noise, the standard median filter remains among the favorites for image processing applications [1]. The median filter, however, often tends to remove fine details in the image, such as thin lines and corners [1]. In recent

---

* This work was supported by an AFOSR grant F49620-98-1-0190 and by ONR-MURI grant JHU-72798-S2 and by NCSU School of Engineering.

M.A.T. Figueiredo, J. Zerubia, A.K. Jain (Eds.): EMMCVPR 2001, LNCS 2134, pp. 19–33, 2001.

years, a variety of median-type filters such as stack filters, weighted median [1], and relaxed median [2] have been developed to overcome this drawback. In spite of an improved performance, these solutions were missing the regularizing power of a prior on the underlying information of interest.

Among Bayesian image estimation methods, the MAP estimator using Markov or maximum entropy random field priors [3–5] has proven to be a powerful approach to image restoration. Among the limitations in using MAP estimation is the difficulty of systematically and easily/reliably choosing a prior distribution and its corresponding optimizing energy function, and in some cases the rsulting computational compexilty.

In recent years, variational methods and partial differential equations (PDE) based methods [6, 7] have been introduced to explicitly account for intrinsic geometry in a variety of problems inluding image segmentation, mathematical morphology and image denoising. The latter will be the focus of the present paper. The problem of denoising has been addressed using a number of different techniques including wavelets [9], order statistics based filters [1], PDE's based algorithms [6, 10, 11], and variational approaches [7]. A large number of PDE based methods have particularly been proposed to tackle the problem of image denoising with a good preservation of the edges. Much of the appeal of PDE-based methods lies in the availability of a vast arsenal of mathematical tools which at the very least act as a key guide in achieving numerical accuracy as well as stability. Partial differential equations or gradient descent flows are generally a result of variational problems using the Euler-Lagrange principle [12]. One popular variational technique used in image denoising is the total variation based approach. It was developed in [10] to overcome the basic limitations of all smooth regularization algorithms, and a variety of numerical methods have also been recently developed for solving total variation minimization problems [10, 13, 14].

In this paper, we present a variational approach to MAP estimation. The key idea behind this approach is to use geometric insight in helping construct regularizing functionals and avoiding a subjective choice of a prior in MAP estimation. Using tools from robust statistics and information theory, we propose two gradient descent flows for image denoising to illustrate the resulting overall methodology.

In the next section we briefly recall the MAP estimation formulation. In Section 3, we formulate a variational approach to MAP estimation. Section 4 is devoted to a robust variational formulation. In section 5, an entropic variational approach to MAP estimation is given. An improved entropic gradient descent flow is proposed in Section 6. Finally, in Section 7, we provide experimental results to show a much improved performance of the proposed gradient descent flows in image denoising.

2   Problem Formulation

Consider an additive noise model for an observed image

$$u_0 = u + \eta, \tag{1}$$

where u is the original image $u : \Omega \to \mathbb{R}$, and Ω is a nonempty, bounded, open set in $\mathbb{R}^2$ (usually Ω is a rectangle in $\mathbb{R}^2$). The noise process η is i.i.d., and u_0 is the observed image. The objective is to recover u, knowing u_0 and also some statistics of η. Throughout, $\boldsymbol{x} = (x_1, x_2)$ denotes a pixel location in Ω, $|\cdot|$ denotes the Euclidean norm and $||\cdot||$ denotes the L^2-norm.

Many image denoising methods have been proposed to estimate u, and among these figure Bayesian estimation schemes [3], wavelet based methods [9], and PDE based techniques [6, 10, 11].

One commonly used Bayesian approach in image denoising is the maximum a posteriori (MAP) estimation method which incorporates prior information. Denote by $p(u)$ the prior distribution for the unknown image u. The MAP estimator is given by

$$\hat{u} = \arg \max_u \{ \log p(u_0|u) + \log p(u) \}, \tag{2}$$

where $p(u_0|u)$ denotes the conditional probability of u_0 given u.

A general model for the prior distribution $p(u)$ is a Markov random field (MRF) which is characterized by its Gibbs distribution given by [3]

$$p(u) = \frac{1}{Z} \exp \left\{ -\frac{\mathcal{F}(u)}{\lambda} \right\},$$

where Z in the partition function, λ is a constant known as the temperature in the terminology of physical systems. For large λ, the prior probability becomes flat, and for small λ, the prior probability has sharp modes. $\mathcal{F}$ is called the *energy function* and has the form $\mathcal{F}(u) = \sum_{c \in \mathcal{C}} V_c(u)$, where $\mathcal{C}$ denotes the set of cliques for the MRF, and V_c is a potential function defined on a clique. Markov random fields have been extensively used in computer vision particularly for image restoration, and it has been established that Gibbs distributions and MRF's are equivalent [3], in other words, if a problem can be defined in terms of local potentials then there is a simple way of formulating the problem in terms of MRF's.

If the noise process η is i.i.d. Gaussian, then we have

$$p(u_0|u) = K \exp \left(-\frac{|u - u_0|^2}{2\sigma^2} \right),$$

where K is a normalizing positive constant, and σ^2 is the noise variance. Thus, the MAP estimator in (2) yields

$$\hat{u} = \arg \min_u \left\{ \mathcal{F}(u) + \frac{\lambda}{2} |u - u_0|^2 \right\}. \tag{3}$$

Image estimation using MRF priors has proven to be a powerful approach to restoration and reconstruction of high-quality images. A major problem limiting its utility is, however, the lack of a practical and robust method for systematically selecting the prior distribution. The Gibbs prior parameter λ is also of particular importance since it controls the balance of influence of the Gibbs prior and that of the likelihood. If λ is too small, the prior will tend to have an over-smoothing effect on the solution. Conversely, if it is too large, the MAP estimator may be unstable, reducing to the maximum likelihood solution as λ goes to infinity.

Another difficulty in using a MAP estimator is the non-uniqueness of the solution when the energy function $\mathcal{F}$ is not convex.

3   A Variational Approach to MAP Estimation

According to noise model (1), our goal is to estimate the original image u based on the observed image u_0 and on any knowledge of the noise statistics of η. This leads to solving the following noise-constrained optimization problem

$$
\begin{aligned}
\min_{u} \ &\mathcal{F}(u) \\
\text{s.t.} \ &\|u - u_0\|^2 = \sigma^2
\end{aligned}
\tag{4}
$$

where $\mathcal{F}$ is a given functional which is often a criterion of smoothness of the reconstructed image.

Using Lagrange's theorem, the minimizer of (4) is given by

$$
\hat{u} = \arg\min_{u} \left\{ \mathcal{F}(u) + \frac{\lambda}{2}\|u - u_0\|^2 \right\}.
\tag{5}
$$

where λ is a nonnegative parameter chosen so that the constraint $\|u_0 - u\|^2 = \sigma^2$ is satisfied. In practice, the parameter λ is often estimated or chosen *a priori*.

Equations (3) and (5) show a close connection between image recovery via MAP estimation and image recovery via optimization of variational integrals. Indeed, Eq. (3) may be written in integral form as Eq. (5).

A critical issue is the choice of the variational integral $\mathcal{F}$. The classical functionals (also called *variational integrals*) used in image denoising are the Dirichlet and the total variation integrals defined respectively as follows

$$
\mathcal{D}(u) = \frac{1}{2}\int_{\Omega} |\nabla u|^2 d\boldsymbol{x}, \quad \text{and} \quad TV(u) = \int_{\Omega} |\nabla u| d\boldsymbol{x},
\tag{6}
$$

where ∇u stands for the gradient of the image u.

A generalization of these functionals is the variational integral given by

$$
\mathcal{F}(u) = \int_{\Omega} F(|\nabla u|) d\boldsymbol{x},
\tag{7}
$$

where $F : \mathbb{R}^+ \to \mathbb{R}$ is a given smooth function called *variational integrand* or *Lagrangian* [12].

The total variation method [10] basically consists in finding an estimate $\hat{u}$ for the original image u with the smallest total variation among all the images satisfying the noise constraint $\|u - u_0\|^2 = \sigma^2$, where σ is assumed known. Note that the regularizing parameter λ controls the balance between minimizing the term which corresponds to fitting the data, and minimizing the regularizing term.

The intuition behind the use of the total variation integral is that it incorportes the fact that discontinuities are present in the original image u (it measures the jumps of u, even if it is discontinuous). The total variation method has been used with success in image denoising, especially for denoising images with piecewise constant features while preserving the location of the edges exactly [15, 16].

Using Eq. (7), we define the following functional

$$\mathcal{L}(u) = \mathcal{F}(u) + \frac{\lambda}{2}\|u - u_0\|^2 = \int_\Omega \left(F(|\nabla u|) + \frac{\lambda}{2}|u - u_0|^2 \right) d\boldsymbol{x}. \tag{8}$$

Thus, the optimization problem (5) becomes

$$\hat{u} = \arg\min_{u \in X} \mathcal{L}(u) = \arg\min_{u \in X} \left\{ \mathcal{F}(u) + \frac{\lambda}{2}\|u - u_0\|^2 \right\}, \tag{9}$$

where X is an appropriate image space of smooth functions like $C^1(\overline{\Omega})$, or the space $BV(\Omega)$ of image functions with bounded variation[1], or the Sobolev space[2] $H^1(\Omega) = W^{1,2}(\Omega)$.

3.1   Properties of the Optimization Problem

A problem is said to be *well-posed* in the sense of Hadamard if (i) a solution of the problem exists, (ii) the solution is unique, (iii) and the solution is stable, i.e. depends continuously on the problem data. It is *ill-posed* when it fails to satisfy at least one of these criteria. To guarantee the well-posedness of our minimization problem (9), the following result provides some conditions.

Theorem 1. *Let the image space X be a reflexive Banach space, and let $\mathcal{F}$ be*
(i) weakly lower semicontinuous, i.e. if for any sequence (u^k) in X converging weakly to u, we have $\mathcal{F}(u) \le \liminf_{k\to\infty} \mathcal{F}(u^k)$.
(ii) coercive, i.e. $\mathcal{F}(u) \to \infty$ as $\|u\| \to \infty$.
Then the functional $\mathcal{L}$ is bounded from below and possesses a minimizer, i.e. there exists $\hat{u} \in X$ such that $\mathcal{L}(\hat{u}) = \inf_X \mathcal{L}$. Moreover, if $\mathcal{F}$ is convex and $\lambda > 0$, then the optimization problem (9) has a unique solution, and it is stable.

Proof. From (i) and (ii) and the weak lower semicontinuity of the L^2-norm, the functional $\mathcal{L}$ is weak lower semicontinuous, and coercive.
Let u^n be a minimizing sequence of $\mathcal{L}$, i.e. $\mathcal{L}(u^n) \to \inf_X \mathcal{L}$. An immediate consequence of the coercivity of $\mathcal{L}$ is that u^n must be bounded. As X is reflexive, thus u^n converges weakly to $\hat{u}$ in X, i.e $u^n \rightharpoonup \hat{u}$. Thus $\mathcal{L}(\hat{u}) \le \liminf_{n\to\infty} \mathcal{L}(u^n) = \inf_X \mathcal{L}$. This proves that $\mathcal{L}(\hat{u}) = \inf_X \mathcal{L}$.
It is easy to check that convexity implies weakly lower semicontinuity. Thus the solution of the optimization problem (9) exists and it is unique because the L^2-norm is strictly convex. The stability follows using the semicontinuity of $\mathcal{L}$ and the fact that u^n is bounded.   □

---

[1] $BV(\Omega) = \{u \in L^1(\Omega) : TV(u) < \infty\}$ is a Banach space with the norm $\|u\|_{BV} = \|u\|_{L^1(\Omega)} + TV(u)$.
[2] $H^1(\Omega) = \{u \in L^2(\Omega) : \nabla u \in L^2(\Omega)\}$ is a Hilbert space with the norm $\|u\|^2_{H^1(\Omega)} = \|u\|^2 + \|\nabla u\|^2$.

3.2   Gradient Descent Flows

To solve the optimization problem (9), a variety of iterative methods may be applied such as gradient descent [10], or fixed point method [13, 16].

The most important first-order necessary condition to be satisfied by any minimizer of the functional $\mathcal{L}$ given by Eq. (8) is that its first variation $\delta\mathcal{L}(u; v)$ vanishes at u in direction of v, that is

$$\delta\mathcal{L}(u; v) = \frac{d}{d\epsilon}\mathcal{L}(u + \epsilon v)\bigg|_{\epsilon=0} = 0, \tag{10}$$

and a solution u of (10) is called a *weak extremal* of $\mathcal{L}$ [12].

Using the fundamental lemma of the calculus of variations, relation (10) yields the Euler-Lagrange equation as a necessary condition to be satisfied by minimizers of $\mathcal{L}$. This Euler-Lagrange equation is given by

$$-\nabla \cdot \left(\frac{F'(|\nabla u|)}{|\nabla u|}\nabla u\right) + \lambda(u - u_0) = 0, \quad \text{in } \Omega, \tag{11}$$

with homogeneous Neumann boundary conditions. An image u satisfying (11) (or equivalently $\nabla\mathcal{L}(u) = 0$) is called an *extremal* of $\mathcal{L}$.

Note that $|\nabla u|$ is not differentiable when $\nabla u = 0$ (e.g. flat regions in the image u). To overcome the resulting numerical difficulties, we use the following slight modification

$$|\nabla u|_\epsilon = \sqrt{|\nabla u|^2 + \epsilon},$$

where ϵ is positive sufficiently small.

By further constraining λ, we may be in a position to sharpen the properties of the minimizer, as given in the following.

Proposition 1. *Let $\lambda = 0$, and S be a convex set of an image space X. If the Lagrangian F is nonegative convex and of class C^1 such that $F'(0) \geq 0$, then the global minimizer of $\mathcal{L}$ is a constant image.*

Proof. Since F is convex and $F'(0) \geq 0$, it follows that $F(|\nabla u|) \geq F(0)$. Thus the constant image is a minimizer of $\mathcal{L}$. Since S is convex, it follows that this minimizer is global. □

Using the Euler-Lagrange variational principle, the minimizer of (9) can be interpreted as the steady state solution to the following nonlinear elliptic PDE called *gradient descent flow*

$$u_t = \nabla \cdot (g(|\nabla u|)\nabla u) - \lambda(u - u_0), \quad \text{in } \Omega \times \mathbb{R}_+, \tag{12}$$

where $g(z) = F'(z)/z$, with $z > 0$, and assuming homogeneous Neumann boundary conditions.

The following examples illustrate the close connection between minimizing problems of variational integrals and boundary value problems for partial differential equations in the case of no noise constraint (i.e. setting $\lambda = 0$):

(a) Heat equation: $u_t = \Delta u$ is the gradient descent flow for the Dirichlet variational integral

$$D(u) = \frac{1}{2} \int_\Omega |\nabla u|^2 dx, \tag{13}$$

(b) Perona-Malik PDE: It has been shown in [17] that the anisotropic diffusion PDE of Perona and Malik [6] given by $u_t = \nabla \cdot (g(|\nabla u|)\nabla u)$, is the gradient descent flow for the variational integral

$$\mathcal{F}_c(u) = \int_\Omega F_c(|\nabla u|) dx,$$

with Lagrangians

$$F_c(z) = \frac{c^2}{2} \log\left(1 + \frac{z^2}{c^2}\right) \quad \text{or} \quad F_c(z) = \frac{c^2}{2}\left(1 - \exp\left(-\frac{z^2}{c^2}\right)\right),$$

where $z \in \mathbb{R}^+$ and c is a tuning positive constant.

The key idea behind using the diffusion functions proposed by Perona and Malik is to encourage smoothing in flat regions and to diffuse less around the edges, so that small variations in the image such as noise is smoothed and edges are preserved. However, it has been noted that the anisotropic diffusion is ill-posed and it becomes well-posed under certain conditions on the diffusion function or equivalently on the Lagrangian [17].

(c) Curvature flow: $u_t = \nabla \cdot (\frac{\nabla u}{|\nabla u|})$ corresponds to the total variation integral

$$TV(u) = \int_\Omega |\nabla u| dx. \tag{14}$$

4 Robust Variational Approach

Robust estimation addresses the case where the distribution function is in fact *not* precisely known [18, 9]. In this case, a reasonable approach would be to assume that the density is a member of some set, or some family of parametric families, and to choose the *best* estimate for the *least favorable* member of that set. Huber [18] proposed an ϵ-contaminated normal set $\mathcal{P}_\epsilon$ defined as

$$\mathcal{P}_\epsilon = \{(1 - \epsilon)\Phi + \epsilon H : \quad H \in \mathcal{S}\},$$

where Φ is the standard normal distribution, $\mathcal{S}$ is the set of all probability distributions symmetric with respect to the origin (i.e. such that $H(-x) = 1 - H(x)$) and $\epsilon \in [0, 1]$ is the known fraction of "contamination". Huber found that the least favorable distribution in $\mathcal{P}_\epsilon$ which maximizes the asymptotic variance (or, equivalently, minimizes the Fisher information) is Gaussian in the center and Laplacian in the tails, and switches from one to the other at a point whose value depends on the fraction of contamination ϵ, larger fractions corresponding to smaller switching points and vice versa.

For the set $\mathcal{P}_\epsilon$ of ϵ-contaminated normal distributions, the least favorable distribution has a density function f_H given by [18, 9]

$$f_H(z) = \frac{(1-\epsilon)}{\sqrt{2\pi}} \exp(-\rho_k(z)), \tag{15}$$

where ρ_k is the Huber M-estimator cost function given by

$$\rho_k(z) = \begin{cases} \dfrac{z^2}{2} & \text{if } |z| \leq k \\ k|z| - \dfrac{k^2}{2} & \text{otherwise} \end{cases} \tag{16}$$

and k is a positive constant related to the fraction of contamination ϵ by the equation [18]

$$2\left(\frac{\phi(k)}{k} - \Phi(-k) \right) = \frac{\epsilon}{1-\epsilon}, \tag{17}$$

where Φ is the standard normal distribution function and ϕ is its probability density function. It is clear that ρ_k is a convex function, quadratic in the center and linear in the tails.

Motivated by the robustness of the Huber M-filter in the probabilistic approach of image denoising [1], we define the Huber variational integral as

$$\mathcal{R}_k(u) = \int_\Omega \rho_k(|\nabla u|)d\boldsymbol{x}. \tag{18}$$

It is worth noting that the Huber variational integral is a hybrid of the Dirichlet variational integral ($\rho_k(|\nabla u|) \propto |\nabla u|^2/2$ as $k \to \infty$) and the total variation integral ($\rho_k(|\nabla u|) \propto |\nabla u|$ as $k \to 0$). One may check that the Huber variational integral $\mathcal{R}_k : H^1(\Omega) \to \mathbb{R}^+$ is well defined, convex, and coercive. It follows from Theorem 1 that the minimization problem

$$\hat{u} = \arg \min_{u \in H^1(\Omega)} \int_\Omega \left(\rho_k(|\nabla u|) + \frac{\lambda}{2}|u - u_0|^2 \right) d\boldsymbol{x} \tag{19}$$

has a solution. This solution is unique when $\lambda > 0$

Proposition 2. *The optimization problem (19) is equivalent to*

$$\hat{u} = \arg \min_{(u,\theta) \in H^1(\Omega) \times \mathbb{R}} \left\{ \frac{\theta^2}{2} + \int_\Omega \left(k\big||\nabla u| - \theta\big| + \frac{\lambda}{2}|u - u_0|^2 \right) d\boldsymbol{x} \right\}. \tag{20}$$

Proof. For z fixed, define $\Psi(\theta) = \frac{1}{2}\theta^2 + k|z - \theta|$ on $\mathbb{R}$. It is is clear that Ψ is convex on $\mathbb{R}$. It follows that Ψ attains its minimum at θ_0 such that $\Psi'(\theta_0) = 0$ and $\Psi''(\theta_0) > 0$, that is $\theta_0 = k \, \text{sign}(z - k)$. Thus we have

$$\Psi(\theta_0) = \begin{cases} kz - \dfrac{k^2}{2} & \text{if } z > k \\ \dfrac{z^2}{2} & \text{if } z = k \\ -kz - \dfrac{k^2}{2} & \text{if } z < -k \end{cases}$$

It follows that $\rho_k(z) = \arg\min_{\theta \in \mathbb{R}} \Psi(\theta)$. This concludes the proof. □

Using the Euler-Lagrange variational principle, it follows that the Huber gradient descent flow is given by

$$u_t = \nabla \cdot (g_k(|\nabla u|)\nabla u) - \lambda(u - u_0), \quad \text{in } \Omega \times \mathbb{R}_+, \tag{21}$$

where g_k is the Huber M-estimator weight function [18]

$$g_k(z) = \frac{\rho_k'(z)}{z} = \begin{cases} 1 & \text{if } |z| \le k \\ \dfrac{k}{|z|} & \text{otherwise} \end{cases}$$

and with homogeneous Neumann boundary conditions.

For large k, the Huber gradient descent flow results in the isotropic diffusion (heat equation when $\lambda = 0$), and for small k, it corresponds to total variation gradient descent flow (curvature flow when $\lambda = 0$).

It is worth noting that in the case of no noise constraint (i.e. setting $\lambda = 0$), the Huber gradient descent flow yields the robust anisotropic diffusion [19] obtained by replacing the diffusion functions proposed in [6] by robust M-estimator weight functions [18, 1].

Chambolle and Lions [14] proposed the following variational integral

$$\Phi_\epsilon(u) = \int_\Omega \phi_\epsilon(|\nabla u|)dx,$$

where the Lagrangian ϕ_ϵ is defined as

$$\phi_\epsilon(z) = \begin{cases} \dfrac{z^2}{2\epsilon} & \text{if } |z| \le \epsilon \\ |z| - \dfrac{\epsilon}{2} & \text{if } \epsilon \le |z| \le \frac{1}{\epsilon} \\ \dfrac{\epsilon z^2}{2} - \dfrac{1 - \epsilon^2}{2\epsilon} & \text{if } |z| \ge \frac{1}{\epsilon} \end{cases} \tag{22}$$

As mentioned in [14], the case $|z| \ge 1/\epsilon$ may be dropped when dealing with discrete images since in this case the image gradients have bounded magnitudes. Hence, the variational integral Φ_ϵ becomes the Huber variational integral $\mathcal{R}_k$.

5 Entropic Variational Approach

The maximum entropy criterion is an important principle in statistics for modelling the prior probability $p(u)$ of an unknown image u, and it has been used with success in numerous image processing applications [4]. Suppose the available information by way of moments of some known functions $m_r(u), r = 1, \ldots, s$. The maximum entropy principle suggests that a good choice of the prior probability $p(u)$ is the one that has the maximum entropy or equivalently has the minimum negentropy [20]

$$\begin{aligned} &\min_u \int p(u) \log p(u) du \\ &\text{s.t.} \int p(u) du = 1 \\ &\quad\; \int m_r(u)p(u) du = \mu_r, \quad r = 1, \ldots, s \end{aligned} \tag{23}$$

Using Lagrange's theorem, the solution of (23) is given by

$$p(u) = \frac{1}{Z} \exp\left\{ -\sum_{r=1}^{s} \lambda_r m_r(u) \right\}, \tag{24}$$

where λ_r's are the Lagrange multipliers, and Z is the partition function. Thus, the maximum entropy distribution $p(u)$ given by Eq. (24) can be used as a model for the prior distribution in MAP estimation.

5.1   Entropic Gradient Descent Flow

Motivated by the good performance of the maximum entropy method in the probabilistic approach to image denoising, we define the negentropy variational integral as

$$\mathcal{H}(u) = \int_\Omega H(|\nabla u|)d\boldsymbol{x} = \int_\Omega |\nabla u| \log |\nabla u| d\boldsymbol{x}, \tag{25}$$

where $H(z) = z\log(z)$, $z \geq 0$. Note that $-H(z) \to 0$ as $z \to 0$.

It follows from the inequality $z\log(z) \leq z^2/2$ that

$$|\mathcal{H}(u)| \leq \int_\Omega |\nabla u|^2 d\boldsymbol{x} \leq \|u\|_{H^1(\Omega)}^2 < \infty, \quad \forall u \in H^1(\Omega),$$

Thus the negentropy variational integral $\mathcal{H} : H^1(\Omega) \to \mathbb{R}$ is well defined. Clearly, the Lagrangian H is strictly convex, and coercive, i.e. $H(z) \to \infty$ as $|z| \to \infty$. The following result follows from Theorem 1.

Proposition 3. *Let $\lambda > 0$. The minimization problem*

$$\hat{u} = \arg\min_{u \in H^1(\Omega)} \int_\Omega \left(|\nabla u| \log |\nabla u| + \frac{\lambda}{2}|u - u_0|^2 \right) d\boldsymbol{x}$$

has a unique solution provided that $|\nabla u| \geq 1$.

Using the Euler-Lagrange variational principle, it follows that the entropic gradient descent flow is given by

$$u_t = \nabla \cdot \left(\frac{1 + \log|\nabla u|}{|\nabla u|} \nabla u \right) - \lambda(u - u_0), \quad \text{in } \Omega \times \mathbb{R}_+, \tag{26}$$

with homogeneous Neumann boundary conditions.

Proposition 4. *Let u be an image. The negentropy variational integral and the total variation satisfy the following inequality*

$$\mathcal{H}(u) \geq TV(u) - 1.$$

Proof. Since the negentropy H is a convex function, the Jensen inequality yields

$$\int_\Omega H(|\nabla u|)d\boldsymbol{x} \geq H\left(\int_\Omega |\nabla u| d\boldsymbol{x} \right)$$
$$= H\big(TV(u)\big)$$
$$= TV(u) \log TV(u),$$

and using the inequality $z\log(z) \geq z - 1$ for $z \geq 0$, we conclude the proof.   □

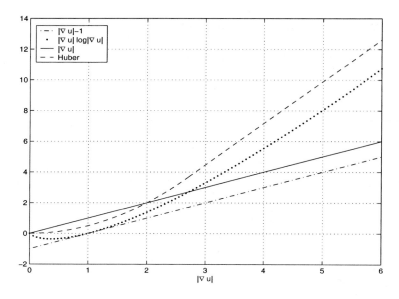

Fig. 1. Visual comparison of some variational integrands.

5.2 Improved Entropic Gradient Descent Flow

Some variational integrands discussed in this paper are plotted in Fig. 1. From these plots, one may define a hybrid functional between the negentropy variational integral and the total variation as follows

$$\widetilde{\mathcal{H}}(u) = \begin{cases} \mathcal{H}(u) & \text{if } |\nabla u| \leq e \\ TV(u) & \text{otherwise.} \end{cases}$$

Note that the functional $\widetilde{\mathcal{H}}$ is not differentiable when the Euclidean norm of ∇u is equal to e (i.e. Euler number: $e = \lim_{n \to \infty}(1 + 1/n)^n \approx 2.71$). This difficulty is overcome if we replace $\widetilde{\mathcal{H}}$ with the following functional $\mathcal{H}_{TV}$ defined as

$$\mathcal{H}_{TV}(u) = \int_\Omega H_{TV}(|\nabla u|)d\boldsymbol{x} = \begin{cases} \mathcal{H}(u) & \text{if } |\nabla u| \leq e \\ 2\,TV(u) - |\Omega|e & \text{otherwise} \end{cases} \qquad (27)$$

where $H_{TV} : \mathbb{R}^+ \to \mathbb{R}$ is defined as

$$H_{TV}(z) = \begin{cases} z\log(z) & \text{if } z \leq e \\ 2z - e & \text{otherwise} \end{cases}$$

and $|\Omega|$ denotes the Lebesque measure of the image domain Ω. In the numerical implementation of our algorithms, we may assume without loss of generality that $\Omega = (0,1) \times (0,1)$, so that $|\Omega| = 1$. Note that $\mathcal{H}_{TV} : H^1(\Omega) \to \mathbb{R}$ is well defined, differentiable, weakly lower semicontinuous, and coercive. It follows from

Theorem 1 that the minimization problem

$$\hat{u} = \arg \min_{u \in H^1(\Omega)} \left\{ \mathcal{H}_{TV}(u) + \frac{\lambda}{2}\|u - u_0\|^2 \right\} \tag{28}$$

has a solution.

Using the Euler-Lagrange variational principle, it follows that the improved entropic gradient descent flow is given by

$$u_t = \nabla \cdot \left(\frac{H'_{TV}(|\nabla u|)}{|\nabla u|} \nabla u \right) - \lambda(u - u_0), \quad \text{in } \Omega \times \mathbb{R}_+, \tag{29}$$

with homogeneous Neumann boundary conditions.

6   Simulation Results

This section presents simulation results where Huber, entropic, total variation and improved entropic gradient descent flows are applied to enhance images corrupted by Gaussian and Laplacian noise.

The performance of a filter clearly depends on the filter type, the properties of signals/images, and the characteristics of the noise. The choice of criteria by which to measure the performance of a filter presents certain difficulties, and only gives a partial picture of reality. To assess the performance of the proposed denoising methods, a mean square error (MSE) between the filtered and the original image is evaluated and used as a quantitative measure of performance of the proposed techniques. The regularization parameter (or Lagrange multiplier) λ for the proposed gradient descent flows is chosen to be proportional to signal-to-noise ratio (SNR) in all the experiments.

In order to evaluate the performance of the proposed gradient descent flows in the presence of Gaussian noise, the image shown in Fig. 2(a) has been corrupted by Gaussian white noise with SNR = 4.79 db. Fig. 2 displays the results of filtering the noisy image shown in Fig. 2(b) by Huber with optimal $k = 1.345$, entropic, total variation and improved entropic gradient descent flows. Qualitatively, we observe that the proposed techniques are able to suppress Gaussian noise while preserving important features in the image. The resulting mean square error (MSE) computations are also tabulated in Fig. 2.

The Laplacian noise is somewhat heavier than the Gaussian noise. Moreover, the Laplace distribution is similar to Huber's least favorable distribution [9] (for the no process noise case), at least in the tails. To demonstrate the application of the proposed gradient descent flows to image denoising, qualititive and quantitative comparisons are performed to show a much improved performance of these techniques. Fig. 3(b) shows a noisy image contaminated by Laplacian white noise with SNR = 3.91 db. The MSE's results obtained by applying the proposed techniques to the noisy image are shown in Fig. 3 with the corresponding filtered images. Note that the improved entropic gradient descent flow outperforms the other flows in removing Laplacian noise. Comparison of these images clearly indicates that the improved entropic gradient descent flow preserves well the image structures while removing heavy tailed noise.

Gradient descent flows	MSE		
	SNR = 4.79	SNR = 3.52	SNR = 2.34
Huber	234.1499	233.7337	230.0263
Entropic	205.0146	207.1040	205.3454
Total Variation	247.4875	263.0437	402.0660
Improved Entropic	121.2550	137.9356	166.4490

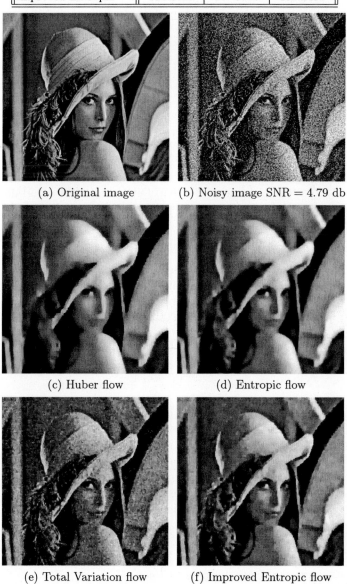

(a) Original image

(b) Noisy image SNR = 4.79 db

(c) Huber flow

(d) Entropic flow

(e) Total Variation flow

(f) Improved Entropic flow

Fig. 2. Filtering results for Gaussian noise.

Gradient descent flows	MSE		
	SNR = 6.33	SNR = 3.91	SNR = 3.05
Huber	237.7012	244.4348	248.4833
Entropic	200.5266	211.4027	217.3592
Total Variation	138.4717	176.1719	213.1221
Improved Entropic	104.4591	170.2140	208.8639

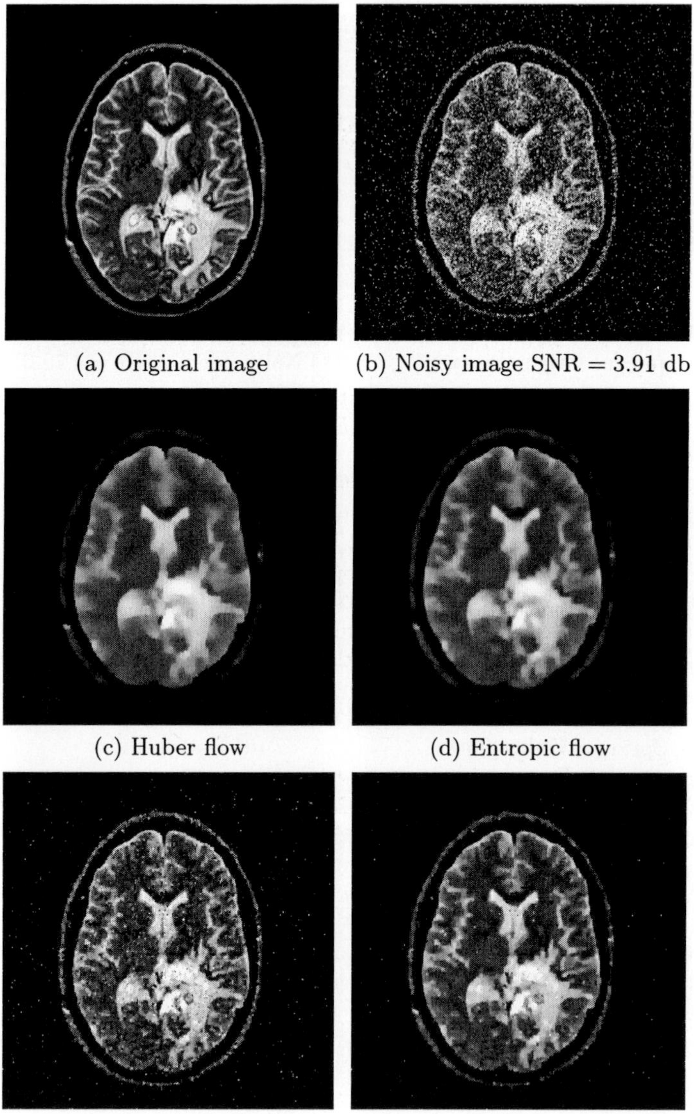

(a) Original image   (b) Noisy image SNR = 3.91 db

(c) Huber flow   (d) Entropic flow

(e) Total Variation flow   (f) Improved Entropic flow

Fig. 3. Filtering results for Laplacian noise.

References

1. J. Astola and P. Kuosmanen, *Fundamentals of Nonlinear Digital Filtering*, CRC Press LLC, 1997.
2. A. Ben Hamza, P. Luque, J. Martinez, and R. Roman, "Removing noise and preserving details with relaxed median filters," *Journal of Mathematical Imaging and Vision*, vol. 11, no. 2, pp. 161-177, October 1999.
3. S. Geman and D. Geman, "Stochastic relaxation, Gibbs distributions and the Bayesian restoration of images," *IEEE Trans. Pattern Analysis and Machine intelligence*, vol. 6, no. 7, pp. 721-741, July 1984.
4. H. Stark, Ed., *Image Recovery: Theory and Application*, New York: Academic, 1987.
5. S.C. Zhu and D. Mumford, "Prior learning and Gibbs reaction-diffusion," *IEEE Trans. Pattern Analysis and Machine intelligence*, vol. 19, no. 11, pp. 1236-1244, November 1997.
6. P. Perona and J. Malik, "Scale space and edge detection using anisotropic diffusion," *IEEE IEEE Trans. Pattern Analysis and Machine intelligence*, vol. 12, no. 7, pp. 629-639, July 1990.
7. J Morel and S. Solemini, *Variational Methods in Image Segmentation*, Birkhauser, Boston, 1995.
8. C. Samson, L. Blanc-Feraud, G. Aubert, and J. Zerubia, "A variational model for image classification and restoration," *IEEE Trans. Pattern Analysis and Machine intelligence*, vol. 22, no. 5, pp. 460-472, May 2000.
9. H. Krim and I.C. Schick, "Minimax description length for signal denoising and optimized representation," *IEEE Trans. Information Theory*, vol 45, no. 3, pp. 898-908, April 1999.
10. L. Rudin, S. Osher, and E. Fatemi, "Nonlinear total variation based noise removal algorithms," *Physica D*, vol. 60, pp. 259-268, 1992.
11. I. Pollak, A.S. Willsky, and H. Krim, "Image Segmentation and Edge Enhancement with Stabilized Inverse Diffusion Equations," *IEEE Trans. Image Processing*, vol. 9, no. 2, pp. 256-266, February 2000.
12. M. Giaquinta and S. Hildebrandt, *Calculus of Variations I: The Lagrangian Formalism*, Springer-Verlag, 1996.
13. C. Vogel and M. Oman, "Iterative methods for total variation denoising," *SIAM J. Sci. Stat. Comput.*, vol. 17, pp. 227-238, 1996.
14. A. Chambolle and P.L. Lions, "Image Recovery via total variation minimization and related problems," *Numerische Mathematik*, 76, pp. 167-188, 1997.
15. T.F. Chan and C.K. Wong, "Total variation blind deconvolution", *IEEE Trans. Image Processing*, vol. 7, no. 3, pp. 370-375, March 1998.
16. K. Ito and K. Kunisch, "Restoration of Edge-Flat-Grey Scale Images," *Inverse Problems*, vol 16, no.4, pp. 909-928, August 2000.
17. Y.L. You, W. Xu, A. Tannenbaum, and M. Kaveh, "Behavioral Analysis of anisotropic diffusion in image processing," *IEEE Trans. Image Processing*, vol. 5, no. 11, pp. 1539-1553, November 1996.
18. P. Huber, *Robust Statistics*. John Wiley & Sons, New York, 1981.
19. M.J. Black, G. Sapiro, D.H. Marimont, and D. Heeger, "Robust anisotropic diffusion," *IEEE Trans. Image Processing*, vol. 7, no. 3, pp. 421-432, March 1998.
20. H. Krim, "On the distributions of optimized multiscale representations," *ICASSP-97*, vol. 5, pp. 3673-3676, 1997.

Maximum Likelihood Estimation
of the Template of a Rigid Moving Object

Pedro M.Q. Aguiar[1] and José M.F. Moura[2]

[1] Instituto de Sistemas e Robótica, Instituto Superior Técnico, Lisboa, Portugal
aguiar@isr.ist.utl.pt, www.isr.ist.utl.pt/~aguiar
[2] Electrical and Computer Eng., Carnegie Mellon University, Pittsburgh PA, USA
moura@ece.cmu.edu, www.ece.cmu.edu/~moura

Abstract. Motion segmentation methods often fail to detect the motions of low textured regions. We develop an algorithm for segmentation of low textured moving objects. While usually current motion segmentation methods use only two or three consecutive images our method refines the shape of the moving object by processing successively the new frames as they become available. We formulate the segmentation as a parameter estimation problem. The images in the sequence are modeled taking into account the *rigidity* of the moving object and the *occlusion* of the background by the moving object. The segmentation algorithm is derived as a computationally simple approximation to the *Maximum Likelihood* estimate of the parameters involved in the image sequence model: the motions, the template of the moving object, its intensity levels, and the intensity levels of the background pixels. We describe experiments that demonstrate the good performance of our algorithm.

1 Introduction

The segmentation of an image into regions that undergo different motions has received the attention of a large number of researchers. According to their research focus, different scientific communities addressed the motion segmentation task from distinct viewpoints.

Several papers on image sequence coding address the motion segmentation task with computation time concerns. They reduce temporal redundancy by predicting each frame from the previous one through motion compensation. See reference [16] for a review on very low bit rate video coding. Regions undergoing different movements are compensated in different ways, according to their motion. The techniques used in image sequence coding attempt to segment the moving objects by processing only two consecutive frames. Since their focus is on compression and not in developing a high level representation, these efforts have not considered low textured scenes, and regions with no texture are considered unchanged. As an example, we applied the algorithm of reference [8] to segmenting a low textured moving object. Two consecutive frames of a traffic road video clip are shown in the left side of Figure 1. In the right side of Figure 1, the template of the moving car was found by excluding from the regions

M.A.T. Figueiredo, J. Zerubia, A.K. Jain (Eds.): EMMCVPR 2001, LNCS 2134, pp. 34–49, 2001.

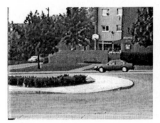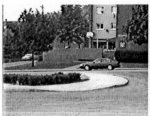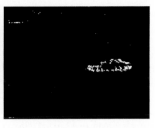

Fig. 1. Motion segmentation in low texture.

that changed between the two co-registered frames the ones that correspond to uncovered background areas, see reference [8]. The small regions that due to the noise are misclassified as belonging to the car template can be discarded by an adequate morphological post-processing. However, due to the low texture of the car, the regions in the interior of the car are misclassified as belonging to the background, leading to a highly incomplete car template.

High level representation in image sequence understanding, such as layered models [14, 18, 3], has been considered in the computer vision literature. Their approach to motion-based segmentation copes with low textured scenes by coupling motion-based segmentation with prior knowledge about the scenes as in statistical regularization techniques, or by combining motion with other atributtes. For example, reference [7] uses a *Markov Random Field* (MRF) prior and a *Bayesian Maximum a Posteriori* (MAP) criterion to segment moving regions. The authors suggest a multiscale MRF modeling to resolve large regions of uniform intensity. In reference [9], the contour of a moving object is estimated by fusing motion with color segmentation and edge detection. In general, these methods lead to complex and time consuming algorithms.

References [10, 11] describe one of the few approaches using temporal integration by averaging the images registered according to the motion of the different objects in the scene. After processing a number of frames, each of these integrated images is expected to show only one sharp region corresponding to the tracked object. This region is found by detecting the stationary regions between the corresponding integrated image and the current frame. Unless the background is textured enough to blur completely the averaged images, some regions of the background can be classified as stationary. In this situation, their method overestimates the template of the moving object. This is particularly likely to happen when the background has large regions with almost constant color or intensity level.

1.1 Proposed Approach

We formulate image sequence analysis as a parameter estimation problem by using the analogy between a communications system and image sequence analysis, see references [15] and [17]. The segmentation algorithm is derived as a computationally simple approximation to the *Maximum Likelihood* (ML) estimate of the parameters involved in the two-dimensional (2D) image sequence model: the motions, the template of the moving object, its intensity levels (the object texture), and the intensity levels of the background pixels (the background texture). The joint ML estimation of the complete set of parameters is a very complex task. Motivated by our experience with real video sequences, we decouple the estimation of the motions (moving objects and camera) from that of the remaining parameters. The motions are estimated on a frame by frame basis and then used in the estimation of the remaining parameters. Then, we introduce the motion estimates into the ML cost function and minimize this function with respect to the remaining parameters.

The estimate of the object texture is obtained in closed form. To estimate the background texture and the moving object template, we develop a fast two-step iterative algorithm. The first step estimates the background for a fixed template – the solution is obtained in closed form. The second step estimates the template for a fixed background – the solution is given by a simple binary test evaluated at each pixel. The algorithm converges in a few iterations, typically three to five iterations.

Our approach is related to the approach of references [10, 11], however, we model explicitly the *occlusion* of the background by the moving object and we use all the frames available rather than just a single frame to estimate the moving object template. Even when the moving object has a color very similar to the color of the background, our algorithm has the ability to resolve accurately the moving object from the background, because it integrates over time those small differences.

1.2   Paper Organization

In section 2, we state the segmentation problem. We define the notation, develop the observation model, and formulate the ML estimation. In section 3, we detail the two-step iterative method that minimizes the ML cost function. In section 4, we describe two experiments that demonstrate the performance of our algorithm. Section 5 concludes the paper.

For the details not included in this paper, see reference [1]. A preliminary version of this work was presented in reference [2].

2   Problem Formulation

We discuss motion segmentation in the context of *Generative Video* (GV), see references [13, 14]. GV is a framework for the analysis and synthesis of video sequences. In GV the operational units are not the individual images in the original sequence, as in standard methods, but rather the world images and the ancillary data. The world images encode the non-redundant information about the video sequence. They are augmented views of the world – background world image – and complete views of moving objects – figure world images. The ancillary data registers the world images, stratifies them at each time instant, and positions the camera with respect to the layering of world images. The world images and the ancillary data are the GV representation, the information that is needed to regenerate the original video sequence. We formulate the moving object segmentation task as the problem of generating the world images and ancillary data for the GV representation of a video clip.

2.1   Notation

An image is a real function defined on a subset of the real plane. The image space is a set $\{\mathbf{I} : \mathcal{D} \to \mathcal{R}\}$, where $\mathbf{I}$ is an image, $\mathcal{D}$ is the domain of the image, and $\mathcal{R}$ is the range of the image. The domain $\mathcal{D}$ is a compact subset of the real plane $\mathbb{R}^2$, and the range $\mathcal{R}$ is a subset of the real line $\mathbb{R}$. Examples of images are the frame f in the video sequence, denoted by $\mathbf{I}_f$, the background world image, denoted by $\mathbf{B}$, the moving object world image, denoted by $\mathbf{O}$, and the moving object template, denoted by $\mathbf{T}$. The images $\mathbf{I}_f$, $\mathbf{B}$, and $\mathbf{O}$ have range $\mathcal{R} = \mathbb{R}$. They code intensity gray levels[1]. The template of the moving object is a binary image, i.e., an image with range $\mathcal{R} = \{0, 1\}$, defining the region occupied by the moving object. The domain of the images $\mathbf{I}_f$ and $\mathbf{T}$ is a rectangle corresponding to the support of the frames. The domain of the background world image $\mathbf{B}$ is a subset $\mathcal{D}$ of the plane whose shape and size depends on the camera motion, i.e., $\mathcal{D}$ is the region of the background observed in the entire sequence. The domain $\mathcal{D}$ of the moving object world image is the subset of $\mathbb{R}^2$ where the template $\mathbf{T}$ takes the value 1, i.e., $\mathcal{D} = \{(x, y) : \mathbf{T}(x, y) = 1\}$.

In our implementation, the domain of each image is rectangular shaped with size fitting the needs of the corresponding image. Although we use a continuous spatial dependence for commodity, in practice the domains are discretized and the images are stored as matrices. We index the entries of each of these matrices by the pixels (x, y) of each image and refer to the value of image $\mathbf{I}$ at pixel (x, y) as $\mathbf{I}(x, y)$. Throughout the text, we refer to the image product of two images $\mathbf{A}$ and $\mathbf{B}$, i.e., the image whose value at pixel (x, y) equals $\mathbf{A}(x, y)\mathbf{B}(x, y)$, as the image $\mathbf{AB}$. Note that this product corresponds to the Hadamard product, or elementwise product, of the matrices representing images $\mathbf{A}$ and $\mathbf{B}$, not their matrix product.

We consider two-dimensional (2D) parallel motions, i.e., all motions (translations and rotations) are parallel to the camera plane. We represent this kind of motions by specifying time varying position vectors. These vectors code rotation-translation pairs that take values in the group of rigid transformations of the

---

[1] The intensity values of the images in the video sequence are positive. In our experiments, these values are coded by a binary word of eight bits. Thus, the intensity values of a gray level image are in the set of integers in the interval $[0, 255]$. For simplicity, we do not take into account the discretization and the saturations, i.e., we consider the intensity values to be real numbers and the gray level images to have range $\mathcal{R} = \mathbb{R}$. The analysis in the thesis is easily extended to color images. A color is represented by specifying three intensities, either of the perceptual attributes *brightness*, *hue*, and *saturation*; or of the primary colors *red*, *green*, and *blue*, see reference [12]. The range of a color image is then $\mathcal{R} = \mathbb{R}^3$.

plane, the special Euclidean group SE(2). The image obtained by applying the rigid motion coded by the vector $\mathbf{p}$ to the image $\mathbf{I}$ is denoted by $\mathcal{M}(\mathbf{p})\mathbf{I}$. The image $\mathcal{M}(\mathbf{p})\mathbf{I}$ is also usually called the registration of the image $\mathbf{I}$ according to the position vector $\mathbf{p}$. The entity represented by $\mathcal{M}(\mathbf{p})$ is seen as a motion operator. In practice, the (x, y) entry of the matrix representing the image $\mathcal{M}(\mathbf{p})\mathbf{I}$ is given by $\mathcal{M}(\mathbf{p})\mathbf{I}(x, y) = \mathbf{I}(f_x(\mathbf{p}; x, y), f_y(\mathbf{p}; x, y))$ where $f_x(\mathbf{p}; x, y)$ and $f_y(\mathbf{p}; x, y)$ represent the coordinate transformation imposed by the 2D rigid motion. We use bilinear interpolation to compute the intensity values at points that fall in between the stored samples of an image.

The motion operators can be composed. The registration of the image $\mathcal{M}(\mathbf{p})\mathbf{I}$ according to the position vector $\mathbf{q}$ is denoted by $\mathcal{M}(\mathbf{q}\mathbf{p})\mathbf{I}$. By doing this we are using the notation $\mathbf{q}\mathbf{p}$ for the composition of the two elements of SE(2), $\mathbf{q}$ and $\mathbf{p}$. We denote the inverse of $\mathbf{p}$ by $\mathbf{p}^{\#}$, i.e., the vector $\mathbf{p}^{\#}$ is such that when composed with $\mathbf{p}$ we obtain the identity element of SE(2). Thus, the registration of the image $\mathcal{M}(\mathbf{p})\mathbf{I}$ according to the position vector $\mathbf{p}^{\#}$ obtains the original image $\mathbf{I}$, so we have $\mathcal{M}(\mathbf{p}^{\#}\mathbf{p})\mathbf{I} = \mathcal{M}(\mathbf{p}\mathbf{p}^{\#})\mathbf{I} = \mathbf{I}$. Note that, in general, the elements of SE(2) do not commute, i.e., we have $\mathbf{q}\mathbf{p} \neq \mathbf{p}\mathbf{q}$, and $\mathcal{M}(\mathbf{q}\mathbf{p})\mathbf{I} \neq \mathcal{M}(\mathbf{p}\mathbf{q})\mathbf{I}$. Only in special cases is the composition of the motion operators not affected by the order of application, as for example when the motions $\mathbf{p}$ and $\mathbf{q}$ are pure translations or pure rotations.

The notation for the position vectors involved in the segmentation problem is as follows. The vector $\mathbf{p}_f$ represents the position of the background world image relative to the camera in frame f. The vector $\mathbf{q}_f$ represents the position of the moving object relative to the camera in frame f.

2.2   Observation Model

The observation model considers a scene with a moving object in front of a moving camera with two-dimensional (2D) parallel motions. The pixel (x, y) of the image $\mathbf{I}_f$ belongs either to the background world image $\mathbf{B}$ or to the object world image $\mathbf{O}$. The intensity $\mathbf{I}_f(x, y)$ of the pixel (x, y) is modeled as

$$\mathbf{I}_f(x, y) = \mathcal{M}(\mathbf{p}_f^{\#})\mathbf{B}(x, y) \left[1 - \mathcal{M}(\mathbf{q}_f^{\#})\mathbf{T}(x, y)\right]$$
$$+ \mathcal{M}(\mathbf{q}_f^{\#})\mathbf{O}(x, y)\,\mathcal{M}(\mathbf{q}_f^{\#})\mathbf{T}(x, y) + \mathbf{W}_f(x, y). \qquad (1)$$

In equation (1), $\mathbf{T}$ is the moving object template, $\mathbf{p}_f$ and $\mathbf{q}_f$ are the camera pose and the object position, and $\mathbf{W}_f$ stands for the observation noise, assumed Gaussian, zero mean, and white.

Equation (1) states that the intensity of the pixel (x, y) on frame f, $\mathbf{I}_f(x, y)$, is a noisy version of the true value of the intensity level of the pixel (x, y). If the pixel (x, y) of the current image belongs to the template of the object, $\mathbf{T}$, after the template is compensated by the object position, i.e., registered according to the vector $\mathbf{q}_f^{\#}$, then $\mathcal{M}(\mathbf{q}_f^{\#})\mathbf{T}(x, y) = 1$. In this case, the first term of the right hand side of (1) is zero, while the second term equals $\mathcal{M}(\mathbf{q}_f^{\#})\mathbf{O}(x, y)$, the intensity of the pixel (x, y) of the moving object. In other words, the intensity $\mathbf{I}_f(x, y)$

equals the object intensity $\mathcal{M}(\mathbf{q}_f^{\#})\mathbf{O}(x,y)$ corrupted by the noise $\mathbf{W}_f(x,y)$. On the other hand, if the pixel (x,y) does not belong to the template of the object, $\mathcal{M}(\mathbf{q}_f^{\#})\mathbf{T}(x,y) = 0$, and this pixel belongs to the background world image $\mathbf{B}$, registered according to the inverse $\mathbf{p}_f^{\#}$ of the camera position. In this case, the intensity $\mathbf{I}_f(x,y)$ is a noisy version of the background intensity $\mathcal{M}(\mathbf{p}_f^{\#})\mathbf{B}(x,y)$. We want to emphasize that rather than modeling simply the two different motions, as usually done when processing only two consecutive frames, expression (1) models the *occlusion* of the background by the moving object explicitly.

Expression (1) is rewritten in compact form as

$$\mathbf{I}_f = \left\{ \mathcal{M}(\mathbf{p}_f^{\#})\mathbf{B} \left[\mathbf{1} - \mathcal{M}(\mathbf{q}_f^{\#})\mathbf{T} \right] + \mathcal{M}(\mathbf{q}_f^{\#})\mathbf{O}\,\mathcal{M}(\mathbf{q}_f^{\#})\mathbf{T} + \mathbf{W}_f \right\} \mathbf{H}, \quad (2)$$

where we assume that $\mathbf{I}_f(x,y) = 0$ for (x,y) outside the region observed by the camera. This is taken care of in equation (2) by the binary image $\mathbf{H}$ whose (x,y) entry is such that $\mathbf{H}(x,y) = 1$ if pixel (x,y) is in the observed images $\mathbf{I}_f$ or $\mathbf{H}(x,y) = 0$ if otherwise. The image $\mathbf{1}$ is constant with value 1.

2.3   Maximum Likelihood Estimation

Given F frames $\{\mathbf{I}_f, 1 \le f \le F\}$, we want to estimate the background world image $\mathbf{B}$, the object world image $\mathbf{O}$, the object template $\mathbf{T}$, the camera poses $\{\mathbf{p}_f, 1 \le f \le F\}$, and the object positions $\{\mathbf{q}_f, 1 \le f \le F\}$. The quantities $\{\mathbf{B}, \mathbf{O}, \mathbf{T}, \{\mathbf{p}_f\}, \{\mathbf{q}_f\}\}$ define the GV representation, the information that is needed to regenerate the original video sequence.

Using the observation model of expression (2) and the Gaussian white noise assumption, ML estimation leads to the minimization over all GV parameters of the functional[2]

$$C_2 = \iint \sum_{f=1}^{F} \left\{ \mathbf{I}_f(x,y) - \mathcal{M}(\mathbf{p}_f^{\#})\mathbf{B}(x,y) \left[\mathbf{1} - \mathcal{M}(\mathbf{q}_f^{\#})\mathbf{T}(x,y) \right] \right.$$
$$\left. - \mathcal{M}(\mathbf{q}_f^{\#})\mathbf{O}(x,y)\,\mathcal{M}(\mathbf{q}_f^{\#})\mathbf{T}(x,y) \right\}^2 \mathbf{H}(x,y)\, dx\, dy, \quad (3)$$

where the inner sum is over the full set of F frames and the outer integral is over all pixels.

The estimation of the parameters of expression (2) using the F frames rather than a single pair of images is a distinguishing feature of our work. Other techniques usually process only two or three consecutive frames. We use all frames available as needed. The estimation of the parameters through the minimization of a cost function that involves directly the image intensity values is another distinguishing feature of our approach. Other methods try to make some type

---

[2] We use a continuous spatial dependence for commodity. The variables x and y are continuous while f is discrete. In practice, the integral is approximated by the sum over all the pixels.

of post-processing over incomplete template estimates. We process directly the image intensity values, through ML estimation.

The minimization of the functional C_2 in equation (3) with respect to the set of GV constructs $\{\mathbf{B}, \mathbf{O}, \mathbf{T}\}$ and to the motions $\{\{\mathbf{p}_f\}, \{\mathbf{q}_f\}, 1 \leq f \leq F\}$ is a highly complex task. To obtain a computationally feasible algorithm, we simplify the problem. We decouple the estimation of the motions $\{\{\mathbf{p}_f\}, \{\mathbf{q}_f\}, 1 \leq f \leq F\}$ from the determination of the GV constructs $\{\mathbf{B}, \mathbf{O}, \mathbf{T}\}$. This is reasonable from a practical point of view and is well supported by our experimental results with real videos.

The rationale behind the simplification is that the motion of the object (and the motion of the background) can be inferred without having the knowledge of the exact object template. When only two or three frames are given, even humans find it much easier to infer the motions present in the scene than to recover an accurate template of the moving object. To better appreciate the complexity of the problem, the reader can imagine an image sequence for which there is not prior knowledge available, except that there is a background and an ocluding object that moves differently from the background. Since there are no spatial cues, consider, for example, that the background texture and the object texture are spatial white noise random variables. In this situation, humans can easily infer the motion of the background and the motion of the object, even from only two consecutive frames. With respect to the template of the moving object, we are able to infer much more accurate templates if we are given a higher number of frames because in this case we easily capture the *rigidity* of the object across time. This observation motivated our approach of decoupling the estimation of the motions from the estimation of the remaining parameters.

We perform the estimation of the motions on a frame by frame basis by using a known motion estimation method [5], see reference [1] for the details. After estimating the motions, we introduce the motion estimates into the ML cost function and minimize with respect to the remaining parameters. The solution provided by our algorithm is sub-optimal, in the sense that it is an approximation to the ML estimate of the entire set of parameters, and it can be seen as an initial guess for the minimizer of the ML cost function given by expression (3). Then, we can refine the estimate by using a greedy approach. We must emphasize, however, that the key problem here is to find the initial guess in an expedite way, not the final refinement.

3   Minimization Procedure

In this section, we assume that the motions have been correctly estimated and are known. We should note that, in reality, the motions are continuously estimated. Assuming the motions are known, the problem becomes the minimization of the ML cost function with respect to the remaining parameters, i.e., with respect to the template of the moving object, the texture of the moving object, and the texture of the background.

3.1   Two-Step Iterative Algorithm

Due to the special structure of the ML cost function C_2, we can express explicitly and with no approximations involved the estimate $\widehat{\mathbf{O}}$ of the object world image in terms of the template $\mathbf{T}$. Doing this, we are left with the minimization of C_2 with respect to the template $\mathbf{T}$ and the background world image $\mathbf{B}$, still a non-linear minimization. We approximate this minimization by a two-step iterative algorithm: (i) in step one, we solve for the background $\mathbf{B}$ while the template $\mathbf{T}$ is kept fixed; and (ii) in step two, we solve for the template $\mathbf{T}$ while the background $\mathbf{B}$ is kept fixed. We obtain closed-form solutions for the minimizers in each of the steps (i) and (ii). The two steps are repeated iteratively. The value of the ML cost function C_2 decreases along the iterative process. The algorithm proceeds till every pixel has been assigned unambiguously to either the moving object or to the background.

To initialize the segmentation algorithm, we need an initial estimate of the background. A simple, often used, estimate for the background is the average of the images in the sequence, including or not a robust statistic technique like outlier rejection, see for example reference [6]. The quality of this background estimate depends on the occlusion level of the background in the images processed. Depending on the particular characteristics of the image sequence, our algorithm can recover successfully the template of the moving object when using the average of the images as the initial estimate of the background. This is the case with the image sequence we use in the experiments reported in section 4. In reference [1], we propose a more elaborate initialization that leads to better initial estimates of the background.

3.2   Estimation of the Moving Object World Image

We express the estimate $\widehat{\mathbf{O}}$ of the moving object world image in terms of the object template $\mathbf{T}$. By minimizing C_2 with respect to the intensity value $\mathbf{O}(x, y)$, we obtain the average of the pixels that correspond to the point (x, y) of the object. The estimate $\widehat{\mathbf{O}}$ of the moving object world image is then

$$\widehat{\mathbf{O}} = \mathbf{T} \frac{1}{F} \sum_{f=1}^{F} \mathcal{M}(\mathbf{q}_f)\mathbf{I}_f. \tag{4}$$

This compact expression averages the observations $\mathbf{I}$ registered according to the motion $\mathbf{q}_f$ of the object in the region corresponding to the template $\mathbf{T}$ of the moving object.

We consider now separately the two steps of the iterative algorithm described above.

3.3   Step (i): Estimation of the Background for Fixed Template

To find the estimate $\widehat{\mathbf{B}}$ of the background world image, given the template $\mathbf{T}$, we register each term of the sum of the ML cost function C_2 in equation (3) according to the position of the camera $\mathbf{p}_f$ relative to the background. This is a valid operation because C_2 is defined as a sum over all the space $\{(x, y)\}$. We get

$$C_2 = \int\!\!\int \sum_{f=1}^{F} \left\{ \mathcal{M}(\mathbf{p}_f)\mathbf{I}_f - \mathbf{B}\left[1 - \mathcal{M}(\mathbf{p}_f\mathbf{q}_f^{\#})\mathbf{T}\right]\right.$$
$$\left. - \mathcal{M}(\mathbf{p}_f\mathbf{q}_f^{\#})\mathbf{O}\,\mathcal{M}(\mathbf{p}_f\mathbf{q}_f^{\#})\mathbf{T}(x, y)\right\}^2 \mathcal{M}(\mathbf{p}_f)\mathbf{H}\,dx\,dy. \qquad (5)$$

Minimizing the ML cost function C_2 given by expression (5) with respect to the intensity value $\mathbf{B}(x, y)$, we get the estimate $\widehat{\mathbf{B}}(x, y)$ as the average of the observed pixels that correspond to the pixel (x, y) of the background. The background world image estimate $\widehat{\mathbf{B}}$ is then written as

$$\widehat{\mathbf{B}} = \frac{\sum_{f=1}^{F}\left[1 - \mathcal{M}(\mathbf{p}_f\mathbf{q}_f^{\#})\mathbf{T}\right]\mathcal{M}(\mathbf{p}_f)\mathbf{I}_f}{\sum_{i=f}^{F}\left[1 - \mathcal{M}(\mathbf{p}_f\mathbf{q}_f^{\#})\mathbf{T}\right]\mathcal{M}(\mathbf{p}_f)\mathbf{H}}. \qquad (6)$$

The estimate $\widehat{\mathbf{B}}$ of the background world image in expression (6) is the average of the observations $\mathbf{I}_f$ registered according to the background motion $\mathbf{p}_i$, in the regions $\{(x, y)\}$ not ocluded by the moving object, i.e., when $\mathcal{M}(\mathbf{p}_f\mathbf{q}_f^{\#})\mathbf{T}(x, y) = 0$. The term $\mathcal{M}(\mathbf{p}_f)\mathbf{H}$ provides the correct averaging normalization in the denominator by accounting only for the pixels seen in the corresponding image.

If we compare the moving object world image estimate $\widehat{\mathbf{O}}$ given by equation (4) with the background world image estimate $\widehat{\mathbf{B}}$ in equation (6), we see that $\widehat{\mathbf{O}}$ is linear in the template $\mathbf{T}$, while $\widehat{\mathbf{B}}$ is nonlinear in $\mathbf{T}$. This has implications when estimating the template $\mathbf{T}$ of the moving object, as we see next.

3.4   Step (ii): Estimation of the Template for Fixed Background

Let the background world image $\mathbf{B}$ be given and replace the object world image estimate $\widehat{\mathbf{O}}$ given by expression (4) in expression (3). The ML cost function C_2 becomes linearly related to the object template $\mathbf{T}$. Manipulating C_2 as described next, we obtain

$$C_2 = \int\!\!\int \mathbf{T}(x, y)\,\mathbf{Q}(x, y)\,dx\,dy + \text{Constant}, \qquad (7)$$

$$\mathbf{Q}(x, y) = \mathbf{Q}_1(x, y) - \mathbf{Q}_2(x, y), \qquad (8)$$

$$\mathbf{Q}_1(x, y) = \frac{1}{F}\sum_{f=2}^{F}\sum_{g=1}^{f-1}\left[\mathcal{M}(\mathbf{q}_f)\mathbf{I}_f(x, y) - \mathcal{M}(\mathbf{q}_g)\mathbf{I}_g(x, y)\right]^2, \qquad (9)$$

$$\mathbf{Q}_2(x, y) = \sum_{f=1}^{F}\left[\mathcal{M}(\mathbf{q}_f)\mathbf{I}_f(x, y) - \mathcal{M}(\mathbf{q}_f\mathbf{p}_f^{\#})\mathbf{B}(x, y)\right]^2. \qquad (10)$$

We call $\mathbf{Q}$ the *segmentation matrix.*

Derivation of expressions (7) to (10)

Replace the estimate $\widehat{\mathbf{O}}$ of the moving object world image, given by expression (4), in expression (3), to obtain

$$C_2 = \iint \sum_{f=1}^{F} \left\{ \mathbf{I} - \mathcal{M}(\mathbf{p}_f^{\#})\mathbf{B} \left[1 - \mathcal{M}(\mathbf{q}_f^{\#})\mathbf{T} \right] \right.$$
$$\left. - \frac{1}{F} \sum_{g=1}^{F} \mathcal{M}(\mathbf{q}_f^{\#}\mathbf{q}_g)\mathbf{I}_g \, \mathcal{M}(\mathbf{q}_f^{\#})\mathbf{T} \right\}^2 \mathbf{H} \, dx \, dy. \qquad (11)$$

Register each term of the sum according to the object position $\mathbf{q}_f$. This is valid because C_2 is defined as an integral over all the space $\{(x,y)\}$. The result is

$$C_2 = \iint \sum_{f=1}^{F} \left\{ \left[\mathcal{M}(\mathbf{q}_f)\mathbf{I}_f - \mathcal{M}(\mathbf{q}_f\mathbf{p}_f^{\#})\mathbf{B} \right] \right.$$
$$\left. + \left[\mathcal{M}(\mathbf{q}_f\mathbf{p}_f^{\#})\mathbf{B} - \frac{1}{F} \sum_{g=1}^{F} \mathcal{M}(\mathbf{q}_g)\mathbf{I}_g \right] \mathbf{T} \right\}^2 \mathcal{M}(\mathbf{q}_f)\mathbf{H} \, dx \, dy. \qquad (12)$$

In the remainder of the derivation, the spatial dependence is not important here, and we simplify the notation by omitting (x, y). We rewrite the expression for C_2 in compact form as

$$C_2 = \iint \mathbf{C} \, dx \, dy, \quad \mathbf{C} = \sum_{f=1}^{F} \left\{ \left[\mathcal{I}_f - \mathcal{B}_f \right] + \left[\mathcal{B}_f - \frac{1}{F} \sum_{g=1}^{F} \mathcal{I}_g \right] \mathbf{T} \right\}^2 \mathcal{H}_f, \qquad (13)$$

$$\mathcal{I}_f = \mathcal{M}(\mathbf{q}_f)\mathbf{I}_f(x,y), \quad \mathcal{B}_f = \mathcal{M}(\mathbf{q}_f\mathbf{p}_f^{\#})\mathbf{B}(x,y), \quad \mathcal{H}_f = \mathcal{M}(\mathbf{q}_f)\mathbf{H}(x,y). \qquad (14)$$

We need in the sequel the following equalities

$$\left[\sum_{g=1}^{F} \mathcal{I}_g \right]^2 = \sum_{f=1}^{F} \sum_{g=1}^{F} \mathcal{I}_f\mathcal{I}_g \quad \text{and} \quad \sum_{f=2}^{F} \sum_{g=1}^{f-1} \left[\mathcal{I}_i^2 + \mathcal{I}_g^2 \right] = (F-1) \sum_{g=1}^{F} \mathcal{I}_g^2. \qquad (15)$$

Manipulating $\mathbf{C}$ under the assumption that the moving object is completely visible in the F images ($\mathbf{T}\mathcal{H}_f = \mathbf{T}, \forall_f$), and using the left equality in (15), we obtain

$$\mathbf{C} = \mathbf{T} \left\{ \sum_{f=1}^{F} \left[2\mathcal{I}_f\mathcal{B}_f - \mathcal{B}_f^2 \right] - \frac{1}{F} \left[\sum_{g=1}^{F} \mathcal{I}_g \right]^2 \right\} + \sum_{f=1}^{F} \left[\mathcal{I}_f - \mathcal{B}_f \right]^2 \mathcal{H}_f. \qquad (16)$$

The second term of $\mathbf{C}$ in expression (16) is independent of the template $\mathbf{T}$. To show that the sum that multiplies $\mathbf{T}$ is the segmentation matrix $\mathbf{Q}$ as defined by expressions (8), (9), and (10), write $\mathbf{Q}$ using the notation introduced in (14):

$$\mathbf{Q} = \frac{1}{F} \sum_{f=2}^{F} \sum_{g=1}^{f-1} \left[\mathcal{I}_f^2 + \mathcal{I}_g^2 - 2\mathcal{I}_f\mathcal{I}_g \right] - \sum_{f=1}^{F} \left[\mathcal{I}_f^2 + \mathcal{B}_f^2 - 2\mathcal{I}_f\mathcal{B}_f \right]. \qquad (17)$$

Manipulating this equation, using the two equalities in (15), we obtain

$$\mathbf{Q} = \sum_{f=1}^{F} \left[2\mathcal{I}_f\mathcal{B}_f - \mathcal{B}_f^2 \right] - \frac{1}{F} \left[\sum_{g=1}^{F} \mathcal{I}_g^2 + 2 \sum_{f=2}^{F} \sum_{g=1}^{f-1} \mathcal{I}_f\mathcal{I}_g \right]. \qquad (18)$$

The following equality concludes the derivation:

$$\left[\sum_{g=1}^{F} \mathcal{I}_g \right]^2 = \sum_{g=1}^{F} \mathcal{I}_g^2 + 2 \sum_{f=2}^{F} \sum_{g=1}^{f-1} \mathcal{I}_f\mathcal{I}_g. \qquad (19)$$

□

We estimate the template $\mathbf{T}$ by minimizing the ML cost function given by expression (7) over the template $\mathbf{T}$, given the background world image $\mathbf{B}$. It is clear from expression (7), that the minimization of C_2 with respect to each spatial location of $\mathbf{T}$ is independent from the minimization over the other locations. The template $\widehat{\mathbf{T}}$ that minimizes the ML cost function C_2 is given by the following test evaluated at each pixel:

$$\mathbf{Q}_1(x,y) \begin{array}{c} \widehat{\mathbf{T}}(x,y) = 0 \\ \gtrless \\ \widehat{\mathbf{T}}(x,y) = 1 \end{array} \mathbf{Q}_2(x,y). \qquad (20)$$

The estimate $\widehat{\mathbf{T}}$ of the template of the moving object in equation (20) is obtained by checking which of two accumulated square differences is greater. In the spatial locations where the accumulated differences between each frame $\mathcal{M}(\mathbf{q}_f)\mathbf{I}_f$ and the background $\mathcal{M}(\mathbf{q}_g\mathbf{p}_g^{\#})\mathbf{B}$ are greater than the accumulated differences between each pair of co-registered frames $\mathcal{M}(\mathbf{q}_f)\mathbf{I}_f$ and $\mathcal{M}(\mathbf{q}_g)\mathbf{I}_g$, we estimate $\widehat{\mathbf{T}}(x,y) = 1$, meaning that these pixels belong to the moving object. If not, the pixel is assigned to the background.

The reason why we did not replace the background world image estimate $\widehat{\mathbf{B}}$ given by (6) in (3) as we did with the object world image estimate $\widehat{\mathbf{O}}$ is that it leads to an expression for C_2 in which the minimization with respect to each different spatial location $\mathbf{T}(x,y)$ is not independent from the other locations. Solving this binary minimization problem by a conventional method is extremely time consuming. In contrast, the minimization of C_2 over $\mathbf{T}$ for fixed $\mathbf{B}$ results in a local binary test. This makes our solution computationally very simple.

It may happen that, after processing the F available frames, the test (20) remains inconclusive at a given pixel (x,y) ($\mathbf{Q}_1(x,y) \simeq \mathbf{Q}_2(x,y)$): in other words, it is not possible to decide if this pixel belongs to the moving object or to the background. We modify our algorithm to address this ambiguity by defining the modified cost function

$$C_{2\text{MOD}} = C_2 + \alpha \operatorname{Area}(\mathbf{T}) = C_2 + \alpha \iint \mathbf{T}(x,y) \, dx \, dy, \qquad (21)$$

where C_2 is as in equation (3), α is non-negative, and Area($\mathbf{T}$) is the area of the template. Minimizing $C_{2\text{MOD}}$ balances the agreement between the observations and the model (term C_2), with minimizing the area of the template. Carrying out the minimization, first note that the second term in expression (21) does not depend on $\mathbf{O}$, neither on $\mathbf{B}$, so we get $\widehat{\mathbf{O}}_{\text{MOD}} = \widehat{\mathbf{O}}$ and $\widehat{\mathbf{B}}_{\text{MOD}} = \widehat{\mathbf{B}}$. By replacing $\widehat{\mathbf{O}}$ in $C_{2\text{MOD}}$, we get a modified version of equation (7),

$$C_{2\text{MOD}} = \int\!\!\int \mathbf{T}(x,y)\left[\mathbf{Q}(x,y) + \alpha\right] \, dx \, dy + \text{Constant}, \tag{22}$$

where $\mathbf{Q}$ is defined in equations (8), (9), and (10). The template estimate is now given by the following test, that extends test (20),

$$\mathbf{Q}(x,y) \begin{array}{c} \widehat{\mathbf{T}}(x,y) = 0 \\ \gtrless \\ \widehat{\mathbf{T}}(x,y) = 1 \end{array} - \alpha \; . \tag{23}$$

The parameter α may be chosen by experimentation, by using the *Minimum Description Length* (MDL) principle, see reference [4], or made adaptive by a annealing schedule like in stochastic relaxation.

4   Experiments

We describe two experiments. The first one uses a challenging computer generated image sequence to illustrate the convergence of the two-step iterative algorithm and its capability to segment complex shaped moving objects. The second experiment segments a real life traffic video clip.

4.1   Synthetic Image Sequence

We synthesized an image sequence according to the model described in section 2. Figure 2 shows the world images used. The left frame, from a real video, is the background world image. The moving object template is the logo of the *Instituto Superior Técnico* (IST) which is transparent between the letters. Its world image, shown in the right frame, is obtained by clipping with the IST logo a portion of one of the frames in the sequence. The task of reconstructing the object template is particularly challenging with this video sequence due to the low contrast between the object and the background and the complexity of the template. We synthesized a sequence of 20 images where the background is static and the IST logo moves arround.

Figure 3 shows three frames of the sequence obtained according to the image formation model introduced in section 2, expression (2), with noise variance $\sigma^2 = 4$ (the intensity values are in the interval $[0, 255]$). The object moves from the center (left frame) down by translational and rotational motion. It is difficult to recognize the logo in the right frame because its texture is confused with the texture of the background.

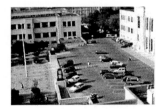
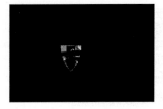

Fig. 2. Background and moving object.

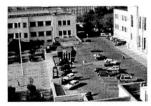
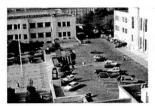
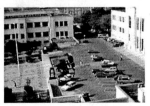

Fig. 3. Three frames of the synthesized image sequence.

Figure 4 illustrates the four iterations it took for the two-step estimation method of our algorithm to converge. The template estimate is initialized to zero (top left frame). Each background estimate in the right hand side was obtained using the template estimate on the left of it. Each template estimate was obtained using the previous background estimate. The arrows in Figure 4 indicate the flow of the algorithm. The good template estimate obtained, see bottom left image, illustrates that our algorithm can estimate complex templates in low contrast background.

Note that this type of complex templates (objects with transparent regions) is much easier to describe by using a binary matrix than by using contour based descriptions, like splines, Fourier descriptors, or snakes. Our algorithm over-comes the difficulty arising from the higher number of degrees of freedom of the binary template by integrating over time the small intensity differences between the background and the object. The two-step iterative algorithm performs this integrations in an expedite way.

4.2   Road Traffic

In this experiment we use a road traffic video clip. The road traffic video sequence has 250 frames. Figure 5 shows frames $15, 166$, and 225. The example given in section 1 to motivate the study of the segmentation of low textured scenes, see Figure 1, also uses frames 76 and 77 from the road traffic video clip.

In this video sequence, the camera exhibits a pronounced panning motion, while four different cars enter and leave the scene. The cars and the background have regions of low texture. The intensity of some of the cars is very similar to the intensity of parts of the background.

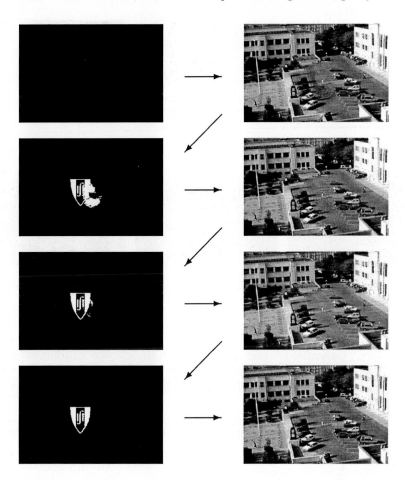

Fig. 4. Two-step iterative method: template estimates and background estimates.

Figures 6 and 7 show the good results obtained after segmenting the sequence with our algorithm. Figure 7 displays the background world image, while Figure 6 shows the world images of each of the moving cars. The estimates of the templates for the cars in Figure 6 becomes unambiguous after 10, 10, and 14 frames, respectively.

5 Conclusion

We develop an algorithm for segmenting 2D rigid moving objects from an image sequence. Our method recovers the template of the 2D rigid moving object by processing directly the image intensity values. We model both the *rigidity* of the moving object over a set of frames and and the *occlusion* of the background by the moving object.

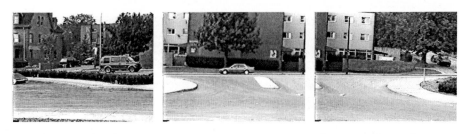

Fig. 5. Traffic road video sequence. Frames 15, 166, and 225.

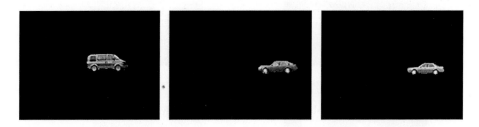

Fig. 6. Moving objects recovered from the traffic road video sequence.

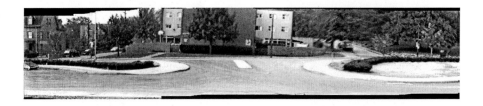

Fig. 7. Background world image recovered from the traffic road video sequence.

We motivate our algorithm by looking for a feasible approximation to the ML estimation of the unknowns involved in the segmentation problem. Our methodology introduces the 2D motion estimates into the ML cost function and uses a two-step iterative algorithm to approximate the minimization of the resultant cost function. The solutions for both steps result computationally very simple. The two-step algorithm is computationally efficient because the convergence is achieved in a small number of iterations (typically three to five iterations).

Our experiments show that the algorithm proposed can estimate complex templates in low contrast scenes.

References

1. P. M. Q. Aguiar. *Rigid Structure from Video.* PhD thesis, Instituto Superior Técnico, Lisboa, Portugal, 2000. Available at www.isr.ist.utl.pt/~aguiar.
2. Pedro M. Q. Aguiar and José M. F. Moura. Detecting and solving template ambiguities in motion segmentation. In *ICIP'97*, Santa Barbara, CA, USA, 1997.

3. S. Baker, R. Szeliski, and P. Anandan. Hierarchical model-based motion estimation. In *CVPR'99*, Santa Barbara CA, USA, 1998.

4. A. Barron, J. Rissanen, and B. Yu. The minimum description length principle in coding and modeling. *IEEE Trans. on Information Theory*, 44(6), 1998.

5. J. R. Bergen, P. Anandan, K. J. Hanna, and R. Hingorani. Hierarchical model-based motion estimation. In *ECCV'92*, Santa Margherita Ligure, Italy, 1992.

6. M. J. Black and A. Rangarajan. On the unification of line processes, outlier rejection, and robust statistics with applications in early vision. *IJCV*, 19(1), 1996.

7. Patrick Bouthemy and Edouard François. Motion segmentation and qualitative dynamic scene analysis from an image sequence. *IJCV*, 10(2), 1993.

8. Norbert Diehl. Object-oriented motion estimation and segmentation in image sequences. *Signal Processing: Image Communication*, 3(1):23–56, February 1991.

9. Marie-Pierre Dubuisson and Anil K. Jain. Contour extraction of moving objects in complex outdoor scenes. *IJCV*, 14(1), 1995.

10. Michal Irani and Shmuel Peleg. Motion analysis for image enhancement: Resolution, occlusion, and transparency. *Journal of Visual Communications and Image Representation*, 4(4):324–335, December 1993.

11. Michal Irani, Benny Rousso, and Shmuel Peleg. Computing occluding and transparent motions. *IJCV*, 12(1), February 1994.

12. Anil K. Jain. *Fundamentals of Digital Image Processing*. Prentice Hall Information and Sciences Series. Prentice-Hall International Inc., 1989.

13. R. S. Jasinschi and J. M. F. Moura. *Generative Video: Very Low Bit Rate Video Compression*. U.S. Patent and Trademark Office, S.N. 5,854,856, issued, 1998.

14. Radu S. Jasinschi and José M. F. Moura. Content-based video sequence representation. In *ICIP'95*, Washigton D.C., USA, September 1995.

15. D. C. Knill, D.l Kersten, and A. Yuille. A Bayesian formulation of visual perception. In *Perception as Bayesian Inference*. Cambridge University Press, 1996.

16. Haibo Li, Astrid Lundmark, and Robert Forchheimer. Image sequence coding at very low bitrates: A review. *IEEE Trans. on Image Processing*, 3(5), 1994.

17. Joseph A. O'Sullivan, Richard E. Blahut, and Donald L. Snyder. Information-theoretic image formation. *IEEE Trans. on Information Theory*, 44(6), 1998.

18. H. S. Sawhney and S. Ayer. Compact representations of videos through dominant and multiple motion estimation. *IEEE PAMI*, 18(8), 1996.

Metric Similarities Learning through Examples: An Application to Shape Retrieval

Alain Trouvé and Yong Yu[*]

University Paris 13
LAGA/L2TI
93430 Villetaneuse, France
{trouve,yuyong}@zeus.math.univ-paris13.fr

Abstract. The design of good features and good similarity measures between features plays a central role in any retrieval system. The use of *metric* similarities (i.e. coming from a real distance) is also very important to allow fast retrieval on large databases. Moreover, these similarity functions should be flexible enough to be tuned to fit users behaviour. These two constraints, *flexibility* and *metricity* are generally difficult to fulfill. Our contribution is two folds: We show that the kernel approach introduced by Vapnik, can be used to generate metric similarities, especially for the difficult case of planar shapes (invariant to rotation and scaling). Moreover, we show that much more flexibility can be added by non-rigid deformation of the induced feature space. Defining an adequate Bayesian users model, we describe an estimation procedure based on the maximisation of the underlying log-likelihood function.

1 Introduction

The selection of good features from objects and the design of efficient similarity measures appear to play a central role for any retrieval algorithm for searching a database (see [17] for a recent survey on content-based retrieval). Moreover, similarity functions should come from true distances, hereafter called *metric similarities*, between objects to allow content-based databases using similarity-based retrieval to scale to large databases (several thousands up to several millions of objects) [21]. However, this last property appears to be a hard constraint for the usual "home cooked" similarity functions, especially when dealing with objects defined up to the action of some group of transformations (as planar shapes). These metric similarities should also ideally be seen as Euclidean distances between points in some vector space. The usual way to achieve such a result is to define some feature vector for each object and to identify the similarity with a possibly weighted Euclidean distance, or more suitably, to extract first some principal components from a PCA analysis of the feature vectors.

More formally, a huge amount of distance can be obtained by a simple embedding procedure: Let $\phi : \mathcal{X} \to \mathcal{Z}$ be a one to one function from the object

---

[*] This work was partially supported by the CNRS

M.A.T. Figueiredo, J. Zerubia, A.K. Jain (Eds.): EMMCVPR 2001, LNCS 2134, pp. 50–62, 2001.
© Springer-Verlag Berlin Heidelberg 2001

space or so called *image space*, to some *feature space* equipped with a structure of Hilbert space. Then

$$d_\phi(x, x') \doteq |\phi(x) - \phi(x')|_Z \qquad (1)$$

defines a distance on the object space. Now, defining the kernel $k_\phi(x, x') \doteq \langle \phi(x), \phi(x') \rangle_Z$, we get for the distance

$$d_\phi(x, x') = (k_\phi(x, x) + k_\phi(x', x') - 2k_\phi(x, x'))^{1/2} \ . \qquad (2)$$

The recent development of kernel methods, is based essentially on the fact (the so called *kernel trick*) that instead of defining explicitly the embedding ϕ, it can be enough to start from a closed expression of an admissible kernel (satisfying the famous Mercer's conditions) so that all the computations can be done without the need of any explicit expression of ϕ. This approach has been followed successfully in statistical learning, through the so called support vector machines and their extensions [20, 5] but also in data mining through nonlinear principal component analysis [15]. When objects are planar shapes, this kernel approach can be quite interesting to generate real distance between shapes. One difficulty arises if rotation, scale and translation invariance is required. In [19], we propose a construction of an invariant polynomial kernel for planar shapes. The first contribution of this paper will be to show an important extension of the previous invariant kernel into a large family of kernels which can still be computed in a very fast way.

However, concerning distance functions families, and the derivation of metric similarities, despite the fact a quite large family of different kernels are known (polynomial kernel, radial basis functions kernels, etc), all theses families appear to be of low dimensional parametrically (often one or two parameters), allowing in fact a restricted flexibility. Moreover, this flexibility is highly required for at least two main reasons. The first one is that simple retrieval processes based on the retrieval of the k-nearest objects around the query-example, can be very inefficient if the metric similarity does not fit the user's "implicit" similarity (if exists!). The second one is that efficient retrieval systems should provided some feedback mechanism to improve the relevance of retrieved objects, through inter-action with the user. This interaction should be built around a good user model allowing to predict for a given target and two displayed objects, which will be chosen as the most similar and with what probability. The entropy reduction scheme has been advocated by the PicHunter's group in [4] and Geman *et al* in [7, 8] and strongly depends, according to the terminology in [8], on the "synchro-nisation" between the actual user behaviour and the predicted user behaviour on a given target hypothesis. Now, it appears that some partial learning of the metric similarities should be done in a sufficiently large set of metric similarities.

In some recent work in [3], Chapelle *et al* introduce some flexibility in the kernel through scaling parameters between different features. Their basic idea is to tune the variance parameters σ_i according to some estimation of the test error $T((\sigma_i))$ given by a SVM built on the kernel $k_\sigma(x, x') = \exp(-\sum_i |x_i - x'_i|^2/2\sigma_i^2))$ (a similar version is provided for polynomial kernels). In some sense, independently of them, we have followed some common route, but with different means and in a different framework. In this paper, we want to show how one can improve in a surprising way a similarity measure by non-rigid deformation of a finite dimensional subspace of the feature space. Starting from the feature mapping ϕ induced by a chosen "primary" kernel k, the basic idea is to try to learn a perturbation $\tilde{\phi} = \phi + u(\phi)$ of the feature mapping by successive presentation to the user of triplets of objects $\tilde{x} = (x_1, x_2, x_3)$. For each of them, the user is asked to give the position y of the most similar pair, by mental comparison of the individual similarity of the three possible pairs $\{x_2, x_3\}$ ($y = 1$), $\{x_1, x_3\}$ ($y = 2$) and $\{x_1, x_2\}$ ($y = 3$). Hence, the user answers $y = j$ if $\{x_{j+1}, x_{j+2}\}$ is the most similar pair (the sums $j+1$ and $j+2$ are mod 3). Let $\tilde{X}_1^N \doteq (\tilde{X}_1, \cdots, \tilde{X}_N)$ be N triplets independently generated and $\tilde{Y}_1^N \doteq (\tilde{Y}_1, \cdots, \tilde{Y}_N)$ be the corresponding users answers. We will use $(\tilde{X}_1^N, Y_1^N)$ as a learning set for the selection of $\tilde{\phi}$ through a Bayesian inference presented in section 3. If for any distance d, and any triple $\tilde{X}$, we denote

$$Y^{(d)} = \mathrm{argmin}_j d(X_{j+1}, X_{j+2}) \ , \tag{3}$$

the goal is to select the perturbation $\tilde{\phi}$ such that for the distance $d = d_{\tilde{\phi}}$ (see (1)), the classification rule $Y^{(d)}$ gives good generalisation performance on a new triplet $\tilde{X}$.

The paper is organised as following: in section 2, we present a new family of invariant kernels for planar shapes. These kernels can be used as primary kernels inducing different features space $\mathcal{Z}$. Then, in section 3, we present our Bayesian inference framework and the derivation of the deformation process driven by a variational formula. Finally, in section 4, we report some learning experiments in the case of planar shapes.

2   Rotation and Shift Invariant Kernels for Planar Shapes

2.1   Shape-Based Search

We focus our experiments on planar shapes, since we believe that in such a case, keywords are not very useful for non expert users (possibly speaking different languages), to describe and select a shape in a retrieval process. Note that some existing retrieval and indexing systems perform shape-based search, such as the IBM's QBIC [6] but still in a limited way (see [10] for an extended review). A notable exception is the Shape Query Using Image Database (SQUID) prototype developed by University of Surrey which entirely relies on shapes similarities (but without the usual functionalities of a real retrieval system). However, many issues on that field are still open such as the design of good similarity functions between shapes and efficient retrieval strategies for big database as well. It is commonly accepted that rotation, translation and scale invariance are highly recommended for any shape similarity function. Moreover, as said in the introduction, metric similarities based on real distances (satisfying the triangle inequality) are much more suited for big databases since there exists faster search procedures in that

case. Several such similarity functions are available from the literature, based on
Fourier descriptors [14], on curvature scale space [12], on modal representation
[16, 9] and other features (see [10] and references therein). All of them appear
to have good reported features, but none of them is a real metric similarity. As
far as we know, the first real rotation and scale invariant metric similarity for
arbitrary shapes has been proposed by Younes in [22] as a geodesic distance for
a special Riemannian structure on a shape manifold. However, the computation
time for this distance penalised its use for large databases. Another common
drawback to the previous reported distances is that they can not be deduced
from any obvious kernel as defined in the introduction. Therefore, no principal
component analysis of the shape database can be performed (in this special case,
the use of kernel PCA is unavoidable if one want a rotation scale and even shift
(choice of the starting point in the curve representation of a shape) invariant
analysis).

2.2   A New Family of Invariant Kernels for Planar Shapes

We want to show in this section a systematic way to get a family of shift and
rotation invariant kernel. Note that we are interested in the case of closed curves
defined as functions $c : \mathbb{T} \to \mathbb{R}^2$ where $\mathbb{T}$ is the one dimensional torus $\mathbb{R}/\mathbb{Z}$.
Since we want also the translation invariance, for any pair of curves c and c',
we will define $K(c, c') = k(f, g)$ where $f = \dot{c}$ and $g = \dot{c}'$ are the time derivative
of c and c'. Moreover, since we are interested in the shapes of the curves and
not really in the actual parameterisation of these shapes, we will assume that
$|f| = 1$ and $|g| = 1$ i.e. that the curves are parametrised by arc-length. Hence,
we can focus on shift and rotation invariant kernel defined on the closed ball
$B = \left\{ f \in L^2(\mathbb{T}, \mathbb{R}^2) | \int_{\mathbb{T}} |f(x)|^2 \, dx \leq 1 \right\}$.

Definition 1. *For any $\theta \in [0, 2\pi]$, we denote r_θ the rotation in $\mathbb{R}^2$ defined by
the 2×2 matrix $r_\theta = \begin{pmatrix} \cos(\theta) & -\sin(\theta) \\ \sin(\theta) & \cos(\theta) \end{pmatrix}$.*

We denote by F the set of all the functions from $\mathbb{T}$ to $\mathbb{R}^2$.

Definition 2. *For any $u \in [0, 1]$ and $\theta \in [0, 2\pi]$ we define the shift $\tau_u : F \to F$
and $R_\theta : F \to F$ by $\tau_u(f)(x) = f(x + u)$ and $R_\theta(f)(x) = r_\theta(f(x))$.*

Definition 3. *We say that $k : B \times B \to \mathbb{R}$ is a shift and rotation invariant
kernel if*

1. *For any $u \in [0, 1]$, any $\theta \in [0, 2\pi]$ and any f and $g \in B$, we have*

$$k(R_\theta \circ \tau_u(f), g) = k(f, g) .$$

2. *For any finite family $(f_i)_{1 \leq i \leq n}$ of points in B, and any family $(\alpha_i)_{1 \leq i \leq n}$ of
real valued numbers, we have $\sum_{ij} \alpha_i \alpha_j k(f_i, f_j) \geq 0$*
3. *The kernel k is symmetric*

We can now state the main result of this section

Theorem 1. *Let $(a_n)_{n \in \mathbb{N}}$ be a sequence of non-negative real valued numbers such that $\sum_{n \in \mathbb{N}} a_n < +\infty$. Then let us define $\psi(x) = \sum_{n \geq 0} a_n x^n$ for any $x \in [-1, 1]$ and define for any f and g in B*

$$k(f, g) = \int_{[0,1]} \psi(|\rho_{f,g}(u)|^2) du \ ,$$

where $\rho_{f,g}(u) = \int_{\mathbb{T}} f(x + u)\overline{g(x)}dx$ (here we identify $\mathbb{R}^2$ with $\mathbb{C}$ and $\overline{g}$ denotes the complex conjugate). Then, k is a shift and rotation invariant kernel on B and

$$k(f, g) = \frac{1}{4\pi^2} \int_{[0,1]^2 \times [0,2\pi]^2} \varphi(\langle \tau_u \circ R_\theta(f), \tau_v \circ R_{\theta'}(g) \rangle) du \, dv \, d\theta \, d\theta' \ , \quad (4)$$

where $\varphi(x) = \sum_{q \geq 0} a_q \frac{q! q!}{(2q)!} x^{2q}$ and $\langle \ , \ \rangle$ denotes the usual dot product on $L^2(\mathbb{T}, \mathbb{R}^2)$.

Proof. First one can remark that, thanks to the Stirling formula, φ is well defined and C^∞ on $]-2, 2[$. Moreover, if we prove equality (4), then the shift and rotation invariance is deduced immediately. By linearity, it is sufficient to prove the inequality for $\psi(x) = x^d$ for an arbitrary $d \in \mathbb{N}$, which is proved by theorem 2 given in appendix A.

As a consequence, one can build easily a full range of kernels choosing for instance

1. $\psi(x) = x^d$ for any positive integer d,
2. $\psi(x) = \exp(\gamma x)$ for any $\gamma > 0$,
3. $\psi(x) = 1/(1 - \gamma x)^d$ for any $\gamma \in]0, 1[$ and any positive integer d.

Remark 1. Let us remark that if we start from a closed formula for ψ, the computation of k can be achieved in an efficient way. Indeed, if we consider two discrete version f_N and g_N in N steps of f and g by $f_N(k) = f(k/N)$ and $g_N(k) = g(k/N)$, we define

$$k_N(f_N, g_N) = \frac{1}{N} \sum_{k=0}^{N-1} \psi(|\rho_{N,f,g}(k)|^2) \ ,$$

where $\rho_{N,f,g}(k) = \frac{1}{N} \sum_{j=0}^{N-1} f_N(j + k)\overline{g_N}(j)$. Hence, if we consider the Fourier decomposition of f_N and g_N, we get

$$\rho_{N,f,g}(k) = \frac{1}{N^3} \sum_{j,l,m=0}^{N-1} \hat{f}_{N,l} \overline{\hat{g}_{N,m}} e^{i\frac{2\pi}{N}((j+k)l - jm)} = \frac{1}{N^2} \sum_{l=0}^{N-1} \hat{f}_{N,l} \overline{\hat{g}_{N,l}} e^{i\frac{2\pi}{N}kl} \ .$$

Hence, using discrete FFT, the computation of $\rho_{N,f,g}$ can be achieved in $N \log(N)$ steps.

An interesting application is where $\varphi(x) = (1+x)^2$ which corresponds to $\psi(x) = 1 + 2x$. In that case, we get

$$k_N(f_N, g_N) = 1 + \frac{2}{N} \sum_{k=0}^{N-1} |\rho_{N,f,g}(k)|^2 = 1 + \frac{2}{N^2} \sum_{k=0}^{N-1} |\hat{f}_{N,l}|^2 |\hat{g}_{N,l}|^2 \ .$$

In [19], we show that this kernel can be used to build an unsupervised hierarchical clustering tree based on kernel PCA. Here this kernel will be used as a good starting point to define a well suited feature space $\mathcal{Z}$. The associated distance will be denoted d_C. We report in fig. 1, a comparison of our kernel distance for $\varphi(x) = (1 + x)^d$, $d = 4$, and the more involved approach using curvature scale space developed in [12]. The remarkable fact is that we get comparable results but with a simple real metric similarity, still rotation and shift invariant. Moreover, in the feature space, this distance is just a usual Hilbert distance, so we can tune it to fit users behaviour as described now.

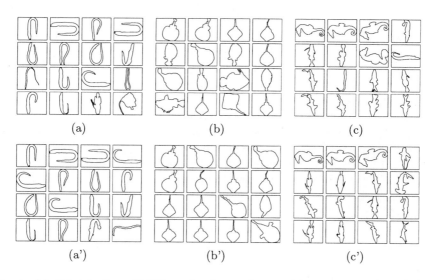

Fig. 1. (a) (b) (c): three K-NN retrieval experiments (the query is the upper-left shape) using the kernel distance for $\varphi(x) = (1 + x)^4$; (a') (b') (c'), corresponding K-NN retrieval according to the CSS matching values from the SQUID demo site http://www.ee.surrey.ac.uk/Research/VSSP/imagedb/demo.html

3 Deformation Process

As developed in the introduction, we believe that there is no reason that the first selected metric similarity should fit perfectly the implicit similarity underlying users decision processes. We agree with the discussion developed by Cox *et al* in

[4] and Geman and Moquet in [8] about the need of psychophysical experiments to improve similarity functions and ultimately the users model. We develop our approach in this section. From now on, the space $\mathcal{Z}$ will denote the feature space underlying the choice of the initial kernel, called the *primary* kernel.

Let E be a finite dimensional affine subspace of $\mathcal{Z}$ with direction $\boldsymbol{E}$ (for any $z_0 \in E$, $E = z_0 + \boldsymbol{E}$) and p_E be the orthogonal projection on E. For any displacement field $u : E \to \boldsymbol{E}$, we can define

$$\phi_u(x) \doteq \phi(x) + u(p_E(\phi(x))) \ . \tag{5}$$

3.1   Probabilistic Model

We assume that users answers are driven by the choice of a random U drawn according to a Gaussian model and that given U, the different answers are independent so that

$$\mathcal{L}(\tilde{X}_1^N, Y_1^N \mid U) = \otimes_{i=1}^N \mathcal{L}(\tilde{X}_i, Y_i \mid U) \ . \tag{6}$$

For a given choice of U and a given experiment $\tilde{X}$, the answer Y of the user is assumed to follow the probabilistic model

$$P(Y = j \mid \tilde{X}, U) \propto \exp(-\gamma d_{\phi_U}(X_{j+1}, X_{j+2})^2) \ . \tag{7}$$

In [7, 8], this kind of Bayesian model has been proposed but with some important differences. On one hand, they assume that the user selects a distance according to a law which could depend also on the triplet itself which is a more general model. One the other hand, the model for the choice of the distance is simpler than our, and based on the random selection of a point in the convex set of the mixture of a small set of predefined distances.

Now, the Bayesian estimator for the answer $\hat{Y}$ to a new experiment $\tilde{X}$ is given by $\hat{Y} \doteq \operatorname{argmax} P(Y = j \mid \tilde{X}_1^N, Y_1^N, \tilde{X})$. Denoting $Z_1^N = (\tilde{X}_1^N, Y_1^N)$, we deduce that

$$P(Y = j \mid Z_1^N, \tilde{X}) = E(P(Y = j \mid U, \tilde{X}) \mid Z_1^N, \tilde{X}) \ ,$$

so that we get for $\tilde{X} = \tilde{x}$

$$\hat{Y} = \operatorname{argmax} E(\varphi_{\tilde{x}}(j, U) \mid \tilde{X}_1^N, Y_1^N) \tag{8}$$

with $\varphi_{\tilde{x}}(j, U) = P(Y = j \mid \tilde{X} = \tilde{x}, U)$. The integration (8) over the posterior law of U given the observations $\tilde{X}_1^N, Y_1^N$ could be computed by Monte Carlo simulations [2]. However, this approach may lead to prohibitive CPU time so that we focus on a simpler approximation for which the a posteriori law is replaced by the Dirac measure δ_{U_*}, where U_* is the maximum a posteriori of U [11]

$$U_* = \operatorname{argmax} P(U = u \mid \tilde{X}_1^N, Y_1^N). \tag{9}$$

Note here, that the previous definition of U_* is ambiguous in this infinite dimensional setting. This should be understood in a limit sense from finite dimension

approximations [13]. Finally, the Bayesian decision is approximated by the maximisation in j of $P(Y = j \mid \tilde{X}, U_*)$, so that using (7), we get our approximate
estimator

$$Y^* = \operatorname{argmin}_j d_{\phi U_*}(X_{j+1}, X_{j+2}). \qquad (10)$$

3.2   Variationnal Formulation

From equation (9), since the prior on U is Gaussian, if $\mathcal{H}$ is its reproducing
kernel Hilbert space with norm $\| \ \|_V$ (which can be understood by the formal
expression $dP(U = u) \propto \exp(-\frac{1}{2}\|u\|_V^2)du$), then U_* is the defined as the element
$u \in V$ achieving the maximum value of

$$W(u) = -\frac{1}{2}\|u\|_V^2 + \sum_{i=1}^N \log\left(P(Y_i \mid \tilde{X}_i, U = u)\right) \qquad (11)$$

Here again, the equation (11) cannot be derived rigorously from the Bayesian
formulation but this could be done in a limit sense on finite dimensional approximations [13]. Another way is to start directly from (11) as variational formulation
of the problem.

To specify the Gaussian prior, we choose an orthonormal basis $(e_1, \cdots, e_p)$
of $\boldsymbol{E}$, such that $U(z) = \sum_{k=1}^p U^k(z)e_k$, and we assume that the coordinates are
independent and that the covariance structure is given by

$$E(U^k(z)U^{k'}(z')) = \lambda \mathbf{1}_{k=k'} g_{\sigma^2}(z - z')$$

for any $z, z' \in E$, where $g_{\sigma^2}(\boldsymbol{z}) = \exp(-|z|_{\mathcal{Z}}^2/2\sigma^2)/(2\pi\sigma^2)^{p/2}$ is defined from
$\boldsymbol{E}$ to $\mathbb{R}$ (other covariance structure could be used but this one induces smooth
random fields and depends on a single parameter σ). Then the associated reproducing kernel Hilbert space is defined by ($*$ is the convolution)

$$V = \left\{ u(z) = \sum_{k=1}^p (g_{\sigma^2/2} * h^k)(z)e_k \mid h_k \in L^2(E, \mathbb{R}, dz) \right\}$$

and $\|u\|_V = \sqrt{\sum_{k=1}^p \int_E |h^k(z)|^2 dz}$. To perform the computation, we use a finite
element V_L approximation of the space V, where

$$V_L = \{u(z) = \sum_{k,l} a_l^k g_{\sigma^2}(t_l - z)e_k \mid a_l^k \in \mathbb{R}\}$$

where $(t_l)_{1 \leq l \leq L}$ is a family of control points chosen in E. We have $V_L \subset V$ and

$$\|u\|_V^2 = \sum_{l,l',k} a_l^k a_{l'}^k g_{\sigma^2}(t_l - t_{l'})$$

for $u \in V_L$. The problem of optimisation of W on V_L is now an optimisation
problem in dimension $L \times \dim(E)$ for which we use a gradient descent. The

existence of a maximizer for W in V could be proved easily by showing the continuity of $\sum_{i=1}^{N} \log \left(P(Y_i \mid \tilde{X}_i, U = u) \right)$ for the weak topology on V but in finite dimension, this existence is straightforward. Importantly, the gradient should be computed with respect to the dot product on V, the so called "natural gradient" [1, 18]. This allows in particular a good stability of the solution with respect to the number of control points.

4   Experiments

We have performed our experiment on two databases, the LaTeX database[1] and the African database[2]. We fix a random sequence of 220 triplets of shapes. Five members of the L2TI laboratory have been asked to decide the most similar pair among the three possible pairs as described previously with a friendly GUI interface. The same sequence of triplets is presented to each user. In many cases,

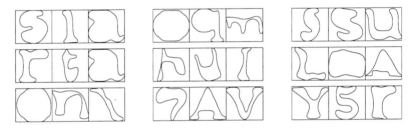

Fig. 2. Examples of triplets presented to the users from the LaTeX database

for example when the three curves seem to have nothing in common, different users make different choices. We denote $Y_i^{(k)}$ the answer of the kth user to the ith experiment in the sequence. The sequence is then split in two subsets $\mathcal{L}$ (learning set) and $\mathcal{T}$ (test set). We start from the primary kernel k_C presented in section 2 with $(\varphi(x) = (1 + x)^2)$, and we keep only the 10 first principal nonlinear components (we have checked that the remaining squared variation on the orthogonal space is negligible) dealing with a reduced feature space $\mathcal{Z}$ of dimension 10. Now, choose for E, the affine subspace going through the mean value $\bar{z}$ of the features vectors in the database and with direction $\boldsymbol{E}$ given by the first p principal (nonlinear) axes (the reported results have been obtained with $p = 3$ and 60 controls points). We use the learning set to learn a deformation as defined in the previous section, and we get a new distance $d_* \doteq d_{\phi_{u_*}}$ (see (1) and (5)). On the test set, we compare the prediction $Y^{(d)}$ (see (3)) for a given

---

[1] This database contains outlines of randomly deformed LaTeX symbols
[2] This database contains outlines of homogeneous ecological regions from the inner delta of the River Niger in Mali (14000 different shapes)

distance d with the answers $Y^{(k)}$ given by the users leading to the empirical score

$$J_d = \frac{1}{5|\mathcal{T}|} \sum_{k=1}^{5} \sum_{i \in \mathcal{T}} \mathbf{1}_{(Y_i^{(d)} = Y_i^{(k)})} \tag{12}$$

For comparison to the human performance, we compute the mean cross-prediction score on the test set between the different humans:

$$J_{\text{hum}} = \frac{1}{20|\mathcal{T}|} \sum_{k \neq k'} \sum_{i \in \mathcal{T}} \mathbf{1}_{(Y_i^{(k)} = Y_i^{(k')})} \tag{13}$$

To see the improvement of the "learning" process in the selection of the distance, we propose different comparison against various "home cooked" (or not) distances. The first distance is the usual L^2 "distance" defined by $d_1(c, c')^2 = \inf_{\theta,s} \int |e^{i\theta}\dot{c}(u+s) - \dot{c}'(u)|^2 du$. The second one is a *geodesic distance* between curves defined in [22]. The third one is the distance d_C deduced from the primary kernel k_C (see (2)). For all the presented results, the size of the test set $|\mathcal{T}| = 100$ and the size of the learning set $|\mathcal{L}| = 120$. The following table is the output of the experiment.

Table 1. First column: the different distances used for prediction; second column: LaTeX database; third column: African database.

Database	LaTeX $J_{\text{hum}} = 77.5\%$		African $J_{\text{hum}} = 70\%$	
Distances d	J_d	J_d/J_{hum}	J_d	J_d/J_{hum}
L^2 distance	57.2%	73.8%	48.8%	71.4%
geodesic distance	59.2%	76.4%	50%	71.43%
kernel distance d_C	58.6%	75.6%	59%	84.4%
deformed distance d_*	77.2%	**99.6%**	70%	**100%**

Concerning the experiments on the LaTeX database, one remarkable fact is that the first three distances have very close scores about 75% of the human performance. We also test other kernels distances through optimisation of the coefficients in the ψ expansion without getting really important improvements. After the learned deformation, the performance is very close to the human's one. We think that the gap between 75% and 99.6% could not be filled by any existing parametric family of kernel. However, our approach needs basically only two continuous parameters σ, λ to be tuned (in the reported results $\sigma = 0.3$ and $\lambda = 20$). Same comments could be done for the African database.

We display in figure 3 the effect of the deformation on the representation in the feature space of the shapes involved in the experiment (we display only the first two components). We can see strong effect on the deformation process. To have a better visualisation of it, we display in figure 4 the 3D deformation of the 2D subspace corresponding to the first two principal axes.

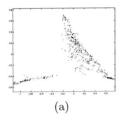
(a)

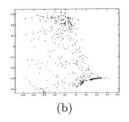
(b)

Fig. 3. The first two principal components distribution. (a) directly from KPCA projection with kernel k_C, (b) after "learning"process (LaTeX database)

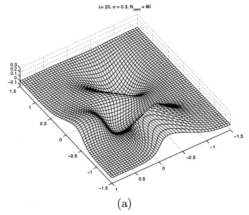
(a)

Fig. 4. Deformations effect on a 2D subspace of the feature space (LaTeX database)

5   Conclusion

The previous experiments show that we can efficiently tune a primary designed kernel to fit the human behaviour. Our feeling is that the choice of the primary kernel should be done in order to embed in the feature space all the invariance properties we need (as the rotation and scale invariance in our case). However, one can not expect a fine tuning without feedback through examples. The introduction of non-rigid deformation driven by a well chosen subspace of the feature space gives the necessary flexibility. Moreover, the Bayesian framework we have developed shows that the information given by the experiments with the users can be used to define the good deformations. The complexity of the learning algorithm remains low (the learning time does not exceed few seconds on a standard PC). Such approach could be used in many context and allow to define fitted similarity measures which still are distances. This is an important fact for speed and efficiency in all subsequent steps in a retrieval process.

A   Appendix

In this appendix, we prove a preliminary result (Theorem 2) which is the core result for the proof of theorem 1. The central idea, will be to extend the framework to functions with values in $\mathbb{C}^2$.

Let us consider 2-dimensional space $\mathbb{C}^2$ and denotes $e = (e_1, e_2)$ the canonical basis. Note that the rotation r_θ can be extended straightforwardly on $\mathbb{C}^2$ (with the same matrix representation in the new canonical basis) as well as the definition of R_θ and τ_u. We define on $\mathbb{C}^2$ the usual hermitian product define for any $z = (z_1, z_2)$ and $z' = (z'_1, z'_2)$ in $\mathbb{C}^2$ by $\langle z, z' \rangle_{\mathbb{C}^2} = z_1 \overline{z'_1} + z_2 \overline{z'_2}$. We define now the new orthonormal basis $t = (t_1, t_2)$ by $t_1 = (e_1 + ie_2)/\sqrt{2}$ and $t_2 = (e_1 - ie_2)/\sqrt{2}$. Moreover, as usual, for any f and g in $L^2(\mathbb{T}, \mathbb{C}^2)$, we denote $\langle f, g \rangle$ the hermitian product on $L^2(\mathbb{T}, \mathbb{C}^2)$ defined by $\langle f, g \rangle = \int_\mathbb{T} \langle f(x), g(x) \rangle_{\mathbb{C}^2} \, dx$.

Let $d \in \mathbb{N}$. We consider for any functions $f, g \in L^2(\mathbb{T}, \mathbb{C}^2)$,

$$k(f,g) = \frac{1}{4\pi^2} \int_{[0,1)^2 \times [0,2\pi]^2} (\langle \tau_u \circ R_\theta(f), \tau_v \circ R_{\theta'}(g) \rangle)^d \, du \, dv \, d\theta \, d\theta'$$

For any $f \in L^2(\mathbb{T}, \mathbb{C}^2)$, we define f_1 and f_2 in $L^2(\mathbb{T}, \mathbb{C})$ by $f_1(x) = \langle f(x), t_1 \rangle_{\mathbb{C}^2}$ and $f_2(x) = \langle f(x), t_2 \rangle_{\mathbb{C}^2}$ so that $f = f_1 t_1 + f_2 t_2$. In the sequel, we identify $\mathbb{R}^2$ with the subspace $\mathbb{R}e_1 \oplus \mathbb{R}e_2$.

Lemma 1. *Assume that $d = 2q$ is even. Then, for any $f, g \in L^2(\mathbb{T}, \mathbb{R}^2)$ we have* $k(f,g) = \int_{[0,1]} C_{2q}^q \left| \int_\mathbb{T} \tau_u f_2(x) \overline{g_2}(x) dx \right|^{2q} du$ *. If d is odd, then $k(f,g) = 0$.*

Proof. First, we notice that for any $\theta \in [0, 2\pi]$, $r_\theta(t_1) = e^{-i\theta} t_1$ and $r_\theta(t_2) = e^{i\theta} t_2$ so that $R_\theta(f) = e^{-i\theta} f_1 t_1 + e^{i\theta} f_2 t_2$. Hence, one get that $\langle R_\theta(f), g \rangle = \int_\mathbb{T} e^{-i\theta} f_1 \overline{g_1}(x) + e^{i\theta} f_2 \overline{g_2}(x) dx$ so that, raising to the power of d and integrating over $\theta \in [0, 2\pi]$, we obtain finally $\frac{1}{2\pi} \int \langle R_\theta(f), g \rangle^d d\theta = \frac{1}{2\pi} \int \sum_{k=0}^d C_d^k e^{i(d-2k)\theta} \left(\int_\mathbb{T} f_1 \overline{g_1} \right)^k \left(\int_\mathbb{T} f_2 \overline{g_2} \right)^{d-k} d\theta$. Using the fact that $\int e^{i(d-2k)\theta} d\theta = 0$ if $d \neq k$, we get the result for d odd. If $d = 2q$ then we have $\frac{1}{2\pi} \int_{[0,2\pi]} \langle R_\theta(f), g \rangle^d d\theta = C_{2q}^q \left(\int_\mathbb{T} f_1(x) \overline{g_1}(x) dx \right)^q \left(\int_\mathbb{T} f_2(x) \overline{g_2}(x) dx \right)^q$. Now, noticing that $f_2 = \overline{f_1}$, we get $\frac{1}{2\pi} \int \langle R_\theta(f), g \rangle^d d\theta = C_{2q}^q \left| \int_\mathbb{T} f_2(x) \overline{g_2}(x) dx \right|^{2q}$. The proof is ended since $\langle \tau_u \circ R_\theta(f), \tau_v \circ R_{\theta'}(g) \rangle = \langle \tau_{u-v} \circ R_{\theta-\theta'}(f), g \rangle$.

Now, for $f : \mathbb{T} \to \mathbb{R}^2$, we get that $f_2 = j(f)$ where j is the canonical injection of $\mathbb{R}^2$ in $\mathbb{C}$ given by $j((x,y)) = x + iy$ for any $x, y \in \mathbb{R}^2$. Hence, one get the following theorem

Theorem 2. *Let f and g be two measurable functions in $L^2(\mathbb{T}, \mathbb{R}^2)$. Let d be a positive integer and assume that $\varphi(x) = x^d$. Then we have $k(f,g) = \int_{[0,1]} C_{2q}^q \left| \int_\mathbb{T} f(x+u) \overline{g}(x) dx \right|^{2q} du$ where we identify f and g with $j(f)$ and $j(g)$.*

References

1. S.-I. Amari. Natural gradient works efficiently in learnig. *Neural Computation*, 10:251–276, 1998.
2. Y. Amit and M. Piccioni. A non-homogeneous Markov process for the estimation of Gaussian random fields with non-linear observations. *Annals of probability*, 19(4):1664–1679, 1991.

3. O. Chapelle, V. Vapnik, B. O, and S. Mukherjee. Choosing multiple parameters for support vectors machines. submited to Machine Learning, 2000.

4. I. Cox, M. Miller, T. Minka, and P. Papathomas, Thomas ans Yianilos. The bayesian image retrieval system, pichunter: Theory, implementation and psychophysical experiments. *IEEE Trans. Image Processing*, 9:20–37, 2000.

5. N. Cristianini and J. Shawe-Taylor. *An Introduction to Support Vector Machines.* Cambridge University Press, Cambridge, UK, 2000.

6. M. Flickner, H. Sawhney, W. Niblack, J. Ashley, Q. Huang, B. Dom, M. Gorkani, J. Hafner, D. Lee, D. Petkovic, D. Steele, and P. Yanker. Query by image and video content: the qbic system. *IEEE Computer*, 28(9):23–32, 1995.

7. D. Geman and R. Moquet. A stochstic feedback model for image retrieval. In *Proc. RFIA, Paris*, 2000.

8. D. Geman and R. Moquet. Q & A models for interactive search. Preprint, December, 2000.

9. B. Gunsel and M. Tekalp. Shape similarity matching for query-by-example. *Pattern Recognition*, 31(7):931–944, 1998.

10. A. K. Jain and Vailaya. Shape-based retrieval: A case study with tramework image database. *Pattern Recognition*, 31(9):1369–1390, 1998.

11. MacKay and D. J. C. Bayesian interpolation. *Neural Computation*, 4:415–447, 1992.

12. F. Mokhtarian, S. Abbasi, and J. Kittler. Robust and efficient shape indexing through curvature scale space. In *Proc. British Machine Vision Conference*, pages 53–62, 1996.

13. D. Mumford. *Goemetry-Driven Diffusion in Computer Vision*, chapter The Bayesian rationale for Energy Functionals, pages 141–153. Kluwer Academic, 1994.

14. Y. Rui, A. She, and T. Huang. *Image Databases and Multimedia Search*, volume 8 of *Series on Software Engineering and Knowledge Engineering*, chapter A Modified Fourier Descriptor For Shape Matching in MARS, pages 165–180. World Scientific Publishing House in Singapore, 1998.

15. B. Schölkopf, A. Smola, and K.-R. Müller. Nonlinear component analysis as a kernel eigenvalue problem. *Neural Computation*, 10:1299–1319, 1998. Technical Report No. 44, 1996, Max Planck Institut für biologische Kybernetik, Tübingen.

16. S. Sclaroff and A. Pentland. Modal mathing for correspondence and recognition. *IEEE Trans. Pattern Analysis Mach. Intell.*, 17:545–561, 1995.

17. A. Smeulders, M. Worring, S. Santini, A. Gupta, and R. Jain. Content-based image retrieval at the end of the eraly years. *IEEE Trans. PAMI*, 22:1348–1375, 2000.

18. A. Trouvé. Diffeomorphisms groups and pattern matching in image analysis. *Int. J. of Comp. Vis.*, 28:213–221, 1998.

19. A. Trouvé and Y. Yu. Unsupervised clustering trees by non-linear principal component analysis. *Pattern Recognition and Image Analysis*, II:108–112, 2001.

20. V. Vapnik. *The Nature of Statistical Learning Theory.* Springer, N.Y., 1995.

21. D. White and R. Jain. Similarity indexing: Algorithms and performance. In *Proc. SPIE, San Diego*, volume 2670, 1996.

22. L. Younes. Computable distance between shapes. *SIAM J. Appl. Math*, 58:565–586, 1998.

A Fast MAP Algorithm for 3D Ultrasound

João M. Sanches* and Jorge S. Marques

IST/ISR, Torre Norte, Av. Rovisco Pais, 1049-001, Lisbon, Portugal

Abstract. Bayesian methods have been avoided in 3D ultrasound. The multiplicative type of noise which corrupts ultrasound images leads to slow reconstruction procedures if Bayesian principles are used. Heuristic approaches have been used instead in practical applications.

This paper tries to overcome this difficulty by proposing an algorithm which is derived from sound theoretical principles and fast. This algorithm is based on the expansion of the noise probability density function as a Taylor series, un the vicinity of the maximum likelihood estimates, leading to a linear set of equations which are easily solved by standard techniques. Reconstruction examples with synthetic and medical data are provided to evaluate the proposed algorithm.

1 Introduction

This paper addresses the problem of 3D ultrasound. 3D ultrasound aims to reconstruct the human anatomy from a set of ultrasound images, corresponding to cross-sections of the human body. Based on this information, the idea is to estimate a volume of interest for diagnosis proposes. This technique is wide spread due essentially to its non invasive and non ionizing characteristics [1]. Furthermore, the ultrasound equipment is less expensive than other medical modalities, such CT, MRI or PET [2, 3]. One way to perform 3D ultrasound is by using 2D ultrasound equipment with a spatial locator attached to the ultrasound probe, giving the position and orientation of the cross-section along the time(see Fig.1). The estimation algorithm should fuse these information, image and position, to estimate the volume.

Traditionally ultrasound imaging technique is made in real time using the B-scan mode. The inspections results are visualized in real time being allowed to the medical doctor to choose the best cross sections for the diagnosis. In 3D ultrasound this goal is much more difficult to achieve since the amount of data is much higher. However, reconstruction time should be kept as small as possible. This is the reason why a lot of algorithms used in 3D ultrasound are designed in ad hoc basis [4, 5], aiming to be as simple and fast as possible.

Bayesian approaches in 3D ultrasound have been avoided since these methods are usually computationally demanding. In this paper we present an algorithm for 3D ultrasound designed in a Bayesian framework. Its theoretical foundation is

---

* Correspondent author: to João Sanches, IST/ISR, Torre Notre, Av. Rovisco Pais, 1049-001 Lisboa, Portugal, Email:jmrs@alfa.ist.utl.pt, Phone:+351 21 8418195

M.A.T. Figueiredo, J. Zerubia, A.K. Jain (Eds.): EMMCVPR 2001, LNCS 2134, pp. 63–74, 2001.

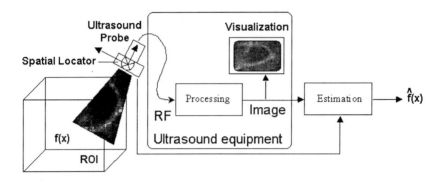

Fig. 1. 3D ultrasound acquisition system

presented as well the simplification procedures and justifications in order to speed up the reconstruction process. Our goal is to designed an efficient reconstruction algorithm to work in a quasi real time basis, while keeping a solid theoretical foundation.

This paper is organized as follows. Section 2 describes the problem of 3D reconstruction and the notation adopted in this paper. Sections 3 and 4 present two algorithms for 3D reconstruction: the standard solution and a fast algorithm. Section 5 present experimental results with synthetic and real data using both algorithms. Finally section 6 concludes the paper.

2   Problem Formulation

This section describes the reconstruction of a 3D function f from a set of ultrasound images. Additional details can be found in [6].

Let us consider a scalar function $f(x)$ defined in $\Omega \subset R^3$, i.e., $f : \Omega \to R$. We assume that this function is expressed as a linear combination of known basis functions, i.e.,

$$f(x) = \sum_g b_g(x) u_g \qquad (1)$$

where $u_1, u_2, ..., u_N$ are the unknown coefficients to be estimated and $b(x_i)$ are known basis functions centered at the nodes of a 3D regular grid. Let $\{y_i\}$ be a set of intensity data points, measuring $f(x)$ at locations $\{x_i\}$, belonging to one of the inspection planes. It is assumed that intensity measurements, y_i, are corrupted by multiplicative noise and the goal is to estimate $f(x)$ based on the observations $\{y_i\}$.

This estimation problem can be formulated in a Bayesian framework using a MAP criterion, as follows: given a set of data $Y = \{y_i\}$ with a distribution $p(Y|U)$ which depends on the unknown parameters, $U = \{u_g\}$ with a prior distribution $p(U)$, estimate U in order to maximize the joint probability density function of the data and parameters, $p(Y, U)$, i.e.,

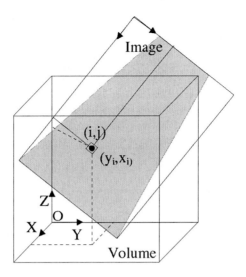

Fig. 2. Volume and image coordinates

$$\hat{U} = arg \max_{U} \log(p(Y|U)p(U)) \tag{2}$$

In this paper we assume that all the elements of Y are i.i.d. (independent and identically distributed) [8] with a Rayleigh distribution, i.e.,

$$\log p(Y|U) = \sum_{i} \{\log(\frac{y_i}{f(x_i)}) - \frac{y_i^2}{2f(x_i)}\} \tag{3}$$

where $f(x_i)$ is the value of the function f to be reconstructed at x_i.

The Rayleigh distribution is achieved in [9] from physical principles that the human tissue consists of a large number of independent scatters with different orientations.

The prior used is gaussian [10], i.e.,

$$p(U) = \frac{1}{Z} e^{-\psi \sum_g \sum_i (u_g - u_{gi})^2} \tag{4}$$

where u_{gi} is a neighbor of u_g and Z is a normalization factor.

Therefore, the objective function can be expressed as

$$L(U) = l(U) + q(U) \tag{5}$$

where $l = \log p(Y/U)$ is the log likelihood function of the data and $q = \log p(U)$ is the logarithm of the prior associated to the unknown parameters.

To optimize (5) the ICM algorithm proposed by Besag [7] is used. The ICM algorithm simplifies the optimization process by optimizing the objective function with respect to a single variable at a time, keeping the other variables constant. Each step is a 1D optimization problem which can be solved in a number of

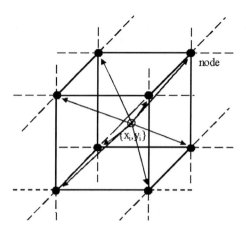

Fig. 3. Neighboring nodes of a data point.

ways. This step is repeated for all the unknown coefficients in each iteration of
the ICM algorithm.

To optimize (5) with respect to a single coefficient u_p the stationary equation,

$$\frac{\partial l(U)}{\partial u_p} + \frac{\partial q(U)}{\partial u_p} = 0 \qquad (6)$$

is numerically solved.

The next sections present two approaches to compute (6). Section 3 attempts
to solve this equation using nonlinear optimization methods. Section 4 presents a
fast algorithm based on the solution of a linear set of equations. The second perform some simplifications in order to speed up the computations. Both methods
are iterative.

3   Nonlinear Method

Let us first compute the derivatives of l and q.

After straightforward manipulation it can be concluded that

$$\frac{\partial l(U)}{\partial u_p} = \frac{1}{2} \sum_i \left(\frac{y_i^2 - 2f(x_i)}{f(x_i)^2} b_p(x_1) \right) \qquad (7)$$

where the sum is performed for all data points that are in the neighborhood
$[-\Delta, \Delta]^3$ of the p-th node. In fact, each data point contributes to the estimation
of its 8 neighboring coefficients (see Fig.3).

It is also easy to concluded that

$$\frac{\partial q(U)}{\partial u_p} = -2\psi N_v(u_p - \bar{u}_p) \qquad (8)$$

where N_v is the number of neighbors of u_p ($N_v = 6$) and $\bar{u}_p$ is the average intensity computed using the N_v neighbors.

To optimize the objective function a set of non-linear equations should be solved,

$$\frac{1}{2} \sum_i (\frac{y_i^2 - 2f(x_i)}{f(x_i)^2} b_p(x_1)) - 2\psi N_v (u_p - \bar{u}_p) = 0 \qquad (9)$$

This is an huge optimization problem, which must be solved using numerical methods. The ICM algorithm proposed by Besag [7] is used and each equation is numerically solved by using the Newton-Rapson method assuming that the other coefficients, $u_k, k \neq p$ are known. The computation of the solution of (9) is computationally heavy, presenting some undesirable difficulties.

First, it would be nice to factorize the equation in two terms, one depending only on the data and the other depending on the unknown to estimate,

$$h(u_p)g_1(Y)r_1(U \setminus \{u_p\}) + g_2(Y)r_2(U \setminus \{u_p\}) + C = 0 \qquad (10)$$

where $g_1(Y)$ and $g_2(Y)$ are sufficient statistics. This formulation would allow to concentrate the influence of the observed data on a small set of coefficients, computed once for all at the first iteration and kept unchanged during the optimization process. Data processing would be done only once speeding up the estimation process.

Unfortunately, it is not possible to write (9) in the form of (10), i.e., there are no sufficient statistics for the estimation of the interpolating function f. This means that all the data must be read from the disk and processed in each iteration of the nonlinear reconstruction algorithm. This is a strong limitation when a large number of cross-sections is involved, e.g., 1000 images with 640×480 pixels will lead to 3072×10^5 pixels, preventing a wide spread use of this algorithm.

Another important difficulty concerns the stability of the convergence process. The system of equations (9) is non-linear. The stability of the numerical methods used to solve it, strongly depends on the data and on the regularization parameter, ψ, and on the initial estimates of U. The process of finding the right parameters to obtain acceptable reconstructions is in general often done by trial and error.

To overcome these difficulties an approximation approach is proposed in the next section.

4   Linear Solution

Let us develop $l(U)$ in Taylor series about the maximum likelihood estimates, U_{ML},

$$l(u_p) = l(u_p^{ML}) + \frac{\partial l(u_p^{ML})}{\partial u_p}(u_p - u_p^{ML}) + \frac{1}{2}\frac{\partial^2 l(u_p^{ML})}{\partial u_p^2}(u_p - u_p^{ML})^2 + \epsilon \qquad (11)$$

the first derivative of $l(U)$ with respect to u_p is

$$\frac{\partial l(U)}{\partial u_p} \approx \frac{\partial^2 l(u_p^{ML})}{\partial u_p^2}(u_p - u_p^{ML}) \tag{12}$$

where it was assumed that $\frac{\partial l(u_p^{ML})}{\partial u_p} = 0$ since by definition U_{ML} is a stationary point of $l(U)$. The residue ϵ was discarded for convenience.

Thus (6) takes the form

$$\frac{\partial L(U)}{\partial u_p} \approx \frac{\partial^2 l(u_p^{ML})}{\partial u_p^2}(u_p - u_p^{ML}) - 2\psi N_v(u_p - \bar{u}_p) = 0 \tag{13}$$

leading to

$$u_p = \frac{1}{1 + \tau_p}u_p^{ML} + \frac{\tau_p}{1 + \tau_p}\bar{u}_p \tag{14}$$

where $\tau_p = -\frac{2\psi N_v}{\partial^2 l(u_p^{ML})\backslash \partial u_p^2}$

Equations show that the MAP estimation can be seen as a linear combination of the ML estimates with the average intensity computed in the neighborhood of each node.

Let us compute the maximum likelihood estimation of U.

Assuming that $f(x)$ changes slowly in the neighborhood of each node, i.e., $f(x_i) \approx u_p$ will be used in (7) to obtain

$$\frac{\partial l(U)}{\partial u_p} = \frac{1}{2u_p^2}\sum_i(y_i^2 b_p(x_i)) - \frac{1}{u_p}\sum_i(b_p(x_i)) = 0 \tag{15}$$

Solving with respect to u_p^{ML} leads to

$$u_p^{ML} = \frac{1}{2}\frac{\sum_i(y_i^2 b_p(x_i))}{\sum_i b_p(x_i)} \tag{16}$$

and by deriving (15) in order to u_p leads to

$$\frac{\partial^2 l(u_p^{ML})}{\partial u_p^2} = -\frac{\sum_i b_p(x_i)}{(u_p^{ML})^2} \tag{17}$$

This expression for the second derivative of the log likelihood function, obtained by deriving (15) with respect to u_p, can be more accurately computed if (7) is used. By deriving two times (7) with respect to u_p and after replacing $f(x_i)$ by u_p it obtains:

$$\frac{\partial^2 l(u_p^{ML})}{\partial u_p^2} = -\frac{\sum (y_i b_p(x_i))^2}{(u_p^{ML})^3} + \frac{\sum b_p^2(x_i)}{(u_p^{ML})^2} \tag{18}$$

We have used expression (17) in the reconstruction using synthetic data and (18) in the case of real data.

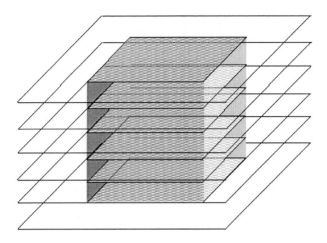

Fig. 4. Cross sections extracted from a synthetic 3D cube

Therefore, the MAP estimate of the volume of interest is obtained by solving a system of linear equations given by (14) where $\tau_p = \frac{2\psi N_v}{\sum_i b_p(x_i))}(u_p^{ML})^2$ and where u_p^{ML} is given by(16).

For sake of simplicity (14) can be rewrite as

$$u_p = k_p + c_p \bar{u}_p \tag{19}$$

where $k_p = \frac{u_p^{ML}}{1+\tau_p}$ and $c_p = \frac{\tau_p}{1+\tau_p}$. These parameters, k_p and c_p are computed once for all during the initialization phase. The solution of (14) can be done by standard algorithms for the solution of linear sets of equations.

5   Experimental Results

This section presents two 3D reconstruction examples using synthetic and real data.

The synthetic data consists of a set of 100 images of 128×128 pixels corresponding to parallel cross sections of the 3D interval $[-1, 1]^3$ (see Fig.4). The function to be reconstructed is assumed to be binary: $f(x) = 5000, x \in [-0.5, 0.5]^3, f(x) = 2500$ otherwise. The cross sections were corrupted with Rayleigh noise according to (3). The histogram of the whole set of images is shown in Fig.5 and is a mixture of two Rayleigh densities. Both reconstruction algorithm were used to reconstruct f in the interval $[-1, 1]^3$ using a regularization parameter $\psi = 16.10^{-6}$.

Fig.6 shows the profiles extracted from the estimated volumes using both methods. These two profiles are quite similar which means that both methods lead to similar results in this problem. The SNR of 21.4dB for the nonlinear method and 20.8dB for the fast algorithm proposed in this paper stresses the

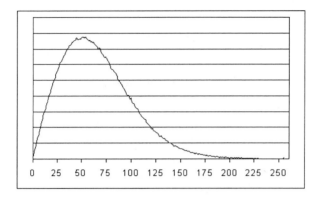

Fig. 5. Synthetic data set histogram

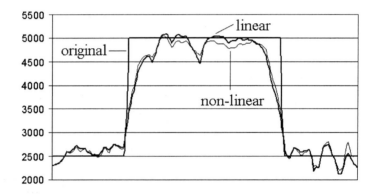

Fig. 6. Profiles extracted from the original volume and from the estimated volumes using the nonlinear and linear methods

ability of the linear algorithm to produce similar results as those obtained with the nonlinear method.

It should be stressed that the linear method is less heavy in computational terms. Fig.7 and Fig.8 show the evolution of the posteriori distribution function, $\log(p(Y, U))$ along the iterative process. Fig.7 displays $\log(p(Y, U))$ as function of the index of the iteration while Fig.8 displays the same values as function of the time.

The nonlinear algorithm converges in less iterations(62) than the linear algorithm(97) in this example. However, since each iteration of the nonlinear method is slower and it involves processing all (millions) of the observations, the convergence is slower in terms of computation time (see Fig.8) (in this case about 6 times slower than the linear method[1]).

---

[1] These values depend on the number and dimensions of the images and on the desired accuracy for the solution. For very accurate solutions it is need more iterations and the linear method becomes more efficient

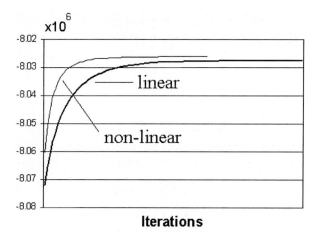

Fig. 7. L(U) along the iterative process

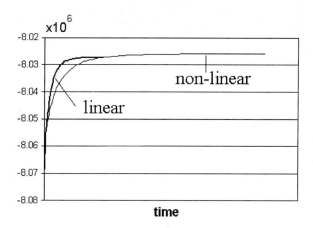

Fig. 8. L(U) along the iterative process in function of time

Fig. 9 shows cross sections of the 3D volume (left) as well as the 3D surface of the cube displayed using rendering methods (right). The results are again similar, the nonlinear method performing slightly better at the transitions.

The real data if formed by a set of 100 images of a human thyroid with 128×128 pixels. Fig.10 shows the corresponding histogram. This histogram reveals some significant differences from the one of the synthetic data. In the case of the synthetic data the underlying 3D object is binary while in the case of the real data a continuous range of reflectivity values are admissible.

Profiles extracted from both estimated volumes are shown in Fig.11. In this figure are also shown images belonging to the initial data set. The profiles were computed from images extracted from the estimated volumes with dimensions and positions equivalent to the cross-sections shown in the figure. In this graph it

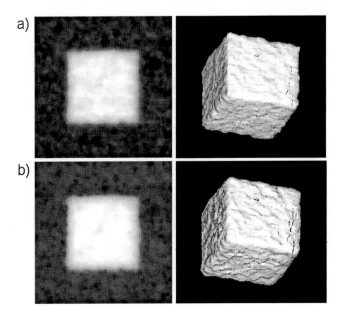

Fig. 9. Reconstructed volumes, a)using the nonlinear method and b) using the linear method

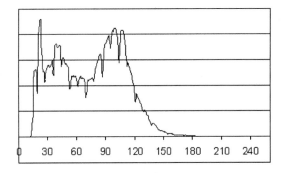

Fig. 10. Real data histogram

is also shown a profile extracted from a maximum likelihood estimates computed by using the expression (16). Here, the difference between both methods are more visible which is related with the deviation of the real data from the true Rayleigh model. However, we conclude once more that the linear method leads to acceptable results, similar to the ones obtained with the nonlinear algorithm.

6   Conclusion

This paper presents an algorithm to estimate the acoustic reflectivity in a given region of interest from a set of ultrasound images. The images are complemented

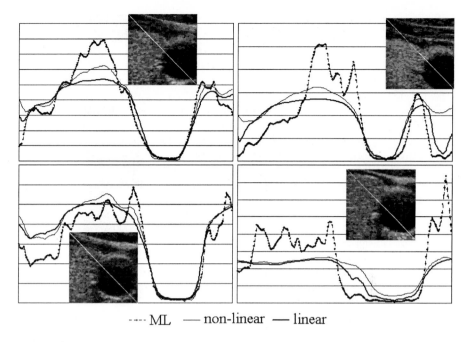

---- ML   —— non-linear   —— linear

Fig. 11. Profiles extracted from the estimated volumes using the nonlinear and linear method

with the position and orientation of the ultrasound probe. The proposed algorithm is formulated in a Bayesian framework using a MAP criterion. To speed the reconstruction time a simplified (linear) algorithm was proposed based on the concept of sufficient statistics.

The goal is obtain a fast and efficient MAP algorithm to estimate volumes in a quasi real time basis. Reconstruction results obtained with both methods are presented, one using a set of images extracted from a synthetic 3D cube and the other using a set of real cross-sections of a human thyroid. Both examples show that the fast(linear) algorithm performs almost as well as the nonlinear version. Profiles extracted from the estimated volumes are quite similar and the signal to noise ration (for the synthetic case only) computed with the original volume reenforce this similarity. It is concluded that the linear algorithm needs more iterations to reconstruct the volume than the nonlinear one but it spend mutch less time. This is explained by the fact that the linear method only has to process the huge amount of data only once, while the nonlinear method must read and process the data in each iteration. A final note should be provide. The formulation of the linear method is more simple than the nonlinear method. The estimation process in the first case is obtained by solving a set of linear equations while in the non simplified case a set of non-linear equations should be solved. The nonlinear method present problems of convergence and stability, that are not addressed in this paper, which are also solved by using the linear reconstruction method proposed in this paper.

References

1. T. Nelson, D. Downey, D. Pretorius, A. Fenster, Three-Dimensional Ultrasound, Lippincott, 1999.
2. J. Quistgaard, Signal Acquisition and Processing in Medical Diagnostics Ultrasound, IEEE Signal Processing Magazine, vol.14, no.1, pp 67-74, January 1997.
3. G.T.Herman, A.Kuba, Discrete Tomography, Foundations, Algorithms, and Applications, Birkhauser, 1999.
4. R.N.Rohling, A. H. Gee and L. Berman, A comparation of freehand three-dimensional ultrasound reconstruction techniques, Medical Image Analysis, vol.4, no.4, pp.339-359, 1999.
5. S. Ogawa et al., Three Dimension Ultrasonic Imaging for Diagnosis of Beast Tumor,Ultrasonics Symp., 1998.
6. J. Sanches, J.Marques, A Rayleigh reconstruction/interpolation algorithm for 3D ultrasound, Pattern Recognition Letters, 21, pp. 917-926, 2000.
7. J. Besag, On the Statistical Analysis of Dirty Pictures, J. R. Statist. Soc. B, vol.48, no. 3, pp. 259-302, 1986.
8. J. Dias and J. Leitão, Wall position and thickness estimation from sequences of echocardiograms images, IEEE Transactions on Medical Imaging, vol.15, pp.25-38, February 1996.
9. C. Burckhardt, Speckle in Ultrasound B-Mode Scans, IEEE Trans. on Sonics and Ultrasonics, vol. SU-25, no.1, pp.1-6, January 1978.
10. S.Z.Li, Close-Form Solution and Parameter Selection for Convex Minimization-Based Edge-Preserving Smoothing, IEEE Trans. on PAMI, vol. PAMI-20, no.9, pp.916-932, September 1998.

Designing the Minimal Structure
of Hidden Markov Model by Bisimulation

Manuele Bicego, Agostino Dovier, and Vittorio Murino

Dip. di Informatica, Univ. di Verona
Strada Le Grazie 15, 37134 Verona, Italy
{bicego,dovier,murino}@sci.univr.it

Abstract. Hidden Markov Models (HMMs) are an useful and widely utilized approach to the modeling of data sequences. One of the problems related to this technique is finding the optimal structure of the model, namely, its number of states. Although a lot of work has been carried out in the context of the model selection, few work address this specific problem, and heuristics rules are often used to define the model depending on the tackled application. In this paper, instead, we use the notion of probabilistic bisimulation to automatically and efficiently determine the minimal structure of HMM. Bisimulation allows to merge HMM states in order to obtain a minimal set that do not significantly affect model performances. The approach has been tested on DNA sequence modeling and 2D shape classification. Results are presented in function of reduction rates, classification performances, and noise sensitivity.

1 Introduction

Hidden Markov Models (HMMs) represent a widespread approach to the modeling of sequences: they attempt to capture the underlying structure of a set of symbol strings. HMMs can be viewed as stochastic generalizations of finite-state automata, when both transitions between states and generation of output symbols are governed by probability distributions [1].

The basic theory of HMMs was developed by Baum *et al.* [2, 3] in the late 1960s, but only in the last decade it has been extensively applied in a large number of problems. A non-exhaustive list of such problems consists of speech recognition [1], handwritten character recognition [4], DNA and protein modelling [5], gesture recognition [6] and, more in general, behavior analysis and synthesis [7].

HMMs fit very well in a large number of situations, in particular where the state sequence structure of the process examined can be assumed to be Markovian. Unfortunately, there are some drawbacks [8]. First, the iterative technique for the HMM learning (*Baum-Welch re-estimation*) converges to a local optimum, not necessarily the global one, and the choice of appropriate initial parameters' estimates is crucial for convergence. Second, a large amount of training data

M.A.T. Figueiredo, J. Zerubia, A.K. Jain (Eds.): EMMCVPR 2001, LNCS 2134, pp. 75–90, 2001.

is generally necessary to estimate HMM parameters. Finally, the HMM topology and number of states have to be determined prior to learning, and usually heuristic rules are pursued for this purpose (e.g., [9]). This paper proposes a novel approach for resolving this final problem, in particular to determine the number of states. This issue could be tackled by using traditional methods of model selection; numerous paradigms have been proposed in this context, a non-exhaustive list includes [10]: *Minimum Description Length* (MDL), *Bayesian Inference Criterion* (BIC), *Minimum Message Length* (MML), *Mixture Minimal Description Length* (MMDL), *Evidence Based Bayesian* (EBB) etc.. More computational intensive approaches are stochastic approaches (e.g., *Markov Chain Monte Carlo* (MCMC)), re-sampling based schemes, and cross-validation methods. Although principally derived for fitting mixture models, many of these techniques could be applied also in the HMM context, as proposed in [11] and [12]. It is worth noting that these approaches are devoted to find the optimal model on the basis of a criterion function by exploring all (or a large part of) the search space. Our work proposes instead a direct method to identify the model without searching the whole space, resulting less computationally intensive. In [11], starting with redundant configuration, an optimal structure can be obtained by repeated Bayesian merging of states in an incremental way, as far as new evidence arrives. In [12], a method for simultaneous learning of HMM structure and parameters is proposed. Parameters' uncertainty is minimized by introducing an entropic prior and Maximum a Posteriori Probability (MAP) estimation. In this way, redundant parameters are eliminated and the model becomes sparse; moreover posterior probability increases, and an easier interpretation of resulting architecture is allowed.

Our approach consists in eliminating syntactic redundancy of an Hidden Markov Model using a technique called bisimulation. Bisimulation is a notion of equivalence between graphs whose usefulness has been demonstrated in various fields of Computer Science. In Concurrency it is used for testing process equivalence [18], in Model-Checking as a notion of equivalence between Kripke Structures [20], in Web-like databases for providing operational semantics to query languages [17], in Set Theory, for replacing extensionality in the context of non well-founded sets [13].

With our approach, the structure of an HMM is reduced by computing bisimulation equivalence relation between states of the model, so that equivalent states can be collapsed. We employed both the notions of probabilistic and standard bisimulation. We will prove that bisimulation reduces the number of states without significant loss in term of likelihood and classification accuracy. We will test this approach reporting experiments on DNA sequence modelling and 2D shape recognition using chain code. We will show that the proposed procedure is fully automatic, efficient, and provides promising results. We also compare our approach with BIC (Bayesian Inference Criterion) method, which is equivalent to MDL [10], showing that this technique is nearly as acceptable as our, as far as classification accuracy is concerned, but is more computationally demanding.

The rest of the paper is organized as follows: Sect. 2 contains formal description of HMM. In Sect. 3, the notion of bisimulation and the algorithm to compute equivalence classes are described. In Sect. 4 we detail our strategy and in Sect. 5 experiments and results are presented. Finally, Sect. 6 contains conclusions and future perspectives.

2   Hidden Markov Models

An HMM is formally defined by the following elements (see [1] for further details):

- A set $S = \{S_1, S_2, \cdots, S_N\}$ of (hidden) states.
- A state transition probability distribution, also called transition matrix $A = \{a_{ij}\}$, representing the probability to go from state S_i to state S_j.

$$a_{ij} = P[q_{t+1} = S_j | q_t = S_i] \qquad 1 \leq i, j \leq N \qquad (1)$$

with $a_{ij} \geq 0$ and $\sum_{j=1}^{N} a_{ij} = 1$.
- A set $V = \{v_1, v_2, \cdots, v_M\}$ of observation symbols.
- An observation symbol probability distribution, also called emission matrix $B = \{b_j(k)\}$, indicating the probability of emission of symbol v_k when system state is S_j.

$$b_j(k) = P[v_k \text{ at time } t \,|q_t = S_j] \qquad 1 \leq j \leq N, 1 \leq k \leq M \qquad (2)$$

with $b_i(k) \geq 0$ and $\sum_{j=1}^{M} b_j(k) = 1$.
- An initial state probability distribution $\pi = \{\pi_i\}$, representing probabilities of initial states.

$$\pi_i = P[q_1 = S_i] \qquad 1 \leq i \leq N \qquad (3)$$

with $\pi_i \geq 0$ and $\sum_{i=1}^{N} \pi_i = 1$. For convenience, we denote an HMM as a triplet $\lambda = (A, B, \pi)$, which determines uniquely the model.

3   Bisimulation

Bisimulation is a notion of equivalence between graphs useful in several fields of Computer Science. The notion was introduced by Park for testing process equivalence, extending a previous notion of automata simulation by Milner. Milner then employed bisimulation as the core for establishing observational equivalence of the Calculus of Communicating Systems [18].

Kanellakis and Smolka in [16] relate the bisimulation problem with the general (relational) coarsest partition problem and pointed out that the partition refinement algorithm in [19] solves this task. More precisely, in [19] Paige and Tarjan solve the problem in which the stability requirement is relative to a relation E (edges) on a set N (nodes) with an algorithm whose complexity is $O(|E| \log |N|)$.

Standard Bisimulation. Bisimulation can be equivalently formulated as a relation between two graphs and as a relation between nodes of a single graph. We adopt the latter definition since we are interested in reducing states of a unique graph.

Definition 1. *Given a graph $G = \langle N, E \rangle$ a bisimulation on G is a relation $b \subseteq N \times N$ s.t. for all $u_0, u_1 \in N$ s.t. $u_0 \, b \, u_1$ and for $i = 0, 1$: if $\langle u_i, v_i \rangle \in E$, then there exists $\langle u_{1-i}, v_{1-i} \rangle \in E$ s.t. $v_0 \, b \, v_1$.*

In order to minimize the number of nodes of a graph, we look for the maximal bisimulation $\equiv$ on G. Such a maximal bisimulation always exists, it is unique, and it is an equivalence relation over the set of nodes of G [13]. The minimal representation of $G = \langle N, E \rangle$ is therefore the graph:

$$\langle N/\equiv, \{\langle [m]_\equiv, [n]_\equiv \rangle : \langle m, n \rangle \in E\} \rangle$$

which is usually called the *bisimulation contraction of G*. Using the algorithm in [19] the problem can be solved in time $O(|E| \log |N|)$; for acyclic graphs and for some classes of cyclic graphs it can be solved in linear time w.r.t. $|N| + |E|$ [15].

Bisimulation on labeled graphs. If the graphs are such that nodes and/or edges are labeled, the notion can be reformulated as follows:

Definition 2. *Let $G = \langle N, E, \ell \rangle$ be a graph with a labeling function ℓ for nodes, and labeled edges of the form $m \overset{a}{\to} n$ (a belongs to a set of labels). A bisimulation on G is a relation $b \subseteq N \times N$ s.t. for all $u_0, u_1 \in N$ s.t. $u_0 \, b \, u_1$ it holds that: $\ell(u_1) = \ell(u_2)$ and for $i = 0, 1$, if $u_i \overset{a}{\to} v_i \in E$, then there exists $u_{1-i} \overset{a}{\to} v_{1-i} \in E$ s.t. $v_0 \, b \, v_1$.*

If only the nodes are labeled, the procedure in [19] can be employed to find the bisimulation contraction, provided that in the initialization phase nodes with the same labels are put in the same class. The case in which edges are labeled can be reduced to the last one by replacing a labeled edge $m \overset{a}{\to} n$ by a new node ν labeled by a and by the edges $\langle m, \nu \rangle$ and $\langle \nu, n \rangle$. Therefore, finding the bisimulation contraction also in this case can be done using the algorithm of [19]; moreover, the procedure of [19] can be modified in order to deal directly (i.e., without preprocessing) with the general case described.

Probabilistic Bisimulation The notion of bisimulation over labeled graphs (Def. 2) has been introduced in a context where labels denote actions executed (e.g. a symbol is emitted) by processes during their run. Labels can also store pairs of values $\langle x, y \rangle$: an action x and a probability value y (that could be read as: this edge can be crossed with probability y and in this case an action x is done). In this case another notion of bisimulation is perhaps more suitable. Consider, for instance, the graph of Fig. 1 (we use n_1–n_8 to refer to the nodes: they are not labels). n_7 and n_8 are trivially equivalent since they have no outgoing edges. Nothing can be done in both the cases. The four nodes n_2, n_3, n_5, n_6 are in the same equivalence class, since they have equivalent successors (reachable performing the same action b, with probability 1). The nodes n_1 and n_4 are instead not

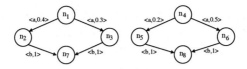

Fig. 1. n_1 and n_4 are not bisimilar, but probabilistically bisimilar.

equivalent, since, for instance, there is the edge $n_1 \overset{\langle a,0.4 \rangle}{\to} n_3$ but no edges labeled $\langle a, 0.4 \rangle$ starts from n_4. However, both from n_1 and n_4 it can be reached one of the equivalent states, performing action a with probability 0.7: the two nodes should be considered equivalent. These graphs are called *Fully Probabilistic Labelled Transition System* (FPLTS).

The notion of *probabilistic bisimulation* [14] is aimed at formally justifying this intuitive concept. We start by providing two auxiliary notions: Given a graph $G = \langle N, E \rangle$ with edge labeled by pairs as above, and $b \subseteq N \times N$ a relation, then for two nodes $m, n \in N$ and a symbol a, we define the functions B and S as follows

$$B(m,n,a) = \{\mu : \exists q (m \overset{\langle a,q \rangle}{\to} \mu \in E \land \mu \, b \, n)\} \text{ and } S(m,n,a) = \sum_{m \overset{\langle a,q \rangle}{\to} \mu \in E, \mu b n} q$$

Definition 3. *Let $G = \langle N, E \rangle$ be a graph with edge labeled by pairs consisting of symbols and probability values, a probabilistic bisimulation on G is a relation $b \subseteq N \times N$ s.t.: for all $u_0, u_1 \in N$, if $u_0 \, b \, u_1$ then for $i = 0, 1$ if $u_i \overset{\langle a,p \rangle}{\to} v_i \in E$, then then there exists $v_{1-i} \in N$ s.t.:*

— $u_{1-i} \overset{\langle a,p' \rangle}{\to} v_{1-i} \in E$,
— $S(u_i, v_i, a) = S(u_{1-i}, v_{1-i}, a)$, and
— and for all $m \in B(u_i, v_i, a)$ and $n \in B(u_{1-i}, v_{1-i}, a)$ it holds that $m \, b \, n$.

In [14] a modification of the Paige-Tarjan procedure is presented in this case and proved to correctly return the probabilistic contraction of a graph $G = \langle N, E \rangle$ in time $O(|N||E| \log |N|)$. In the example of Fig. 1 the two nodes n_1 and n_4 are put in the same class.

In this paper we will further extend the possible labels for edges. We admit triplets $\langle p_1, a, p_2 \rangle$ where a is a symbol while p_1 and p_2 are probabilistic values. We extend the notion of the above Definition 3 point to point. In other words, we reason as if the edge $\langle p_1, a, p_2 \rangle$ is replaced by the two edges $\langle a, p_1 \rangle, \langle \hat{a}, p_2 \rangle$ and $\hat{a}$ can not be confused with a (see Fig. 2).

4   The Strategy

HMM as labeled graphs. Probabilistic bisimulation is defined on FPLTS, which are slightly different from HMMs. Neglecting notation, the real problem is represented by emission probability of each state, which has not counterpart in

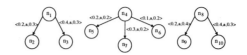

Fig. 2. n_1 and n_4 are probabilistically bisimilar. n_1 and n_8 are not.

FPLTS. As described in Sect. 3, we can solve the problem by choosing an appropriate initial partition, whose sets contains states with same emission probability and then run the algorithm of [19]. This approach is correct, but it is too restrictive with respect to the concept of probabilistic bisimulation. In other words, using this initialization we create classes of bisimulation equivalence using concept of syntactic labelling, loosing instead the semantic labeling concept, which is the kernel of the probabilistic bisimulation.

Thus, we propose another method, a bit more expensive in terms of memory allocation and computational cost, but offering a better semantic characterization.

Definition 4. *Given a HMM* $\lambda = (A, B, \pi)$, *trained with a set of strings from an alphabet* $V = \{v_1, v_2, \cdots, v_M\}$, *the equivalent FPLTS is obtained as follows. For each state* S_i:

− *Let* A_i *be the set of edges outgoing from the state* S_i, *defined as*

$$A_i = \{\langle S_i, S_j \rangle : a_{ij} \neq 0, \ 1 \leq j \leq N\}$$

− *each edge* e *in* A_i *is replaced by* M *edges, whose labels are* $\langle a_{ij}, v_k, B_i(k) \rangle$, *where, for* $1 \leq i, j \leq N$, $1 \leq k \leq M$:
  • a_{ij} *is probability of* e;
  • v_k *is* k-th *symbol of* V;
  • $B_i(k)$ *is probability of emission of* v_k *from state* S_i.

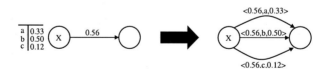

Fig. 3. Basic idea of procedure to represent HMM as a FPLTS.

Given an HMM with N states, K edges and M symbols, with this approach the complexity of bisimulation contraction grows from $O(KN log N)$ to $O(MKN log N)$ for time, and from $O(KN)$ to $O(MKN)$ for space.

By applying bisimulation to a HMM we have to face another important issue: the partial control of compression rate of our strategy. To this end, we introduce the concept of *quantization* of probability: given a set of quantization level values (prototypes) in the interval $[0, 1]$, we approximate each probability with the closest prototype. A uniform quantization is adopted on interval $[0, 1]$. To control this approximation we define a *reduction factor*, representing the number of levels that subdivide the interval: it is calculated as *(number of prototypes - 2)*. For example, reduction factor 3 means that probability are approximated with the values $\{0, 0.25, 0.5, 0.75, 1\}$. Thus, the notion of equivalent labels is governed by the test of equality of their quantization, where $quant(p)$ is define as the prototype j closest to p.

As a final consideration, the reduction factor represents a tuning parameter for deciding the degree of compression adopted. Obviously, for a low value of the factor, information lost in approximation is high, and the resulting model can be a very poor representation of the original one.

Algorithm. Given a problem, determining optimal number of HMM states is performed following the following steps:

1. Training of HMM with a number of states that is reasonably large with respect to the problem considered. This number strongly depends from available data, and it can be determined using some heuristics.
2. Transform HMM in labelled graph (FPLTS), using procedure described in Def. 4 of Sect. 4. In this step we have to choose a reduction factor, that provides a measure of accuracy adopted in the conversion. It also gives a rough meaning of reduction rate: lower precision likely means higher compression.
3. Run bisimulation algorithm on such graph, obtaining equivalence classes. Optimal number of states N' is represented by cardinality of the quotient set (i.e. the number of different classes determined by bisimulation).
4. Retraining of the HMM using N' states.

This method is designed for discrete HMM, but can be generalized for other typologies by working on Step 2 of the procedure.

5   Experimental Results

The aim of the following experiments is to show that this method reduces HMM states without significant loss in terms of likelihood and classification accuracy. We tested these two properties on two distinct problems: DNA modeling, i.e. using HMM to model and recognize different DNA sequences (typically, fragments of genes), and 2D shape classification using chain code (modeled by HMM). In all tests, each HMM was trained in three learning sessions, using Baum-Welch re-estimation and choosing the one presenting the maximum likelihood. Each learning started using random initial estimates of A, B and π and ended when likelihood is converged or after 100 training cycles. Performances are measured in terms of some indices:

- *Compression Rate*, representing a percentage measure of the number of states eliminated by bisimulation: $CR = 100 \left(\frac{N_{orig} - N_{reduct}}{N_{orig}} \right)$, where N_{reduct} are the number of states after bisimulation on a HMM with N_{orig} states;

- *Log Likelihood Loss*, estimating the difference in LL between original and re-duced HMM: $LLL = 100 \left(\frac{LL_{orig} - LL_{reduct}}{LL_{orig}} \right)$, where LL_{reduct} and LL_{orig} are log likelihood of HMM with N_{reduct} and N_{orig} number of states, respectively.

5.1 DNA Modeling

Genomics offers tremendous challenges and opportunities for computational sci-entists. DNA are sequences of various lengths formed by using 4 symbols: *A*, *T*, *C*, and *G*. Each symbol represent a base, *Adenine, Thymine, Cytosine*, and *Guanine* respectively. Recent advances in biotechnology have produced enormous volumes of DNA related information, needing suitable computational techniques to manage them [21].

From a machine learning point of view [22], there are three main problems to deal with : *genome annotation*, including identification of genes and classification into functional categories, *computational comparative genomics*, for comparing complete genomic sequences at different levels of detail, and *genomic patterns*, including identification of regular pattern in sequence data. Hidden Markov Mod-els are widely used in resolving these problems, in particular for classification of genes, protein family modeling, and sequence alignment. This is because they are very suitable in modeling strings (as DNA or protein sequences), and can provide useful measures of similarity (LL) in comparing genes.

In this paper, we employ HMM to model gene sequences for classification pur-poses. This simple example is nevertheless significant to demonstrate HMM abil-ity in recognizing genes, also in conditions of noise (as biological mutations). Data were obtained extracting a 200 bp (base pair) fragment of *recA* gene sequence of a lactobacillus. We trained 95 HMMs on this sequence, where N (number of states) grows from 10 to 200 (step 2). We applied the bisimulation contraction algorithm on each HMM, with reduction factor varying from 1 to 9 (step 2), computing the number of resulting states. We then compared Log Likelihood (LL) of original sequence produced by original and reduced HMMs, obtaining results plotted on Fig. 4(b). One can notice that the two curves are very similar, in particular when reduction factor is high. In Table 1, average and maximum loss of likelihood (LLL) are presented for each value of resolution factor, with maximum compression rate: loss of Log Likelihood is fairly low, decreasing when augmenting precision of bisimulation (reduction factor). This kind of analysis is performed to show the graceful evolution of the HMM likelihood when number of states is decreased using bisimulation.

In Fig. 4(a) original number of states vs. reduced number of states are plotted, at varying number of states. More precisely, for a generic value N on abscissa, ordinate represents the number of states obtained after running bisimulation on N-states HMM. It is worth noting that compression rate increases when the number of states grows: this is reasonable, because small structures cannot have a large redundancy.

The second part of this experiment tries to exploit performance of our al-gorithm regarding classification accuracy. To perform this step we trained two

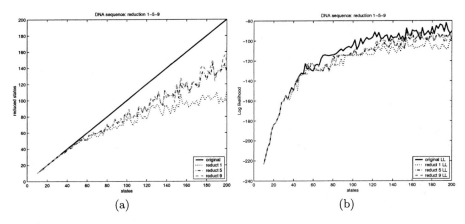

(a)   (b)

Fig. 4. Compression rate (a) and comparison of Likelihood curve for original and reduced HMM (b) on DNA modeling experiment. Reduction factor are 1, 5 and 9.

Table 1. Maximum compression rate, average and maximum Log Likelihood loss for DNA modeling experiment at varying reduction factors.

Reduction factor	Maximum CR (%)	Average LLL (%)	Maximum LLL (%)
1	50.00	9.57	32.20
3	38.16	6.69	20.07
5	33.14	5.45	20.31
7	34.87	5.91	18.90
9	34.04	5.77	22.30

HMMs with 150 states on 200 bases fragments of two different *recA* genes: one was from *glutamicum bacillus* and second was from *tubercolosis bacillus*. Each HMM was then reduced using bisimulation, varying reduction factor from 1 to 9 (step 2). Then, HMMs were retrained with reduced number of states, resulting in 10 reduced HMMs (5 for each sequence). Compression rate varies from 32% for reduction factor 1 to 22% for reduction factor 9 (see Table 2). We tested classification accuracy of HMMs using 300 sequences, obtained by adding synthetic noise to the original two. The noising procedure is the following: each base is changed with fixed probability p (ranging from 0.3 to 0.4), and following determined biological rules (for examples, A becomes T with probability higher than G). Each sequence of this set was evaluated using both models, and classified as belonging to the class whose model showed highest LL. Error rate was then calculated counting misclassified trials and dividing by the total number of trials. Figure 5 shows error rate for original and reduced HMMs, varying the probability of noise. One can notice that error rate trend is quite similar, and that error is very low, always below 5%, proving that HMMs work very well on this type of problems. In Table 2 (a–b), average errors on original and reduced HMMs are presented, respectively, varying noise level and reduction factor value. For the latter, maximum compression rate and maximum LL loss are also pre-

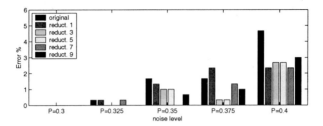

Fig. 5. Error rate for different noise level for DNA modeling experiment.

Table 2. Error on original and reduced HMMs for DNA modeling experiments in function of (a) varying noise level, and (b) varying reduction factor value.

<table>
<tr><td colspan="3" align="center">(a)</td><td colspan="5" align="center">(b)</td></tr>
<tr><td>Noised Level</td><td>Error on Original (%)</td><td>Error on Reduced (%)</td><td>Reduction Factor</td><td>Average CR (%)</td><td>Average LLL (%)</td><td>Error on Original (%)</td><td>Error on Reduced (%)</td></tr>
<tr><td>0.3</td><td>0.00</td><td>0.00</td><td>1</td><td>32.00</td><td>3.89</td><td>1.67</td><td>1.27</td></tr>
<tr><td>0.325</td><td>0.33</td><td>0.13</td><td>3</td><td>25.33</td><td>1.72</td><td>1.67</td><td>0.80</td></tr>
<tr><td>0.35</td><td>1.67</td><td>0.80</td><td>5</td><td>22.00</td><td>4.15</td><td>1.67</td><td>0.80</td></tr>
<tr><td>0.375</td><td>1.67</td><td>1.07</td><td>7</td><td>21.33</td><td>5.61</td><td>1.67</td><td>0.80</td></tr>
<tr><td>0.4</td><td>4.67</td><td>2.60</td><td>9</td><td>21.66</td><td>2.14</td><td>1.67</td><td>0.93</td></tr>
</table>

sented. One can notice that the difference between two errors grows with noise level, i.e., error value becomes higher when noise level increases, and differences can be more significant. Nevertheless, LL losses are very low if compared with compression rate and amount of noise. Actually, classification errors remain below 5%, even on experiments with 40% noise level. Moreover, error level seems to be lower in the reduced case than in the original one. Reasonably, HMMs with less states are able to generalize better, so as recognize also sequences with higher noise, even if we expect a breakdown point, causing a reversing behavior between original and reduced HMMs.

5.2   2D Shape Recognition

Object recognition, shape modeling, and classification are related issues in computer vision. A lot of three-dimensional (3-D) object recognition techniques are based on the analysis of two-dimensional (2-D) aspects (images) and several work can be found in literature on the analysis of 2-D shape or presenting methods devoted to planar object recognition.

A key issue is the kind of image feature used to describe an object, and its representation. Object contours are widely chosen as features, and their representation is basic to the design of shape analysis techniques. Different types of approaches have been proposed in the previous years, like, e.g., Fourier descriptors, chain code, curvature-based techniques, invariants, auto-regressive coefficients, Hough-based transforms, associative memories, and others, each one featured

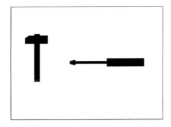

Fig. 6. Toy images for 2D shape recognition using Chain Code.

by different characteristics like robustness to noise and occlusions, invariance to translation, rotation and scale, computational requirements, and accuracy.

In this paper, HMMs are proposed as a tool for shape classification. This preliminary experiment aims at presenting a simple example on the capability of HMM on discriminating object classes, showing its robustness in terms of partial views and, in minor way, of noise. Shape is modeled using chain code, a well-known method to represent contours, which presents some inherent characteristic like the invariance to rotation (if code local differences are considered), and translation.

Although a large literature addresses these issues, the use of HMM for shape analysis has not been widely addressed. To our knowledge, only the work of He and Kundu [9] has been found to have some similarities with our approach. They utilize HMMs to model shape contours represented as auto-regressive (AR) coefficients. Results are quite interesting and presented in function of the number of HMM states ranging from 2 to 6. Moreover, shapes are constrained to be a closed contour.

In our experiment, although limited to a pair of similar objects, the degree of occlusion is quite large, and noise has been included to affect object coding, (without heavily degrading classification performances). Due to lack of space, we will not present results on rotational and scale invariance. Let us only state that scale is not a problem, as the HMM structure can manage it due to the possibility of permanence in the same state. Actually, simple tests on some differently scaled and noised objects have confirmed that HMMS behave correctly in this case. A detailed description of our approach with extensive experiments is not in the scope of this paper, and will be the subject of our future work. In this paper, we would only like to show the capabilities of the HMM to discriminate (also similar) shapes and its stable performances when the minimal structure is obtained by bisimulation with respect to the redundant topology.

In our experiment, given an image of 2D objects, data are gathered assigning at each object its chain code, calculated on object contours. Edges are extracted using *Canny edge detector* [23], while chain code is calculated as described in [24]. Fig. 6 shows the two simple objects, a stylized hammer and a screwdriver, used in the experiment. We train one HMM for each object, varying the number of states from 4 to 20. After applying bisimulation contraction, with reduction factor from 1 to 9, we re-trained HMMs with reduced number of states and compared

Table 3. Maximum compression rate, average and maximum Log Likelihood loss for 2D shape recognition test, at varying reduction factor.

Reduction factor	Maximum CR	Average LLL	Maximum LLL
1	16.74	4.91	72.20
3	9.43	0.55	29.39
5	6.33	2.30	72.26
7	6.40	1.72	72.85
9	4.71	1.28	68.73

them in term of Log Likelihood. Average and maximum Log Likelihood loss are calculated, and results are shown in Table 3, with maximum compression rate for different reduction factor values. Average LLL values are confortantly low: bisimulation does not seem to affect HMM characteristics. Nevertheless, we can also observe that average loss is very low compared with related maximum LLL. This is because compression is not so strong, as evident in Table 3, and therefore some learning session on reduced HMM can produce better results in terms of Log Likelihood. LL of an HMM on a sequence typically grows with N. On the other hand, LL depends on how well the training algorithm worked on the data. Baum-Welch re-estimation ensures to reach the nearest local optimum, without any information about global optimum. So, it is possible that for closed N_1, N_2, with $N_1 < N_2$, a HMM with N_1 states shows larger LL than those with N_2 states, because the training algorithm worked better. To partially solve the problem of convergence, each HMM was trained three times, starting with different random initial conditions. The case of so high LL loss may be explained by a low compression rate (the HMMs have the similar number of states) and very bad training (in this case three trials seems to be insufficient to ensure correct learning).

For testing classification accuracy, we synthetically create two test sets. The first set is obtained considering, for each object, fragments of their chain code of variable length, expressed as percentage rate of the whole length. It varies from 20 to 90 percent, and the point where fragment starts was randomly chosen. The second set is obtained by adding synthetic noise to the two chain codes, using a procedure similar to that used for DNA noising procedure. Each code is changed with fixed probability P, i.e. if cc_i is the original code, with probability P, $(((cc_i - 1) \pm 1) \bmod 8) + 1$ is carried out. Probability ranges from 0.05 to 0.35, and, for each value, 60 sequences are generated. As usual, a sequence is assigned to the class whose model shows the highest Log Likelihood, and error rate is estimated counting misclassified patterns. For each of the two test sets, we calculate performance using original and reduced HMMs and varying reduction factor from 1 to 9. In Table 4, average error for original and reduced HMMs on set of pieces are presented varying reduction factor from 1 to 9. We can see that the difference between two errors is very low.

The same results are presented in Table 5 for a set of noisy sequences, varying reduction factor (Table 5(a)) and noise level (Table 5(b)).

Table 4. Error on original and reduced HMMs for 2D shape recognition experiment (fragments set): (a) varying resolution factor; (b) varying fragment length.

(a)

Reduction factor	Error on Original (%)	Error on Reduced (%)
1	2.52	2.91
3	2.52	2.19
5	2.52	1.51
7	2.52	0.44
9	2.52	2.70

(b)

Fragment Length (%)	Error on Original (%)	Error on Reduced (%)
20 %	4.50	4.33
30 %	3.60	3.28
40 %	2.77	2.32
50 %	3.23	2.31
60 %	3.23	1.75
70 %	2.83	1.36
80 %	0.00	0.23
90 %	0.00	0.01

Table 5. Error on original and reduced HMMs for 2D shape recognition experiment (noised set): (a) varying resolution factor; (b) varying noise level (b).

(a)

Reduction factor	Error on Original (%)	Error on Reduced (%)
1	29.08	24.83
3	29.08	29.05
5	29.08	21.14
7	29.08	28.23
9	29.08	25.97

(b)

Noise level (%)	Error on Original (%)	Error on Reduced (%)
5	11.33	9.64
10	20.5	17.24
15	27.11	23.61
20	31.67	28.21
25	35.24	31.70
30	37.78	34.16
35	39.95	36.33

A consideration can be made on performance of HMMs applied to this problem: average error in recognizing the fragment sequence is 1.21%, a very low value. This means that a simple HMM can be invariant of some type of object occlusions. Nevertheless, noise seems to be a more serious problem, but working on topology and training algorithms classification accuracy may be less affected by this problem.

Another point regards the similarity of the two objects which may seriously affect performances. Using very different objects this problems may be attenuated. More extensive tests on invariance on scale and rotation should be carried out to better evaluate HMM performance for shape classification.

5.3   Comparison with Other Methods

Regarding the model selection approaches present in literature and listed in Section 1, an interesting comparative evaluation is presented in [25]. In that paper, a comparison between MDL/BIC, EBB and MDL for gaussian mixture model is reported, showing comparable performances and proving their superiority with respect to other methods. For convenience, we choose the BIC method [26] for our comparative analysis. BIC is a likelihood criterion penalized by the model complexity, i.e., in our case, the number of HMM states. Let $X = \{x_i, i = 1, \cdots, N\}$ be the data set we are modeling and $M = \{M_i, i = 1, \cdots, K\}$ be the candidate models. Let us denote as $|M_i|$ the number of parameters of the model M_i, and assuming to maximize the likelihood function $\mathcal{L}(X, M_i)$ for each possible model structure M_i, the BIC criterion is defined as:

$$BIC(M_i) = \log \mathcal{L}(X, M_i) - \frac{1}{2}|M_i| \log(N)$$

This strategy selects the model for which the BIC criterion is maximized.

We compare our strategy with this approach related to the 2D shape experiment. We train 18 HMMs, with states number varying from 3 to 20, and for each model we compute the BIC value. BIC vs number of states curves are plotted in Fig. 7, for the two objects. We then choose the HMM showing the highest

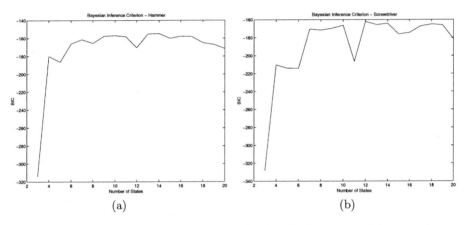

Fig. 7. BIC value vs number of states curves for the 2D shape recognition experiment with (a) the hammer and (b) the screwdriver.

BIC value (corresponding to 12 and 14 states, respectively for screwdriver and hammer).

With our bisimulation approach we train one HMM with 20 states, apply bisimulation and train another HMM with calculated number of states, varying reduction factor fro 1 to 9 (step 2). To compare the two methods we create a test set by adding synthetic noise (of various entity) to the two chain codes, in a way similar to that presented in the previous section, obtaining, for each noise level, 120 sequences to be classified. We then calculate the classification error applying the two approaches, presenting results in Table 6, in function of variable noise level. We can notice that, on the average, classification accuracy is quite similar: in fact BIC method needs 18 training session, while our method only two, plus the time for determining bisimulation contraction (that is $O(MKN \log N)$, given an HMM with N states, K edges and M symbols). In problems with a short

Table 6. Comparison between BIC method and our approach.

Method	States		Classification Error						
	Screw.	Hammer	Noise 0.05	Noise 0.10	Noise 0.15	Noise 0.20	Noise 0.25	Noise 0.30	Noise 0.35
BIC	12	14	13.33	25.00	32.50	36.88	39.83	41.81	42.98
Bisim RF 1	14	15	20.00	30.00	33.89	36.25	42.67	44.44	48.57
Bisim RF 3	15	16	21.67	34.17	39.44	42.08	43.67	44.72	45.48
Bisim RF 5	18	18	10.00	10.83	22.78	29.17	34.67	40.28	35.71
Bisim RF 7	17	19	28.33	38.33	42.22	44.17	45.33	46.11	46.67
Bisim RF 9	20	20	31.67	37.50	37.22	37.08	37.00	34.17	30.24

alphabet (as DNA modeling and chain code problems), our method is definitively faster than BIC, giving approximately the same classification accuracy.

6 Conclusions

In this paper, probabilistic bisimulation is used to estimate the minimal structure of a HMM. It has been shown that starting from a redundant configuration, bisimulation allows to merge equivalent states while preserving classification performances. Redundant and minimal HMM architectures have been tested on two different cases, DNA modeling and 2D shape classification, showing the usefulness of the approach. Moreover, our method has been compared with a classic model selection scheme, showing comparative performances but with a less computational complexity.

References

1. Rabiner, L.R.: A tutorial on Hidden Markov Models and Selected Applications in Speech Recognition. Proc. of IEEE **77(2)** (1989) 257–286.
2. Baum, L.E., Petrie, T.E, Soules, G., Weiss, N.: A maximization technique occurring in the statistical analysis of probabilistic functions of Markov chains. Annals of Math. Statistics. **41(1)** (1970) 164–171.
3. Baum, L.E.: An inequality and associated maximization technique in statistical estimation for probabilistic functions of Markov processes. Inequality **3** (1970) 1–8.
4. Veltman, S.R., Prasad, R.: Hidden Markov Models applied to on-line handwritten isolated character recognition. IEEE Trans. Image Proc., **3(3)** (1994) 314–318.
5. Churchill, G.A.: Hidden Markov Chains and the analysis of genome structure. Computers & Chemistry **16** (1992) 107–115.
6. Eickeler, S., Kosmala, A., Rigoll, G.: Hidden Markov Model based online gesture recognition. Proc. Int. Conf. on Pattern Recognition (ICPR) (1998) 1755–1757.
7. Jebara, T., Pentland, A.: Action Reaction Learning: Automatic Visual Analysis and Synthesis of interactive behavior. In 1st Intl. Conf. on Computer Vision Systems (ICVS'99) (1999).
8. Theodoridis, S., Koutroumbas, K.: Pattern recognition. Academic Press (1999).
9. He, Y., Kundu, A.: 2-D shape classification using Hidden Markov Model. IEEE Trans. Pattern Analysis Machine Intelligence. **13(11)** (1991) 1172–1184.

10. Figueiredo, M.A.T., Leitao, J.M.N., Jain, A.K.: On Fitting Mixture Models, in E. Hancock and M. Pellilo(Editors), Energy Minimization Methods in Computer Vision and Pattern Recognition, 54–69, Springer Verlag, 1999.

11. Stolcke, A., Omohundro, S.:Hidden Markov Model Induction by Bayesian Model Merging. Hanson, S.J., Cowan, J.D., Giles, C.L. eds. Advances in Neural Information Processing Systems **5** (1993) 11–18.

12. Brand, M.: An entropic estimator for structure discovery. Kearns, M.S., Solla, S.A., Cohn, D.A. eds. Advances in Neural Information Processing Systems **11** (1999).

13. Aczel, P.: Non-well-founded sets. Lecture Notes, Center for the Study of Language and Information **14** (1988).

14. Baier, C., Engelen, B., Majster-Cederbaum, M.: Deciding Bisimilarity and Similarity for Probabilistic Processes. J. Comp. and System Sciences **60** (1999) 187–231.

15. Dovier, A., Piazza, C., Policriti, A.: A Fast Bisimulation Algorithm. In proc. of *13th Conference on Computer Aided Verification, CAV'01*, 2001. Paris, France.

16. Kanellakis, P.C., Smolka, S.A.: CCS Expressions, Finite State Processes, and Three Problems of Equivalence. Information and Computation, **86(1)** (1990) 43–68.

17. Lisitsa, A., Sazanov, V.: Bounded Hyperset Theory and Web-like Data Bases. In 5th Kurt Gödel Colloquium. LNCS**1289** (1997) 172–185.

18. Milner, R.: Operational and Algebraic Semantics of Concurrent Processes. In J. van Leeuwen, editor, Handbook of Theoretical Computer Science (1990).

19. Paige, R., Tarjan, R. E.: Three Partition refinement algorithms. SIAM Journal on Computing **16(6)** (1987) 973–989.

20. Van Benthem, J.: Modal Correspondence Theory. PhD dissertation, Universiteit van Amsterdam, Instituut voor Logica en Grondslagenonderzoek van Exacte Wetenschappen, (1978) 1-148.

21. Salzberg, S.L.: Gene discovery in DNA sequences. IEEE Intelligent Systems **14(6)** (1999) 44–48.

22. Salzberg, S.L., Searls, D., Kasif, S.: Computational methods in Molecular Biology. Elsevier Science (1998).

23. Canny, J.F.: A computational approach to edge detection. IEEE Trans. Pattern Analysis Machine Intelligence **8(6)** (1986) 679–698.

24. Jain, R., Kasturi, R., Schunck, B.G.: Machine Vision. McGraw-Hill (1995).

25. Roberts, S., Husmeier, D., Rezek, I., Penny, W.: Bayesian Approaches to gaussian mixture modelling, IEEE Trans. on P.A.M.I., **20(11)** (1998) 1133–1142.

26. Schwarz, G.: Estimating the dimension of a model, The Annals of Statistics, **6(2)** (1978) 461–464.

Relaxing Symmetric Multiple Windows Stereo Using Markov Random Fields

Andrea Fusiello[1], Umberto Castellani[1], and Vittorio Murino[1]

Dipartimento di Informatica, Università di Verona
Strada le Grazie 15, 37134 Verona, Italy
{fusiello,castellani,murino}@sci.univr.it

Abstract. This paper introduces R-SMW, a new algorithm for stereo matching. The main aspect is the introduction of a Markov Random Field (MRF) model in the Symmetric Multiple Windows (SMW) stereo algorithm in order to obtain a non-deterministic relaxation. The SMW algorithm is an adaptive, multiple window scheme using left-right consistency to compute disparity. The MRF approach allows to combine in a single functional the disparity values coming from different windows, the left-right consistency constraint and regularization hypotheses. The optimal estimate of the disparity is obtained by minimizing an energy functional with simulated annealing. Results with both synthetic and real stereo pairs demonstrate the improvement over the original SMW algorithm, which was already proven to perform better than state-of-the-art algorithms.

1   Introduction

Three-dimensional (3D) reconstruction is a fundamental issue in Computer Vision, and in this context, structure from stereo algorithms play a major role. The process of stereo reconstruction aims at recovering the 3D scene structure from a pair of images by searching for *conjugate points*, i.e., points in the left and right images that are projections of the same scene point. The difference between the positions of conjugate points is called *disparity*.

Stereo is a well known issue in Computer Vision, to which many articles have been devoted (see [4] for a survey). In particular, the search for conjugate points in the two images is one of the main problem, and several techniques have been proposed to make this task more reliable. The search is based on a matching process that estimates the "similarity" of points in the two images on the basis of local or punctual information. Actually, feature-based methods try to associate image features (e.g., corners) in the image pair, whereas area-based methods try to find point correspondences by comparing local information. The main difference lies in the fact the the former approach produces a sparse (i.e., only in correspondence of features) disparity map, whereas, the latter generates a dense disparity image. In particular, the area-based matching process is typically based on a similarity measure computed between small windows in two images (left and

M.A.T. Figueiredo, J. Zerubia, A.K. Jain (Eds.): EMMCVPR 2001, LNCS 2134, pp. 91–104, 2001.

right). The match is normally found in a deterministic way, in correspondence of the highest similarity value.

In this paper, a novel probabilistic stereo method is proposed, which is based on the *Symmetric Multi-Window*(SMW) algorithm presented in [7, 8]. In this algorithm, matching is performed by correlation between different kinds of windows in the two images, and by enforcing the so-called *left-right consistency* constraint. This imposes the uniqueness of the conjugate pair, i.e., each point on one image can match at most one point on the other image. This algorithm is fully deterministic and exhibits good performances, as compared with the state of the art, namely [15, 23]. Still, there is margin for improvement (as our results show) by implementing a probabilistic SMW using Markov Random Fields (MRFs). To this end, SMW has been re-designed in a probabilistic framework by defining a random field evolving according to a suitable energy function.

Literature about MRFs is large and covers many topics of image processing, like restoration, segmentation, and image reconstruction considering both intensity (video) [3] and range images [1]. In addition, different approaches, closer in spirit to ours, were proposed aimed at integrating additional information in the MRF model, like, for instance, edges to guide the line extraction process [10], or confidence data to guide the the reconstruction of underwater acoustic images [19].

More specifically, MRFs are also frequently used in computer vision applications in the context of stereo or motion. For example, in [14] the motion vector is computed adopting a stochastic relaxation criterion, or, in [16], MRFs are used to detect occlusions in image sequences. Stereo disparity estimation methods using MRFs have been proposed in several papers. In [21], a stereo matching algorithm is presented as a regularized optimization problem. Only a simple correspondence between single pixels in the image pair is considered that leads to an acceptable photometric error, without exploiting local information for disparity estimation. In [17], matching is based on a fixed single correlation window, shifted along raster scan lines, and disparity is calculated by integrating gradient information in both left and right images. In this way, a mix between area- and feature-based matching is obtained, but occlusions are not managed by the algorithm. In [22], an MRF model was designed to take into account occlusions defining a specific dual field, so that they can be estimated in a similar way as in a classic *line process* similar to that presented in [12].

In our approach, for each pixel, different windows are (ideally) considered to estimate the Sum of Squared Differences (SSD) values and related disparities. When using area-based matching, the disparity is correct only if the area covered by the matching window has constant depth. The idea is that a window yielding a smaller SSD error is more likely to cover a constant depth region; in this way, the disparity profile itself drives the selection of an appropriate window.

The main contribution of this paper lies in the definition of a MRF model for a non-deterministic implementation of the SMW algorithm, in order to consider in a probabilistic way the contributions associated to the several windows, also introducing a local smoothness criterion. The initial disparity is computed for each window with SSD matching, then the *Winner-Take-All* approach of the SMW algorithm is relaxed by exploiting the MRF optimization.

The rest of the paper is organized as follow. In Section 2, the stereo process is described, and the MRF basic concepts are reported in Section 3. The actual MRF model is detailed in Section 4, and results are presented in Section 5. Finally, in Section 6, conclusions are drawn.

2   The Stereo Process

Many algorithms for disparity computation assume that conjugate pairs lie along raster lines. In general this is not true, therefore stereo pairs need to be *rectified* – after appropriate camera calibration – to achieve epipolar lines parallel and horizontal in each image [9].

A customary assumption, moreover, is that the image intensity of a 3D point is the same on the two images. If this is not true, the images must be *normalized*. This can be done by a simple algorithm [2] which computes the parameters of the gray-level transformation

$$I_l(x, y) = \alpha I_r(x, y) + \beta \qquad \forall (x, y)$$

by fitting a straight line to the plot of the left cumulative histogram versus the right cumulative histogram.

The matching process consist in finding the element (a point, region, or generic feature) in the right image which is most similar, according to a similarity metric, to a given element in the left image.

In the simple correlation stereo matching, similarity scores are computed, for each pixel in the left image, by comparing a fixed window centered on the pixel, with a window in the right image, shifting along the raster line. It is customary to use the Euclidean distance, or Sum of Squared Differences (SSD), as a (dis)similarity measure. The computed disparity is the one that minimizes the SSD error.

Even under simplified conditions, it appears that the choice of the window size is critical. A too small window is noise-sensitive, whereas an exceedingly large one acts as a low-pass filter, and is likely to miss depth discontinuities. This problem is addressed effectively – although not efficiently – by the Adaptive Window algorithm [15], and by the simplified version of the multiple window approach, introduced by [13, 11].

Several factors make the correspondence problem difficult. A major source of errors in computational stereo are occlusions, although they help the human visual system in detecting object boundaries. Occlusions create points that do not belong to any conjugate pairs (Figure 1). There are two key observations to address the occlusions issue: (i) matching is not a symmetric process. When searching for corresponding elements, only the visible points in the reference image (usually, the left image) are matched; (ii) in many real cases a disparity discontinuity in one image corresponds to an occlusion in the other image. Some

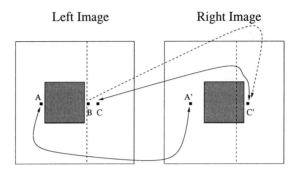

Fig. 1. Left-right consistency in the case of the random-dot stereogram of Figure 3. Point B is given C' as a match, but C' matches $C \neq B$.

authors [6, 5] use the observation (i) to validate matching (left-right consistency); others [11, 2] use (ii) to constrain the search space.

Recently, a new algorithm has been proposed [8] that computes disparity by exploiting both the multiple window approach and the left-right consistency constraint. For each pixel, SSD matching is performed with nine 7×7 windows with different centers: the disparity with the smallest SSD error value is retained.

The idea is that a window yielding a smaller SSD error is more likely to cover a constant depth region. Consider the case of a piecewise-constant surface: points within a window covering a surface discontinuity come from two different planes, therefore a single "average" disparity cannot be assigned to the whole window without making a manifest error. The multiple windows approach can be regarded as a robust technique able to fit a constant disparity model to data consisting of piecewise-constant surface, that is, capable of discriminate between two different populations. Occlusions are also detected, by checking the left-right consistency and suppressing unfeasible matches accordingly.

In this work we introduce a relaxation of the SMW algorithm using MRF. Both the multiple windows and the left-right consistency constraint features are kept but, in some sense, they are relaxed.

As for the multiple windows, one may note that correlation needs to be computed only once, because an off-centered window for a pixel is the on-centered window for another pixel. Therefore, the multiple windows technique used by the SMW reduces to assign a given pixel the disparity computed for one of its neighbors with an on-centered window, namely, the neighbour with the smallest SSD error. The nine 7×7 windows scheme gives forth to a sparse neighbourhood of nine pixels. The idea is to relax this scheme, and consider the pixel with the smallest SSD error in a full $n \times n$ neighbourhood (Figure 2).

As for the left-right consistency, we noticed that in presence of large amount of noise or figural distortion, the left-right consistency could fail for true conjugate pairs, and points could be wrongly marked as occluded. In this respect, it would be useful to relax the constraint, allowing for small errors.

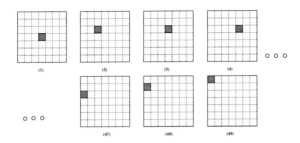

Fig. 2. The 49 asymmetric correlation windows for a 7×7 neighbourhood. The pixel for which disparity is computed is highlighted. The off-centered window for the highlighted pixel is the on-centered window for another pixel.

All these requests can be cast in terms of cost functions to be minimized over a disparity field, and this points strongly to Markov Random Fields.

3   Markov Random Fields

In this section will shall briefly review some basic concepts regarding MRF, in order to introduce our notation.

A MRF is defined on a finite lattice field I of elements i called sites (in our case, image pixels). Let us define a family of random variables $D=\{D_i= d_i, i \in I\}$, and let us suppose that each variable may assume values taken from a discrete and finite set (e.g., grey levels set). The image is interpreted as a realization of the discrete stochastic process in which pixel i is associated to a random variable D_i (being d_i its realization), and where, owing to the Markov property, the conditional probability $P\left(d_i \mid d_{I-\{i\}}\right)$ depends only on the value on the neighboring set of i, N_i (see [12]).

The Hammersley-Clifford theorem establishes the Markov-Gibbs equivalence between MRFs and Gibbs Random Fields [18], so the probability distribution takes the following form:

$$P\left(d\right) = Z^{-1} \cdot e^{-\beta \cdot U(d)} \tag{1}$$

where Z is a normalization factor called partition function, β is a parameter called temperature and $U(d)$ is the energy function, which can be written as a sum of local energy potentials dependent only on the cliques $c \in C$ (local configurations) relative to the neighboring system [12]:

$$U\left(d\right) = \sum_{c \in C} V_c\left(d\right) \tag{2}$$

In general, given the observation g, the posterior probability $P(d \mid g)$ can be derived from the Bayes rule by using the a-priori probability $P(d)$ and the conditional probability $P(g \mid d)$. The problem is solved computing the estimate d according to a Maximum A-Posteriori (MAP) probability criterion. Since the posterior probability is still of the Gibbs type, we have to minimize $U(d \mid g)$ $= U(g \mid d) + U(d)$, where $U(g \mid d)$ is the *observation model* and $U(d)$ is the *a-priori model* [12]. Minimization of the functional $U(d \mid g)$ is performed by a simulated annealing algorithm with Metropolis sampler [20][18].

When the MRF model is applied to image processing the observation model describes the noise that degrades the image and the a-priori model describes the a-priori information independent from the observations, like, for instance, the smoothness of the surfaces composing the scene objects.

4   Model Description

To deal with the stereo problem the scene is modeled as composed by a set of planes located at different distances to the observer, so that each disparity value corresponds to a plane in scene. Therefore, the a-priori model is piecewise constant [18]. The observation model is harder to define because the disparity map is not produced by a process for which a noise model can be devised.

Whilst the a-priori model imposes a smoothness constraint on the solution, the observation model should describe how the observations are used to produce the solution. In fact, it is the observation term that encodes the **multiple windows** heuristic. For each site, we take into account all the disparity values in the neighbourhood, favouring the ones with the smallest SSD.

First a disparity map is computed using the simple SSD matching algorithm outlined in Sec. 2, taking in turn the left and the right images as the reference one. This produces two disparity maps, which we will call left and right, respectively. The **left-right consistency** constraint is implemented by coupling the left disparity and the right disparity values.

In order to define the MRF model, we introduce two random fields D^l and D^r to estimate the left and the right disparity map, two random fields G^l and G^r to model the left and the right observed disparity map, and two random field S^l and S^r to model the SSD error. The field D^l (or equivalently D^r) will yield the output disparity.

In the following we shall describe the MRF functional, by defining the the a-priori model, the observation model, and the left-right consistency constraint term. In the next two subsections, will shall omit superscript l and r in the field variables. It is understood that the a-priori model and the observation model applies to both left and right fields.

4.1   A-priori Model

With the a-priori term we encode the hypothesis that the surfaces in the scene are locally flat. Indeed, we employ a piecewise constant model, defined as:

$$U(d) = \sum_{i \in I} \sum_{j \in N_i} [1 - \delta(d_i, d_j)] \qquad (3)$$

where d_i and d_j are the estimate disparities value (the realization of the field D) and the function $\delta(x,y)$ is defined as:

$$\delta(x,y) = \begin{cases} 1 & if \quad x = y \\ 0 & otherwise \end{cases} \tag{4}$$

This term introduces a regularization constraint, imposing that all pixels assume the same value in a region, thereby smoothing out isolated spikes.

4.2   Observation Model

In order to mimic the behaviour of the SMW algorithm, the observation model term introduces a local non-isotropic relaxation, favouring the neighbour observations with the lower SSD value:[1]

$$U(g, s \mid d) = \sum_{i \in I} \sum_{j \in N_i \cup \{i\}} [1 - \delta(d_i, g_j)] \cdot \left(\frac{1}{s_j}\right) \tag{5}$$

where g is the observation disparity map (the realization of the field G), s is the observed SSD values (the realization of the field S), and d is the disparity estimate (the realization of the field D). Following [18] the term $1 - \delta(x,y)$ represent a generalization of the sensor model for binary surface (derived by the binary symmetric channel theory).

In this term, the estimate value at site i, d_i, is compared with all its observed neighbours $\{g_j\}_{j \in N_i}$ and with g_i. When d_i takes the disparity of one (or more) of its neighbours, one (or more) term(s) in the sum vanishes. The lower is the SSD error of the chosen disparity, the higher is the cost reduction.

Please note that we are not relating the SSD value to the matching likelihood: the rationale behind this energy term is the multiple windows idea.

4.3   Left-Right Consistency Constraint Term

In our MRF model, besides an observation term and an a-priori term for both left and right disparity fields, we define a coupling term that settles the left-right constraint.

Let d_i^l be the left disparity (i.e., the disparity computed taking the left image as the reference) at site i, and d_i^r the right disparity at site i. The left-right consistency constraint states that:

$$d_i^l = -d_{i+d_i^l}^r. \tag{6}$$

The corresponding energy term is:

$$V(d^l, d^r) = \sum_{i \in I} \theta\left(d_i^l + d_{i+d_i^l}^r\right) \tag{7}$$

---

[1] Please note that SSD is an *error* measure, not a correlation or similarity measure.

where $\theta(x)$ is define as:

$$\theta(x) = \begin{cases} 0 & if \quad x = 0 \\ 1 & otherwise \end{cases} \tag{8}$$

In this way we introduces a payload when the left-right constraint is violated.

4.4 Final Model

The final MRF writes:

$$U\left(d_{i}^{l}, d^{r} \mid g_{i}^{l}, s_{i}^{l}, g_{i}^{r}, s^{r}\right) = k_{1} \cdot \left[U\left(g_{i}^{l}, s^{l} \mid d^{l}\right) + U\left(g_{i}^{r}, s^{r} \mid d^{r}\right)\right] +$$
$$+ k_{2} \cdot \left[U\left(d^{l}\right) + U\left(d^{r}\right)\right] +$$
$$+ k_{3} \cdot V\left(d_{i}^{l}, d^{r}\right) \tag{9}$$

where $U\left(g_{i}^{l}, s^{l} \mid d^{l}\right)$ and $U\left(g^{r}, s^{r} \mid d^{r}\right)$ are the observation model applied to the left and right disparity reconstruction, $U\left(d^{l}\right), U\left(d^{r}\right)$ are the a-priori models and $V\left(d_{i}^{l}, d^{r}\right)$ is the left-right constraint term. Please note that these terms are all weighted by the coefficients k_{1}, k_{2}, k_{3} heuristically chosen.

This model performs both simultaneously the left and right disparity reconstruction and the two estimates influence each other in a *cooperative* way. We call our algorithm Relaxed SMW (R-SMW).

5 Results

This section reports the main results of the experimental evaluation of our algorithm. Numerical and visual comparison with other algorithms are shown.

We first performed experiments on noise-free random-dot stereograms (RDS), shown in Figure 3. In the disparity maps, the gray level encodes the disparity, that is the depth (the brighter the closer). Images have been equalized to improve readability.

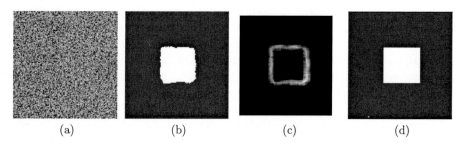

(a)   (b)   (c)   (d)

Fig. 3. Random-dot stereograms (RDS). The right image of stereogram (not shown here) is computed by warping the left one (a), which is a random texture, according to given disparity pattern: the square has disparity 10 pixel, the background 3 pixel. Disparity map computed with SSD matching (b), SSD values (c) and R-SMW disparity map.

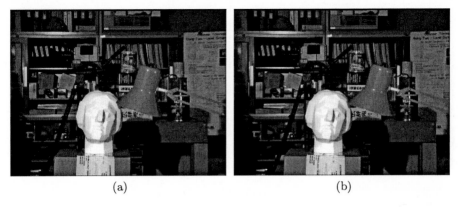

Fig. 4. "Head" stereo pairs from the Multiview Image Database, University of Tsukuba.

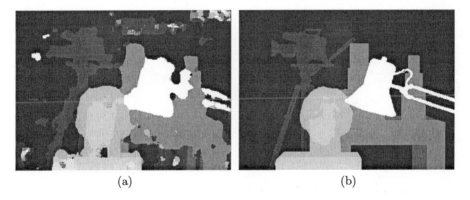

Fig. 5. R-SMW disparity map (a) and ground truth (b).

Figure 3.b shows a disparity map computed by SSD matching with 7×7 fixed window. The negative effect of disparity jumps (near the borders of the square patch) is clearly visible. Accordingly, Figure 3.c shows that along the borders the SSD error is higher. R-SMW yields the correct disparity map, shown in Figure 3.d. This replicates exactly the result obtained by SMW [7]. We expect to appreciate the improvement brought by the MRF when noise affects the images, like in the real cases.

As a real example, we used the "Head" stereo pair shown in Figure 4, for which the disparity ground truth is given. The output of R-SMW is reported in Figure 5. The error image (Figure 6.a) shows in black the pixels where the disparity is different from the ground truth. For the others, the disparity value is shown as a gray level (the brighter the closer).

The R-SMW algorithms outputs two optimal disparity maps, the left and the right. By checking the left-right consistency against these two maps, one can detect occluded points. Figure 6 shows the occlusions map. It is worth noting that most of the wrong pixels of Figure 6.a comes from occlusions.

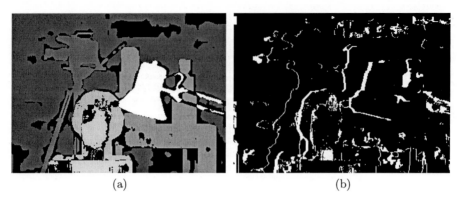

Fig. 6. Error map (a): the wrong pixels are black, the other take the right disparity value. Occlusions map (b).

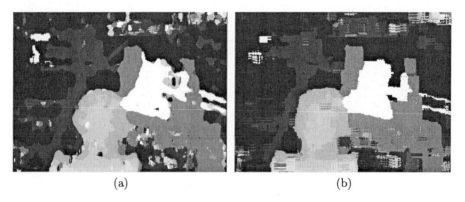

Fig. 7. Disparity map calculated by Zabih and Woodfill algorithm (a) and through SMW algorithm (b).

We compared R-SMW with SMW and our implementation of the Zabih and Woodfill algorithm (Figure 7). In the R-SMW result, the regions are more homogeneous and the edge are better defined. Moreover a lot of spurious points are cleared. Please note that there is a large wrong area, corresponding to a box on the shelf (top right). The ground truth disparity for that box is the same as the background, but all the stereo algorithms we tested agree in detecting a different disparity for the box. We suspect that the ground truth could be incorrect for that area.

For quantitative comparison, two error measures have been used: the Mean Absolute Error (MAE), i.e, the mean of absolute differences between estimated and ground true disparities, and the Percentage Error (PE), i.e., the percentage of pixel labeled with a wrong disparity. Table 1 reports the MAE and PE errors obtained on the "Head" stereo pair by SSD matching, Zabih and Woodfill algorithm, SMW, and by R-SMW. Results are ordered by decreasing errors: R-SMW exhibit the best performance, improving over the SMW. The Zabih and Woodfill

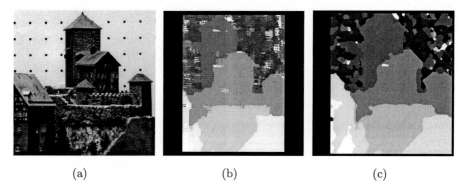

(a)   (b)   (c)

Fig. 8. "Castle" left image (a), SMW disparity (b), and R-SMW disparity (c).

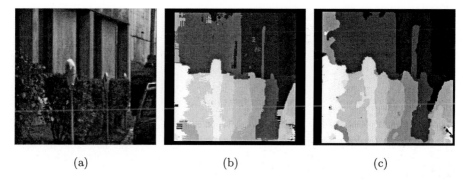

(a)   (b)   (c)

Fig. 9. "Parking meter" left image (a), SMW disparity (b), and R-SMW disparity (c).

algorithm is very fast (it reaches 30 frames per second on dedicated hardware), but results suggest that accuracy is not its best feature. We did not compared R-SMW with the Adaptive Windows (AW) algorithm by Okutomi and Kanade [15], but in [7] SMW was already proven to be more accurate than AW.

Table 1. Error values obtained by the different disparity reconstruction algorithm.

Algorithm	MAE	PE
SSD with fixed window	0.8569	30.73%
Zabih and Woodfill	0.8012	31.56%
SMW	0.6194	24.98%
R-SMW	0.5498	21.33%

We also report in Figures 8, 9, 10,and 12 the results of our algorithm on standard image pairs from the JISCT (JPL-INRIA-SRI-CMU-TELEOS) stereo test set, and from the CMU-CIL (Carnegie-Mellon University—Calibrated Imaging

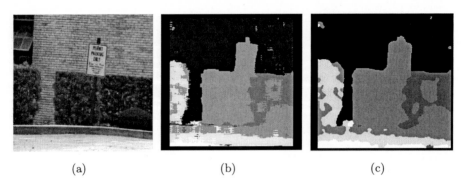

Fig. 10. "Shrub" left image (a), SMW disparity (b), and R-SMW disparity (c).

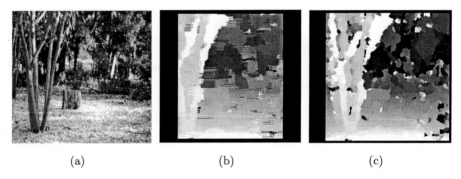

Fig. 11. "Trees" left image (a), SMW disparity (b), and R-SMW disparity (c).

Laboratory). Although a quantitative evaluation was not possible on this image, the quality of our results seems to improve over SMW, especially because spurious points and artifacts are smoothed out.

6   Conclusions

We have introduced a relaxation of the SMW algorithm by designing a Markov Random Field where both the multiple windows scheme and the left-right consistency are embedded. Moreover, a regularization constraint is introduced, as customary, to bias the solution toward piecewise constant disparities. Thanks to the MRF versatility, all these constraints are easily expressed in terms of energy, and the final solution benefits from the trade off between a-priori model and observations. Indeed, results showed that R-SMW performs better than state-of-the-art algorithms, namely SMW, Zabih and Woodfill and (indirectly) AW.

A sequential implementation of a MRF is computational intensive, of course: our algorithm took several minutes to converge to a solution, on the examples shown in the previous section. On the other hand, it reaches a high accuracy, and

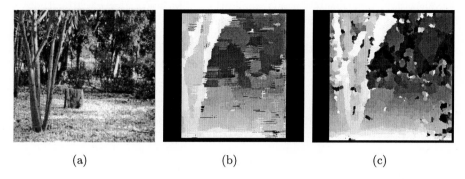

(a) (b) (c)

Fig. 12. "Trees" left image (a), SMW disparity (b), and R-SMW disparity (c).

in some applications (eg. model acquisition), one might want to trade accuracy for time.

A drawback of R-SMW is that coefficients in the energy functional need to be adjusted heuristically, and their value is fairly critical for the overall quality of the result. Work is in progress to implement a procedure for selecting the best coefficients automatically.

Acknowledgements

The authors thank Daniele Zini who wrote the implementation in C of the Zabih and Woodfill algorithm. The "Castle" images were provided by the Calibrated Imaging Laboratory at Carnegie Mellon University (CMU-CIL), supported by ARPA, NSF, and NASA. The "Head" images with ground truth, from the Multiview Image Database, are courtesy of Dr. Y. Otha, University of Tsukuba. Thanks to the anonymous referees who made useful comments.

References

1. G.S Nadabar A.K. Jain. Range image segmentation using MRF models. In A.K. Jain and R. Chellappa, editors, *Markov Random Fields Theory and Application*, pages 542–572. Academic Press, 1993.
2. I. J. Cox, S. Hingorani, B. M. Maggs, and S. B. Rao. A maximum likelihood stereo algorithm. *Computer Vision and Image Understanding*, 63(3):542–567, May 1996.
3. H. Derin and H. Elliot. Modeling and segmentation of noisy and textured images using Gibbs random fields. *IEEE Trans. on Pattern Analysis and Machine Intelligence*, 9(1):39–54, 1987.
4. U. R. Dhond and J. K. Aggarwal. Structure from stereo – a review. *IEEE Transactions on Systems, Man and Cybernetics*, 19(6):1489–1510, November/December 1989.
5. O. Faugeras, B. Hotz, H. Mathieu, T. Viéville, Z. Zhang, P. Fua, E. Théron, L. Moll, G. Berry, J. Vuillemin, P. Bertin, and C. Proy. Real-time correlation-based stereo:

algorithm, implementation and applications. Technical Report 2013, Unité de recherche INRIA Sophia-Antipolis, August 1993.

6. P. Fua. Combining stereo and monocular information to compute dense depth maps that preserve depth discontinuities. In *Proceedings of the International Joint Conference on Artificial Intelligence*, pages 1292–1298, Sydney, Australia, August 1991.

7. A. Fusiello, V. Roberto, and E. Trucco. Efficient stereo with multiple windowing. In *Proceedings of the IEEE Conference on Computer Vision and Pattern Recognition*, pages 858–863, Puerto Rico, June 1997. IEEE Computer Society Press.

8. A. Fusiello, V. Roberto, and E. Trucco. Symmetric stereo with multiple windowing. *International Journal of Pattern Recognition and Artificial Intelligence*, 14(8):1053–1066, December 2000.

9. A. Fusiello, E. Trucco, and A. Verri. A compact algorithm for rectification of stereo pairs. *Machine Vision and Applications*, 12(1):16–22, 2000.

10. E. Gamble and T. Poggio. Visual integration and detection of discontinuities: the key role of intensity edge. A.I. Memo 970, Massachusetts Institute of Technology, 1987.

11. D. Geiger, B. Ladendorf, and A. Yuille. Occlusions and binocular stereo. *International Journal of Computer Vision*, 14(3):211–226, April 1995.

12. S. Geman and D. Geman. Stochastic relaxation, Gibbs distribution, and Bayesian restoration of images. *IEEE Trans. on Pattern Analysis and Machine Intelligence*, 6(6):721–741, 1984.

13. S. S. Intille and A. F. Bobick. Disparity-space images and large occlusion stereo. In Jan-Olof Eklundh, editor, *European Conference on Computer Vision*, pages 179–186, Stockholm, Sweden, May 1994. Springer-Verlag.

14. J.Konrad and E.Dubois. Bayesian estimation of motion vector field. *IEEE Transactions on Pattern Analysis and Machine Intelligence*, 14(9):910–927, September 1992.

15. T. Kanade and M. Okutomi. A stereo matching algorithm with an adaptive window: Theory and experiments. *IEEE Transactions on Pattern Analysis and Machine Intelligence*, 16(9):920–932, September 1994.

16. A.Das K.P.Lim, M.N.Chong. A new MRF model for robust estimate of occlusion and motion vector fields. In *International Conference on Image Processing*, 1997.

17. K.G. Lim and R. Prager. Using Markov random field to integrate stereo modules. Technical report, Cambridge University Endineering Department, 1992. Available from http://svr-www.eng.cam.ac.uk/reports.

18. J. K. Marroquine. *Probabilistic Solution of Inverse Problem*. PhD thesis, Massachusetts Institute of Technology, 1985.

19. V. Murino, A. Trucco, and C.S. Regazzoni. A probabilistic approach to the coupled reconstruction and restoration of underwater acoustic images. *IEEE Transactions on Pattern Analysis and Machine Intelligence*, 20(1):9–22, January 1998.

20. C.D. Gellat Jr S. Kirkpatrik and M.P. Vecchi. Optimization by simulated annealing. *Science*, 220(4):671–680, 1983.

21. S.T.Barnard. Stereo matching. In A.K. Jain and R. Chellappa, editors, *Markov Random Fields Theory and Application*, pages 245–271. Academic Press, 1993.

22. W. Woo and A. Ortega. Stereo image compression with disparity compensation using the MRF model. In *Proceedings of Visual Communications and Image Processing (VCIP'96)*, 1996.

23. R. Zabih and J. Woodfill. Non-parametric local transform for computing visual correspondence. In *Proceedings of the European Conference on Computer Vision*, pages 151–158, Stockholm, 1994.

Matching Images to Models – Camera Calibration for 3-D Surface Reconstruction

Robin D. Morris, Vadim N. Smelyanskiy, and Peter C. Cheeseman

NASA Ames Research Center, MS269-2, Moffett Field, CA 94035, USA
{rdm,vadim,cheesem}@ptolemy.arc.nasa.gov

Abstract. In a previous paper we described a system which recursively recovers a super-resolved three dimensional surface model from a set of images of the surface. In that paper we assumed that the camera calibration for each image was known. In this paper we solve two problems. Firstly, if an estimate of the surface is already known, the problem is to calibrate a new image relative to the existing surface model. Secondly, if no surface estimate is available, the relative camera calibration between the images in the set must be estimated. This will allow an initial surface model to be estimated. Results of both types of estimation are given.

1 Introduction

In this paper we discuss the problem of camera calibration, estimating the position and orientation of the camera that recorded a particular image. This can be viewed as a parameter estimation problem, where the parameters are the camera position and orientation. We present two methods of camera calibration, based on two different views of the problem.

1. Using the entire image I, the parameters are estimated by minimizing $(I - \hat{I}(\Theta))^2$, where Θ are the camera parameters and $\hat{I}(\Theta)$ is the image simulated from the (known) surface model.
2. Using features extracted from the image, the parameters are estimated by minimizing $(u - \hat{u}(\Theta))^2$, where $\hat{u}(\Theta)$ is the position of the estimated feature projected into the image plane.

Under the assumption that a surface model is known, the first method has a number of advantages. It makes no assumptions about the size of the displacements between the images; it gives much more accurate estimation as many thousands of pixels are used to estimate a very few camera parameters; most fundamentally for our problem, it does not require feature extraction – images of natural scenes often do not have the sharp corner features required for standard approaches to camera calibration.

In an earlier paper [1] we described a system that inferred the parameters of a high resolution triangular mesh model of a surface from multiple images of that surface. It proceeded by a careful modeling of the image formation process, the process of *rendering*, and showed how the rendering process could be linearized

M.A.T. Figueiredo, J. Zerubia, A.K. Jain (Eds.): EMMCVPR 2001, LNCS 2134, pp. 105–117, 2001.
© Springer-Verlag Berlin Heidelberg 2001

with respect to the parameters of the mesh (in that case, the height and albedo values). This linearization turned the highly nonlinear optimization for the mesh parameters into the tractable solution of a very high dimensional set of sparse linear equations. These were solved using conjugate gradient, using iterative linearization about the estimate from the previous iteration.

The work in [1] required that the camera parameters (both internal and external) were known, and also assumed that the lighting parameters were known. In this paper we continue to assume that the internal parameters are known – NASA mission sensors are extensively calibrated before launch – and that the lighting parameters are known. Here we will describe how the linearization of the rendering process can be performed with respect to the camera parameters, and hence how the external camera parameters can be estimated by minimizing the error between the observed and synthesized images. We assume the usual pinhole camera model [10].

To estimate the camera parameters as described above requires that a surface model is already available. For the initial set of images of a new region, no surface model is available. In principle one could optimize simultaneously over both the surface parameters and the camera parameters. In practice, because the camera parameters are correlated with *all* the surface parameters, the sparseness of the set of equations is destroyed, and the joint solution becomes computationally infeasible. Instead, for the initial set of images we use the standard approach of feature matching, and minimize the sum squared error of the distance on the image plane of the observed feature and the projection of the estimated feature in 3D.

A surface can be inferred using the camera parameters estimated using feature matching. New images can then be calibrated relative to this surface estimate, and used in the recursive update procedure described in [1].

2   Calibration by Minimizing the Whole Image Error

Consider a surface where the geometry is modeled by a triangular mesh, and an albedo value is associated with each vertex of the mesh. A simulated camera produces an image $\hat{I}$ of the mesh. The camera is modeled as a simple pinhole camera, and its location and orientation is determined by six parameters, its location in space (x_c, y_c, z_c), the intersection of the camera axis with the $x - y$ plane, (x_0, y_0), and the rotation of the camera about the camera axis, ϕ. The last three of these parameters can be replaced by the three camera orientation angles, and we will use both representations in different places, depending on which is more convenient. These parameters are collected into a vector Θ.

For a given surface, given lighting parameters, and known internal camera parameters, the image rendered by the synthetic camera is a function of Θ, ie $\hat{I} = \hat{I}(\Theta)$. Making the usual assumption of independent Gaussian errors, and assuming a uniform prior on Θ, reduces the maximum likelihood estimation problem to a least-squares problem

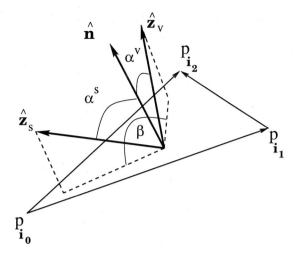

Fig. 1. Geometry of the triangular facet, illumination direction and viewing direction. $\hat{\mathbf{z}}_s$ is the vector to the illumination source; $\hat{\mathbf{z}}_v$ is the viewing direction

$$\hat{\Theta} = \min_{\Theta} \sum_p (I_p - \hat{I}_p(\Theta))^2 \tag{1}$$

where $\hat{\Theta}$ is the maximum-likelihood estimate of the camera parameters. Because $\hat{I}(\Theta)$ is in general a nonlinear function of Θ, to make this estimation practical we linearize $\hat{I}(\Theta)$ about the current estimate Θ_0

$$\hat{I}(\Theta) = \hat{I}(\Theta_0) + \mathbf{D}\mathbf{x}; \quad \mathbf{D} = \frac{\partial \hat{I}_p}{\partial \Theta_i} \tag{2}$$

where $\mathbf{D}$ is the matrix of derivatives evaluated at Θ_0, and $\mathbf{x} = \Theta - \Theta_0$. This reduces the least-squares problem in equation 1 to the minimization of a quadratic form, $F_2(\mathbf{x})$,

$$F_2(\mathbf{x}) = \frac{1}{2}\mathbf{x}\mathbf{D}\mathbf{D}^T\mathbf{x}^T - \mathbf{b}\mathbf{x} \tag{3}$$

$$\mathbf{b} = (I - \hat{I}(\Theta))\mathbf{D} \tag{4}$$

which can be solved using conjugate gradient or similar approaches. In the following section we will describe how an *object space* renderer can also be made to compute $\mathbf{D}$, the derivatives of the pixel values with respect to the camera parameters.

2.1   Forming the Image

As discussed in [1], to enable a renderer to also compute derivatives it is necessary that all computations are done in object space. This implies that the light from a surface triangle, as it is projected into a pixel, contributes to the brightness of that pixel with a weight proportional to the fraction of the area of the triangle which projects into that pixel. The total brightness of the pixel is thus the sum of the contributions from all the triangles whos projection overlaps with the pixel

$$\hat{I}_p = \sum_{\triangle} f_{\triangle}^p \, \Phi_{\triangle} \tag{5}$$

where $f_{\triangle}^p$ is the fraction of the flux that falls into pixel p, and $\Phi_{\triangle}$ is the total flux from the triangle. This is given by

$$\Phi_{\triangle} = \rho \, E(\alpha^s) \cos \alpha^v \cos^\kappa \theta \, \Delta\Omega, \tag{6}$$
$$E(\alpha^s) = \mathcal{A}\left(\mathcal{I}^s \cos \alpha^s + \mathcal{I}^a\right).$$
$$\Delta\Omega = S/d^2.$$

Here ρ is an average albedo of the triangular facet. Orientation angles α^s and α^v are defined in figure 1. $E(\alpha^s)$ is the total radiation flux incident on the triangular facet with area $\mathcal{A}$. This flux is modeled as a sum of two terms. The first term corresponds to direct radiation with intensity $\mathcal{I}^s$ from the light source at infinity (commonly the sun). The second term corresponds to ambient light with intensity $\mathcal{I}^a$. The parameter θ in equation (6) is the angle between the camera axis and the viewing direction (the vector from the surface to the camera); κ is the lens falloff factor. $\Delta\Omega$ in (6) is the solid angle subtended by the camera which is determined by the area of the lens S and the distance d from the centroid of the triangular facet to the camera. If shadows are present on the surface the situation is somewhat more complex. In this paper we assume that there are no shadows or occlusions present.

2.2   Computing Image Derivatives with Respect to Camera Parameters

Taking derivatives of the pixel intensities in equation 5 gives

$$\frac{\partial \hat{I}_p}{\partial \Theta_i} = \sum_{\triangle} \left(f_{\triangle}^p \frac{\partial \Phi_{\triangle}}{\partial \Theta_i} + \Phi_{\triangle} \frac{\partial f_{\triangle}^p}{\partial \Theta_i} \right) \tag{7}$$

Consider first $\partial \Phi_{\triangle}/\partial \Theta_i$. We neglect the derivatives with respect to the falloff angle, as their contribution will be small, and so it is clear from equation 6 that the derivative with respect to any of the camera orientation angles is zero. The derivative with respect to the camera position parameters is given by

$$\frac{\partial \Phi_{\triangle}}{\partial \Theta_i} \propto \frac{\partial}{\partial \Theta_i} \cos \alpha^v \tag{8}$$
$$= \frac{\hat{\mathbf{n}}}{v}(\hat{z}_i - \hat{z}_v(\hat{z}_v.\hat{z}_i))$$

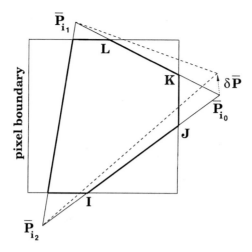

Fig. 2. The intersection of the projection of a triangular surface element (i_0, i_1, i_2) onto the pixel plane with the pixel boundaries. Bold lines corresponds to the edges of the polygon resulting from the intersection. Dashed lines correspond to the new positions of the triangle edges when point $\mathbf{P}_{i_0}$ is displaced by $\delta\mathbf{P}$

where $\mathbf{v}$ is the vector from the triangle to the camera, $v = |\mathbf{v}|$, Θ_i are the three components of the camera position, $\hat{z}_i$ are unit vectors in the three coordinate directions and $\hat{z}_v = \mathbf{v}/v$ (see figure 1).

Now consider $\partial f_\triangle^p / \partial \Theta_i$. For triangles that fall completely within a pixel, the second term in equation 7 is zero, as the derivative of the area fraction is zero. For triangles that intersect the pixel boundary, this derivative must be computed. When the camera parameters change, the positions of the projections of the mesh vertices into the image plane will also move. The derivative of the fractional area is given by

$$\frac{\partial f_\triangle^p}{\partial \Theta_i} = \frac{1}{\bar{A}_\triangle} \sum_{\mathbf{j}=\mathbf{i}_0,\mathbf{i}_1,\mathbf{i}_2} \left(\frac{\partial \bar{A}_{\text{polygon}}}{\partial \bar{\mathbf{P}}_\mathbf{j}} - f_\triangle^p \frac{\partial \bar{A}_\triangle}{\partial \bar{\mathbf{P}}_\mathbf{j}} \right) \frac{\partial \bar{\mathbf{P}}_\mathbf{j}}{\partial \Theta_i}. \tag{9}$$

where $\bar{\mathbf{P}}_\mathbf{j}$ is the projection of point $\mathbf{P}_\mathbf{j}$ onto the image plane, and $\bar{A}_\triangle$ is the area of the projection of the triangle. The point displacement derivatives will be detailed below.

Thus, the task of computing the derivative of the area fraction (9) is reduced to the computation of $\partial \bar{A}_\triangle / \partial \bar{\mathbf{P}}_\mathbf{j}$ and $\partial \bar{A}_{\text{polygon}} / \partial \bar{\mathbf{P}}_\mathbf{j}$. Note that the intersection of a triangle and a pixel for a rectangular pixel boundary can, in general, be a polygon with 3 to 7 edges with various possible forms. However the algorithm for computing the polygon area derivatives that we have developed is general, and does not depend on a particular polygon configuration. The main idea of the algorithm can be described as follows. Consider, as an example, the polygon shown in figure 2 which is a part of the projected surface triangle with indices $\mathbf{i}_0, \mathbf{i}_1, \mathbf{i}_2$. We are interested in the derivative of the polygon area with respect to

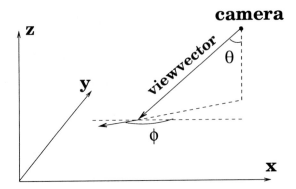

Fig. 3. Illustration of the geometry for determining the rotation between world and camera coordinates

the point $\bar{\mathbf{P}}_{i_0}$ that connects two edges of the projected triangle, $(\mathbf{P}_{i_2}, \mathbf{P}_{i_0})$ and $(\mathbf{P}_{i_0}, \mathbf{P}_{i_1})$. These triangular edges contain segments $(\mathbf{I}, \mathbf{J})$ and $(\mathbf{K}, \mathbf{L})$ that are sides of the corresponding polygon. It can be seen from figure 2 that when the point $\bar{\mathbf{P}}_{i_0}$ is displaced by $\delta\bar{\mathbf{P}}_{i_0}$ the change in the polygon area is given by the sum of two terms

$$\delta\bar{A}_{\text{polygon}} = \delta A_{\mathbf{I},\mathbf{J}} + \delta A_{\mathbf{K},\mathbf{L}}$$

These terms are equal to the areas spanned by the two corresponding segments taken with appropriate signs. Therefore the polygon area derivative with respect to the triangle vertex $\bar{\mathbf{P}}_{i_0}$ is represented as a sum of the two "segment area" derivatives for the 2 segments adjacent to a given vertex. The details of this computation will be given elsewhere.

We now consider the derivatives of the point positions.

Derivatives of the Position of the Projection of a Point on the Image Plane. The pinhole camera model gives

$$\hat{u}_l = \frac{[\mathbf{A}\mathbf{R}(\mathbf{P} - \mathbf{t})]_l}{[\mathbf{R}(\mathbf{P} - \mathbf{t})]_3} \tag{10}$$

where $\mathbf{R}$ is the rotation matrix from world to camera coordinates, $\mathbf{t}$ is the translation of between camera and world coordinates and $\mathbf{A}$ is the matrix of camera internal parameters [13]. In the numerical experiments presented here we assume that the internal camera parameters are known, and further that the image plane axes are perpendicular, and that the principle point is at the origin. This reduces $\mathbf{A}$ to a diagonal matrix with elements $(k_1, k_2, 1)$, where $k_1 = -\mathrm{f}/l_x$, $k_2 = -\mathrm{f}/l_y$. Where f is the focal length of the lens and l_x and l_y are the dimensions of the pixels in the retinal plane.

The rotation matrix $\mathbf{R}$ can be written in terms of the *Rodrigues* vector [10] $\varrho = (\varrho_1, \varrho_2, \varrho_3)$ which defines the axis of rotation, and $\theta = |\varrho|$ is the magnitude of the rotation. (Clearly ϱ can be written in terms of the camera position, the look-at point and the view-up vector.)

$$\mathbf{R} = \mathbf{I} - \mathcal{H}\frac{\sin\theta}{\theta} + \mathcal{H}^2\frac{(1 - \cos\theta)}{\theta^2} \tag{11}$$

where

$$\mathcal{H} = \begin{pmatrix} 0 & -\varrho_3 & \varrho_2 \\ \varrho_3 & 0 & -\varrho_1 \\ -\varrho_2 & \varrho_1 & 0 \end{pmatrix}. \tag{12}$$

Let $H = \mathcal{H}/\theta$ and $r_i = r_i/\theta$ then

$$\frac{\partial \mathbf{R}}{\partial \varrho_i} = -\mathcal{H}_i\frac{\sin\theta}{\theta} + (H\mathcal{H}_i + \mathcal{H}_i H)\frac{(1 - \cos\theta)}{\theta} - H\left(\cos\theta - \frac{\sin\theta}{\theta}\right)r_i \tag{13}$$
$$+ H^2\left(\sin\theta - 2\frac{1 - \cos\theta}{\theta}\right)r_i$$

where $\mathcal{H}_i = \partial\mathcal{H}/\partial\varrho_i$. Then

$$\frac{\partial \hat{u}_l}{\partial \varrho_i} = \left(\frac{\left[\mathbf{A}\frac{\partial \mathbf{R}}{\partial \varrho_i}(\mathbf{P} - \mathbf{t})\right]_l}{[\mathbf{R}(\mathbf{P} - \mathbf{t})]_3} - \frac{[\mathbf{AR}(\mathbf{P} - \mathbf{t})]_l\left[\frac{\partial \mathbf{R}}{\partial \varrho_i}(\mathbf{P} - \mathbf{t})\right]_3}{([\mathbf{R}(\mathbf{P} - \mathbf{t})]_3)^2}\right) \tag{14}$$

The derivatives with respect to the position parameters are

$$\frac{\partial \hat{u}_l}{\partial t_j} = \frac{[\mathbf{AR}(\mathbf{P} - \mathbf{t})]_l[\mathbf{R}]_{3,j}}{([\mathbf{R}(\mathbf{P} - \mathbf{t})]_3)^2} - \frac{[\mathbf{AR}]_{l,j}}{[\mathbf{R}(\mathbf{P} - \mathbf{t})]_3} \tag{15}$$

In practice, optimization using the camera orientation angles directly is inadvisable, as a small change in the angle can move the surface a long distance in the image, and because the minimization in equation 1 is based on a sum over all pixels in the image, this can make for rapid changes in the cost, and failure to converge. Instead we use the "look-at" point (x_0, y_0) which is in the natural length units of the problem. The conversion of the derivatives from angles to look-at is an application of the chain rule, and is not detailed here.

We now consider the second problem, calibration using features detected in the images.

3   Calibration by Minimizing Feature Matching Error

It is well known that camera calibration can be performed using corresponding features in two or more images [4]. This estimation procedure also returns the 3D positions of the corresponding image features. So the parameter space is augmented from Θ^f (where f indexes the frame, or camera parameter set) with $\mathbf{P}_n$, the positions of the 3D points.

If it is assumed that the error between $\mathbf{u}_n^f$, the feature located in image f corresponding to 3D point $\mathbf{P}_n$, and $\hat{\mathbf{u}}_n^f$, the projection of $\mathbf{P}_n$ into image f using camera parameters Θ^f, is normally distributed, then the negative log-likelihood for estimating Θ and $\mathbf{P}$ is

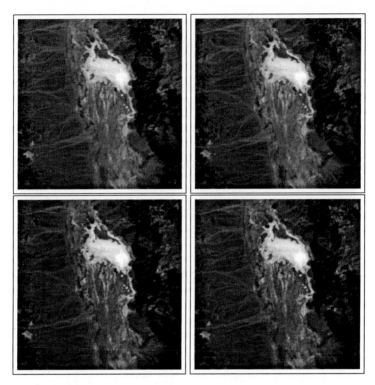

Fig. 4. Four synthetic images of an area of Death Valley

$$L(\Theta, \mathbf{P}) = \sum_{f=1}^{K} \sum_{n \in \Omega_f} \sum_{l=1}^{2} (u_{l,n}^{f} - \hat{u}_{l,n}^{f})^2 \tag{16}$$

$$\mathbf{P} = \{\mathbf{P}_n; \, n = 1 \ldots N\} \tag{17}$$

$$\Theta = \{\Theta_i^f : i = 1 \ldots 6; \quad f = 1 \ldots K\} \tag{18}$$

where Ω_f is the set of features that are detected in image f. Note that the features detected in a given image may well be a subset of all the $\mathbf{P}_n$'s. l indexes the components of $\mathbf{u}$. This form of the likelihood assumes that there is no error in the location of the features in the images.

Typically the non-linear likelihood in equation 18 is minimized using a standard non-linear minimization routine, for example the Levenberg-Marquardt algorithm [11]. The dimensionality of the parameter space in equation 18 is large, equal to 6× (the number of images -1) + 3× the number of 3D points -1, where the parameters of the reference camera are not included, and the overall spatial scale is arbitrary. In general there will be many points, because of this large dimensionality it is important to use exact derivatives, to avoid slow convergence and reduce the need for good initialization. In section 3.2 below we derive the analytic derivatives of the likelihood function, enabling this robust convergence.

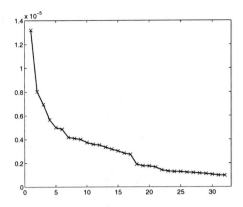

Fig. 5. "Strength" of the features found in image 0

The other practical problem in using feature-based camera calibration is the detection and matching of image features.

3.1   Robust Feature Matching

The maximum likelihood solution to the camera parameter estimation problem is known to be *extremely* sensitive both to mismatches in the feature correspondences, and to even small errors in the localization of the detected features. To reliably estimate the camera parameters we need *reliably located features, reliably matched.* More accurate estimation results from using a smaller set of well localized and well matched features, than a much larger set that includes even a single outlier. Extreme conservatism in both feature detection and matching is needed.

The feature detector most commonly used is the Harris corner detector [2]. This feature detector was developed in the context of images of man-made environments, which contain many strong corners. Remote sensed images of natural scenes of the type we are concerned with (see figure 4) contain some, but much fewer, strong corner features. If the "feature strength" given by the Harris detector is plotted for the features detected on the images in figure 4, it can be seen to fall off rapidly – see figure 5. For this type of image, it is therefore necessary to use only a small number of features, where the associated feature strength is high enough to ensure accurate feature localization. This is a limiting factor in the use of feature based calibration for this type of images, and a motivation for developing the whole image approach described above. Feature detectors more suited to natural scenes are clearly needed, but there will always be particularly mute environments where feature based methods will fail.

Because of the extreme sensitivity to mismatches, it it necessary to ensure that the features found are matched reliably. This is a classic chicken-and-egg problem: to determine reliable matches it is necessary to correctly estimate the camera parameters, and to correctly estimate the camera parameters requires reliable matches. For this reason, feature matching has spawned a number of methods based on *robust estimation* (and one approach which attempts to do away with explicit feature matching altogether [12]).

The RANSAC algorithm [3] finds the largest set of points consistent with a solution based on a minimal set, repeatedly generating trial minimal sets until the concensus set is large enough. Zhang [4] also bases his algorithm on estimation using minimal sets, but uses LMedS (Least Median Squares) to select the optimal minimal set. The estimate of the fundamental matrix [10] generated using that minimal set is used to reject outliers. Zhang also applies a relaxation scheme to disambiguate potential matches. This is a formalization of the heuristic that features nearby in one image are likely be close together in another image, and in the same relative orientation. In our work we use a modification of Zhang's algorithm described below. Torr and co-workers have developed MLESAC [7] and IMPSAC [6] as improvements on RANSAC. IMPSAC uses a multiresolution framework, and propagates the probability density of the camera parameters between levels using importance sampling. This achieves excellent results, but was considered excessive for our application, where prior knowledge of the types of camera motion between frames is known.

Our algorithm proceeds as follows:

1. Use the Harris corner detector to identify features, rejecting those which have feature strength too low to be considered reliable.
2. Generate potential matches using the normalized correlation score between windows centered at each feature point. Use a high threshold (we use $t = 0.9$) to limit the number of incorrect matches.
3. Use LMedS to obtain a robust estimate of the fundamental matrix:
   - Generate an 8 point subsample from the set of potential matches, where the 8 points are selected to be widely dispersed in the image (see [4]).
   - Estimate the fundamental matrix. Zhang uses a nonlinear optimization based approach. We have found that the simple eight point algorithm [9] is suitable, because our features are in image plane coordinates, which correspond closely to the normalization suggested in [8].
   - Compute the residuals, $\mathbf{u}^T \mathbf{F} \mathbf{u}$ for all the potential matches, and store the *median* residual value.
   - Repeat for a new subsample. The number of subsamples required to ensure with a sufficiently high probability that a subset with no outliers has been generated depends on the number of features and the estimated probability that each potential match is an outlier.
   - Identify $\mathbf{F}_{min}$ as the fundamental matrix which resulted in the lowest median residual value.
4. Use $\mathbf{F}_{min}$ to reject outliers by eliminating matches which have residuals greater than a threshold value. (We used $t_{min} = 1.0$ pixels.)
5. Use the following heuristic to eliminate any remaining outliers: because the images are remote sensed images, the variations in heights on the surface are small in comparison to the distance to the camera. So points on the

surface that are close together should move similar amounts, and in similar directions[1]. The heuristic is

- Consider all features within a radius $r = 0.2$ of the image size from the current feature. The match found for that feature is accepted if both of the following conditions hold:
  - (a) The length of the vector between the features is less than a threshold times the length of the largest vector between features in the neighbourhood.
  - (b) The average distance between neighbouring features in one image is less than a threshold times the average distance between the same features in th second image.

  In both cases the threshold used was 1.3.

Features are matches between all pairs of images in the set, and are used in the likelihood minimization (18) to estimate the camera parameters. Note that not all features will be detected in all the images in a set, so the likelihood will only contain terms for the features actually found in that image.

3.2   Computing Derivatives of the Feature Positions

To effectively minimize $L(\Theta, \mathbf{P})$ in equation 18 we need to compute its derivatives, which reduces to computing $\frac{\partial \hat{u}_{l,n}^f}{\partial \Theta_i^f}$ and $\frac{\partial \hat{u}_{l,n}^f}{\partial \mathbf{P}_n}$. In what follows we will concentrate on one frame and drop the f index.

We have already shown in equation 14 the expression for the derivative of the point position with respect to the rotation angles and camera position, which together make up $\frac{\partial \hat{u}_{l,n}^f}{\partial \Theta_i^f}$. It remains only to give the expression for the derivative with respect to the 3D feature point. This is the same as the derivative with respect to the camera position, see equation 15, but with the sign reversed, giving

$$\frac{\partial \hat{u}_{l,n}}{\partial \mathbf{P}_{n,j}} = -\frac{[\mathbf{AR}(\mathbf{P}_n - \mathbf{t})]_l [\mathbf{R}]_{3,j}}{([\mathbf{R}(\mathbf{P}_n - \mathbf{t})]_3)^2} + \frac{[\mathbf{AR}]_{l,j}}{[\mathbf{R}(\mathbf{P}_n - \mathbf{t})]_3} \tag{19}$$

Where the subscript n indexes the features.

4   Results and Conclusions

Figure 4 shows four synthetic images of Death Valley. The images were generated by rendering a surface model from four different viewpoints and with different lighting parameters. The surface model was generated by using the USGS Digital Elevation Model of the area for the heights, and using scaled intensities of a LANDSAT image as surrogate albedos. The size of the surface was approximately

---

[1] This is not true if the camera moves towards the surface, but even then, if the movement towards the surface is not excessive, this heuristic still approximately holds.

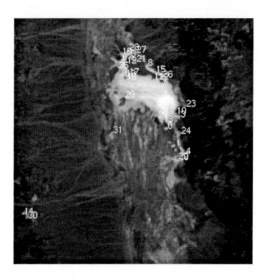

Fig. 6. Features found in image 0

350×350 points, and the distance between grid points was taken as 1 unit. The images look extremely realistic.

Table 1 shows the results of estimating the camera parameters using features detected in the images. These estimates are good, but far from exact. Considering the images in figure 4, it is clear that there are few strong corner features. Figure 6 shows the set of strong features detected in image 0 (the top left image in figure 4). Two things are apparent. Firstly, the features are all due to rapid changes in albedo. Secondly, with two exceptions, the features are clustered. This clustering reduces the accuracy of the estimation. That the features are mostly albedo features confirms that feature based approaches are not applicable to many of the types of image we are interested in.

Table 1 also shows the results for calibration using matching to a pre-existing 3D surface model. The estimation was initialized at the results of the point-matching estimation. The minimization of $(I - \hat{I}(\Theta))^2$ was performed iteratively, re-rendering to compute a new $\hat{I}$ at the value of Θ at the convergence of the previous minimization. As expected, the estimates are very significantly better than the results from point matching, and are very accurate. However, these results are predicated on the existence of a surface model.

These results suggest an approach to camera calibration that is the subject of our current, ongoing, research. Point matching can be used to estimate initial camera parameters, and a very sparse surface representation. A dense surface (shape and albedo) can then be inferred using these camera parameters (see [1]). The whole-image matching approach can be used to re-estimate the camera parameters, and a new surface estimate can be made using the new camera parameter estimates. This process can be iterated. The convergence of this iterative procedure is currently being studied.

Table 1. Results for camera parameter inference. Image 0 was the reference image with parameters camera – $(-300, 1416, 4000)$, look at – $(205, 1416, 0)$ and view up – $(0, 1, 0)$

		true	point-match estimate	whole-image estimate
image 1	camera	$(700, 1416, 4000)$	$(610, 1410, 4030)$	$(685, 1409, 4001)$
	look at	$(205, 1416, 0)$	$205, 1420, 0)$	$(205, 1416, 0)$
	view up	$(0, 1, 0)$	$(-0.005, 1, 0, 002)$	$(0, 1.0, 0.002)$
image 2	camera	$(200, 900, 4000)$	$(200, 968, 4050)$	$(203, 894, 3996)$
	look at	$(205, 1416, 0)$	$(206, 1410, 0)$	$(205, 1416, 0)$
	view up	$(0, 1, 0)$	$(-0.015, 0.994, 0.11)$	$(0, 0.993, 0.129)$
image 3	camera	$(200, 1900, 4000)$	$(176, 1780, 4030)$	$(196, 1881, 4001)$
	look at	$(205, 1416, 0)$	$(206, 1420, 0)$	$(205, 1416, 0)$
	view up	$(0, 1, 0)$	$(-0.007, 0.996, -0.090)$	$(0, 0.993, -0.116)$

References

1. Smelyanskiy, V.N., Cheeseman, P., Maluf, D.A. and Morris, R.D.: Bayesian Super-Resolved Surface Reconstruction from Images. Proceedings of the International Conference on Computer Vision and Pattern Recognition, Hilton Head, 2000
2. Harris, C.: A Combined Corner and Edge Detector. Proceedings of the Alvey Vision Conference, pp 189-192, 1987
3. Fischler, M.A. and Bolles, R.C.: Random Sample Concensus: A Paradigm for Model Fitting with Applications to Image Analysis and Automated Cartography. Communications of the ACM, June 1981, vol. 24, no. 6, pp 381-395
4. Zhang, Z., Deriche, R., Faugeras, O. and Luong, Q.T.: A Robust Technique for Matching Two Uncalibrated Images Through the Recovery of the Unknown Epipolar Geometry. AI Journal, vol. 78, pp 87-119, 1994
5. Rousseeuw, P.J.: Robust Regression and Outlier Detection. Wiley, New York, 1987
6. Torr, P.H.S. and Davidson, C.: IMPSAC: Synthesis of Importance Sampling and Random Sample Consensus. Technical Report, Microsoft Research, Cambridge, UK
7. Torr, P.H.S. and Zisserman, A.: MLESAC: A New Robust Estimator with Application to Estimating Image Geometry. Computer Vision and Image Understanding, vol 1, pp 138-156, 2000
8. Hartley, R.I.: In Defense of the Eight Point Algorithm IEEE Transactions on Pattern Aalysis and Machine Intelligence, vol 19, pp 580-594, June 1997
9. Longuet-Higgins, H.C.: A Computer Algorithm for Reconstructing a Scene from Two Projections. Nature, vol 293, pp 133-135, 1981
10. Faugeras, O.: Three-Dimensional Computer Vision MIT Press, 1993
11. More, J.: The Levenberg-Marquardt Algorithm, Implementation and Theory. In G. A. Watson, editor, Numerical Analysis, Lecture Notes in Mathematics 630. Springer-Verlag, 1977.
12. Dellaert, F., Seitz, S.M., Thorpe, C.E., and Thrun, S.: Structure from Motion Without Correspondences. Proceedings of the International Conference on Computer Vision and Pattern Recognition, Hilton Head, 2000
13. Zhang, Z.: A Flexible New Technique for Camera Calibration. Technical Report MSR-TR-98-71, Microsoft Research, Redmond, Washington

A Hierarchical Markov Random Field Model for Figure-Ground Segregation

Stella X. Yu[1,3], Tai Sing Lee[2,3], and Takeo Kanade[1,2]

[1] Robotics Institute
[2] Department of Computer Science
Carnegie Mellon University
[3] Center for the Neural Basis of Cognition
5000 Forbes Ave, Pittsburgh, PA 15213-3890
{stella.yu,tai,tk}@cs.cmu.edu

Abstract. To segregate overlapping objects into depth layers requires the integration of local occlusion cues distributed over the entire image into a global percept. We propose to model this process using hierarchical Markov random field (HMRF), and suggest a broader view that clique potentials in MRF models can be used to encode any local decision rules. A topology-dependent multiscale hierarchy is used to introduce long range interaction. The operations within each level are identical across the hierarchy. The clique parameters that encode the relative importance of these decision rules are estimated using an optimization technique called learning from rehearsals based on 2-object training samples. We find that this model generalizes successfully to 5-object test images, and that depth segregation can be completed within two traversals across the hierarchy. This computational framework therefore provides an interesting platform for us to investigate the interaction of local decision rules and global representations, as well as to reason about the rationales underlying some of recent psychological and neurophysiological findings related to figure-ground segregation.

1 Introduction

Figure-ground organization is a central problem in perception and cognition. It consists of two major processes: (1) depth segregation - the segmentation and ordering of surfaces in depth and assignment of *border ownerships* to relatively more proximal objects in a scene [15, 26, 27]; (2) figural selection - the extraction and selection of a figure among a number of 'distractors' in the scene. Evidence of both of these processes have been found in the early visual cortex [17, 19, 20, 36].

In computer vision, figure-ground segregation is closely related to image segmentation and has been studied from both contour processing and region processing perspectives. Contour approaches perform contour completion based on good curve continuation [11, 12, 24, 32, 33], whereas region approaches perform image partitioning based on surface properties [28, 30, 37, 39].

M.A.T. Figueiredo, J. Zerubia, A.K. Jain (Eds.): EMMCVPR 2001, LNCS 2134, pp. 118–133, 2001.

Here, we focus on the issue of global depth segregation based on sparse occlusion cues arisen from closed boundaries. The importance of local occlusion cues in determining global depth perception can be appreciated in our remarkable ability in inferring relative depths among objects in cartoon drawings (Fig. 1a). These sparse occlusion cues provide important constraints for the emergent global perception of figure and ground. The formation of global percepts from such local cues and the computation of layer organizations have been modeled as an optimization process with a surface diffusion mechanism [8, 9, 22].

In this paper, we extend these earlier works [8, 9, 22] by embedding explicit decision rules for contour continuation and surface depth propagation in local units of a Hierarchical Markov random field model. The multiscale hierarchy is sensitive to the topology of image structures and is used to facilitate rapid long range propagation of local cues. We also develop a parameter learning method using linear programming to estimate the parameters that encode the relative importance of those decision rules. Results show that parameters learned on a few two-object training samples can generalize successfully to multiple-object images.

The rest of the paper is organized as follows. Section 2 describes the problem and expands our method in detail. Section 3 shows our results on a new test image. Section 4 concludes the paper with a discussion.

2   Methods

2.1   Problem Formulation

For simplicity, we take an edge map (Fig. 1b) with complete and closed contours of rectangular shapes as input to our system. These shapes can overlap and occlude one another. The occluded part of an object is not visible. The system is to produce two complementary maps as output (Fig. 1f): a pixel depth map (Fig. 1d) where a higher depth value is assigned to pixel depth units of a more proximal surface and a lower value to pixel units of a more distant surface; and an edge depth map in which the edge depth units at the border of a more proximal surface assume a higher value. The edge depth units assume the same depth value as the pixel depth units of the surface to which they belong (Fig. 1e). These two representations are sufficient to specify the depth ordering sequence of objects in the scene.

In general, it is not possible to recover the exact depth ordering or overlap sequence in the scene since the solution is not unique. For example, there can be multiple choices when objects do not occlude each other directly (object 1 and 2 in Fig. 1b) and when we cannot tell which object is occluding which (object 3 and 4 in Fig. 1b). If we represent visible pairwise object occlusion relationships in a directed graph (Fig. 1c), these two cases correspond to the existence of unconnected siblings of the same parent. Instead of recovering the overlap sequence, we can sort object depths into layers, ordered by occlusion. This problem is called the 2.1D sketch in [28]. If there is a directed cycle in the graph, then the depth cannot be segregated into layers. We define the depth

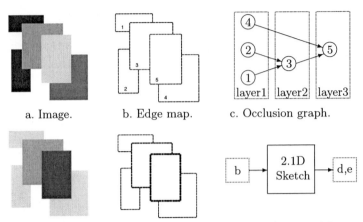

a. Image.   b. Edge map.   c. Occlusion graph.

d. Pixel depth label. e. Edge depth label.   f. Goal of our model.

Fig. 1. Segregate depth into layers. Rectangular objects are numbered in b. Darker object surfaces/edges are in front of lighter object surfaces/edges in d/e. Given an edge map as input, our model produces two complementary depth maps as output.

assignment solution to be the set of smallest depth labels that satisfy all the visible occlusion relationships. For example, object 4 in Fig. 1c is on layer 1 rather than layer 2.

2.2   MRF Model

Segregating depth into layers is a global process which requires the information to be integrated over the entire image. A change of configuration in a small area can influence the depth labeling at a distance. On the other hand, there exist critical local cues such as T and L junctions which give rise to 3D percepts. If each of these cues can be clearly classified and labeled, and there is an unique association between these cues and 3D depth, depth labeling can be solved by logical inference, for example, using the occlusion graph in Fig. 1c. However, there is always uncertainty in identifying local cues in real images and there is no universal rule of association between a low level cue and a high level percept. The ambiguity in this association is reduced with an increase in the range of integration. For example, two L-junctions can be configured to form a T-junction which is not related to occlusion. The meaning of this T-junction can be disambiguated by gathering information from the origins of the arms and stem of the T-junction.

Long range influence can be mediated by local computation using MRF [10, 21]. An MRF is defined over a graph $\mathcal{G}$, which is determined by its site set $\mathcal{S}$ and neighborhood system η. $\mathcal{S} = Z_m \cup Z'_m$, where Z_m is an $m \times m$ pixel lattice and Z'_m is its dual lattice consisting of an $m \times (m-1)$ and an $(m-1) \times m$ interleaved grids for *line sites* [10]. The *coupled neighborhood* of a site includes both its peer sites and dual sites, as illustrated in Fig. 2.

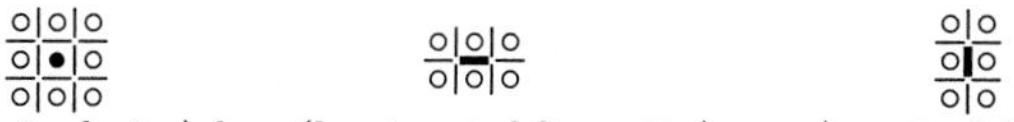

a. η(pixel site) b. η(horizontal line site) c. η(vertical line site)

Fig. 2. The neighborhood system η used in the model.

Given an edge map, $g : Z'_m \mapsto \{0,1\}^{2m(m-1)}$, with 1 and 0 indicating the presence and absence of an edge respectively, we would like to find a depth map on both pixel and line sites, $h : Z_m \cup Z'_m \mapsto \{0,\infty\}^{m^2} \cup \{1,\infty\}^{2m(m-1)}$, with the depth layer numbered from 0 (for background). To model the depth segregation by MRF, we need to specify *clique potentials* $V_c(\omega)$, ω being a particular configuration of an MRF, and c being a *clique* defined as a subset of sites, which consists of either a single site or more sites where any two of them are neighbors. The probability $P(\omega)$ can be written as

$$P(\omega) = \frac{e^{-U(\omega)}}{Z}, \quad Z = \sum_{\omega \in \Omega} e^{-U(\omega)}, \quad U(\omega) = \sum_{c \in \mathcal{C}} V_c(\omega),$$

where Z is called the *partition function* and $U(\omega)$ the *energy function*.

MRF's have been widely used in texture modeling [5], as well as in image segmentation [10, 13]. In texture modeling, the clique potentials are used to model the probability of co-occurrence of subsets of pixels [5] or capture marginal probability distributions in terms of filter responses [38]. In image segmentation, it is closely related to the energy functional approaches [4, 10, 25] and the clique potentials are used to encode smoothness priors [10]. In our formulation below, we generalize the idea of multi-level logistic models, and suggest a broader view that clique potentials can be more general so that they can encode arbitrary local decision rules.

2.3   Encoding Local Decision Rules

To model depth segregation process in MRF, we seek to make correct depth labeling correspond to the most probable configurations or equivalently configurations of the minimum energy.

Let χ and γ denote two indicator functions, which map from {True, False} to $\{1,0\}$ and $\{-1,1\}$ respectively. $\gamma(\cdot) = 1 - 2\chi(\cdot)$. Let ζ denote the *sign* function, which takes on $-1, 0, 1$ for negative, zero and positive numbers respectively. The line site a between pixel i and j is denoted by $a = i \circ j$ and conversely, the set of pixels associated with the line is denoted by $a^\circ = (i,j)$, with i and j ordered from left to right or from top to bottom. In particular, $(i,j) \circ (i,j+1)$ and $(i,j) \circ (i+1,j)$ are abbreviated as $(i,j\circ)$ and $(i\circ,j)$ respectively. Using these symbols and notations, we can define $V_c(h|g)$ to encode our prior knowledge in terms of 10 local rules.

$V_c(h|g)$

$$= \sum_{a=(ioj)\in c} \beta_1 \cdot \gamma(h_i = h_j) \cdot \chi(g_a = 0) \qquad \text{(rule 1)}$$
$$+ \sum_{a=(ioj)\in c} \beta_2 \cdot \gamma(h_i \neq h_j) \cdot \chi(g_a = 1) \qquad \text{(rule 2)}$$
$$+ \sum_{a=(ioj)\in c} \beta_3 \cdot \gamma\Big(h_a = \max(h_i, h_j)\Big) \cdot \chi(g_a = 1) \qquad \text{(rule 3)}$$
$$+ \sum_{(a=ioj,b=kol)\in c^l} \beta_4 \cdot \gamma(h_a = h_b) \cdot \chi(g_a = g_b = 1) \qquad \text{(rule 4)}$$
$$+ \sum_{(a=ioj,b=kol)\in c^l} \beta_5 \cdot \gamma\Big(\zeta(h_i - h_j) = \zeta(h_k - h_l)\Big) \qquad \text{(rule 5)}$$
$$\cdot \chi(h_i \neq h_j, h_k \neq h_l) \cdot \chi(g_a = g_b = 1)$$
$$+ \sum_{(a=iok,b=jok)\in c^c} \beta_6 \cdot \gamma(h_a = h_b) \cdot \chi(g_a = g_b = 1) \qquad \text{(rule 6)}$$
$$+ \sum_{(a=iok,b=jok)\in c^c} \beta_7 \cdot \gamma\Big(\zeta(h_i - h_k) = \zeta(h_j - h_k)\Big) \qquad \text{(rule 7)}$$
$$\cdot \chi(h_a = h_b) \cdot \chi(g_a = g_b = 1)$$
$$+ \sum_{(a=ioj,b=kol,u=jol,v=iok)\in c^t} \beta_8 \cdot \Big(\gamma(h_a > h_u) + \gamma(h_b > h_u)\Big) \qquad \text{(rule 8)}$$
$$\cdot \chi\Big(\zeta(h_i - h_j) = 1 \cup \zeta(h_k - h_l) = 1\Big) \cdot \chi(g_a = g_b = g_u = 1 \cap g_v = 0)$$
$$+ \sum_{(a=ioj,b=kol,u=jol,v=iok)\in c^t} \beta_9 \cdot \Big(\gamma(h_i > h_j) + \gamma(h_k > h_l)\Big) \qquad \text{(rule 9)}$$
$$\cdot \chi\Big(\zeta(h_i - h_j) = 1 \cup \zeta(h_k - h_l) = 1\Big) \cdot \chi(g_a = g_b = g_u = 1 \cap g_v = 0)$$
$$+ \sum_{(a=ioj,b=kol,u=jol,v=iok)\in c^t} \beta_{10} \cdot \gamma(h_i = h_l) \qquad \text{(rule 10)}$$
$$\cdot \chi(g_a = g_u = 0 \cup g_b = g_v = 0)$$

where c^l, c^c, c^t are the sets of cliques for aligned lines, corners and crosses:

$$c^l = \{(a,b) : a = (io, j), b = (io, j+1); a = (i, jo), b = (i+1, jo), a, b \in c\},$$
$$c^c = \{(a,b) : a = (io, j), b = (k, lo), |i - k| \le 1, |j - l| \le 1, a, b \in c\},$$
$$c^t = \{(a, b, u, v) : (a, b) \in c^l, (u, v) \in c^l, \{a, b\} \cap \{u, v\} = \emptyset, a^\circ \cup b^\circ = u^\circ \cup v^\circ\}.$$

The two indicator functions, χ and γ, enable us to embed the conjunction of *if* conditionals into the clique potentials. Let us decode rule 1 as an example. Consider the line site a between pixel i and j. If the clause ($g_a = 0$) is not true, i.e. there is an edge between the two pixels, then this first term is zero, no action will be taken; otherwise, if the clause ($h_i = h_j$) is also true, i.e. the pixel depth values at the two sites are equal, then the term produces a reward of $-\beta_1$, lowering the energy. However, if it is not true, i.e. the depth values at the two pixel sites are different, then $V_c(h|g)$ gets β_1 on this term as a punishment, increasing the energy. Here we require all βs to be positive. These 10 rules are summarized in Table 1 and they can be classified into 6 groups as follows.

Group 1: *Depth continuity within surface.* Rules 1 and 10 assert that surface depth units in adjacent locations should be continuous. Adjacency is defined on two kinds of neighborhood. Rule 1 is concerned with the first order neighborhood (up, down, left and right neighbors), and rule 10 is concerned with the second order neighborhood (diagonally adjacent pixels).

Group 2: *Depth discontinuity across edges.* Rule 2 asserts that when there is an edge between two adjacent locations, the surface depth units in those two locations must have different depth values.

Table 1. Encoding rules in clique potentials. Each of these β terms encodes a logic rule, which in general reads like this: if current clique configuration does not satisfy condition A, it gets a score of 0; otherwise, if condition A is satisfied, pattern B is expected; if B is also satisfied, then it gets a negative score $-C$; otherwise it gets a positive score C. a, b, u and v are labels for line sites while i, j, k, l are labels for pixel sites in the cliques.

Configuration	Condition A	Pattern B	Score C	#	Meaning
o | o i a j	$g_a = 0$	$h_i = h_j$	β_1	1	Depth continues in surface.
	$g_a = 1$	$h_i \neq h_j$	β_2	2	Depth breaks at edges.
	$g_a = 1$	$h_i \neq h_j$	β_3	3	Edges belong to surface in front.
k b l o | o o | o i a j	$g_a = g_b = 1$	$h_a = h_b$	β_4	4	Depth continues along contour.
	$g_a = g_b = 1$ $h_i \neq h_j$ $h_k \neq h_l$	$\zeta(h_i - h_j)$ $=$ $\zeta(h_k - h_l)$	β_5	5	Depth polarity continues along contour.
j o o | o b i a k	$g_a = g_b = 1$	$h_a = h_b$	β_6	6	Depth continues around corners.
	$g_a = g_b = 1$ $h_a = h_b$	$\zeta(h_i - h_k)$ $=$ $\zeta(h_j - h_k)$	β_7	7	Depth polarity continues around corners.
k b l o | o v o | o u i a j	$g_a = g_b = 1$	$h_a > h_u$	β_8	8	Depth breaks on edges at T-junctions.
	$g_u = 1, g_v = 0$	$h_b > h_u$	β_8		
	$\zeta(h_i - h_j) = 1$ or $\zeta(h_k - h_l) = 1$	$h_i > h_j$ $h_k > h_l$	β_9 β_9	9	Depth breaks in surface at T-junctions.
	$g_a = g_u = 0$ or $g_b = g_v = 0$	$h_i = h_l$	β_{10}	10	Depth continues in surface.

Group 3: *Border-ownerships.* Rule 3 specifies that an edge depth unit shares the same depth value as the surface that owns it.

Group 4: *Depth continuity along contour.* Rules 4 and 6 specify the edge depth value along contour or corners should be continuous.

Group 5: *Depth polarity continuity along contour.* Rules 5 and 7 specify the depth polarity of surface units across an edge unit should be continuous along contour and corners.

Group 6: *Occlusion relationships at T-junctions.* At those T-junctions, rule 8 and 9 specify that the arms of the T are in front of the T stem.

In this formulation, the clique potentials no longer simply specify local co-occurrence, smoothness constraints or filter response histograms as in other MRF models, but are generalized to encode a set of local decision rules. From neural modeling perspective, the units in the network are not neurons with linearly weighted inputs and sigmoidal activation functions, but are capable of performing complicated logical computations individually. Recent findings and models in cellular neurophysiology [1, 18, 23] suggest neurons are capable of computations more sophisticated than previously assumed.

The relative importance of the weights βs in the depth segregation can be estimated using a variety of methods. We will describe a particular supervised learning method we use in a later section.

2.4   Multiscale Hierarchy

The MRF model described above suffers from being myopic [14] in local computation and sluggish at propagating constraints between widely separated processing elements [31]. This problem can be overcome by embedding the MRF in a hierarchy using multigrid techniques.

We build an edge map pyramid by down-sampling with a factor of 2(Fig. 3). Assuming $m = 2^k + 1$, we preserve spatial locations at the center and the boundary of the lattices throughout the levels of the hierarchy. Let η^l and Z_m^l denote the neighborhood and lattice at level l. Let $\hat{\ }$ and $\check{\ }$ address the correspondence between pixels at level l and $l+1$, such that $\hat{i} \in Z_m^{l+1}$ and $i \in Z_m^l$, or, $\check{i} \in Z_m^l$ and $i \in Z_m^{l+1}$ point to the same spatial location on the sampling grid (Figure 3c). The edge map at a high level is determined by

$$g_{\hat{i}o\hat{j}}^l = \zeta\big((g_{iok}^{l-1} + g_{koj}^{l-1}) \cdot |\zeta(h_k^{l-1} - h_i^{l-1}) + \zeta(h_j^{l-1} - h_k^{l-1})|\big).$$

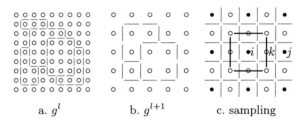

a. g^l b. g^{l+1} c. sampling

Fig. 3. Hierarchical edge maps and illustration of sampling. a. Edge map at some level l. b. Edge map at a higher level $l+1$. c. The hierarchy is built by downsampling pixels (filled circles) by a factor of two and inferring new lines (darker lines) between sampled pixels based on the depth and edge maps at a lower level.

If an edge is considered to disconnect two neighboring pixels, the above operation preserves connectivity when there is only one edge separating two sampled pixels. However, when there are two edges in a local neighborhood, the depth polarity of the edges has to be considered (Fig. 4). When two nearby edges have the same polarity, they can be merged into one edge of the same polarity as in (Fig. 4a). When the two edges have opposite depth polarities as in (Fig. 4b), they would disappear at the next level of the hierarchy. In this way, relaxation at each resolution deals with topologically equivalent diffusion processes and thus the same procedure can be applied.

The intergrid transfer functions involve *restriction* $\Uparrow$ and *extension* $\Downarrow$.

$$h^l = \Uparrow (h^{l-1}, g^{l-1}), \qquad h^l = \Downarrow (h^l, g^l, h^{l+1}).$$

During the restriction, *smoothing* is carried out on *connected* pixel sites. For line sites, the smoothing on aligned horizontal (vertical) edges is blocked by vertical(horizontal) edge neighbors:

$$h_{\hat{i}}^l = \max \left\{ h_k^{l-1} : g_{iok}^{l-1} = 0, k \in Z_m^{l-1} \cap \eta_i^{l-1} \right\}$$

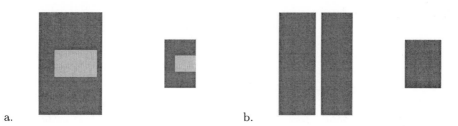

Fig. 4. The operation in the multiscale hierarchy takes edge depth polarity into consideration. a. Edges of overlapping shapes have the same depth polarity and are preserved at a coarser resolution. Edges of abutting shapes that have opposite depth polarities will disappear at a coarser resolution, as indicated by the disappearance of the two edges between the two shapes at the coarser scale. In this way, relaxation at each resolution deals with topologically equivalent diffusion processes and thus the same procedure can be applied. In both a and b, the pictures on the left and right indicate the images at a fine and coarse resolution respectively.

$$h^l_{(\hat{i},\hat{j}o)} = \max\left\{ h^{l-1}_{(p,qo)} : g^{l-1}_{(p,q)o(i,q)} = g^{l-1}_{(p,q+1)o(i,q+1)} = 0, p \in [i-1, i+1], q \in [j, j+1] \right\}.$$

$h^l_{(\hat{i}o,\hat{j})}$ can be defined in a similar fashion. Median filtering can also be used in the above. During the extension, the information is selectively transferred to a fine grid. The dual operation of smoothing is *diffusion*, which is subject to boundary blockage:

$$h^l_i = h^{l+1}_i$$

$$h^l_{(i,\hat{j}o)} = h^{l+1}_{(i,\hat{j}o)}, \text{if } g^{l+1}_{(i,\hat{j}o)} = 1, g^l_{(i,\hat{j}o)} = 1, g^l_{(i,(j+1)o)} = 0 \text{ or } h^l_{(i,j)} > h^l_{(i,j+2)}$$

$$h^l_{(i,(\hat{j}+1)o)} = h^{l+1}_{(i,\hat{j}o)}, \text{if } g^{l+1}_{(i,\hat{j}o)} = 1, g^l_{(i,(j+1)o)} = 1, g^l_{(i,\hat{j}o)} = 0 \text{ or } h^l_{(i,j)} < h^l_{(i,j+2)}$$

$$h^l_i = \max\left\{ h^{l+1}_{\hat{k}} : g^l_{iok} = 0, k \in Z^l_m \cap \eta^l_i, \hat{k} \in Z^{l+1}_m \right\}$$

$$h^l_{(i,\hat{j}o)} = \max\left\{ h^{l+1}_{(\hat{p},\hat{j}o)} : g^l_{(p,j)o(i,j)} = g^l_{(p,j+1)o(i,j+1)} = 0, p \in [i-1, i+1] \right\}.$$

Finally, to complete our HMRF model, we provide site visitation and a multi-level interaction scheme. A complete *sweep* of all the sites includes four checker board update schemes on first pixel sites and then line sites. The separate visitation to pixel sites and line sites allows each of the two MRF's to develop fully in itself so that the resultant configuration provides enough driving force for the other to change accordingly. The hierarchy is visited bottom-up through restriction and then top-down through extension. The MRF at each level carries out a relaxation process until its configuration converges. When the configuration at the lowest level does not change after visiting the entire hierarchy, that configuration is the final result.

In summary, multiscale not only helps to speed up computation, but also helps propagating sparse depth cues at boundary to the interior of the surface by longer range interactions at higher levels of the hierarchy. In addition, at each level of the hierarchy, we repeat the same relaxation operation of local decision rules. This relies on the consistency of topology in the restriction and extension operations.

2.5   Parameter Estimation

The above HMRF model has unknown parameter $\beta = [\beta_1, \cdots, \beta_{10}]^T$. The major difficulty in estimating MRF parameters lies in the evaluation of the partition function. There are several approaches to deal with the problem [21]. One way is to avoid the partition function in the formula, such as pseudo-likelihood [3] and least squares(LS) fit [5]. Another way is to use some estimation techniques such as the coding method, mean field approximation [35] and Markov Chain Monte Carlo maximum likelihood [6]. The approach we take here is to derive a set of constraints on β using a method called *learning from rehearsals* and use linear programming to obtain the β that satisfy these constraints.

This perturbation-based method is most closely related to the LS fit approach [5]. Let $U_k(\omega)$ denote the sum of clique potentials $V_c(\omega)$ over all cliques containing site k. Since $V_c(\omega)$ is a linear function of β, so is $U_k(\omega)$. In general, it can be written as $U_k(\omega) = x(\omega, k) \cdot \beta$, where $x(\omega, k)$ can be obtained by evaluating clique potentials on the configuration ω confined to the neighborhood of k. In the LS approach, the probabilities of training samples are utilized to derive a set of equalities based on the formula below.

$$\ln\left(\frac{P(\omega_k = i|\omega_{\eta_k})}{P(\omega_k = j|\omega_{\eta_k})}\right) = -[U_k(\omega) - U_k(\omega')] = -\left[x(\omega, k) - x(\omega', k)\right] \cdot \beta,$$

where $\omega_k = i, \omega'_k = j, \omega_{S\backslash\{k\}} = \omega'_{S\backslash\{k\}}$ are given. However, this is only applicable to the case where $P(\omega_k = j|\omega_{\eta_k}) > 0$. This condition may not be very restrictive in texture modeling, but it is in our model because when ω_{η_k} is set, ω_k is often determined as well. Another problem concerns numerical stability. When $P(\omega_k = j|\omega_{\eta_k})$ is small, the estimation is not accurate. To relax this condition, we derive inequality constraints on β instead:

$$\left[x(\omega, k) - x(\omega', k)\right] \cdot \beta < 0, \text{if } P(\omega_k = i|\omega_{\eta_k}) > P(\omega_k = j|\omega_{\eta_k}).$$

We do not need to know the exact sizes of the two probabilities, but rather the relative order of the two quantitities. In other words, for a given neighourhood configuration ω_{η_k}, if we know label i is preferred to label j for site k, we obtain a constraint which ensures that site k assuming value of i leads to a lower energy.

We obtain two sets of constraints on β in the form of above inequalities. We generate a set of images which have two randomly positioned rectangular shapes. Both the edge map g and the final depth map h are known for each training image. The first set of constraints come from the fact that given neighbors of a site assuming correct labels, this site prefers its own correct label. This will map the correct labeling into a local minimum in the configuration space. We summarize all such constraints into $A \cdot \beta < 0$, where the rows of A come from the perturbation on the teacher map h at all sites:

$$\left[x(\omega, k) - x(\omega', k) \right] \cdot \beta < 0, \text{for } P(\omega_k | \omega_{\eta_k}) > P(\omega'_k | \omega'_{\eta_k}),$$

where $\omega_k = h_k, \omega'_k = h_k \pm 1, \omega_{\mathcal{S} \setminus \{k\}} = \omega'_{\mathcal{S} \setminus \{k\}} = h_{\mathcal{S} \setminus \{k\}}$. An example on an L-junction is given in Fig. 5. As can be seen in the example, the first set of constraints are usually satisfiable as the correct label is far better than any other choices according to the rules we encode in the energy function.

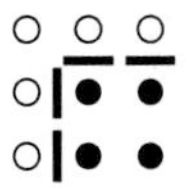

$$\begin{bmatrix} -4 & -4 & -4 & 0 & -2 & 0 & -2 & 0 & 0 & -2 \\ -4 & 0 & -4 & 0 & 0 & 0 & 0 & 0 & 0 & -2 \end{bmatrix} \cdot \beta < 0$$

a. Configuration.   b. Constraints.

Fig. 5. Derive the first set of constraints from teacher depth maps. a. An L-junction at a pixel site's neighborhood. The teacher depth map in this neighborhood is 0 for unfilled circles and 1 for all the line sites and filled circles. b. Two constraints obtained by perturbation on the depth value of the center pixel site. The first constraint comes from the difference in the energy functions for labeling 1 and 0 at the center pixel. The second constraint comes from the difference in the energy functions for labeling 1 and 2 at the center pixel, all its neighbors assuming correct labels. These two constraints on β are trivial as any $\beta > 0$ is feasible.

The first set of constraints only guarantee local behaviors when the system is close to the optimal configuration. They may not be enough to drive an initial configuration toward that final optimal configuration. A second set of constraints are derived for this purpose. This is not easy because there are many possible different paths of evolution from one configuration into another, and we do not necessarily know the intermediate configurations that the system has to go through in order to arrive at the final state. We develop a method called *learning from rehearsals* to overcome this difficulty. Not knowing β in advance or teacher depth maps at intermediate steps, we use the following principle to choose a preferred label during the learning process and to establish its validity by rehearsing. The principle is that a site's depth value should be as close as possible to its final target value at that site subject to the dragging force from its current neighborhood configuration. That is, the derivation of the second set of constraints is based on finding the most effective intermediate states that will move the system from the initial state to the final state with a minimum number of steps. Once a preferred depth label is chosen, we can derive plausible constraints in a similar way as we did in Fig. 5. We build a constraint database during learning. Whenever a new constraint is to be added into the database, we check its own feasibility as well as its compatibility with those already in the database. We implement two simple checks on these two properties by testing if new constraint $\alpha \cdot \beta < 0$ leads to $\beta < 0$, or some other constraint requiring

$-\alpha \cdot \beta < 0$ already exists in the database. If either of these conditions is true, the constraint is removed and accordingly the hypothesized teacher is abandoned and next candidate depth value, which is not so close to the target value as this one, is chosen. When new constraints can be checked into the database, the intermediate teacher is instantiated. We make the depth assignment at the site and continue the learning process as if all the conditions were satisfied. We call this process *rehearsal* because we carry out the relaxation without knowing whether there is a feasible set of β. We summarize the second set of constraints in $\widetilde{A} \cdot \beta < 0$.

The system will rehearse and practice, like a baby learning to walk, trying to reach the final goal from an initial state, while generating constraints on its gaits at each step along the way. Having obtained these two sets of constraints on β, we can proceed to find the set of β that satisfy most constraints by optimizing the following linear programming problem,

$$LP : \text{minimize: } \xi \sum_i \delta_i + \sum_j \tilde{\delta}_j,$$

$$\text{subject to: } A \cdot \beta - \delta \leq -1, \tilde{A} \cdot \beta - \tilde{\delta} \leq -1, \delta \geq 0, \tilde{\delta} \geq 0, \beta \geq 1,$$

where $\xi \geq 1$ is a weighting factor between the two sets of constraints, here we simply set it to 1. Since not every constraint can be satisfied, we introduce slack variable δ and $\tilde{\delta}$ to turn them into soft constraints. Linear programming is used to find the set of β that minimizes the total amount of violation of the constraints.

Once LP yields a set of β, we examine the constraints' slack variables to see which constraint is most severely violated (the largest positive δ or $\tilde{\delta}$). We find that a bad constraint is typically generated by making a hasty jump before the condition is mature, putting an unnecessarily harsh constraint on β. We go back to the constraint database and remove this constraint and choose alternative teachers for all the patterns that give rise to this constraint. This prevents that constraint to be selected again in subsequent rehearsals. We remove enough bad constraints till a feasible β is found. We test its validity by relaxation using this β to see if it can actually drive the system from the initial state to the final state for each training example. The learning and checking processes are iterated until final configurations for all the training images are correct. The learning proceeds from simple to complex images, to gradually build up a set of reasonable constraints. Most time when a new image is learned, only a couple of iterations is sufficient to obtain a new β such that all δ and $\tilde{\delta} = 0$.

3   Results

Learning on a small set of training images containing *two objects* singles out a unique value for β, where $\beta = [18, 9, 97, 23.3, 3.2, 86.7, 3.35, 16.5, 42.5, 137, 20.8]$. With this set of parameters, the model produces reasonable results for a set of test images that the system has never been exposed to before.

Figure 6 shows how the system responds to a test image with *five overlapping rectangles* in the scene. The system generalizes very well in its response to this new input configuration. A sequence of 8 snap shots are taken at different time points during the evolution of the system. Snap shot 1 shows the system detecting T-junctions and starting propagating its initial result one level up the hierarchy. Snap shot 2 shows the information has propagated to the third level, and propagation of depth information within surface is now evident at the second level. Snap shots 3 and 4 show the information has propagated to the fourth and fifth levels respectively. Snap shot 5 shows the information starts to propagate down the hierarchy, introducing rapid filling-in of surface depth and depth segregation in snap shot 6. Snap shots 7 and 8 show the completion of surface/contour depth interpolation and segregation. All these are completed very rapidly in two iterations up and down the hierarchy.

4   Discussion

In this paper, we present a hierarchical MRF model to perform depth segregation of region edge maps. The model is hierarchical rather than simply multiscale because its fine-to-coarse transform is topology-dependent. In this work, we propose a broader view that clique potentials in MRF can be used to encode any local logical decision rules. By introducing a set of rules that asserts continuity of depth assignment values along contour and within surfaces, and discontinuity of depth assignment values across contours, we demonstrate a system that automatically integrates sparse local relative depth cues arisen from T-junctions over long distance into a global ordering of relative depths. Interestingly, because the rules we set are encoding relative relationships between objects, the system trained on scenes containing two objects can actually generalize and perform correctly when a scene containing five objects is first encountered.

We also propose a new method called *learning from rehearsals* for estimating MRF parameters. In this method, we derive a set of constraints based on perturbation of target solutions and the rehearsals of relaxation processes, and then use linear programming to obtain feasible solutions. Conflicting constraints are removed and constraint derivation by rehearsals and parameter solving are repeated until there is a set of parameters that work correctly for every test image. We do not have a theoretical proof that the learning of this system will actually converge. We have restricted our domain of investigation to a world of simple shapes so that we can gain a better understanding of the system and associate constraints with their origins.

Another assumption we made is that the input edge maps are closed contours. There is no technical difficulty here in so far as there exist a number of algorithms such as active contours [16] and region competition algorithms [37, 39] that can produce complete and closed contours. However, depth segregation and ordering can potentially help segmentation by feeding back additional constraints to organize the contour detection and completion process itself. Earlier work by Belhumeur [2] and recent work by Yu and Shi [34] are examples of

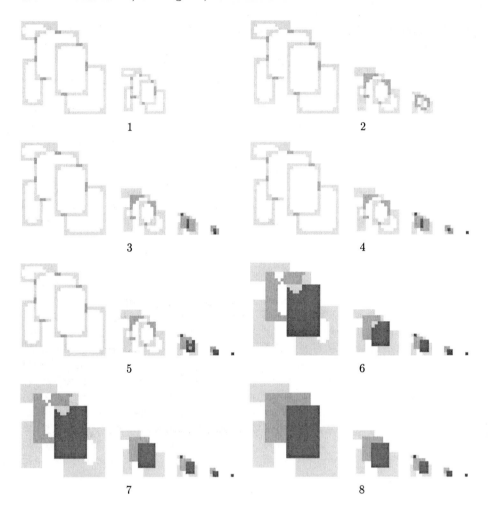

Fig. 6. Dynamics of the HMRF's response to a 5-object test image. The parameters are learned on a few 2-object images. Shown here are a number of snaps shots taken at different time points during the depth segregation computation. The hierarchy is traversed twice till its complete convergence to the correct labeling.

how depth cues and intensity cues can be integrated simultaneously into the segmentation process. These are potential directions for future research.

We think this HMRF model for depth segregation might provide a plausible computational framework for reasoning about and understanding the basic computational constraints and neural mechanisms underlying local and global integration and figure-ground segregation in the brain. This work provides us with several insights to some psychological and neurophysiological phenomena.

First, brightness has been observed to propagate in from the border in the psychophysical experiment by Paradiso and Nakayama [29]. Such phenomenon has been postulated to be mediated by horizontal connections in V1, for example in Grossberg and Mingolla's model [11]. Here, we show that a hierarchical framework can speed up the diffusion of depth assignment process considerably. In fact, traversing up and down the hierarchy twice is sufficient to complete the computation. This suggests that both the brightness perception and the depth segregation could be mediated by the feedback from V2 and V4, which are known to have receptive fields two and four times larger than those of V1 respectively.

Second, while Paradiso and Nakayama's experiment suggests diffusion in the brightness domain, the similarity in dynamics between brightness diffusion and our depth assignment suggests depth segregation and assignment might be the underlying process that carries the brightness diffusion along. By the same reasoning, one would expect other surface cues such as color, texture and stereo disparity should also be accompanying, if not following, the depth assignment process. It will indeed be interesting to examine experimentally whether the propagation of surface cues follows the depth assignment process or occurs simultaneously. That Dobbins et al. [7] found a significant number of V1, V2 and V4 cells sensitive to distance even in monocular viewing conditions suggests that depth assignment might be intertwined with many early visual processes.

Finally, the hierarchy presented is not simply a multiscale network in that, when the information travels up, the topological relationships between different objects are taken into consideration in such a way that the same relaxation procedure can be applied at each level. For example, edges of overlapping shapes are kept (Fig. 4a), whereas the edges of two nearby shapes appearing side by side would disappear at a coarser resolution(Fig. 4b). This operation can be achieved by taking the sum of depth polarities during the down-sampling process. In order to accomplish this in the network, depth polarity of edges needs to be computed and represented explicitly. This might provide a computational rationale for the existence of the depth-polarity sensitive cells von der Heydt and his colleagues found in V1, V2 and V4 [36].

Acknowledgements

Yu and Lee have been supported by NSF LIS 9720350, NSF CAREER 9984706 and NIH core grant EY 08098.

References

1. L. F. Abbott. Integrating with action potentials. *Neuron*, 26:3–4, 2000.
2. P. Belhumeur. A Bayesian approach to binocular stereopsis. *International Journal of Computer Vision*, 19(3):237–260, 1996.
3. J. Besag. Efficiency of pseudo-likelihood estimation of simple Gaussian fields. *Biometrika*, 64:616–8, 1977.
4. A. Blake and A. Zisserman. *Visual Reconstruction*. MIT Press, Cambridge, MA, 1987.

5. H. Derin and H. Elliott. Modeling and segmentation of noisy and textured images using Gibbs random fields. *IEEE Transactions on Pattern Analysis and Machine Intelligence*, 9(1):39–55, 1987.

6. X. Descombes, R. D. Morris, J. Zerubia, and M. Berthod. Estimation of Markov random fields prior parameters using Markov chain Monte Carlo maximum likelihood. *IEEE Transactions on Image Processing*, 8(7):954–62, 1999.

7. A. C. Dobbins, R. M. Jeo, J. Fiser, and J. M. Allman. Distance modulation of neural activity in the visual cortex. *Science*, 281:552–5, 1998.

8. D. Geiger and K. Kumaran. Visual organization of illusory surfaces. In *European Conference on Computer Vision*, Cambridge, England, April 1996.

9. D. Geiger, H. kuo Pao, and N. Rubin. Salient and multiple illusory surfaces. In *IEEE Conference on Computer Vision and Pattern Recognition*. 1998.

10. S. Geman and D. Geman. Stochastic relaxation, Gibbs distributions, and the Bayesian restoration of images. *IEEE Transactions on Pattern Analysis and Machine Intelligence*, 6(6):721–41, 1984.

11. S. Grossberg and E. Mingolla. Neural dynamics of form perception: boundary completion, illusory figures, and neon color spreading. *Psychological Review*, 92:173–211, 1985.

12. F. Heitger and R. von der Heydt. A computational model of neural contour processing: Figure-ground segregation and illusory contours. In *International Conference on Computer Vision*, pages 32–40. 1993.

13. T. H. Hong, K. A. Narayanan, S. Peleg, A. Rosenfeld, and T. Silberberg. Image smoothing and segmentation by multiresolution pixel linking: further experiments and extensions. *IEEE Transactions on Systems, Man, and Cybernetics*, 12:611–22, 1982.

14. T. H. Hong and A. Rosenfeld. Compact region extraction using weighted pixel linking in a pyramid. *IEEE Transactions on Pattern Analysis and Machine Intelligence*, 6(2):222–9, 1984.

15. G. Kanizsa. *Organization in vision*. Praeger Publishers, 1979.

16. M. Kass, A. Witkin, and D. Terzopoulos. Snakes: Active contour models. *International Journal of Computer Vision*, pages 321–331, 1988.

17. J. J. Knierim and D. van Essen. Neuronal responses to static texture patterns in area v1 of the alert macaque monkey. *Journal of Neurophysiology*, 67(4):961–80, 1992.

18. C. Koch. Computation and the single neuron. *Nature*, 385:207–210, 1997.

19. V. Lamme. The neurophysiology of figure-ground segregation in primary visual cortex. *Jounral of neuroscience*, 10:649–69, 1995.

20. T. S. Lee, D. Mumford, R. Romero, and V. Lamme. The role of primary visual cortex in higher level vision. *Vision Research*, 38:2429–54, 1998.

21. S. Z. Li. *Markov random field modeling in computer vision*. Springer-Verlag, 1995.

22. S. Madarasmi, T.-C. Pong, and D. Kersten. Illusory contour detection using MRF models. In *IEEE International Conference on Neural Networks*, volume 7, pages 4343–8. 1994.

23. H. Markram, J. Lubke, M. Frotscher, and B. Sakmann. Regulartion of synaptic efficacy by coincidence of postsynpatic APS and EPSPs. *Science*, 275:213–215, 1997.

24. D. Mumford. Elastica and computer vision. In C. L. Bajaj, editor, *Algebraic geometry and its applications*. Springer-Verlag, 1993.

25. D. Mumford. The bayesian rationale for energy functionals. In B. Romeny, editor, *Geometry-driven diffusion in computer vision*, pages 141–53. Kluwer Academic Publishers, 1994.

26. K. Nakayama and S. Shimojo. Experiencing and perceiving visual surfaces. *Science*, 257:1357–63, 1992.

27. K. Nakayama, S. Shimojo, and G. H. Silverman. Stereoscopic depth: its relation to image segmentation, grouping, and the recognition of occluded objects. *Perception*, 18:55–68, 1989.

28. M. Nitzberg. *Depth from Overlap*. PhD thesis, The Division of Applied Sciences, Harvard University, 1991.

29. M. A. Paradiso and K. Nakayama. Brightness perception and filling-in. *Vision Research*, 31(7/8):1221–36, 1991.

30. J. Shi and J. Malik. Normalized cuts and image segmentation. In *IEEE Conference on Computer Vision and Pattern Recognition*, pages 731–7, June 1997.

31. D. Terzopoulos. Image analysis using multigrid relaxation methods. *IEEE Transactions on Pattern Analysis and Machine Intelligence*, 8(2):129–39, 1986.

32. S. Ullman. Filling-in the gaps: the shape of subjective contours and a model for their generation. *Biological Cybernetics*, 25:1–6, 1976.

33. L. R. Williams and D. W. Jacobs. Stochastic completion fields: A neural model of illusory contour shape and salience. *Neural Computation*, 9(4):837–58, 1997.

34. S. X. Yu and J. Shi. Segmentation with pairwise attraction and repulsion. International Conference on Computer Vision, 2001.

35. J. Zhang. The mean field theory in EM procedures for Markov random fields. *IEEE Transactions on Image Processing*, 40(10):2570–83, 1992.

36. H. Zhou, H. Friedman, and R. von der Heydt. Coding of border ownership in monkey visual cortex. *Journal of Neuroscience*, 20(17):6594–611, 2000.

37. S. C. Zhu, T. S. Lee, and A. Yuille. Region competition: unifying snakes, region-growing and mdl for image segmentation. *Proceedings of the Fifth International Conference in Computer Vision*, pages 416–425, 1995.

38. S. C. Zhu, Y. N. Wu, and D. Mumford. Filters, random field and maximum entropy: — towards a unified theory for texture modeling. *International Journal of Computer Vision*, 27(2):1–20, 1998.

39. S. C. Zhu and A. Yuille. Unifying snake/balloons, region growing and Bayes/MDL/Energy for multi-band image segmentation. *IEEE Transactions on Pattern Analysis and Machine Intelligence*, 18(9), 1996.

Articulated Object Tracking
via a Genetic Algorithm

Jairo Rocha and Arnau Mir

Department of Mathematics and Computer Science
University of the Balearic Islands
{jairo,arnau.mir}@uib.es

Abstract. Within a human motion analysis system, body parts are modeled by simple virtual 3D rigid objects. Its position and orientation parameters at frame $t+1$ are estimated based on the parameters at frame t and the image intensity variation from frame t to $t+1$, under kinematic constraints. A genetic algorithm calculates the 3D parameters that make a goal function that measures the intensity change minimum. The goal function is *robust,* so that outliers located especially near the virtual object projection borders have less effect on the estimation. Since the object's parameters are relative to the reference system, they are the same from different cameras, so more cameras are easily added, increasing the constraints over the same number of variables. Several successful experiments are presented for an arm motion and a leg motion from two and three cameras.

Keywords: Human motion, robust estimation, twist.

1   Introduction

The literature of human motion analysis (e.g., [WADP97,HHD98,WP00]), has reported an important progress. However, the problem of tracking of a human person motion is still unsolved. We present in this paper work in progress, instead of completed research, on a combination and modification of different approaches used before, and some experimental evidence that our more general approach is promising.

Bregler and Malik [BM97] built a system able to track human motion with great precision, including very challenging footage like Muybridge's photograph sequences. They defined a 3D virtual model of the subject and a goal function over body part position parameters that measures the changes in image intensities. Using the twist representation for rigid transformations and the flow constraint equation, they managed to make the goal function lineal in the parameter variables. They could therefore apply an iteration of linear optimization techniques and a warping routine to obtain a very reliable procedure for 3D position estimation. Our system is a modification of this one. The differences are the following: First, our goal function is robust, so that no EM procedure is needed afterwards; instead our optimization directly performs a robust parameter estimation. Second, we do not use the flow constraint equation but direct

M.A.T. Figueiredo, J. Zerubia, A.K. Jain (Eds.): EMMCVPR 2001, LNCS 2134, pp. 134–149, 2001.

difference of pixel intensity, thus fewer assumptions, such as small motion and constant intensity, are assumed and no warping procedure is needed; due to these two previous differences, we cannot apply a linear optimization technique as we will explain below. Third, our parameters are reference-based instead of camera-based, so additional cameras do not increase the number of variables to be estimated. And forth, we handle arbitrary rotations in the articulations, so that a fixed axis for each articulation does not have to be defined by the user, and arbitrary motion can be modeled. Our system is not a finished product and therefore its performance cannot be compared to Bregler and Malik's, but we will try to convey why we think this project is promising.

The *Cardboard People* system [JBY96] performs robust estimation of motion parameters for 2D regions. Assuming the flow constraint equation and a model for the motion of each patch, motion parameters are robustly estimated using a non-linear optimization procedure. This system relies on a good estimation of the flow constraint equation coefficients. We can say that our system is roughly a 3D version of Cardboard People.

Wachter and Nagel [WN97] describe a system in which motion parameters are estimated using a Kalman filter. An optimization procedure finds the parameters that make up the difference between the predicted parameters and the ones that agree with the edges of the next frame minimum. Their results are very impressive. Our system would benefit from a stochastic prediction.

Hunter, Kelly and Jain [HKJ97] present a system for motion tracking in which each step enforces the kinematic constraints by projecting the estimated solution based on the observation processes. The system works well using only black silhouettes because the modified EM algorithm proposed is a robust formulation that makes the recovered motion less sensitive to constraint violations.

All these systems and ours as well assume that a virtual humanoid that matches the real subject in size and initial position can be defined by other means in practice, by user interaction. This is a research subject in itself, and will not be discussed any further.

2   Problem Formulation

Given the film $I_t(x, y)$, we consider two consecutive frames at times t and $t + 1$.

The virtual model of a body part is an ellipsoid of appropriate dimensions. Virtual cameras of the real cameras are defined by a camera calibration routine. Assume that the 3D pose (position and orientation) of the ellipsoid at time t is known. The problem is to find the change in the 3D pose of the ellipsoid so that the motion coincides with the real image'motion. Let ϕ be the pose transformation of the ellipsoid from t to $t + 1$; ϕ is defined by 6 real parameters that will be discussed in detail later.

Let (x, y) be a pixel, and $(u_x(x, y, \phi), u_y(x, y, \phi))$, its displacement vector when a 3D point that is projected onto the camera pixel moves according to ϕ. The goal functional E' is the brightness change sum over the point projections before and after the pose transformation.

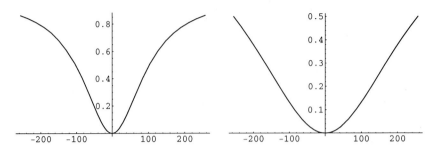

Fig. 1. $\rho(x, 0.4 \times 256)$ and $\rho(x, 1.0 \times 256)$.

We consider the functional E':

$$E'(phi) = \sum_{(x,y)\in\mathcal{R}} \rho(I_t(x,y) - I_{t+1}(x + u_x(\phi), y + u_y(\phi))) = \sum_{(x,y)\in\mathcal{R}} \rho(\Delta I) \quad (1)$$

where $\phi \in R^6$ are the 3-D motion parameters, $I_t(x,y)$ is the image brightness (intensity) function for the initial frame, $I_{t+1}(x,y)$ is the image brightness function for the final frame, $u_x(\phi), u_y(\phi))$ are the horizontal and vertical components of the flow image at the point (x,y), which is the projection from R^3 of the motion associated with the parameters ϕ; $\mathcal{R}$ is the patch to consider, in this case, the projection of the virtual ellipsoid that models that tracked part and, finally,

$$\rho(t) = \frac{t^2}{\sigma^2 + t^2}$$

is the function that reduces the influence of some outlying measurements of the brightness difference and allows an estimation of the dominant parameters; there are other ρ-functions that can be considered as well to obtain a different robust estimation. In the rest of this paper, we will use the one above. See Figure 1 for a representation.

The term $E'(\phi)$ measures how well all pixels of frame t match their corresponding ones in frame $t+1$, and its minimum is used to calculated the new pose of the ellipsoid. For the analysis from frame $t+1$ to $t+2$ this new pose is used, to calculate the pose at $t + 2$. If for any reason (partial occlusion, not finding the optimum, etc.), the new pose at $t + 1$ is not totally correct, the error will persist in the analysis of the rest of the sequence. In order to allow the system to recover from errors during some frames, we add another term that compares the intensity average of each new region with the original region in frame 0.

Assume that $\overline{I_0}$ is the average at frame 0. We define the functional,

$$E''(\phi) = \sum_{(x,y)\in\mathcal{R}} \rho(\overline{I_0} - I_{t+1}(x + u_x(\phi), y + u_y(\phi))). \quad (2)$$

Notice that the each pixel is not compared with another single pixel, but that the average is used.

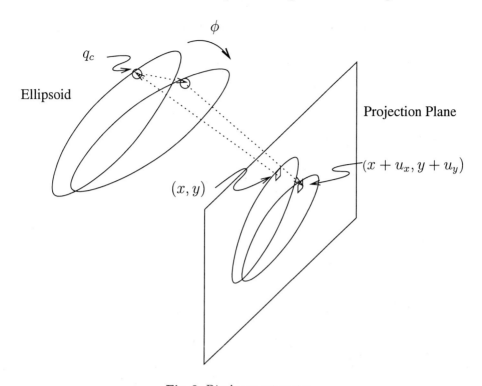

Fig. 2. Displacement vector.

The objective is to minimize $E = E' + E''$ relative to ϕ, for which a precise definition of (u_x, u_y) and its gradient are needed.

3 Motion Projection

The object pose relative to the reference frame can be represented as a rigid body transformation in R^3 using homogeneous coordinates:

$$q_r = G \cdot q_0 = \begin{pmatrix} r_{11} & r_{12} & r_{13} & d_x \\ r_{21} & r_{22} & r_{23} & d_y \\ r_{31} & r_{32} & r_{33} & d_z \\ 0 & 0 & 0 & 1 \end{pmatrix} \cdot q_0,$$

where $q_0 = (x_0, y_0, z_0, 1)^\top$ is a point in the object frame and $q_r = (x_r, y_r, z_r, 1)^\top$ is the corresponding point in the reference frame. $q_c = (x_c, y_c, z_c, 1)^\top$ is the corresponding point in the camera frame: $q_r = M_C \cdot q_c$, where M_C is the transformation matrix associated with the camera frame. See Figure 2.

Using orthographic projection with scale s, the point q_r in the reference frame gets projected onto the image point $(x_{im}, y_{im})^\top = s \cdot (x_c, y_c)^\top$. s is equal to the focal distance divided by the distance of the ellipsoid center to the camera, which happens to be a good approximation for all the points on the ellipsoid.

It can be shown ([MLS94]) that for any arbitrary $G \in SE(3)$, there exists a vector $\xi = (v_1, v_2, v_3, w_x, w_y, w_z)^\top$, called the twist representation, with associated matrix

$$\tilde{\xi} = \begin{pmatrix} 0 & -w_x & w_y & v_1 \\ w_z & 0 & -w_x & v_2 \\ -w_y & w_x & 0 & v_3 \\ 0 & 0 & 0 & 0 \end{pmatrix},$$

such that $G = e^{\tilde{\xi}} = \text{Id} + \tilde{\xi} + \frac{\tilde{\xi}^2}{2} + \frac{\tilde{\xi}^3}{6} + \cdots$

We define the pose of an object as $\xi = (v_1, v_2, v_3, w_x, w_y, w_z)^\top$. A point q_0 in the object frame is projected onto the image location (x_{im}, y_{im}) with:

$$\begin{pmatrix} x_{im} \\ y_{im} \end{pmatrix} = \begin{pmatrix} 1 & 0 & 0 & 0 \\ 0 & 1 & 0 & 0 \end{pmatrix} \cdot s \cdot M_C^{-1} \cdot e^{\tilde{\xi}} \cdot q_0. \tag{3}$$

The image motion of point (x_{im}, y_{im}) from time t to time $t + 1$ is:

$$\begin{pmatrix} u_x \\ u_y \end{pmatrix} = \begin{pmatrix} x_{im}(t+1) - x_{im}(t) \\ y_{im}(t+1) - y_{im}(t) \end{pmatrix}.$$

By using (3) we can write the previous expression as:

$$\begin{pmatrix} u_x \\ u_y \end{pmatrix} = \begin{pmatrix} 1 & 0 & 0 & 0 \\ 0 & 1 & 0 & 0 \end{pmatrix} \cdot M_C^{-1} \left((1 + s') \cdot e^{\tilde{\xi}'} - \text{Id} \right) \cdot s(t) \cdot q_r,$$

with $\xi' = (v_1', v_2', v_3', w_x', w_y', w_z')^\top$ such that $e^{\tilde{\xi}(t+1)} = e^{\tilde{\xi}'} e^{\tilde{\xi}(t)}$ and $s' = \frac{s(t+1)}{s(t)} - 1$.

We assume that the scale change due to the motion is negligible from frame to frame, since the objects are far from the camera. Therefore $s' = 0$.

Assuming that the motion is small, i.e., the ellipsoid center moves a few centimeters and the axis orientation changes a few degrees, we have $\|\xi'\| \ll 1$. We approximate the matrix $e^{\tilde{\xi}'}$ by $\text{Id} + \tilde{\xi}'$. Experimentally, we confirm that the approximation is very good.

We rewrite the previous expression as:

$$\begin{pmatrix} u_x \\ u_y \end{pmatrix} = \begin{pmatrix} 1 & 0 & 0 & 0 \\ 0 & 1 & 0 & 0 \end{pmatrix} \cdot M_C^{-1} \cdot \tilde{\xi}' \cdot s(t) \cdot M_C \cdot q_c. \tag{4}$$

The value of ϕ is $(v_1', v_2', v_3', w_x', w_y', w_z')^\top$, which are the optimization variables of the problem.

Based on (4), for a pixel (x, y), we need only calculate q_c to describe the image motion in terms of the motion parameters ϕ. The 3D point q_c is calculated by intersecting with the ellipsoid a ray orthogonal to the camera image pixel. To do so, we associate with each pixel at t_0 the corresponding z_c of the closest point on the ellipsoid surface that is projected onto that pixel.

The parameters ϕ are independent of the camera. Hence, when we add more cameras, no new variables are needed but more constraints are added.

4   Kinematic Chain

The parameterization of a single body part P_1 has been discussed in the previous section. Assume that a second body part P_2 is attached to the first one in a point and that $E_{P_1}(\phi_1) + E_{P_2}(\phi_2)$ is the new functionals to be minimized that includes both parts. The optimization has to take into account the fact that the parts share a point when they move, by means of a kinematic constraint.

Let p_1 and p_2 be the coordinates of the shared point in the two object frames. Let $\tilde{\xi}_1, \tilde{\xi}_1{}', \tilde{\xi}_2$ and $\tilde{\xi}_2{}'$ be the twist and its change for each part as in the previous section. In order to keep the parts attached, the following equality must be true:

$$e^{\tilde{\xi}_1{}'} e^{\tilde{\xi}_1} \cdot p_1 = e^{\tilde{\xi}_2{}'} e^{\tilde{\xi}_2} \cdot p_2.$$

If the point was shared at frame t, it is true that

$$e^{\tilde{\xi}_1} \cdot p_1 = e^{\tilde{\xi}_2} \cdot p_2 = p_r$$

where p_r are the coordinates of the joint in the reference system. Hence, the constraint simplifies to

$$e^{\tilde{\xi}_1{}'} \cdot p_r = e^{\tilde{\xi}_2{}'} \cdot p_r$$

and using again the first order approximation of the exponential function, it leads to

$$C(\phi_1, \phi_2) = \tilde{\xi}_1{}' \cdot p_r - \tilde{\xi}_2{}' \cdot p_r = 0.$$

The linear equations $C = 0$ above can be used to express three variables in terms of the others, and reduce the number of variables in half. This approach may have the problem that constraints the relative motion to be perfect rotations which, in practice, are not. When n parts are used, the number of variables is $3n + 3$; the last 3 comes from the fact that there is one part (the trunk) that does not depend on any other part, and uses 6 degrees of freedom. This is the approach taken, because the gains of reducing the number of variables are more important that its drawbacks.

5   Multiple Cameras

The use of several cameras reduces the motion ambiguity that comes from having only one camera. The motion parameter ϕ for each part does not depend on a camera, so there is no need to introduce new variables. For each part P and camera c, a term $E_{P,c}$ is added to the functional to be minimized. Therefore, cameras can be easily added or dropped without changing the number of variables or the optimization procedure. For each camera, its associated matrix M must be supplied from calibration.

In fact, at least two cameras are needed if the virtual ellipsoids in the original frame have to be easily positioned by the user without taking real measurements in the recording setting. The user could point to the extreme points of the ellipsoids in two views and the system can easily get their 3D position.

6   The Use of Color

Color also reduces significantly the ambiguity during tracking specially in the absence of textured surfaces.

In the HSL representation, the Hue represents an angle and, therefore, it has a discontinuity between 2π and 0. Following [ROK00], we change coordinates and define:
$$h = S\cos H, \quad s = S\sin H, \quad l = L.$$

The intensity value I used in the previous sections can be one of the three color channels, that we represent as I_h, I_s and I_l. It is well known [PK94] that for tracking purposes the L component is less stable than the others on the same object due to illumination changes; therefore, we give double weight to the other components. In Equation 1, $\rho(\Delta I)$ is replaced for

$$0.4\rho(\Delta I_h) + 0.4\rho(\Delta I_s) + 0.2\rho(\Delta I_l).$$

A similar replacement is done in Equation 2.

When the input images are black and white, H=S=0 and the only channel useful is L. Thus our system handless both color and black and white cameras, and even a mixture of them.

7   Multi-scale Analysis

A multi-scale analysis, as in [WHA93], was implemented. Frame images, and virtual projections are zoomed out with a Gaussian filter. Motion estimation at a rough scale is used as an initial solution(seed) of the optimization procedure at a finer scale. In our approach, the use of a rougher scale has an efficiency advantage: Since images are smaller more iterations and more possibilities (offsprings) can be considered in the search procedure; in a finer scale, the solution should improve according to the improved image precision.

8   Optimization

To minimize the functional E, that includes a term for each part, camera and color channel, we use a genetic algorithm described in [Mic96] that works well on non-linear optimization problems. The representation used for the possible solutions is simply a vector of dimension equal to the number of variables (3 for each part). The fitting function is E.

The system starts with a number of initial values (seeds) for ϕ, for each part, that include some values randomly calculated, and an initial value that is the solution of the previous frame (0 for the first frame) for the rougher scale, and the solution of the scale above for finer scales.

The population of values is replaced by 25%, and there are 10 offsprings for each of the above. The operators used are whole and simple arithmetical crossover, uniform mutation, boundary mutation, non-uniform mutation, whole non-uniform mutation, heuristic crossover, Gaussian mutation and pool recombination. The experiments use between 500 and 1000 iterations. There is, of course, no guaranty that a global optimum is found.

9   Implementation

Using the camera calibration, the user sets the ellipsoid poses at time 0 so that its projections coincide with the three real body parts to be tracked in each view. This is done by calculating the best 3D coordinates for the image positions such as wrist, elbow, knee, etc. The shape parameters of each part are also set manually for the whole film.

The system then tracks each virtual part in 3D: First, the virtual projections are calculated at frame t; for each pixel in the image range, it calculates the 3D position of a point on the ellipsoid that is projected onto the pixel. Frame $t + 1$ is then loaded. An iterative procedure begins that initializes $\phi_0 = 0$. At iteration n, the function is evaluated for certain value of ϕ. The (u_x, u_y) displacement is estimated using the pose change ϕ for each pixel (x, y). The difference of image intensities between the pixel $(x + u_x, y + u_y)$ at frame $t + 1$ and the pixel (x, y) at frame t is accumulated for all pixels, and also the variation of the same pixel in $t + 1$ with respect to the average in $t = 0$ for the corresponding part. For the experiments, The value of ϕ that minimizes the functional within all the iterations is used to calculate the $t + 1$ pose. The procedure starts again for the next frame.

10   Experiments

Experiments were designed to test the system performance. There are several issues to check. First of all, the system should work on different films, with different body parts. Second, we would like to know the importance of color tracking. And third, some comparison is needed with respect to systems that do not use a robust function.

A Pentium II processor at 450 MHz. is used. The frames are 640×480 pixels, and the cameras are situated between three and five meters from the subject. The parameter σ for the robust function is $0.5 \times MaxQ$, where $MaxQ$ is the number of quantization levels for a color channel, in our case 2^{16}.

10.1   A Black and White Film

A subject is filmed by three Black and White cameras. Three ellipsoids are used to track the three parts of an arm. See Figure 3. Several levels of resolution were tried. The system works well using using the finest, first, level or the second. Since, the results on the second level are good enough and we can get them faster, we report only on them. Also, if both levels are used, the results are not significantly better than using only the second level.

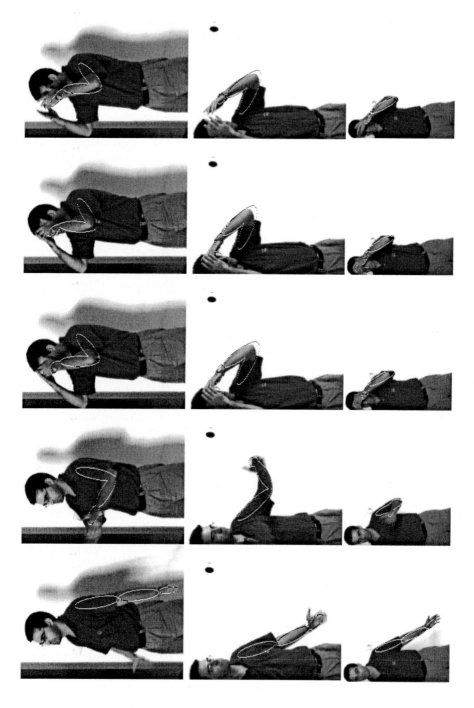

Fig. 3. Arm tracking in Black and White.

The kinematic constraints used keep the articulations connected, and also the shoulder is fixed in space in the virtual model.

50 frames (the whole sequence) can be tracked correctly using the second level. If only the third level is used, only 10 frames are tracked before the ellipsoids loose track of their corresponding body parts. At this level, the motion is not very clear in all the views because of the low resolution. Using two levels the system processes approximately 0.8 frame/min. Using only the second level, the speed is 2 frames/min.

In some frames the virtual elbow does not coincide with the real elbow; it seems that the original position given by the user for the shoulder was not correct, and the upper-arm length does not fit in the corresponding region. Still, the system is able to track the arm.

10.2   Arm Tracking within a Color Film

Another sequence was captured using two color cameras. The arm was selected again because of its visibility and mobility. The results are in Figures 4 and 5. The shoulder is also assumed fixed in space.

Using only the second level, the system starts in frame 0 and tracks 270 frames, which is the length of the whole sequence. After frame 120 (see the previous to the last frame shown) the subject moves the shoulder, so the virtual arm cannot cover the hand. However, 30 frames later the system has recovered the hand because it tries to keep the original colors of the parts. The throughput is 2.8 frames/min.

If the first resolution level is used, no better results are found, since the results at the second level are already very good. It just makes the system slower. If only the third level is used, the system cannot track more than 20 frames, although the arm motion is still very clear at that level; maybe the optimization algorithm is not good enough, but it is still unclear why the system does not work at the lowest level of resolution tried.

If only the black and white information is used (the L component) the ellipsoids loose track of their parts when the subject moves the shoulder and does not recover. This means that the color information makes the system more reliable.

10.3   Leg Tracking

A sequence was filmed with two color cameras and a leg was tracked with three ellipsoids. The tip of the foot is assumed fixed in space.

Figure 6 shows the results. The subject wears very dark clothes so the color information is not very useful. Also, since there is no change of texture or color between the parts, the sequence is really challenging. The system tracks correctly 40 frames. It is clear that if the virtual model includes a part for the trunk the setting would have less ambiguity, i.e., virtual legs could not move freely in the trunk regions.

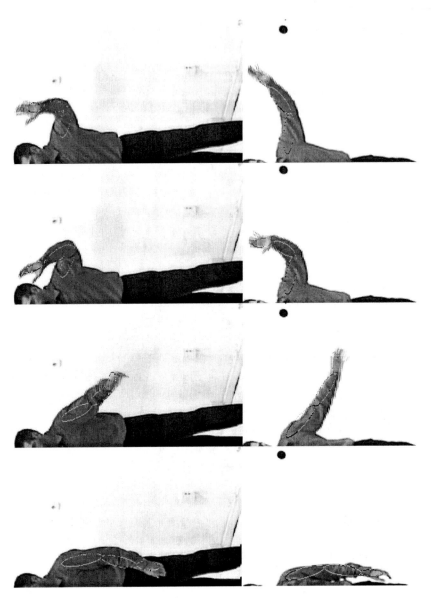

Fig. 4. Arm tracking.

10.4   Robustness

We would like to compare the system performance with respect to systems that
are not robust. To do so, we changed the value of σ in the previous experiments
and compare the results until a fixed frame. If σ is $1.0 \times MaxQ$, ρ is almost
lineal in the range of intensity variation and, therefore, a large variation counts
more than a small one. If σ is $0.5 \times MaxQ$, ρ does not count large variations
necessarily more than small ones, and outliers have less importance.

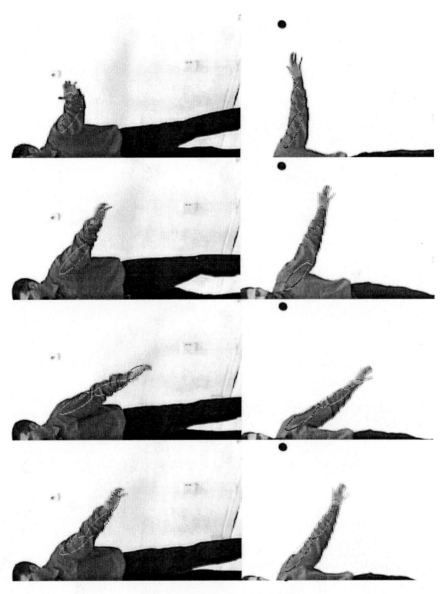

Fig. 5. Arm tracking (cont.).

Figure 7 shows different results for different values of σ: 0.2, 0.4, 0.6, 0.8 and 1.0 of $MaxQ$. We can see that values under 1.0 are better than the others. We also had similar results for the two arm sequences, but are not shown for paper limitations. In the color tracking of the arm, there is not a significant performance difference at that frame (80) when the value of σ is changed.

As we said before, we choose a value in the middle of the above, $\sigma = 0.5 \times MaxQ$, for all the previous experiments.

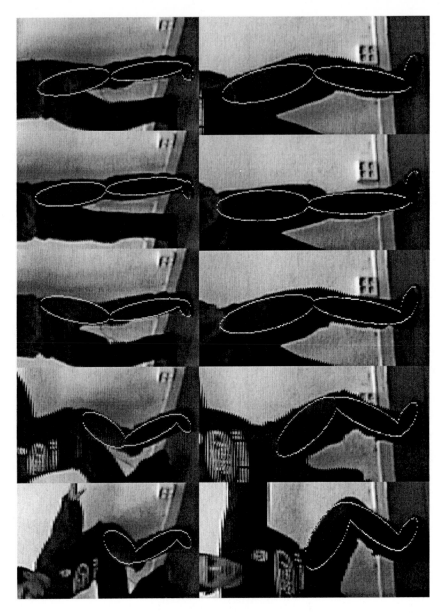

Fig. 6. Leg tracking.

On another experiment with the color tracking of an arm, the function ρ was replaced by a simple absolute value. In this case, the tracking was poorer: Arm and hand were farther from their true directions during most of the sequence, covering background regions. In a sense, the robust function adds tracking stability.

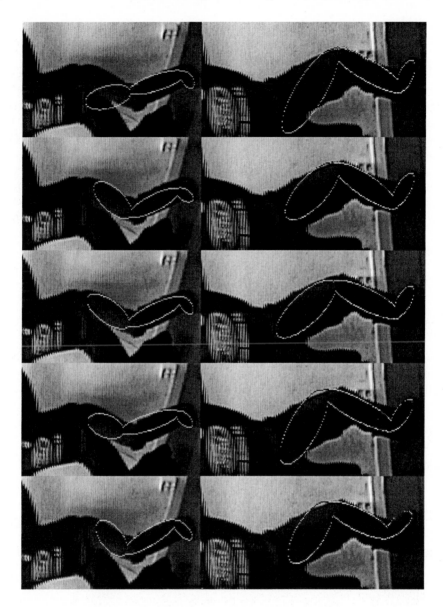

Fig. 7. Robustness comparison of "leg" sequence.

11   Conclusions and Future Work

We have presented a theoretical framework for robust tracking of human parts based on a 3D model. Our experiments show that the robust estimation of motion parameters works better than non-robust estimations, but more testing is needed. Also, the use of color makes the system able to recover easily from tracking errors.

A more reliable global optimization technique may be needed. However, the use of more information from all the body parts may accelerate the convergence in a space of around 45 dimensions.

It is also expected that if more realistic parts are used for the virtual model, less motion ambiguity is allowed and we would get better results. Also better rendering techniques (perspective projection) that usually come with a virtual humanoid may also help. But, if the virtual parts fit better the real parts, less motion flexibility is allowed to compensate for not perfect rotations. It is possible that the robustness be even more important.

Better color representations (e.g. LUV or Lab) can also be used, and different robust parameters for each term of the functional can be tried (difference with frame 0, with previous frame, for each part, and color channel of each camera).

Although the multi-scale analysis was not useful in our experiments, except for finding a resolution level of fast and correct tracking, it may prove to be essential when the full body be tracked.

We consider that our results are promising and that it is worth pursuing further this research.

Acknowledgements

José María Buades calibrated and synchronized the cameras. Isabel Miró helped with the implementation. This research is supported by the Spanish Education and Culture Ministery, under the project TIC98-0302-C0201.

References

[BM97]   C. Bregler and J. Malik. Video motion capture. http://www.cs.berkely.edu/~bregler/digmuy.html, 1997.   UCB-CSD-97-973.

[HHD98]   I. Haritauglu, D. Harwood, and L. Davis. W^4S: A real-time system for detecting and tracking people in $2\frac{1}{2}$D. *Computer Vision- ECCV'98*, 1406:877–892, 1998.

[HKJ97]   E. Hunter, P. Kelly, and R. Jain. Estimation of articulated motion using kinematically constrained mixture densities. In *Proceedings of IEEE Non-Rigid and Articulated Motion Workshop*, pages 10–17, Puerto Rico, USA, 1997.

[JBY96]   S. Ju, M. Black, and Y. Yacoob. Carboard People: A Parameterized model of articulated image motion. In *2nd International Conference on Face and Gesture Analysis*, pages 38–44, Vermont, USA, 1996.

[Mic96]   Z. Michalewicz. *Genetic Algorithms + Data Structures = Evolution Programs*. Springer-Verlag, 1996.

[MLS94]   R. Murray, Z. Li, and S. Sastry. *A Mathematical Introduction to Robotic Manipulation*. CRC Press, 1994.

[PK94]   Frank Perez and Christof Koch.   Toward color image segmentation in analog VLSI:Algorithm and hardware. *Int. Journal of Computer Vision*, 12(1):17–42, Feb. 1994.

[ROK00]   M. Rautiainen, T. Ojila, and H. Kauniskangas. Detecting perceptual color changes from sequential images for scene surveillance. In *Proc. Workshop on Machine Vision Applications*, pages 140–143, Tokyo, Japan, 2000.

[WADP97]   C. Wren, A. Azarbayejani, T. Darrel, and A. Pentland. Pfinder: Real-time tracking of the human body. *IEEE trans. on PAMI*, 19(7):780–785, July 1997.

[WHA93]   J. Weng, T. Huang, and N. Ahuja. *Motion and Structure from Image Sequences*, volume 29 of *Series in Informacion Sciences*. Springer-Verlag, 1993.

[WN97]   S. Wachter and H. Nagel. Tracking of persons in monocular image sequences. In *Proceedings of IEEE Non-Rigid and Articulated Motion Workshop*, pages 2–9, Puerto Rico, USA, 1997.

[WP00]   C. Wren and A. Pentland. Understanding purposeful human motion. In *Fourth IEEE Int. Conf. on Automatic Face and Gesture Recognition*, 2000.

Part II

Image Modelling and Synthesis

Learning Matrix Space Image Representations

Anand Rangarajan[1]

Department of Computer and Information Science and Engineering
University of Florida
Gainesville, FL 32611-6120, US
anand@cise.ufl.edu

Abstract. When we seek to directly learn basis functions from natural scenes, we are confronted with the problem of simultaneous estimation of these basis functions and the coefficients of each image (when projected onto that basis). In this work, we are mainly interested in learning matrix space basis functions and the projection coefficients from a set of natural images. We cast this problem in a joint optimization framework. The Frobenius norm is used to express the distance between a natural image and its matrix space reconstruction. An alternating algorithm is derived to simultaneously solve for the basis vectors and the projection coefficients. Since our fundamental goal is classification and indexing, we develop a matrix space distance measure between images in the training set. Results are shown on face images and natural scenes.

1 Introduction

In recent years, there has been a lot of progress in the mathematical representation of natural scenes [7]. Once it became clear that coding methods using the discrete cosine transform (DCT) [9], Gabor expansions [4], wavelets [3], etc. were quite successful in generating compact codes for images, there was an increased interest in directly *learning* such bases from natural images. Directly learning the basis vectors presents a more challenging computational problem than the usual coding case, because in the former, *both* the bases and the coefficients have to be estimated from the natural images.

The most comprehensive work in this general area of simultaneous estimation of both basis vectors and coefficients is the work of Olshausen and his collaborators [7, 6, 8]. In this body or work, the main interest is in learning compact and (usually) *overcomplete* representations of natural scenes. In this approach, a joint optimization problem is typically constructed on both the basis vectors and the coefficients. A regularization prior is always added to enforce prior knowledge of *sparsity* of the coefficients. Recently, this work has evolved toward adding a mixture of Gaussians prior [8] in order to enforce the constraints of sparsity and distributivity of the coefficients.

In this paper, we are mainly interested in recasting this problem of simultaneous estimation of bases and coefficients in a matrix space. We wish to point out that matrix space representations of natural images has been mostly ignored

M.A.T. Figueiredo, J. Zerubia, A.K. Jain (Eds.): EMMCVPR 2001, LNCS 2134, pp. 153–168, 2001.

despite the fact that it is mostly common knowledge that the singular value decomposition (SVD) [5] is sometimes a good choice for image representation and compression [10]. However, all the previous work (that we are aware of) on SVD-based image representation is focused on single images. There is no previous work on estimating *common matrix space bases* from a set of natural images. To state the goal of this paper, we wish to simultaneously learn a matrix basis set and the projection coefficients of each image. Given a set of 2D grayscale natural images, we represent each of them as matrics and then formulate the learning problem as a *joint optimization* of matrix basis vectors and projection coefficients.

In contrast to earlier work by Olshausen and his collaborators [7], our primary motivation is not to develop a compact *code* based on the statistics of natural scenes. Instead, we are more interested in common matrix space representations for the purposes of recognition, classification and indexing. That is, we believe that matrix space representations can be used to develop new matrix space distance measures for the purposes of classification and indexing. Some of the experimental results presented in the paper aim toward this goal.

2   Grayscale Intensity Images as Matrices

As mentioned in the Introduction, we are mainly motivated by the overall success of image coding. Our principal aim in this paper is to learn a common matrix space representation from a set of images without any *a priori* knowledge of the basis set or of the projection coefficients. The fundamental idea is to express each grayscale intensity image as a matrix and then investigate the extent to which compact coding allows us to extract a common matrix basis from the set of pregiven images. Since coding works and works well, we expect that each image is expressible by a compact set of basis vectors and coefficients. For example, it is well known though not so widely exploited that the SVD representation of a 2D grayscale intensity image has a spectrum that rapidly falls to zero [10].

Denote by X, the matrix corresponding to a grayscale intensity image. The SVD of the image is given by

$$X = USV^T \tag{1}$$

where $U^T U = V^T V = I$. Since the image matrix need not be square, note that the dimensions of the U and V matrices can be different. Reconstructions of the original image using a set of D components can be written as

$$\hat{X} = \sum_{i=1}^{D} s(i,i) u_i v_i^T \tag{2}$$

where u_i and v_i are the ith eigenvectors.

In Figures 1 and 2, we show the spectrum of the well known Lenna image and the SVD-based reconstructions respectively. The first 5 SVD component images (computed as $u_i v_i^T$) are also shown in Figure 2. It is evident from both the

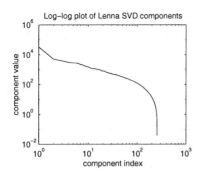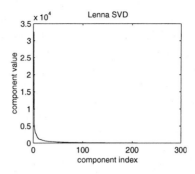

Fig. 1. Spectrum of the Lenna image (256×256). Left: Log-log plot of the spectrum. Right: Spectrum plot. Note the almost linear nature of the log-log spectrum for the dominant singular values.

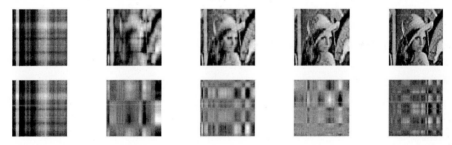

Fig. 2. Lenna reconstructions and components: Top row: Reconstructions using 1, 5, 10, 15 and 20 components. Bottom row: The SVD component images $u_i v_i^T$ corresponding to the first five components.

spectrum plots and the component images that the spatial frequencies tend to vary in inverse proportion to the SVD coefficients; higher the spatial frequencies in a component image, the smaller the SVD coefficient and vice versa. The rapidity with which the SVD coefficients fall off is evident from Figure 2.

3   Learning a Common Reference Frame

We now embark upon the formulation of the problem. Since we wish to represent 2D grayscale intensity images as matrices, the technical challenge is one of finding a common eigen reference basis set of vectors to represent all of the images in the chosen set. Since we have decided to use a matrix space representation for the non-square images, the common eigen reference frame consists of a set of row eigen vectors, each of which has a corresponding counterpart in the set of column eigen vectors. Insofar as only the eigen reference frame is deemed common, the projections of each image in the chosen set onto the basis will be different *and* unknown *a priori*. Consequently, not only do we have to learn the common eigen reference frame, in addition, we have to compute the projections of each image onto the reference in order to determine the representation error.

Let the set $\{X_k, \ k \in \{1, \ldots, K\}\}$ denote the collection of images. The common eigen reference frame is denoted by the pair (U, V) which is intended to invoke the SVD association. The projection of image X_k onto the basis set is denoted by Λ_k with the set $\{\Lambda_k, \ k \in \{1, \ldots, K\}\}$ denoting the set of projections. Each image X_k is of size $M \times N$ and the sizes of the basis sets U and V are $M \times D$ and $N \times D$ respectively. The size of each Λ_k is $D \times D$. Note that each $\Lambda_k, \ k \in \{1, \ldots, K\}$ is *diagonal* since it is a projection onto the basis set. Inequalities, such as $D < \min(M, N)$ hold as a consequence of orthogonality conditions on U and V.

The central technical contribution of this paper is a mathematical unpacking of the following intuition: A reasonable criterion for learning the basis set $(\hat{U}, \hat{V})$ is to minimize the representation error of each image X_k in the set of K images when projected onto the *space* of basis sets (U, V). This criterion is somewhat complicated by the fact that the projections of the images onto the basis set are themselves computed after the basis set is fixed.

We use the Frobenius norm $||A||_F^2 = \sum_{ij} |a_{ij}|^2$ to mathematically characterize the representation error [5]. This norm is chosen because of its close relationship to the matrix spectra. The central cost function used in this paper is

$$(\hat{U}, \hat{V}) = \min_{(U,V)} E_{\text{matrixbasis}}(U, V) = \min_{(U,V)} \sum_{k=1}^{K} ||X_k - U\Lambda_k V^T||_F^2 \qquad (3)$$

with

$$\Lambda_k = \text{diag } (U^T X_k V), \ k \in \{1, \ldots, K\} \qquad (4)$$

and the constraints

$$U^T U = I_D \text{ and } V^T V = I_D. \qquad (5)$$

Equation (4) relates the projection Λ_k with the basis set (U, V). The **diag** operator emphasizes the fact that each Λ_k is diagonal. In this paper, we have elected not to treat the projections as quasi-independent variables. Following [8], it is certainly possible to treat Λ_k as a separate variable and associate a Bayesian regularization prior with it. We have not done so for reasons of simplicity at this preliminary stage. The constraints in (5) express the fact that U and V are orthonormal which in sync with their treatment as SVD-like bases. Note that we have also not chosen to enforce the constraint that each diagonal entry in Λ_k is strictly positive. For $U\Lambda_k V^T$ to be linked to an SVD representation, this constraint has to be active. However, we merely treat the reference basis as "SVD-like" in this paper. This constraint can also be enforced as a Bayesian prior if needed.

We now derive an alternating algorithm to minimize the energy function in (3). First, we enforce the orthogonality constraints in (5) using Lagrange parameters [1]. The Frobenius norm is also rewritten using matrix operators.

$$E_{\text{matrixbasis}}(U, V, \mu, \nu) = \sum_{k=1}^{K} \text{trace } [(X_k - U\Lambda_k V^T)^T (X_k - U\Lambda_k V^T)]$$

$$+ \text{trace } [\mu(U^T U - I_D)] + \text{trace } [\nu(V^T V - I_D)] \qquad (6)$$

with the understanding that $\Lambda_k = \mathrm{diag}\,(U^T X_k V)$. The Lagrange parameter matrices μ and ν are both *symmetric* [1] $D \times D$ matrices. This energy function can be further transformed by dropping terms not involving the basis set (U, V) and by enforcing the orthogonality constraints in the matrix representation error norm.

$$E_{\mathrm{matrixbasis}}(U, V, \mu, \nu) = -2 \sum_{k=1}^{K} \mathrm{trace}\,[X_k^T U \Lambda_k V^T)]$$

$$+\mathrm{trace}\,[\mu(U^T U - I_D)] + \mathrm{trace}\,[\nu(V^T V - I_D)] \tag{7}$$

To derive the alternating algorithm, we first hold V fixed and solve for U in (7). Then we alternate by solving for V given U. Once U and V are updated, Λ_k is updated $\forall k \in \{1, \ldots, K\}$ in order to be in lockstep with the basis set (U, V). Differentiating (7) w.r.t. U and setting the result to zero, we get

$$\sum_{k=1}^{K} X_k V \Lambda_k = \hat{U}\mu \Rightarrow \hat{U} = \sum_{k=1}^{K} X_k V \Lambda_k \mu^{-1}. \tag{8}$$

Enforcing the orthogonality constraint for U, (8) is transformed into

$$\hat{U}^T \hat{U} = \mu^{-1} \left(\sum_{k=1}^{K} X_k V \Lambda_k \right)^T \left(\sum_{k=1}^{K} X_k V \Lambda_k \right) \mu^{-1} = I_D$$

$$\Rightarrow \mu^2 = \left(\sum_{k=1}^{K} X_k V \Lambda_k \right)^T \left(\sum_{k=1}^{K} X_k V \Lambda_k \right)$$

$$\Rightarrow \mu = \left[\left(\sum_{k=1}^{K} X_k V \Lambda_k \right)^T \left(\sum_{k=1}^{K} X_k V \Lambda_k \right) \right]^{\frac{1}{2}}$$

$$\Rightarrow \hat{U} = \sum_{k=1}^{K} X_k V \Lambda_k \left[\left(\sum_{k=1}^{K} X_k V \Lambda_k \right)^T \left(\sum_{k=1}^{K} X_k V \Lambda_k \right) \right]^{-\frac{1}{2}}. \tag{9}$$

The above solution for U is obtained relative to a fixed V. Completely analogous to (8) and (9), we can solve for V relative to a fixed U.

$$\hat{V} = \sum_{k=1}^{K} X_k^T U \Lambda_k \left[\left(\sum_{k=1}^{K} X_k^T U \Lambda_k \right)^T \left(\sum_{k=1}^{K} X_k^T U \Lambda_k \right) \right]^{-\frac{1}{2}}. \tag{10}$$

Once we've obtained a candidate basis set (U, V), we keep each Λ_k in lockstep with the basis by setting

$$\Lambda_k = \mathrm{diag}\,\left(\hat{U}^T X_k \hat{V} \right). \tag{11}$$

The overall algorithm is summarized below.

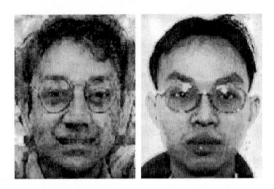

Fig. 3. Original images. Left: Face 1. Right: Face 2.

Learning Matrix Representations

Initialize U, V to random $M \times D$ and $N \times D$ matrices respectively.

Begin A: Do A until $\Delta E < \Delta E_{\mathrm{thr}}$.

$U^{\mathrm{old}} = U$, $V^{\mathrm{old}} = V$, $\Lambda_k^{\mathrm{old}} = \Lambda_k$, $\forall k \in \{1, \ldots, K\}$.

$\Lambda_k = \mathrm{diag}\left(U^T X_k V\right)$, $\forall k \in \{1, \ldots, K\}$.

$$U = \sum_{k=1}^{K} X_k V \Lambda_k \left[\left(\sum_{k=1}^{K} X_k V \Lambda_k\right)^T \left(\sum_{k=1}^{K} X_k V \Lambda_k\right) \right]^{-\frac{1}{2}}.$$

$\Lambda_k = \mathrm{diag}\left(U^T X_k V\right)$, $\forall k \in \{1, \ldots, K\}$.

$$V = \sum_{k=1}^{K} X_k^T U \Lambda_k \left[\left(\sum_{k=1}^{K} X_k^T U \Lambda_k\right)^T \left(\sum_{k=1}^{K} X_k^T U \Lambda_k\right) \right]^{-\frac{1}{2}}.$$

$$\Delta E = \sum_{k=1}^{K} \left(||X_k - U^{\mathrm{old}} \Lambda_k^{\mathrm{old}} (V^{\mathrm{old}})^T||_F^2 - ||X_k - U \Lambda_k V^T||_F^2 \right).$$

End A

A theoretical proof showing that the energy in (6) decreases in each step is not easily forthcoming. This is due to the obvious heuristic device we have employed for updating each Λ_k. In contrast, showing that the energy decreases due to the U and V updates is relatively straightforward due to the updates being constrained least-squares solutions. In all experiments, we have merely executed the above algorithm until an iteration cap is exceeded. We have not encountered any stability problems when executing the above algorithm. This is quite surprising as one would have expected numerical errors to create problems when taking the relevant matrix inverses and square roots. As mentioned in the next section, no effort was made to implement the matrix inverses and square roots in a computationally efficient manner. The matrix routines in Matlab^{TM} 5.3 were used in all computations.

4   Results

Two face images are shown in Figure 3. The images have been registered using a non-rigid registration method [2]. Both images are originally 330×228 and have been down sampled to 150×114.

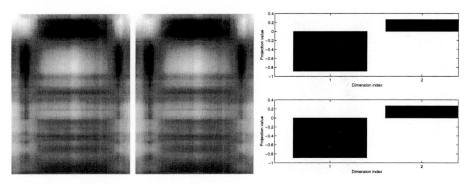

Fig. 4. Reconstructed faces using 2 components Left: Face 1. Middle: Face 2. Right: Projections.

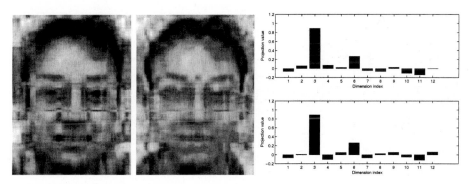

Fig. 5. Reconstructed faces using 12 components Left: Face 1. Middle: Face 2. Right: Projections.

In Figures 4 through 8, we present the results of learning a common matrix space reference frame beginning with two components and moving up to 100 components. In each figure, the reconstructed faces are presented along with the projection coefficients $[\mathrm{diag}(\hat{U}^T X_k \hat{V})]$. The first reconstruction with two components turned out to be identical for both faces, i.e.

$$\hat{U}\Lambda_1\hat{V}^T = \hat{U}\Lambda_2\hat{V}^T.$$

In the reconstructions (which are identical), the hair texture evident in face 1 is clearly discernible. In addition, the reconstruction has the appearance of a fuzzy face. As the number of basis components are increased, the quality of the reconstruction improves as can be seen in the progression from Figure 4 to Figure 8.

Examine the projection bar charts in Figure 4, Figure 5 and Figure 6. The bar charts are a visualization of the projection coefficients. Note the extensive similarities in the projection coefficients. They start out identical in Figure 4 and continue to be strongly related as can be seen in Figure 6. We return to this issue later.

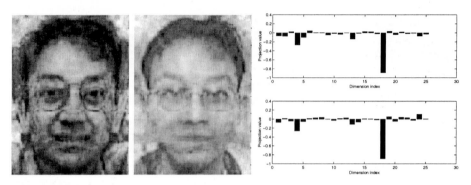

Fig. 6. Reconstructed faces using 25 components Left: Face 1. Middle: Face 2.
Right: Projections.

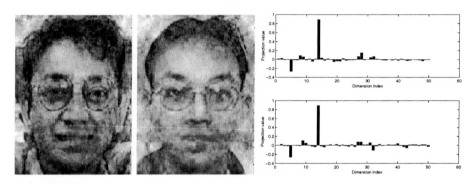

Fig. 7. Reconstructed faces using 50 components Left: Face 1. Middle: Face 2.
Right: Projections.

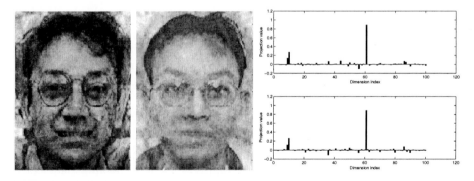

Fig. 8. Reconstructed faces using 100 components Left: Face 1. Middle: Face 2.
Right: Projections.

After reconstructing faces 1 and 2 using 12 basis components, in Figure 9
we visualize six leading common components. This was done by only visualizing
those components for which the projections in *both* face 1 and face 2 were large.
Each image shown in Figure 9 corresponds to a component $u_k v_k^T$ where k is

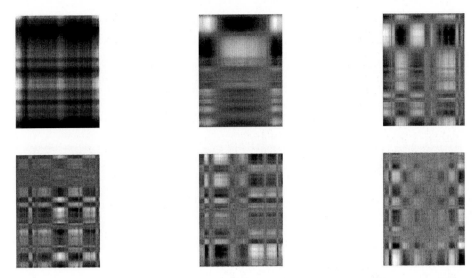

Fig. 9. Reconstruction using 12 components: First six components of the shared representation. Top: Components one through three. Bottom: Components four through six.

the component index. The first component image is not particularly informative but it does correspond to the largest projection value in both face images. The second component image is a different story. It bears a striking resemblence to the reconstruction using two components as shown in Figure 4. The remaining component images show increased spatial frequencies but do not have easily discernible patterns.

Next, we learn a common basis set for three very different images; a baboon, an outdoor scene with a boat and a girl. (Each image is 256×256). Prior to reconstruction, we normalized the spectra of the three images in the following manner. First, we evaluated the number of SVD components necessary to reconstruct each image with minimal loss. Then, we normalized the spectra of each image relative to the mean spectrum. The images before and after normalization are shown below in Figure 10. There are almost no visible perceptible differences.

After normalizing the spectra, we reconstructed the images using 12, 25, 50, 100 and 200 components. The results are shown in Figure 11. Somewhat to our surprise, the original images are discernible in the reconstructions using only 25 components. After about 50 components, there is no clear visual improvement which is also surprising. To take stock of what has been achieved, please note that the 25 component reconstructions use *a common matrix space basis for all three images*. Since the original images are quite different, it is not immediately obvious why the reconstructions should so closely resemble the originals.

For a more quantitative understanding of the above reconstructions, we turn to Table 1. From the table, we see that the reconstruction error $||X_k - \hat{U}\Lambda_k V^T||_F^2$ for the girl image is worse than that of the baboon and the boat images. (Recall

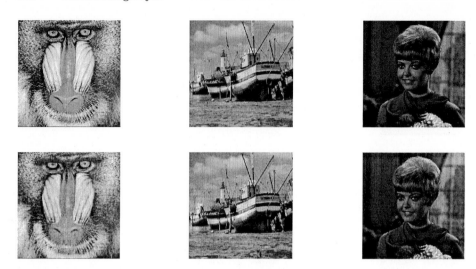

Fig. 10. Top row: Original baboon, boat and girl images. Bottom row: The same images after spectrum normalization.

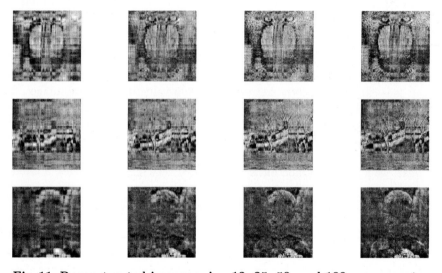

Fig. 11. Reconstructed images using 12, 25, 50, and 100 components

that the images $\{X_k\}$ have normalized spectra with the largest singular value set to one.) In addition to the reconstruction error, in Table 2, we compute the matrix space distances between the three images. The matrix space distance between image k and image l is defined as

$$D_{\text{matrixspace}}(X_k, X_l) \overset{\text{def}}{=} ||\hat{U}\Lambda_k\hat{V}^T - \hat{U}\Lambda_l V^T||_F^2 = ||\Lambda_k - \Lambda_l||_F^2 = \sum_{i=1}^{D}(\lambda_{ki} - \lambda_{li})^2$$

$$(12)$$

Table 1. Reconstruction errors for the baboon, boat and girl images using 50 components. The leading singular value for all three images is unity.

Reconstruction Error		
0.062	0.072	0.104

Table 2. Matrix space distances between the three images using 50 component reconstructions.

	0	0.079	0.115
	0.079	0	0.103
	0.115	0.103	0

Table 3. Reconstruction errors using 100 components.

0.058	0.153	0.217	0.078	0.079	0.048

where λ_{ki} is the ith projection coefficient of the kth reconstruction. Since the reconstructions are in a common matrix space, the image distances are naturally reduced to the distances between the projection coefficients. As before, the integer D denotes the number of components used for the reconstruction.

The next experiment further explores image distances when collapsed onto a single matrix space. We took six images—four faces, an outdoor scene and a fractal image—and reconstructed them using 100 components. Each image is 150×114. We first preprocess the images such that each image has its dominant singular value set to unity and with the rest of spectra normalized as previously

Table 4. Matrix space distances between the six images using 100 component reconstructions.

	0	0.0237	0.0430	0.0293	0.0619	0.0853
	0.0237	0	0.035	0.0212	0.0676	0.0832
	0.043	0.035	0	0.053	0.1146	0.1220
	0.0293	0.0212	0.053	0	0.0667	0.0794
	0.0619	0.0676	0.1146	0.0667	0	0.0817
	0.0853	0.0832	0.122	0.0794	0.0817	0

explained. The reconstruction errors and the matrix space distances are shown in Tables 3 and 4 respectively. From the reconstruction error table, it is clear that face images 2 and 3 have the worst reconstruction errors. Given this empirical fact, we turn to the matrix space distance table in Table 4. The distances from all the face images to the outdoor scene and the Julia set are by far the largest. There is not a single face-face distance which is greater than a face-non face distance. Consequently, the reconstruction error may not be a suitable measure by which to gauge the degree of membership of an image to the estimated matrix space.

Finally, we describe initial experiments in automated filter design using the matrix space representation. The basic idea closely follows the model used in PCA filter design with one crucial difference. From the chosen image, we randomly choose N $K \times K$ blocks where K is the order of the filter mask. Given the N $K \times K$ "images", we learn a common matrix basis as before. Once U and V have been learned, we display $u_i v_i^T$ as a $K \times K$ filter mask. There are a total of K different such filters to choose from for which we implemented the following rank ordering scheme. For each filter, we evaluated the total response over the entire image. The filters were rank ordered using the total response as the metric. The learned filters and the corresponding filtered images are shown

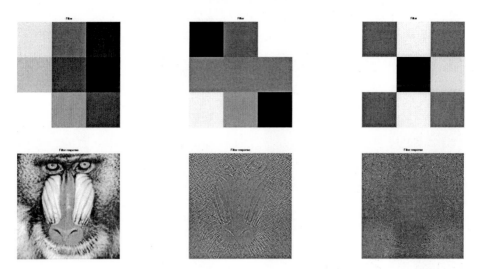

Fig. 12. Top: Learned 3 × 3 filters. Bottom: Corresponding filtered images. From left to right: Filters ranked according to strength of response.

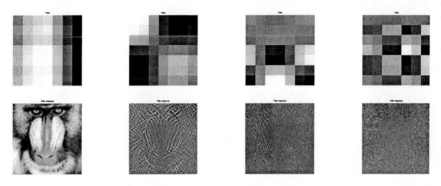

Fig. 13. Top: Learned 7 × 7 filters. Bottom: Corresponding filtered images. From left to right: Top 4 filters ranked according to strength of response.

for 3 × 3, 7 × 7 and 15 × 15 masks in Figures 12, 13 and 14 respectively. We noticed that the first two filters always corresponded to an intensity blur and a first derivative operator respectively. Visual inspection reveals that the filters appear to be ordered according to increasing spatial frequency.

5 Discussion, Extensions and Conclusion

5.1 Isn't This Just Principal Components (PCA)?

Not really. In most versions of PCA, the images are first converted into a vector followed by covariance matrix construction from the pattern vectors. In our approach, there is no covariance matrix formed. Instead, a common *matrix space*

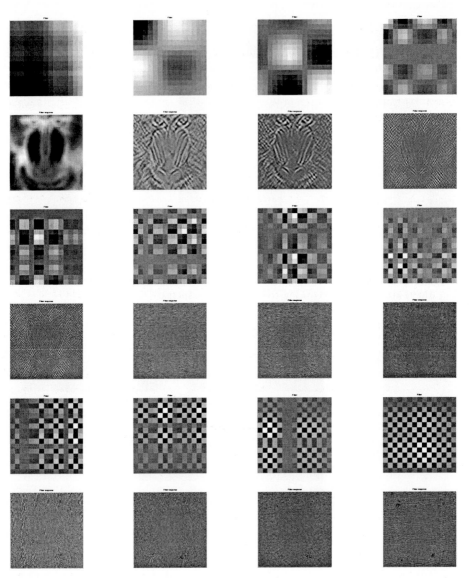

Fig. 14. Top Row: First four learned 15×15 filters. Second Row: Corresponding filtered images. Third Row: Filters 5,7,9 and 10 (15×15). Fourth Row: Corresponding filtered images. Fifth Row: Filters 12,13,14 and 15 (15×15). Sixth Row: Corresponding filtered images.

is estimated from the image intensity matrices. There is no denying the fact that matrix representations are at the heart of our approach as opposed to vector representations in PCA. Also, there is no statistical interpretation of matrix representations in terms of covariance matrices and dimensionality reduction as in PCA.

5.2   Matrix Space Distances

We view our initial experiments with matrix space distances as quite promising. Out of the six images in Table 4, two were non face images. The matrix space distances clearly and unambiguously group the face images together. The distances from each face image to the non-face images are always greater than the face-face image distances. If matrix space distance turns out to be a truly robust distance measure, it could have an impact in pattern clustering, object recognition and classification etc.

There are many ways in which the work presented here can be extended. We stress that the current algorithm is quite preliminary and one of our first goals is to add a regularization prior to better stabilize Λ_k. Once such priors are added, a more proper Bayesian justification (in terms of likelihood and prior) can be given. This would place this work in the context of earlier work by [8]. And there does not seem to be any obvious reason why mixtures of matrix bases cannot be considered in order to provide compact but *overcomplete* representations. Another promising direction of extension is the matrix space distance measure. We have only shown preliminary results of applying the distance measure on the training set. It is certainly possible to estimate basis vectors from different sets of training images and apply the matrix space distance measures to test sets as well.

In sum, we have derived a new learning algorithm for estimating matrix space representations of natural 2D grayscale images. Since the images use a common matrix basis, this allowed us to construct matrix space distances between them. Preliminary results indicate that matrix space image distances possess novel classification properties. While these initial results are promising, it remains to be seen if matrix space representations and distance measures are truly effective in image classification and recognition.

Acknowledgments

We thank Hemant Tagare, Baba Vemuri, Sudeep Sarkar and an anonymous reviewer for useful comments and criticisms. This work is partially supported by an NSF grant (IIS-9906081) to A.R.

References

1. C. Bishop. *Neural Networks for Pattern Recognition*. Oxford University Press, Oxford, 1995.
2. H. Chui and A. Rangarajan. A new algorithm for non-rigid point matching. In *IEEE Conf. on Computer Vision and Pattern Recognition (CVPR)*, volume 2, pages 44–51, 2000.
3. I. Daubechies. *Ten lectures on wavelets*. SIAM, 1992.
4. J. Daugman. Complete discrete 2D Gabor transforms by neural networks for image analysis and compression. *IEEE Trans. Acoustics, SPeech and Signal Proc.*, 7:1169–1179, July 1988.

5. G. Golub and C. Van Loan. *Matrix Computations*. Johns Hopkins University Press, 2nd edition, 1989.

6. M. Lewicki and B. Olshausen. Probabilistic framework for the adaptation and comparison of image codes. *J. Opt. Soc. America*, 16(7):1587–1601, 1999.

7. B. Olshausen and D. Field. Natural image statistics and efficient coding. *Network*, 7:333–339, 1996.

8. B. Olshausen and K. Millmann. Learning sparse codes with a mixture of Gaussians prior. In *Advances in Neural Information Processing Systems (NIPS) 12*, pages 841–847. MIT Press, Cambridge, MA, 2000.

9. K. Rao and P. Yip. *Discrete Cosine Transform—Algorithms, Advantages and Applications*. Academic Press, London, UK, 1990.

10. J. Yang and C. Lu. Combined techniques of singular value decomposition and vector quantization for image coding. *IEEE Trans. Image Proc.*, 4:1141–1146, 1995.

Supervised Texture Segmentation by Maximising Conditional Likelihood

Georgy Gimel'farb

Centre for Image Technology and Robotics
Department of Computer Science
Tamaki Campus, University of Auckland
Private Bag 92019, Auckland 1, New Zealand
g.gimelfarb@auckland.ac.nz
http://www.cs.auckland.ac.nz/~georgy

Abstract. Supervised segmentation of piecewise-homogeneous image textures using a modified conditional Gibbs model with multiple pairwise pixel interactions is considered. The modification takes into account that inter-region interactions are usually different for the training sample and test images. Parameters of the model learned from a given training sample include a characteristic pixel neighbourhood specifying the interaction structure and Gibbs potentials giving quantitative strengths of the pixelwise and pairwise interactions. The segmentation is performed by approaching the maximum conditional likelihood of the desired region map provided that the training and test textures have similar conditional signal statistics for the chosen pixel neighbourhood. Experiments show that such approach is more efficient for regular textures described by different characteristic long-range interactions than for stochastic textures with overlapping close-range neighbourhoods.

1 Introduction

Supervised segmentation is intended to partition a spatially inhomogeneous texture into regions of homogeneous textures after learning descriptions of these latter. Generally, neither textures nor homogeneity have universal formal definitions, so that each statement of the segmentation problem introduces some particular texture descriptions and criteria of homogeneity.

For last two decades, one of most popular approaches is to model textures as samples of a discrete Markov random field on an arithmetic lattice with a joint Gibbs probability distribution of signals (grey levels, or colours) in the pixels [4–6, 10, 11]. The Gibbs model relates the joint distribution that globally describes the images to a geometric structure and quantitative strengths of local pixel interactions. Typically only pixelwise and pairwise pixel interactions are taken into account, and the interaction structure is specified by a spatially invariant subset of pixels interacting with each individual pixel. The subset forms the pixel neighbourhood. The interaction strengths are specified by Gibbs potential functions that depend on signals in the pixel or in the interacting pixel pair.

M.A.T. Figueiredo, J. Zerubia, A.K. Jain (Eds.): EMMCVPR 2001, LNCS 2134, pp. 169–184, 2001.

In this case the texture homogeneity is defined in terms of spatial invariance of certain conditional probability distributions, and a homogeneous texture has its specific spatially invariant interaction structure and potentials. The supervised segmentation has to estimate these model parameters from a given training sample, that is, from a piecewise-homogeneous image with the known map of homogeneous regions or from a set of separate single-region homogeneous textures. Then the parameters are used for taking the optimal statistical decision about the region map of a test image that combines the same homogeneous textures. This approach assumes that the parameters estimated from the training sample are typical for all the images to be segmented.

This paper considers the supervised segmentation using the conditional Gibbs model of piecewise-homogeneous textures proposed in [7, 8]. Here, the model is modified more fully reflect the inter-region relations that usually are quite different in the training and test cases. Previously, the two-pass (initial and final) segmentation had been introduced to implicitly take account of the differences between the training and test inter-region signal statistics. The modified model involves more natural inter-region interactions so that the segmentation can now be achieved in a single pass.

The segmentation process approximates the maximum conditional likelihood of a desired region map providing that the image to be segmented and the training sample have the same or closely similar pixelwise and characteristic pairwise interactions in terms of particular conditional signal statistics. We investigate how precise such a segmentation is for different texture types, in particular, for stochastic and regular textures efficiently described by the Gibbs models of homogeneous textures [8, 9].

The paper is organised as follows. Section 2 describes in brief the modified conditional Gibbs model of piecewise-homogeneous textures and shows how the Controllable Simulated Annealing (CSA) introduced in [7, 8] can be used for maximising the conditional likelihood of the desired region map. Section 3 presents and discusses results of the supervised segmentation of typical piecewise-homogeneous stochastic and regular textures. The concluding remarks are given in Section 4.

2   Gibbs Model of Piecewise-Homogeneous Textures

2.1   Basic Notation

Let $\mathbf{R} = [(m,n) : m = 1,\ldots,M; n = 1,\ldots,N]$ be a finite aritmetic lattice with $M \cdot N$ pixels. Let $\mathbf{Q} = \{0,\ldots,Q-1\}$ be a finite set of grey levels. Let $\mathbf{K} = \{1,\ldots,K\}$ be a finite set of region labels. Let $\mathbf{g} = [g_i : i \in \mathbf{R}; g_i \in \mathbf{Q}]$ and $\mathbf{l} = [l_i : i \in \mathbf{R}; l_i \in \mathbf{K}]$ denote a piecewise-homogeneous digital greyscale texture and its region map, respectively, so that each pixel $i = (m,n) \in \mathbf{R}$ is represented by its grey level g_i and region label l_i.

The spatially invariant geometric structure of pairwise pixel interactions over the lattice is specified by a pixel neighbourhood $\mathbf{A}$. The neighbourhood points up a subset of pixels (neighbours) $\{(i + a) : a \in \mathbf{A}; i + a \in \mathbf{R}\}$ having each a pairwise interaction with the pixel $i \in \mathbf{R}$. Each offset $a = (\xi, \eta) \in \mathbf{A}$ defines a family of interacting pixel pairs, or cliques of the neighbourhood graph [2]. A quantitative strength of pixel interactions in the clique family $\mathbf{C}_a = \{(i, j) : i, j \in \mathbf{R}; \ i - j = a\}$ is given by a Gibbs potential function of grey levels and region labels.

The conditional Gibbs model in [7, 8] specifies the joint probability distribution of the region maps for a given greyscale image in terms of the characteristic neighbourhood $\mathbf{A}$ and the potential $\mathbf{V} = [\mathbf{V}_{\mathrm{p}}; \ \mathbf{V}_a : \ a \in \mathbf{A}]$. Generally, the potential of pixelwise interactions $\mathbf{V}_{\mathrm{pix}} = [V_{\mathrm{p}}(k|q) : \ k \in \mathbf{K}; \ q \in \mathbf{Q}]$ depends on a grey value q and region label k in a pixel. The potential of pairwise interactions $\mathbf{V}_a = [V_a(k, k'|q, q') : \ (k, k') \in \mathbf{K}^2; \ (q, q') \in \mathbf{Q}^2]$ depends on region label and grey level co-occurrences (g_i, l_i, g_j, l_j) in a clique $(i, j) \in \mathbf{C}_a$.

We assume for simplicity that the potential of pairwise interactions depends only on the grey level difference $d = g_i - g_j; \ d \in \mathbf{D} = \{-Q+1, \ldots, 0, \ldots, Q-1\}$. The inter-region grey level differences in the cliques of the same family are quite arbitrary for the various region maps of a piecewise-homogeneous texture. Therefore, the potentials should depend actually only on the region label coincidences $\alpha = \delta(l_i - l_j) \in \{0, 1\}$ so that $V_a(k, k'|q, q') \equiv V_{a,\alpha}(k|q - q')$ where $\alpha = 0$ for the inter-region and $\alpha = 1$ for the intra-region pixel interactions.

Obviously, the intra-region potentials $V_{a,1}(k|d)$ depend both on k and d. But the inter-region potentials $V_{a,0}(k|d)$ actually describe only the region map model and should be independent of region labels and grey level differences: $V_{a,0}(k|d) \equiv V_{a,0}$. In the original model [7, 8] both the intra- and inter-region potentials depend on k and d because the inter-region statistics is assumed to be similar for the training and test images. But in most cases this assumption does not hold.

For the fixed neighbourhood $\mathbf{A}$ and potentials $\mathbf{V}$, the modified conditional Gibbs model of region maps $\mathbf{l}$, given a greyscale texture $\mathbf{g}$, is as follows:

$$\Pr(\mathbf{l}|\mathbf{g}, \mathbf{V}, \mathbf{A}) = \frac{1}{Z_{\mathbf{g}, \mathbf{V}, \mathbf{A}}} \exp\left(E_{\mathrm{p}}(\mathbf{l}|\mathbf{g}, \mathbf{V}_{\mathrm{p}}) + \sum_{a \in \mathbf{A}} E_a(\mathbf{l}|\mathbf{g}, \mathbf{V}_a) \right) \qquad (1)$$

where $Z_{\mathbf{g}, \mathbf{V}, \mathbf{A}}$ is the normalising factor, $E_{\mathrm{p}}(\mathbf{l}|\mathbf{g}, \mathbf{V}_{\mathrm{p}})$ is the total energy of the pixelwise interactions:

$$E_{\mathrm{p}}(\mathbf{l}|\mathbf{g}, \mathbf{V}_{\mathrm{p}}) = \sum_{i \in \mathbf{R}} V_{\mathrm{p}}(l_i|g_i) = |\mathbf{R}| \left(\sum_{q \in \mathbf{Q}} F_{\mathrm{p}}(q|\mathbf{g}) \sum_{k \in \mathbf{K}} V_{\mathrm{p}}(k|q) F_{\mathrm{p}}(k|q, \mathbf{l}, \mathbf{g}) \right) \quad (2)$$

and $E_a(\mathbf{l}|\mathbf{g}, \mathbf{V}_a)$ is the total energy of the pairwise pixel interactions over the clique family $\mathbf{C}_a$:

$$E_a(\mathbf{l}|\mathbf{g}, \mathbf{V}_a) = \sum_{(i,j) \in \mathbf{C}_a} V_{a, \delta(l_i - l_j)}(l_i|g_i - g_j)$$

$$= |\mathbf{R}|\rho_a \left(V_{a,0} F_{a,0}(\mathbf{l}) + \sum_{d \in \mathbf{D}} F_a(d|\mathbf{g}) \sum_{k \in \mathbf{K}} V_{a,1}(k|d) F_{a,1}(k|d, \mathbf{l}, \mathbf{g}) \right) \qquad (3)$$

Here, $F_{\mathrm{p}}(q|\mathbf{g})$ and $F_{\mathrm{p}}(k|q, \mathbf{l}, \mathbf{g})$ denote the relative frequency of the grey level q in the image $\mathbf{g}$ and of the the region label k in the region map $\mathbf{l}$ over the grey level

q in the image $\mathbf{g}$, respectively, and $F_a(d|\mathbf{g})$, $F_{a,0}(\mathbf{l})$, and $F_{a,1}(k|d,\mathbf{l},\mathbf{g})$ denote the relative frequency of the grey level difference d over the clique family $\mathbf{C}_a$ in the image $\mathbf{g}$, of the inter-region label coincidences in the region map $\mathbf{l}$, and of the intra-region label coincidences for the region k in the region map $\mathbf{l}$ over the grey level difference d in the clique family $\mathbf{C}_a$ for the image $\mathbf{g}$, respectively. The factor $\rho_a = \frac{|\mathbf{C}_a|}{|\mathbf{R}|}$ gives the relative size of the clique family $\mathbf{C}_a$.

2.2   Learning the Model Parameters

As shown in [8], the potentials for a given training pair $(\mathbf{l}^\circ, \mathbf{g}^\circ)$ have a simple first approximation of the maximum likelihood estimate. Because of the unified inter-region potential values, this approximation is now as follows:

$$
\begin{aligned}
&\forall k \in \mathbf{K};\ q \in \mathbf{Q};\ d \in \mathbf{D} \\
V_{\mathrm{p}}^{[0]}(k|q) &= \lambda^{[0]} F(q|\mathbf{g}^\circ)\left(F(k|q,\mathbf{l}^\circ,\mathbf{g}^\circ) - \mu\right) \\
V_{a,0}^{[0]} &= \lambda^{[0]} \rho_a \left(F_{a,0}(\mathbf{l}^\circ) - \mu_0\right) \\
V_{a,1}^{[0]}(k|d) &= \lambda^{[0]} \rho_a F_a(d|\mathbf{g}^\circ)\left(F_{a,1}(k|d,\mathbf{l}^\circ,\mathbf{g}^\circ) - \mu_1\right)
\end{aligned}
\tag{4}
$$

where $\mu = \frac{1}{|\mathbf{K}|}$, $\mu_0 = 1 - \mu$, and $\mu_1 = \mu^2$ are the marginal probabilities of region labels and their coincidences, respectively, for the independent random field (IRF) with the equiprobable region labels.

The initial scaling factor $\lambda^{[0]}$ in Eq. (4) is computed as

$$
\lambda^{[0]} = \frac{e_{\mathrm{p}}(\mathbf{l}^\circ, \mathbf{g}^\circ) + \sum\limits_{a \in \mathbf{A}} \left(e_{a,0}(\mathbf{l}^\circ) + e_{a,1}(\mathbf{l}^\circ, \mathbf{g}^\circ)\right)}{e_{\mathrm{p}}(\mathbf{l}^\circ, \mathbf{g}^\circ)\psi + \sum\limits_{a \in \mathbf{A}} \left(e_{a,0}(\mathbf{l}^\circ)\psi_0 + e_{a,1}(\mathbf{l}^\circ, \mathbf{g}^\circ)\psi_1\right)}
\tag{5}
$$

where $e_{\mathrm{p}}(\mathbf{l}^\circ, \mathbf{g}^\circ)$, $e_{a,0}(\mathbf{l}^\circ)$, and $e_{a,1}(\mathbf{l}^\circ, \mathbf{g}^\circ)$ are the normalised first approximations of the Gibbs energies of pixelwise and pairwise pixel interactions:

$$
\begin{aligned}
e_{\mathrm{p}}(\mathbf{l}^\circ, \mathbf{g}^\circ) &= \sum\limits_{q \in \mathbf{Q}} F_{\mathrm{p}}^2(q|\mathbf{g}^\circ) \sum\limits_{k \in \mathbf{k}} F_{\mathrm{p}}(k|q,\mathbf{l}^\circ,\mathbf{g}^\circ)\left(F_{\mathrm{p}}(k|q,\mathbf{l}^\circ,\mathbf{g}^\circ) - \mu\right) \\
e_{a,0}(\mathbf{l}^\circ) &= \rho_a^2 F_{a,0}(\mathbf{l}^\circ)\left(F_{a,0}(\mathbf{l}^\circ) - \mu_0\right) \\
e_{a,1}(\mathbf{l}^\circ, \mathbf{g}^\circ) &= \rho_a^2 \sum\limits_{d \in \mathbf{D}} F_a^2(d|\mathbf{g}^\circ) \sum\limits_{k \in \mathbf{K}} F_{a,1}(k|d,\mathbf{l}^\circ,\mathbf{g}^\circ)\left(F_{a,1}(k|d,\mathbf{l}^\circ,\mathbf{g}^\circ) - \mu_1\right)
\end{aligned}
\tag{6}
$$

and $\psi = \mu(1 - \mu)$ and $\psi_a = \mu_a(1 - \mu_a)$; $\alpha = 0, 1$, are the variances of the region label frequencies for the IRF.

As in [7, 8], most characteristic interaction structure is recovered in this paper by choosing the clique families with the top values of the total energy of pairwise pixel interactions:

$$
e_a(\mathbf{l}^\circ, \mathbf{g}^\circ) = e_{a,0}(\mathbf{l}^\circ) + e_{a,1}(\mathbf{l}^\circ, \mathbf{g}^\circ)
$$

2.3   Supervised Segmentation

When the model of Eq. (1) is used for segmenting piecewise-homogeneous textures, we assume that the first-order and second-order statistics of the images $\mathbf{g}$

to be segmented and the desired region maps l in Eqs. (2) and (3) are similar to those of the training pair (l°, g°). This assumption is crucial because the likelihood maximisation algorithm we use for segmentation actually tries to minimise a (probabilistic) distance between the above statistics for the training pair and segmented image [8].

Because the model of Eq. (1) belongs to the exponential family of distributions, the log-likelihood function $L(\mathbf{V}|l^\circ, g^\circ) = \log \Pr(l^\circ|g^\circ, \mathbf{V}, \mathbf{A})$ with a fixed neighbourhood $\mathbf{A}$ is unimodal [1] with respect to the potential $\mathbf{V}$. The maximum is approached by the stochastic-approximation-based Controllable Simulated Annealing (CSA) [8] that starts from an arbitrary initial region map $l^{[0]}$, e.g., from a sample of the IRF, with the initial Gibbs potentials of Eq. (4). At each step t, the potentials are modified as to approach the conditional pixelwise and pairwise statistics for the training sample (l°, g°) with the like statistics for the current simulated pair $(l^{[t]}, g^\circ)$.

The CSA is easily adapted for approaching the maximum of an arbitrary log-likelihood $L(\mathbf{V}|l, g)$, providing that the pair (l, g) has the same conditional statistics as the training pair. The only change with respect to the maximisation of $L(\mathbf{V}|l^\circ, g^\circ)$ is that the training image g° is replaced with the test image g for generating the successive maps $l^{[t]}$ at each step t.

Using the signal statistics for the training sample (l°, g°) and for the test image g with the region map $l^{[t]}$ generated by stochastic relaxation with the current potential $\mathbf{V}^{[t]}$, the resulting process modifies the potential values as follows:

$$\forall k \in \mathbf{K};\ q \in \mathbf{Q};\ d \in \mathbf{D};\ a \in \mathbf{A}$$

$$
\begin{aligned}
V_{\mathrm{p}}^{[t+1]}(k|q) &= V_{\mathrm{p}}^{[t]}(k|q) + \lambda_t F_{\mathrm{p}}(q|g)\left(F_{\mathrm{p}}(k|q, l^\circ, g^\circ) - F_{\mathrm{p}}(k|q, l^{[t]}, g)\right) \\
V_{a,0}^{[t+1]} &= V_{a,1}^{[t]} + \lambda_t \rho_a \left(F_{a,0}(l^\circ) - F_{a,0}(l^{[t]})\right) \\
V_{a,1}^{[t+1]}(k|d) &= V_{a,1}^{[t]}(k|d) + \lambda_t \rho_a F_a(d|g)\left(F_{a,1}(k|d, l^\circ, g^\circ) - F_{a,1}(k|d, l^{[t]}, g)\right)
\end{aligned}
\tag{7}
$$

3   Experimental Results

3.1   Segmenting an Arbitrary Training Sample

The best results of the above approach should be expected for segmenting just the training image. For instance, the training sample in Figure 1,a–b, contains five arbitrary chosen but spatially homogeneous natural and artificial textures.

In this case the segmentation results in the region maps having from 17.12% to 0.0% of errors when the model of Eq. (1) contains, respectively, from one to six clique families with the top total energies (Figure 1,c–h, and Table 1).

In these experiments the search window for choosing the characteristic interaction structures has 60 clique families with the short-range offsets ($|\xi| \le 5; |\eta| \le 5$). All the segmentation maps are obtained after 300 steps of the CSA with the scaling factor in Eq. (7) that is changing as follows:

$$\lambda^{[t]} = \lambda^{[0]} \frac{1}{1 + 0.001 \cdot t}$$

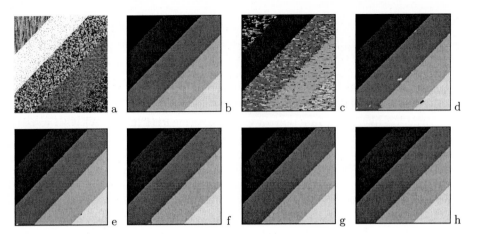

Fig. 1. Training five-region texture (a), its ideal region map (b), and segmentation maps obtained with 1–6 clique families (c–h), respectively.

Table 1. Characteristic clique families included successively into the model of Eq. (1), their Gibbs energies, and the relative segmentation errors ε in Figure 1,c–h.

$|\mathbf{A}|$	1	2	3	4	5	6
$a = (\xi, \eta)$	[1,0]	[-1,1]	[0,1]	[-2,2]	[-3,3]	[-4,4]
$e_a(1°, \mathbf{g}°)$	478.4	440.3	427.7	407.4	400.4	395.4
$\varepsilon, \%$	17.12	0.54	0.15	0.27	0.0	0.0

The same number of steps and the same schedule for changing $\lambda^{[t]}$ is used in all the experiments below.

3.2   Segmenting Collages of Stochastic and Regular Textures

To investigate the above segmentation in more detail, we use two types of homogeneous textures, namely, stochastic and regular textures that can be efficiently simulated by the Gibbs models with multiple pairwise pixel interactions [8, 9]. Figures 2 and 3 present collages of stochastic textures D4, D9, D29, and D57 and regular textures D1, D6, D34, and D101 from [3].

The former four textures have the characteristic short-range interactions whereas the latter ones have mostly the characteristic long-range interactions. In both cases three textures from each group (the stochastic textures D4, D9, and D29 and the regular textures D1, D6, and D34) possess similar statistics of the close-range pairwise pixel interactions (in terms of the relative frequency distributions of grey level differences).

Below we use the collages in Figures 2,a and 2,e with the same region map in Figure 2,i as the training samples for each group of the textures. The search

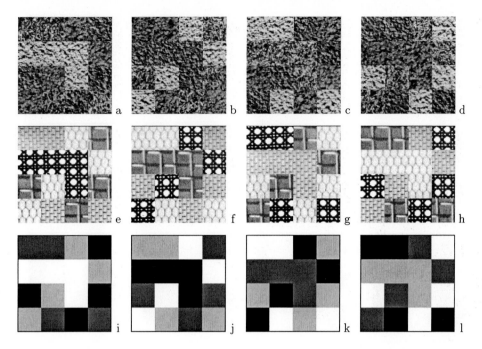

Fig. 2. Four-region training (a,e) and test collages (b–d,f–h) of stochastic textures D4, D9, D29, D57 (a–d) and regular textures D1, D6, D34, D101 (e–h) with their ideal region maps (i–l).

Table 2. Characteristic clique families with the top Gibbs energies $e_a(1°, \mathbf{g}°)$ selected for the training four-region collage of stochastic textures in Figures 2,a and 2,i.

$a = (\xi, \eta)$	(1,0)	(0,1)	(1,1)	(-1,1)	(2,0)	(2,1)	(0,2)	(-2,1)
$e_a(1°, \mathbf{g}°)$	413.1	330.2	277.2	262.9	240.6	209.7	202.1	198.5
$a = (\xi, \eta)$	(1,2)	(3,0)	(-1,2)	(3,1)	(2,2)	(0,3)	(-3,1)	(-2,2)
$e_a(1°, \mathbf{g}°)$	189.8	182.3	182.1	169.7	168.4	167.1	162.4	159.9

window for choosing the characteristic interaction structure contains 3240 clique families with the short- and long-range offsets ($|\xi| \leq 40; |\eta| \leq 40$).

Piecewise-Homogeneous Stochastic Textures. In this case, relative errors of segmenting the training image using four, eight, or 16 characteristic clique families with the top-rank Gibbs energies are, respectively, 21.36%, 16.44%, and 13.88%. Here, the ranking of the clique families by their Gibbs energies results in only the close-range interaction structures. The corresponding 16 clique families in terms of their offsets $a = (\xi, \eta)$ are shown in Table 2.

The relative errors of segmenting the training sample are slowly decreasing with the neighbourhood size (for instance, 10.15% for $|\mathbf{A}| = 36$). Segmentation

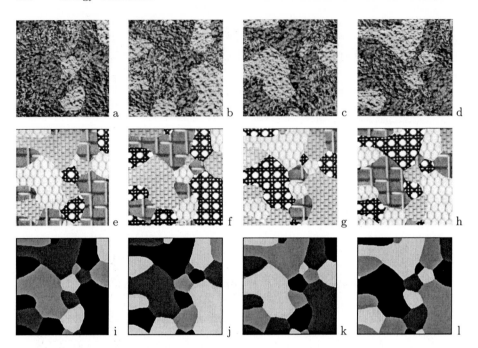

Fig. 3. Four-region test collages of stochastic textures D04, D09, D29, D57 (a–d) and regular textures D1, D6, D34, D101 (e–h) with their ideal region maps (i–l).

errors for the test images in Figure 2,b–d and 3,a–d depend in a similar way on the neighbourhood size so that most of the experiments below are conducted with the same fixed characteristic neighbourhood of size $|\mathbf{A}| = 16$.

Segmentation of the test images yields larger error rates (23.39–32.43%) caused mostly by misclassified parts of the textures D4 and D9 (Figure 4). The main reason is that the stochastic textures D4, D9, and D29 have very similar signal statistics over the chosen characteristic short-range neighbourhood. Thus the individual regions produced by segmentation (Figures 6 and 7) differ from the ideal maps although they are quantitatively, in terms of the chi-square distances between the training and test statistics, and even visually quite homogeneous. Table 3 demonstrates how the segmentation separates the individual textures.

These experiments demonstrate the basic difficulty in segmenting stochastic textures by taking account of characteristic conditional pairwise statistics. The close-range characteristic neighbourhoods selected by ranking the total Gibbs energies for the clique families may not be adequate for separating these textures because the conditional signal statistics similar to the training ones can be obtained for regions that differ much from the ideal ones.

Piecewise-Homogeneous Regular Textures. In this case we can expect more efficient segmentation using the conditional model in Eq. (1) because simulations of these textures involve usually characteristic long-range interactions [9].

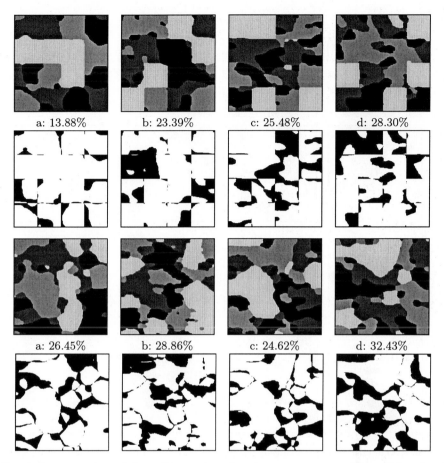

Fig. 4. Segmentation of the collages of stochastic textures using the neighbourhood of size 16; the top and the bottom region maps a–d are obtained for the collages in Figures 2,a–d, and 3,a–d, respectively. Black regions under each map indicate the segmentation errors.

Table 3. Segmentation results (in %) for the training and test collages of stochastic textures (the rows correspond to the ideal regions, and the columns show how many pixels of each ideal region are actually assigned to a particular texture).

	Training collage				Test collages			
	D4	D9	D29	D57	D4	D9	D29	D57
D4	75.4	15.9	8.5	2.0	47.3–73.0	20.3–44.4	5.5–21.0	0.0–5.3
D9	11.6	82.6	4.2	1.6	6.3–31.7	58.3–73.8	4.9–30.4	0.4–27.2
D29	9.2	2.6	87.4	0.8	4.4–25.6	3.4–9.2	64.5–89.6	0.0–2.1
D57	0.4	0.2	0.3	99.0	0.1–1.0	0.0–9.4	0.0–2.7	89.2–99.6

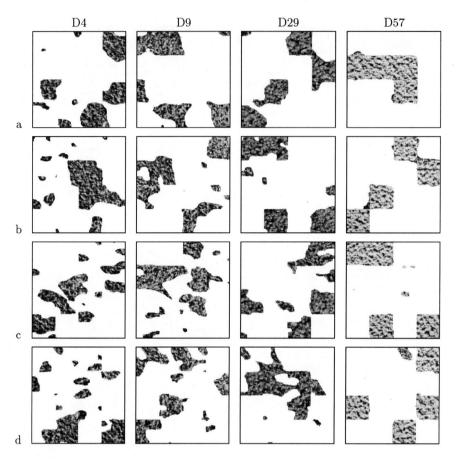

Fig. 5. Homogeneous regions found by segmenting the training and test collages of stochastic textures (the top row of the maps a–d in Figure 4).

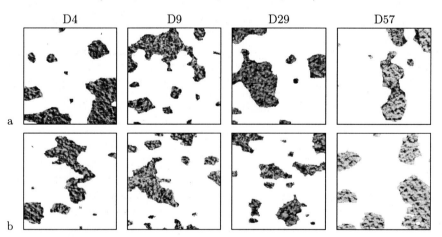

Fig. 6. Homogeneous regions found by segmenting the test collages of stochastic textures (the bottom row of the maps in Figure 4,a,b).

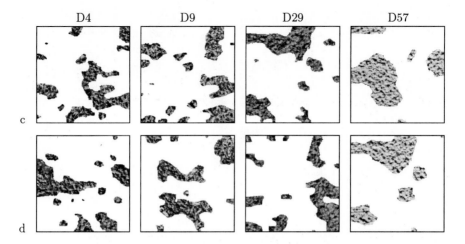

Fig. 7. Homogeneous regions found by segmenting the test collages of stochastic textures (the bottom row of the maps in Figure 4,c,d).

Table 4. Characteristic clique families with the top Gibbs energies $e_a(1°, \mathbf{g}°)$ selected for the training four-region collage of regular textures in Figures 2,e and 2,i.

$a = (\xi, \eta)$	(1,0)	(0,1)	(1,1)	(-1,1)	(2,0)	(0,2)	(2,1)	(1,2)
$e_a(1°, \mathbf{g}°)$	613.7	549.2	360.8	353.5	325.6	323.2	189.8	189.3
$a = (\xi, \eta)$	(0,2)	(-2,1)	(3,0)	(0,3)	(2,2)	(3,1)	(-2,2)	(-3,1)
$e_a(1°, \mathbf{g}°)$	183.3	182.1	173.0	159.9	66.8	64.5	60.1	59.0

Actually, the relative error of segmenting the training collage in Figure 2,e is 2.67% with the same neighbourhood size of 16 although once again the top-rank total energies correspond to only the close-range interactions (Table 4).

Figure 8 shows results of segmenting the training collage and test collages of regular textures in Figures 2,e–h and 3,e–h, respectively, using the characteristic neighbourhood of size 16. The relative errors for the test collages are 1.66–14.09%. The test collages in Figure 3,e–h result in less precise segmentation because of many small subregions in these textures that effect the collected conditional statistics.

The individual homogeneous regions found by segmentation are shown in Figures 9–11, and Table 5 demonstrates the separation of these textures. Most of the errors are caused by the textures D6 and D34 with very similar uniform backgrounds resulting in close similarity between their conditional statistics of short-range grey level differences.

The desired distinctions between the close-range conditional statistics may exist also for certain spatially inhomogeneous textures. For example, the collages of regular textures in Figure 12,a,c contain both the homogeneous regular textures D20, D55, D77 and the weakly inhomogeneous texture D36 from [3]. The

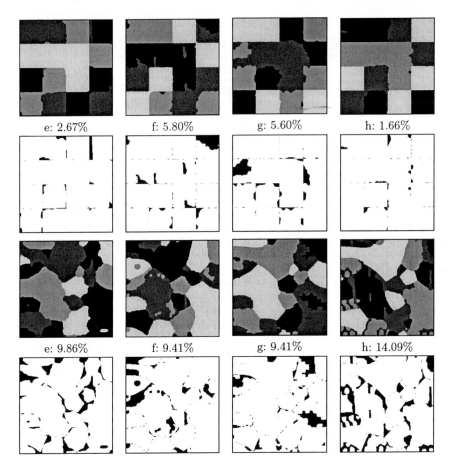

Fig. 8. Segmentation of the training and test collages of regular textures using the neighbourhood of size 16: the top and bottom region maps e–h are obtained for the collages in Figures 2,e–h, and 3,e–h, respectively. Black regions under each map indicate the segmentation errors.

error rate of segmenting the training image with the characteristic short-range neighbourhood of size 16 is 28.63%. When the size is extended to 36 then the error rates of segmenting the training and test collages are 5.15% and 16.71%, respectively. The resulting region maps for the neighbourhood of size 36 are shown in Figure 12,b,d. The main errors in this case are due to assigning small border parts of the textures D20 and D55 to the texture D77 having similar statistics of the close-range grey level differences.

4   Concluding Remarks

These and other our experiments show that the supervised segmentation by approaching the maximum conditional likelihood is efficient for textures with

Table 5. Segmentation results (in %) for the training and test collages of regular textures (the rows correspond to the ideal regions, and the columns show how many pixels of each ideal region are actually assigned to a particular texture).

	Training collage				Test collages			
	D1	D6	D34	D101	D1	D6	D34	D101
D1	96.0	4.0	0.0	0.0	81.9–99.9	0.1–17.7	0.0–0.8	0.0–7.7
D6	1.6	97.0	1.4	0.0	1.0–16.5	75.7–97.6	0.0–17.9	0.0–5.0
D34	0.8	2.4	96.4	0.4	0.0–4.2	1.0–16.7	78.5–99.0	0.0–2.1
D101	0.1	0.0	0.0	99.9	0.0–0.4	0.0–0.3	0.0–1.6	97.7–99.9

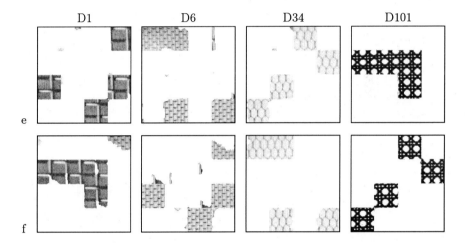

Fig. 9. Homogeneous regions found by segmenting the training and test collages of regular textures (the top row of the maps in Figure 8,e,f).

different characteristic interaction structures. But the overlapping close-range structures and similar pairwise signal statistics of individual homogeneous textures may result in a segmentation map that differs considerably from the ideal one although both the maps possess conditional signal statistics similar to the training ones and have visually homogeneous textured regions.

The modified conditional Gibbs model allows to accelerate segmentation comparing to the previous two-stage scheme [7, 8] by obviating the need for the initial stage. This latter sets to zero the inter-region potentials in order to roughly approximate the desired homogeneous regions even though their inter-region signal statistics are different in the test and training samples. Then the initial (and usually quite "noisy") region map is refined at the final stage by using both the intra- and inter-region potentials.

The one-stage process of Eq. (7) forms the final region map starting directly from a sample of the IRF. Simultaneously the accuracy of segmentation is slightly

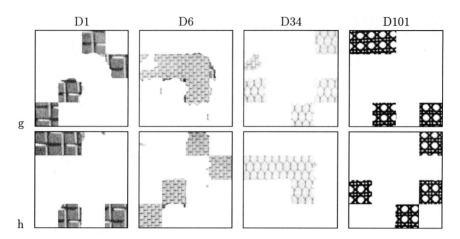

Fig. 10. Homogeneous regions found by segmenting the test collages of regular textures (the top row of the maps in Figure 8,g,h).

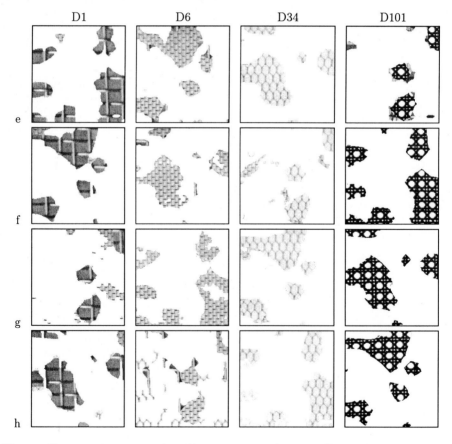

Fig. 11. Homogeneous regions found by segmenting the test collages of regular textures (the bottom row of the maps e–h in Figure 8).

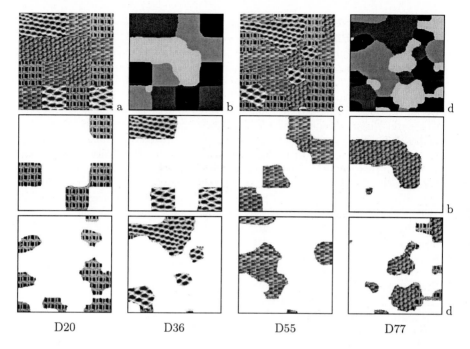

D20   D36   D55   D77

Fig. 12. Region maps (b) and (d) and the corresponding homogeneous regions obtained by segmenting the training (a) and test (c) collages of regular textures D20, D36, D55, and D77, respectively.

improved in that the modified model yields smaller differences between the error rates for the training and test images. For instance, the two-stage segmentation in [8] results in the error rates of 2.6% and 29.0–35.2% for the training and test collages of the textures D3–D4–D5–D9 from [3], respectively, or 1.9% and 15.3–33.0% for the like collages of the textures D23–D24–D29–D34, and so forth. The one-stage segmentation based on the modified Gibbs model produces more predictable results for the test and training samples like 13.9% vs. 23.4–32.4% for the stochastic textures with very similar close-range pairwise signal statistics or 2.7% vs. 1.7–14.1% for the regular textures, respectively.

Our experiments show that the choice of most characteristic pixel neighbourhoods should be based not only on partial Gibbs energies of pairwise pixel interactions but also on the accuracy of segmentation. If the top-rank Gibbs energies correspond mostly to the close-range neighbourhoods then these latter can be efficient only for segmenting the textures with sufficiently different close-range pairwise signal statistics of the homogeneous regions.

References

1. Barndorff-Nielsen, O.: Information and Exponential Families in Statistical Theory. John Wiley and Sons: New York, 1978.

2. Besag, J.E.: Spatial interaction and the statistical analysis of lattice systems. J. Royal Stat. Soc. **B36** (1974) 192–236.
3. Brodatz, P.: Textures: A Photographic Album for Artists and Designers. Dover Publications: New York, 1966.
4. Cross, G.R., Jain, A.K.: Markov random field texture models. IEEE Trans. Pattern Analysis and Machine Intelligence. **5** (1983) 25–39.
5. Derin, H., Cole, W.S.: Segmentation of textured images using Gibbs random fields. Computer Vision, Graphics, and Image Processing. **35** (1986) 72–98.
6. Dubes, R.C., Jain, A.K., Nadabar, S.G., Chen, C.C.: MRF model-based algorithms for image segmentation. Proc. 10th Int. Conf. Pattern Recognition, 16–21 June 1990, Atlantic City, N.J., USA. Vol. 1. IEEE Computer Soc. Press (1990) 808–814.
7. Gimel'farb, G.L.: Gibbs models for Bayesian simulation and segmentation of piecewise-uniform textures. Proc. 13th Int. Conf. Pattern Recognition, August 1996, Vienna, Austria. Vol. 2. IEEE Computer Soc. Press (1996) 760–764.
8. Gimel'farb, G.: Image Textures and Gibbs Random Fields. Kluwer Academic: Dordrecht, 1999.
9. Gimel'farb, G.: Quantitative description of spatially homogeneous textures by characteristic grey level co-occurrences. Australian Journal of Intelligent Information Processing Systems **6** (2000) 46–53.
10. Hassner, M., Sklansky, J.: The use of Markov random fields as models of texture. Computer Graphics and Image Processing **12** (1980) 357–370.
11. Krishnamachari, S., Chellappa, R.: Multiresolution Gauss–Markov random field models for texture segmentation. IEEE Trans. Image Processing **6** (1997) 251–267.

Designing Moiré Patterns

Guy Lebanon[1] and Alfred M. Bruckstein[1]

[1] School of Computer Science, Carnegie Mellon University
[2] Department of Computer Science, Technion – Israel Institute of Technology

Abstract. Moiré phenomena occur when two or more images are non-linearly combined to create a new "superposition image". Moiré patterns are patterns that don't exist in any of the original images but appear in the superposition image for example as the result of a multiplicative superposition rule. The topic of moiré pattern synthesis deals with creating images that, when superimposed, will reveal certain desired moiré patterns. Conditions ensuring that a desired moiré pattern will be present in the superposition of two images are known, however they do not specify these images uniquely. The freedom in choosing the superimposed images can be exploited to produce various degrees of visibility and ensure desired properties. Performance criteria for the images that measure when one superposition is better than another are introduced. These criteria are based on the visibility of the moiré patterns to the human visual system and on the digitization which takes place when presenting the images on discrete displays. We here propose to resolve the freedom in moiré synthesis by choosing the images that optimize the chosen criteria.

1 Introduction

The term moiré comes from French where it refers to watered silk. The moiré silk consists of two layers of fabric pressed together. As the silk bends and folds, the two layers shift with respect to each another, causing the appearance of interfering patterns. The moiré technique for manufacturing clothes was developed in China a long time ago, and later introduced to France in 1754 by the English manufacturer Badger.Natural moiré phenomena can be seen in daily life, for example in the folds of a moving nylon curtain or when looking through parallel wire-mesh fences. The first scientific observations were made by Lord Rayleigh [1] who suggested to use the moiré phenomenon for testing quality of gratings.

Two goals exist in moiré patterns research. The first is the analysis of moiré patterns. This usually involves some physical situation in which moiré patterns appear either naturally or by human intervention. The task is to analyze and characterize the patterns. Most of the research in moiré patterns analysis deals with finding equations describing the moiré patterns. In moiré pattern synthesis the generation of certain moiré patterns is required. The synthesis process involves producing two images such that when these images are superimposed the required moiré patterns emerge. Moiré synthesis and analysis are tightly linked and understanding one task gives insight into the other.

M.A.T. Figueiredo, J. Zerubia, A.K. Jain (Eds.): EMMCVPR 2001, LNCS 2134, pp. 185–200, 2001.

Over the years different methods to model and analyze the moiré phenomenon have been suggested. We shall describe two main approaches to model the moiré phenomenon in the next section. Section 3 presents the moiré pattern synthesis problem and in section 4, criteria for measuring the performance of moiré patterns in a superposition are introduced. Section 5 discusses the integrability constraint which ensures that a certain vector field is a gradient field. Section 6 reviews some basic results from variational calculus and their use in moiré synthesis and section 7 addresses the problem of recovering the potential function of a gradient field. Section 8 concludes with some results and closing remarks.

Throughout this paper we will discuss the case of superposition of two images for the sake of simplicity. It is not too difficult to extend the results to several superimposed images. We will assume a multiplicative superposition rule. Such a rule is motivated by the multiplication effect implicit in laying transparencies on one another. It is, however, possible to consider other superposition rules [2]. The nonlinearity of the multiplicative superposition allows new frequencies, which do not exist in the original image to appear in the superimposed image. In fact nonlinearity is at the heart of the moiré phenomenon and linear superposition like addition does not elicit it (see Fig. 1).

2 Moiré Pattern Analysis

Two models for moiré pattern analysis are reviewed. The indicial equation method operates in the image plane and the Fourier domain method operates in the frequency plane. The following model description follow closely [3] in which more detailed descriptions appear.

2.1 The Indicial Equation Method

The simplest and oldest model for analyzing the geometric shape of moiré patterns in the superposition of two curvilinear gratings is the indicial (or parametric) equation method surveyed in [4] and [5]. This model is based on the curve equations of the original curvilinear gratings. If each of the original layers is regarded as an indexed family of curves, the moiré pattern of the superposition forms a new indexed family of curves, whose equations can be inferred from the equations of the original gratings.

According to this model the original images consist of black curves on a white background. The curves in each image are assumed to be the equal height contours of two dimensional functions. We thus have two images which consist of black curved gratings whose centerlines are the equal height contours of two functions $\psi(x, y)$ and $\phi(x, y)$ as follows

$$\psi(x, y) = m \quad m \in \mathbb{Z}$$
$$\phi(x, y) = n \quad n \in \mathbb{Z} \tag{1}$$

Since the images are binary the multiplicative superposition is also an AND operator. Each of the curves in both images has an index given by the height

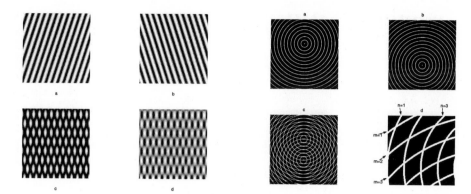

Fig. 1. The two gratings in a and b are multiplied in c and added in d. Image brightness is scaled

Fig. 2. Subtractive and additive moiré in the indicial equation model

of the respective contour. As a result adjacent curves get adjacent integers as indices. We denote the indices of the curves on one image by an integer variable m and the indices of the curves in the second image by the integer variable n. The coordinates m, n define an (m, n) net. In each point of the (m, n) net, an m and an n curve intersect. The (k_1, k_2) moiré curves are defined as the curves joining the intersection points of m and n curves whose indices obey $k_1 m + k_2 n = l$ where k_1, k_2 are constant integers and l runs over the set of integers.

Conceptually by letting m and n vary continuously, the (k_1, k_2) moiré curves obeying

$$k_1 m + k_2 n = l \quad l \in \mathbb{Z} \tag{2}$$

become continuous curves, that may be regarded as equal-height contours of a new bivariate function $g(x, y)$.

The order of the (k_1, k_2) moiré is defined to be the highest absolute value of k_1, k_2. The first order moirés are therefore the additive moiré $u + v = l$ and the subtractive moiré $u - v = l$. The first order moiré patterns are the curves connecting the intersection points of constant sum and constant difference of the curves index values. In Figure 2, (a) and (b) show two binary images whose curves correspond to equal height contours of a round summit. In (c) the superposition of (a) and (b) is exhibited and in (d) the superposition image is zoomed in. The subtractive moiré in (d) is described by the short diagonals of the curved parallelograms and the additive moiré is described by the long diagonals. Clearly, not all the (k_1, k_2) moirés visually stand out. The visibility of the moiré patterns will be discussed in greater length later. Usually only first order moirés stand out - if at all. In the case of first order moirés sometimes only the additive or only the subtractive moiré stand out and sometimes no moiré is apparent. Substituting (1) in (2) results in eliminating the indices m, n

$$k_1 \psi(x, y) + k_2 \phi(x, y) = l \quad l \in \mathbb{Z}. \tag{3}$$

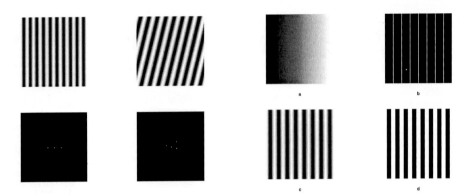

Fig. 3. The two raised cosine gratings and their spectra

Fig. 4. Periodic profiles of a linear function

We can thus state that the centerlines of the (k_1, k_2) moiré corresponds to the equal height contours of $g(x, y) = k_1\psi(x, y) + k_2\phi(x, y)$. The indicial equation methods enables a complete geometric specification of the moiré curves based on the implicit geometric specification of the curves in the two original images as equal-height contours of bivariate functions. The indicial equation method has several drawbacks. In order to use the indicial equation we need explicit analytic expressions for the curves which may not be readily available. Although the method gives us a condition for the possible moiré curves , it does not tell us whether the moiré pattern will indeed be visible to the human eye. For example, consider the superposition of a family of horizontal lines and a family of vertical lines. The superposition will consist of small squares. There will not be any visible pattern although the first order moiré patterns are diagonal lines connecting the opposite vertices of each square.

2.2   The Fourier Domain Method

So far we assumed that the original images were binary images showing the equal height contours of $\psi(x, y)$ and $\phi(x, y)$ as black curves on a white background. We now generalize this setting through the concept of periodic profile.

The original images are allowed to be $p(\psi(x, y))$ and $p(\phi(x, y))$ where $p(z)$ is a periodic function of one variable with period of one. If $p(z)$ is taken to be a discrete impulse train: $p(z) = 1$ when $z \in \mathbb{Z}$ and $p(z) = 0$ else, the images $p(\psi(x, y))$ and $p(\phi(x, y))$ reduce to binary images with curves representing equal-height contours of ψ and ϕ.

In this section we will restrict ourselves to linear ψ and ϕ: $\psi(x, y) = p_1 x + q_1 y$, $\phi(x, y) = p_2 x + q_2 y$ $p_1, p_2, q_1, q_2 \in \mathbb{R}$. Note that $p(\psi(x, y))$ and $p(\phi(x, y))$ will be periodic images. In Figure 4 (a), a linear function $\psi(x, y)$ is shown. In (b) (c) and (d), $p(\psi(x, y))$ is shown, where the periodic profile p is a discrete impulse train, cosine and square wave grating respectively.

Although we here restrict ourselves to linear functions, results obtained in this case are useful since many functions can locally be approximated by a linear function (the first two terms of the 2D Taylor expansion).

The Fourier domain method analyzes the moiré pattern in the frequency[1] domain. According to the convolution theorem, the multiplicative superposition rule in the image domain transforms to a two dimensional convolution between the spectra of the original images

$$g(x,y) = p(\psi(x,y)) \cdot p(\phi(x,y)) \iff G(u,v) = \mathcal{F}[p(\psi(x,y))] * \mathcal{F}[p(\phi(x,y))]. \quad (4)$$

The Fourier transform of $p(x) = e^{2\pi jfx}$ is $P(u) = \delta(u-f)$. In the two dimensional domain the Fourier transform of $p(x,y) = e^{2\pi j(f_1 x + f_2 y)}$ is $P(u,v) = \delta(u - f_1, v - f_2)$. Since p is a periodic function, it can be expanded to a Fourier series $p(x,y) = \sum_{m=-\infty}^{\infty} \sum_{n=-\infty}^{\infty} c_{m,n} e^{2\pi j(mu_0 x + nv_0 y)}$ The Fourier transform of $p(x,y)$ is readily obtained from the Fourier series decomposition and linearity of the Fourier transform $P(u,v) = \sum_{m=-\infty}^{\infty} \sum_{n=-\infty}^{\infty} c_{m,n} \delta(u - mu_0, v - nv_0)$. Furthermore, by the convolution theorem, $G(u,v)$ consists of translated and scaled impulses as well.

Since $\psi(x,y) = p_1 x + q_1 y \quad \phi(x,y) = p_2 x + q_2 y$, $p(\psi(x,y))$ and $p(\phi(x,y))$ have frequency components only in the direction of the gradients $\nabla\psi$ and $\nabla\phi$. This means that the frequency domain representation of $p(\psi(x,y))$ and $p(\phi(x,y))$ will have impulses only along the lines $p_1 u + q_1 v = 0$ and $p_2 u + q_2 v = 0$. This can also be seen from the fact that $p(\psi)$ and $p(\phi)$ are rotated 1D periodic functions on the x axis. Therefore, $\mathcal{F}[p(\psi(x,y))]$ and $\mathcal{F}[p(\phi(x,y))]$ are obtained by rotating the 1D spectra from the u axis by the same angles. In the case of a raised cosine profile $p(\cdot)$ is given by $p(\psi(x,y)) = \frac{1}{2}\cos(2\pi\psi(x,y)) + \frac{1}{2}$, and only three impulses will exist in the frequency domain. Two impulses at either sides of the origin are contributed by the cosine function. These two impulses are at distance one from the origin and lie along the line $p_1 u + q_1 v$ where $\phi = p_1 x + q_1 y$. The third impulse is contributed by the constant term and lies at the origin (see Figure 3).

The convolution of the impulse spectra is performed as a discrete convolution. The location of each impulse in the superposition spectrum will be the vectorial sum of the locations of two impulses, one from each original image. We will label the (k_1, k_2) superposition impulse as the impulse whose location is created by the vectorial sum of the k_1 impulse in the first original spectrum and the k_2 impulse in the second original spectrum. The amplitude of the (k_1, k_2) impulse is the product of the amplitudes of the k_1 impulse in the first original spectrum and the k_2 impulse in the second original spectrum.

Each impulse in the 2D spectrum is characterized by three main properties: its label, its geometric location and its amplitude. To the geometric location of an impulse, a frequency vector $\boldsymbol{f}$ is attached (in the frequency domain). This vector can be expressed in polar coordinates (f, θ) where f is the distance of $\boldsymbol{f}$ from the origin and θ is the angle of $\boldsymbol{f}$. In terms of the image domain, the geometric location of an impulse in the spectrum determines the frequency f

---

[1] In this paper we adopt the following Fourier transform convention (see [6]) $F(u,v) = \iint_{-\infty}^{\infty} f(x,y) e^{-j2\pi(ux+vy)} dx dy$, $f(x,y) = \iint_{-\infty}^{\infty} F(u,v) e^{j2\pi(ux+vy)} du dv$

and the direction θ of the corresponding periodic component in the image. The amplitude of the impulse represents the intensity of that periodic component in the image.

The geometric locations which include impulses in the superposition spectrum but do not include impulses in the original spectra represent the moiré patterns. These impulses represent new frequency components created by the superposition and not by one of the original images alone. Impulses which are labeled $f_{(0,i)}$ or $f_{(i,0)}$ for some i exist in one of the original images since f_0 represent the DC term.

In the case of other profiles such as square wave, we will have also higher order moiré impulses. The spectrum of a linear square wave grating is an infinite set of impulses along the frequency direction. Convolution of two such impulse trains will result in an infinite lattice covering the entire frequency plane.

However, we will show that the amplitude of impulses away from the origin tend to zero. We can disregard impulses with low amplitude since their effect on the image is small.

More formally, let $p(z)$ be a periodic function whose values are bounded between 0 and 1. Then all its Fourier series coefficients (impulse amplitudes) have absolute values between 0 and 1: $p(x) = \sum_{m=-\infty}^{\infty} c_m e^{2\pi jmfx}$, $0 \le |c_m| = \left| \frac{1}{T} \int_T p(x) e^{2\pi jmfx} dx \right| \le \left| \frac{1}{T} \int_T e^{2\pi jmfx} dx \right| \le 1$

Furthermore, it is true for any convergent Fourier series that $|c_m| \to 0$ as $|m|$ tend to ∞. Moreover, if $p(x)$ has n continuous derivatives, then its Fourier transform $P(u)$ tend to 0 as $|u| \to \infty$ at least as fast as $1/u^{n+1}$ (see [7] page 74): $\lim_{|u| \to \infty} |P(u)| = O\left(\frac{1}{u^{n+1}}\right)$. Thus, the smoother the function, the more rapidly the coefficients of the series tend to zero.

Recall that the spectra of the original images is given by $P(u)$ rotated along the frequency directions. Also, the amplitude of the (k_1, k_2) impulse is the product of the amplitudes of the k_1 and k_2 impulses in the original images spectra. Therefore, the amplitude of the (k_1, k_2) impulse in the superposition will tend to 0 faster than $\left(\frac{1}{u_1 u_2}\right)^{n+1}$ where u_1 and u_2 are the locations of the k_1 and k_2 impulses.

The Fourier approach has the advantage that it enables to analyze the moiré patterns in the frequency domain which is a suitable domain for deciding the response of the visual system. In the case of nonlinear gratings, the spectrum of the gratings no longer consists of impulses and may be continuous. It is then impossible to analyze the superposition spectrum with the same ease as before. However, a local frequency analysis can use the above results since any smooth function can be approximated by a linear function in a small enough region.

3   The Problem of Moiré Synthesis

Synthesis of moiré patterns is the generation of two images that when superimposed will reveal the intended moiré pattern. We restate the condition for the generation of a certain moiré pattern. Let $\psi(x,y), \phi(x,y)$ be two 2-D functions and let $p(z)$ be a 1-D periodic function with period of unity. The superposition $p(\psi(x,y)) \cdot p(\phi(x,y))$ will contain the (k_1, k_2) moiré pattern whose geometric layout is the equal height contours of $g(x,y)$ if the following condition holds

$$g(x,y) = k_1\psi(x,y) + k_2\phi(x,y). \tag{5}$$

This condition determines ϕ completely from g and ψ. There is, however, a degree of freedom in choosing ψ or ϕ. The moiré pattern described by g will stand out visually for some choices of ψ and yet it may be hidden for other choices due to the inherent filtering process of the human visual system.

We will first determine criteria for evaluating the superposition image. Based on these criteria we will choose ψ and ϕ that will satisfy (5) and optimize our performance criteria.

From here on, we will deal with synthesis of first order $(1, -1)$ moiré patterns since higher order moiré patterns are generally less dominant (see section 2.2). Synthesis of the $(1, 1)$ or higher order moiré patterns requires some straightforward modifications.

4   Performance Criteria

When synthesizing moiré patterns we have to choose ψ and ϕ from an infinite set of functions which satisfy (5). In this section we propose criteria to estimate the visual performance of the moiré. Based on these criteria we can decide whether one choice of ψ and ϕ that satisfy (5) is better than another. In section 7 we use these criteria to optimally choose ψ and ϕ.

We will first consider performance criteria for linear moiré. We assume that the superposition image and the resulting moiré patterns are approximately linear in a small enough region. Based on local analysis and the results for linear moiré performance we will formulate criteria for general moiré patterns.

4.1   Linear Moiré Performance

The filtering process of the human visual system is nicely demonstrated in two simple experiments. A figure of cosine vertical bars with continuously varying frequencies and amplitudes (see [8] Figure 2.4-3 p. 35) demonstrates sensitivity to the spatial frequency of the cosine bars. Comparing a figure of a checkerboard with a rotated duplicate (see [9] Fig. 5.2 p. 83) demonstrates the non-isotropy of the visual system filtering: The human visual system is more sensitive at 0 and 90 degrees than at 45 degrees to changes with equal contrast and frequency.

The contrast of a pattern I is defined by $C = \frac{I_{max}-I_{min}}{I_{max}+I_{min}}$ where I_{max} and I_{min} are the maximum and minimum intensities in the pattern respectively. For an absolute uniform image, $I_{max} = I_{min}$ and $C = 0$. For a square wave gratings, $I_{max} = 1, I_{min} = 0, C = 1$. Since the denominator is proportional to the mean intensity, contrast can also be considered as the degree of modulation of intensity above the mean. For sinusoidal gratings the contrast is proportional to the amplitude.

The contrast sensitivity function (CSF) of a system is defined as $CSF = \dfrac{\text{output contrast}}{\text{input contrast}}$. It is not always feasible to measure the output for humans in a completely controlled fashion. Necessarily, psychological experiments are used, requiring many assumptions about the system behavior.

The experimental procedure for measuring the CSF involves presenting each of a set of vertical sinusoidal gratings on a visual display to a viewer who can vary the contrast control while maintaining constant average luminance. For a given pattern coarseness, the viewer is asked to adjust the contrast until the grating is just barely distinguishable. The threshold of contrast perception $c(u)$ is obtained at different spatial frequencies and the contrast sensitivity function is $CSF(u) = \frac{\alpha}{c(u)}$ (the constant α is assigned to barely distinguishable contrast).

Dooley (see [10] p. 118) has provided the following equation to fit the data from the above experiments $CSF(u) = \left|5.05\left(e^{-0.138u}\right)\left(1 - e^{0.1u}\right)\right|$ Where $u = 2\pi f$, f is the spatial frequency along the x axis in cycles per degrees and $\alpha = 0.005$.

A review of the non-isotropy of the visual system [11], describes results of the following experiment. Gratings were presented to a viewer at different angles and different distances. The distances at which the gratings were barely visible represent the sensitivity of the visual system to orientations.

As a measure of the visibility of an impulse whose location on the frequency plane is $\boldsymbol{f}$ we take

$$V(\boldsymbol{f}) = H_1(\|\boldsymbol{f}\|) \cdot H_2(\text{angle}(\boldsymbol{f})) \tag{6}$$

Where H_1 and H_2 are the functions obtained from the above two experiments.

Recall that for the raised cosinusoidal profile we have only the first order moiré. In moiré pattern synthesis, we receive the desired pattern $p(g(x,y)) = p(p_1 x + q_1 y)$ as input. The gradient of the desired pattern $\nabla g = (p, q)$ points at the required frequency direction. In addition, $1/\|\nabla g\|$ is the distance between two adjacent periods of $p(g(x,y))$. Therefore the magnitude of the spatial frequency of $p(g(x,y))$ is $\|\nabla g\|$. In other words, for $p(g(x,y))$ to appear as the $(1,-1)$ moiré, $\boldsymbol{f}_{(1,-1)}$ should be equal to ∇g. Since in moiré synthesis we receive g as input, the location of $\boldsymbol{f}_{(1,-1)}$ is set by ∇g when (5) is satisfied.

The freedom in choosing different ψ and ϕ that satisfy (5) allows controlling the location of $\boldsymbol{f}_{(1,1)}$. For the $(1,-1)$ moiré to be visible, we should minimize the visibility of the $(1,1)$ moiré. The optimal ϕ_{opt}, ψ_{opt} for this minimization is

$$\phi_{opt} = \arg\min_{\phi} H_1(\|\boldsymbol{f}_{(1,1)}\|) \cdot H_2(\text{angle}(\boldsymbol{f}_{(1,1)})) \tag{7}$$

$$\psi_{opt} = g + \phi_{opt} \tag{8}$$

$\boldsymbol{f}_{(1,1)}$ can be computed by $\boldsymbol{f}_{(1,1)} = \boldsymbol{f}_\phi + \boldsymbol{f}_\psi = \nabla\phi + \nabla\psi = 2\nabla\phi + \nabla g$ where we used the following result $g = \psi - \phi \Rightarrow \nabla\psi = \nabla g + \nabla\phi$.

As $\|\nabla\phi\|$ is increased, the frequency vector that corresponds to the $(1,1)$ moiré becomes larger in magnitude. According to the visibility function (6) this means that the visual system will be less responsive to this frequency, hence the performance will improve as $\|\nabla\phi\|$ is increased.

Such uncontrolled improvement in the performance becomes problematic when we use digital media to represent the images. As we further increase $\|\nabla\phi\|$ we will get an additional strong unwanted moiré between the grating and the pixel frequency of the display due to aliasing.

To account for this effect in the performance criteria, another term M, will be added to (6) as follows

$$V(\boldsymbol{f}_{(1,1)}) = H_1(\|\boldsymbol{f}_{(1,1)}\|) \cdot H_2(\text{angle}(\boldsymbol{f}_{(1,1)})) + M(\|\boldsymbol{f}_{(1,1)}\|) \tag{9}$$

This term will become dominant for very high frequencies and prevent the unbounded decrease in (9). This digitization term $M(\|\boldsymbol{f}_{(1,1)}\|)$ should be negligible for low frequencies and dominant for high frequencies. In addition to choosing M with these properties, we should choose the crossing point

$$M(\|\boldsymbol{f}_{(1,1)}\|) = H_1(\|\boldsymbol{f}_{(1,1)}\|) \cdot \min H_2(\text{angle}(\boldsymbol{f}_{(1,1)})) \tag{10}$$

with care. To do so the function $M(\cdot)$ was chosen to be of the form $M(\cdot) = m\tilde{M}(\cdot)$ where $\tilde{M}(\cdot)$ is an increasing polynomial and m is a parameter. m is determined in order to set the crossing point (10) as described below. We define the digitization threshold T_f as the frequency at which two periods of the gratings ψ and ϕ start to merge on the display. We denote $\tilde{\phi}$ and $\tilde{\psi}$ as the functions computed by equations (7) and (8). We would like $\|\nabla\tilde{\phi}\|$ and $\|\nabla\tilde{\psi}\|$ to be smaller than the digitization threshold by $\epsilon_1 > 0$: $\|\nabla\tilde{\phi}\| < T_f - \epsilon_1$, $\|\nabla\tilde{\psi}\| < T_f - \epsilon_1$ Since the choice of M affects the choice of $\tilde{\phi}$ and only then $\tilde{\psi}$ is computed, we will explore the relation between $\|\nabla\phi\|$ and $\|\nabla\psi\|$: $g = \psi - \phi$, $\nabla\psi = \nabla g + \nabla\phi$, $\|\nabla\psi\| = \|\nabla g + \nabla\phi\| \leq \|\nabla g\| + \|\nabla\phi\|$ If the condition $\|\nabla\tilde{\phi}\| < T_f - \epsilon_1$ holds, we have $\|\nabla\tilde{\psi}\| \leq T_f - \epsilon_1 + \|\nabla g\|$

We denote the frequency of the crossing point as f_{cp}. If we assume that $\|\nabla\tilde{\phi}\| \leq f_{cp} + \epsilon_2$, $\epsilon_2 > 0$ we arrive at the following result: If we choose the crossing point frequency f_{cp} according to $f_{cp} \leq T_f - \|\nabla g\| - \epsilon_1 - \epsilon_2$, $\tilde{\phi}$ and $\tilde{\psi}$ will satisfy $\|\nabla\tilde{\phi}\| \leq T_f - \epsilon_1 - \|\nabla g\|$, $\|\nabla\tilde{\psi}\| \leq T_f - \epsilon_1$. Intuitively, the value of ϵ_1 represents how much we would like to stay away from the digitization threshold and ϵ_2 represents the possibility that the minimization procedure will carry $\|\nabla\tilde{\phi}\|$ beyond the crossing point.

4.2   Performance of Non-linear Moiré Patterns

The visibility of the $(1,1)$ moiré in a general superposition over a region Ω is defined as $W(\boldsymbol{f}_{(1,1)})(\Omega) = \iint_\Omega V(\boldsymbol{f}_{(1,1)}(x,y))dxdy$ were $V(\boldsymbol{f}_{(1,1)}(x,y))$ is the function defined in (9). Over a discrete image I of size $M \times N$ we have

$$W(\boldsymbol{f}_{(1,1)})(I) = \sum_{i=1}^{M}\sum_{j=1}^{N} V(\boldsymbol{f}_{(1,1)}(i,j)) \tag{11}$$

5   The Integrability Constraints

When minimizing the visibility of the $(1,1)$ moiré equation (11) depends on $\boldsymbol{f}_{(1,1)}(x,y) = 2\nabla\phi(x,y) + \nabla g(x,y)$. Since (11) depends explicitly on $\nabla\phi$, we may state the optimization problem as

$$\text{for each } (i,j) \text{ find } \nabla\phi_{opt}(i,j) \text{ that will minimize } V(\boldsymbol{f}_{(1,1)}(i,j)).$$

The problem with such a scheme is that the obtained vector field $\nabla\phi_{opt}$ may not be a conservative field. This means that no function can be found, that $\nabla\phi_{opt}$ will be its gradient.

Enforcing the integrability test for $\nabla\phi$, we are led to the following problem:

$$\nabla\phi_{opt} = \arg\min_{\nabla\phi} W(\boldsymbol{f}_{(1,1)})(I) \tag{12}$$

$$\text{subject to:} \quad \phi_{xy} = \phi_{yx}$$

As we shall see in the next section our variational solution will not impose integrability as a hard constraint, but we shall enforce it approximately via a penalty term.

6   Results from Variational Calculus

In this section we will state some results from variational calculus that are used in the following sections. For the cases below see also [12] and for a more complete description with derivations refer for example to [13] or [7].

The calculus of variations deals with minimizing functionals. A functional is a function from a set of functions to the real line. A fundamental result of the calculus of variations is that the extrema of functionals must satisfy an associated differential equation called the Euler equation over the domain.

The Euler equation is a necessary but not sufficient condition for the existence of an extremum. By extrema we mean local minima, maxima and inflection points. We assume that all functions and functionals are continuous and have derivatives. Another assumption is that the functional values are positive.

For example a functional I_1 which depends on a bivariate function $z(x,y)$ as follows $I_1[z] = \iint_\Omega F(x,y,z,z_x,z_y)dxdy$ yields the following Euler equation $F_z - \frac{\partial}{\partial x}F_{z_x} - \frac{\partial}{\partial y}F_{z_y} = 0$.

The functional I_2 which depends on the gradient of $z(x,y)$, i.e. $\nabla z(x,y) = (p(x,y), q(x,y))$ as follows $I_2[p,q] = \iint_\Omega F(x,y,p,q,p_x,p_y,q_x,q_y)dxdy$ yields a coupled set of differential Euler equations $F_p - \frac{\partial}{\partial x}F_{p_x} - \frac{\partial}{\partial y}F_{p_y} = 0$, $F_q - \frac{\partial}{\partial x}F_{q_x} - \frac{\partial}{\partial y}F_{q_y} = 0$. The Euler differential equations require boundary conditions to have a specified solution. However, in many problems there are no imposed prior conditions on the boundary values or the behavior of the function at the boundary may be restricted by some general conditions. In such cases, the variational calculus supplies us with further conditions for the boundary values. These conditions are also necessary conditions for the functional to be stationary with respect to variations (see [7] page 208). Such conditions are called natural boundary conditions. In the case of I_1, the natural boundary condition is $(F_{z_x}, F_{z_y}) \cdot \boldsymbol{n} = 0$ where $\boldsymbol{n}$ is the normal to the parametric curve representing the boundary of Ω. For I_2, the natural boundary conditions are $(F_{p_x}, F_{p_y}) \cdot \boldsymbol{n} = 0, \quad (F_{q_x}, F_{q_y}) \cdot \boldsymbol{n} = 0$

Recall that the visibility of the $(1, 1)$ moiré in a small area surrounding (x, y) is expressed by $V(p(x, y), q(x, y))$ where $(p(x, y), q(x, y)) = \nabla \phi$. Adding a penalty term which represent the integrability constraint and squaring V results in the following functional

$$I[p, q] = \iint_\Omega \left(V^2(p, q) + \lambda(p_y - q_x)^2 \right) \mathrm{d}x \mathrm{d}y. \tag{13}$$

Equation (13) is in I_2 form and its Euler equations are

$$-VV_p + \lambda(p_{yy} - q_{xy}) = 0, \quad -VV_q + \lambda(q_{xx} - p_{yx}) = 0 \tag{14}$$

By discretizing (14) the following iterative scheme is obtained

$$p_{i,j}^{k+1} = \bar{p}_{i,j}^k - \frac{1}{2}\tilde{q}_{i,j}^k - \frac{1}{2\lambda}V(p_{i,j}^k, q_{i,j}^k)V_p(p_{i,j}^k, q_{i,j}^k)$$

$$q_{i,j}^{k+1} = \bar{q}_{i,j}^k - \frac{1}{2}\tilde{p}_{i,j}^k - \frac{1}{2\lambda}V(p_{i,j}^k, q_{i,j}^k)V_q(p_{i,j}^k, q_{i,j}^k)$$

$$\bar{p}_{i,j} = \frac{p_{i,j+1} + p_{i,j-1}}{2}, \quad \bar{q}_{i,j} = \frac{q_{i+1,j} + q_{i-1,jx}}{2}$$

$$\tilde{p}_{i,j} = \frac{p_{i+1,j+1} + p_{i-1,j-1} - p_{i+1,j-1} - p_{i-1,j+1}}{4}$$

$$\tilde{q}_{i,j} = \frac{q_{i+1,j+1} + q_{i-1,j-1} - q_{i+1,j-1} - q_{i-1,j+1}}{4}$$

The choice of including the integrability constraints as a penalty term works better than other approaches that try to strictly enforce the integrability constraints [12]. The parameter λ enables control of the trade-off between a "smoother" vector field that will enable better recovery of ϕ and a vector field which reaches lower visibility.

As initial conditions, we took an arbitrary vector field. The boundary conditions are described in section 9. Note that the natural boundary conditions in this case reduce to the integrability condition $p_y = q_x$ on boundary.

7   Recovering Height from Gradient

7.1   Height from Gradient Problem

The height from gradient problem deals with following problem: Given a vector field $\boldsymbol{F}(x, y)$, find a function $\phi(x, y)$ such that $\nabla \phi(x, y) = \boldsymbol{F}(x, y)$.

Note that the solution ϕ is not unique since adding a constant term to ϕ will result in another solution to the problem. This problem can therefore be classified as an initial value problem: Given an initial value at some location $\phi(x_0, y_0)$ and $\boldsymbol{F}(x, y)$, find $\phi(x, y)$ for all the region.

A simple solution to this problem is

$$\phi(x, y) = \phi(x_0, y_0) + \int_C \nabla\phi \cdot d\boldsymbol{l}. \tag{15}$$

Where C is a curve from (x_0, y_0) to (x, y). This method allows us to compute ψ completely once an initial value $\psi(x_0, y_0)$ is determined. The problem with equation (15) is that it is numerically unstable. A height value at some point would, in the presence of noise, depend on the integration path that was taken. It is better to find a best fit surface $\phi^\star$ to ϕ. This can be accomplished by a variational calculus setting [12]. The variational approach to height from gradient is discussed in the next subsection.

7.2 Variational Calculus Setting for Height from Gradient

Given the vector field $\boldsymbol{F}(x, y) = (p(x, y), q(x, y))$ and a possible approximate solution $\phi^\star$ we wish to minimize the following functional

$$\iint_\Omega (\phi_x^\star - p)^2 + (\phi_y^\star - q)^2 dx dy \tag{16}$$

Calculating the Euler equation for (16) yields $\Delta\phi^\star = p_x + q_y$ Where $\Delta\phi^\star$ is the Laplacian of $\phi^\star$: $\frac{\partial^2 \phi^\star}{\partial x^2} + \frac{\partial^2 \phi^\star}{\partial y^2}$. This equation is a second order elliptic PDE called Poisson equation. The Poisson equation is widely studied and many procedures for numerical solutions exist. In our experiments we used two methods to solve this equation. One is a multigrid method and the other is based on sine transforms and tridiagonal solutions [14].

Once again, note that this equation does not uniquely specify a solution without further constraints. In fact, we can add any function h that satisfy $\Delta h = 0$ to the solution. For this particular problem, the natural boundary conditions are $(\phi_x^\star, \phi_y^\star) \cdot \boldsymbol{n} = (p, q) \cdot \boldsymbol{n}$ where $\boldsymbol{n}$ is the normal to the boundary $\boldsymbol{n} = \left(-\frac{dy}{ds}, \frac{dx}{ds}\right)$. With these boundary conditions, the solution is still not unique, since an arbitrary constant can be added to $\phi^\star$ without changing the functional. To get a unique solution, one can fix arbitrary height at some point.

8   Experimental Results and Conclusions

When solving (14) we have to specify a boundary condition and an initial value. The initial value is $p_{i,j}^0, q_{i,j}^0$ for all i, j in the domain. The boundary condition is the update rule from one iteration to the next along the boundary of the domain. Since we have no apriori knowledge of the boundary values, we will consider two methods for updating the boundary values between iterations.

If we have additional knowledge on the desired p and q we may be able to incorporate this knowledge into the boundary condition. For example, if the desired pattern can be rolled along the x and y axis up to form the surface of a three dimensional torus or donut, periodic boundary conditions can be used.

In periodic boundary conditions, the boundary value in the next iteration is taken from the computed values along the opposite boundary. For the case of an image I of size $N \times N$, the update rule is $p_{i,1}^{k+1} = p_{i,N-1}^{k}, p_{i,N}^{k+1} = p_{i,2}^{k}, p_{1,i}^{k+1} = p_{N-1,i}^{k}, p_{N,i}^{k+1} = p_{2,i}^{k}$. and the boundary of $q_{i,j}^{k}$ is updated in a similar manner. Periodic boundary conditions will perform well for periodic shapes, but this is hardly the general case. In the general case, if we knew p_y, q_x on the boundary we could update the boundary values by integration $p(1,j) = p(1, j-1) + \int_{j-1}^{j} p_y(1, t) \mathrm{dt}$, $p(N, j) = p(N, j-1) + \int_{j-1}^{j} p_y(N, j) \mathrm{dt}$, $p(i, 1) = p(i, 2) - \int_{2}^{1} p_y(i, t) \mathrm{dt}$, $p(i, N) = p(i, N-1) + \int_{N-1}^{N} p_y(i, t) \mathrm{dt}$. The values of q can be similarly updated. The integration can be numerically approximated by the trapezoidal rule.

We now turn to the problem of approximating the derivatives in the update equations. We can approximate $q_x(i, 1), q_x(i, N), i = 2 \ldots N - 1$ by central difference formula. The values of $q_x(1, j), q_x(N, j)$ can be approximated by forward or backward formulas. We can now use the fact that p and q satisfy $p_y = q_x$ on the boundary to compute p_y needed for the above computation.

To evaluate the algorithm it would be desirable to synthesize moiré patterns whose optimal ϕ and ψ is known. We could then compare the optimal ϕ and ψ with the functions found by the minimization process.

Finding optimal ϕ and ψ for arbitrary moiré patterns require exhaustive search over a function space. Such search is, in the general case, clearly impractical. However, for certain moiré patterns, optimal synthesis can be computed without exhaustive search. An example of such moiré patterns is linear patterns. From the structure of the optimality criterion it is clear that the optimal $\nabla \phi$ should be constant throughout the image. The optimal ϕ should therefore be a linear image.

To find the optimal ϕ we proceed as follows. Every linear function ϕ is characterized by two parameters $(p, q) = \nabla \phi$. Finding the optimal ϕ reduces in this case to evaluating the performance criteria over $\mathbb{R}^2$. The optimal ϕ is not unique since the performance criteria is symmetric with respect to reflection around the lines $x = 0, y = 0, y = x, y = -x$. In other words, $V(p_0, q_0) = V(p_0, -q_0) = V(-p_0, q_0)$ and so on. We then check the solution found by the iterative scheme. Starting from an initial condition of $(p, q) = (0, 1)$ and using the boundary conditions we arrive at the solution whose gradient is identical to one of the optimal gradients. The initial values are shown in Fig. 5 and the values at iteration 20 are shown in Fig. 6. The dashed vector represent the gradient of the original linear image and the solid vectors represent the computed $\nabla \phi$.

It is interesting to start with two functions, create a superposition and feed this superposition to the iterative procedure. In general, the solution will not be the same as the two original functions. The reason for this is that probably the superposition we started with was not optimal or that the algorithm converge to a different local minimum.

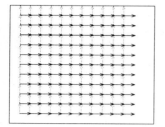
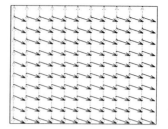

Fig. 5. Linear moiré, initial condition   **Fig. 6.** Linear moiré, iteration 20

However, we succeeded in calculating the two original functions in the following case. We start with two ellipses whose centers are shifted along the x axis. The equations for two such ellipses are $\frac{(x-s)^2}{a^2} + \frac{y^2}{b^2} = h^2$, $\frac{(x+s)^2}{a^2} + \frac{y^2}{b^2} = k^2$. The indicial equation is $h - k = p$ By elimination of h and k from these equations and after some rearrangements the following equation is obtained [4] $\frac{4x^2}{a^2p^2} - \frac{y^2}{(b^2p^2/4)-b^2s^2} = 1$ which represents a hyperbola parameterized by p. Indeed, when we used the synthesis algorithm to produce hyperbolic moiré patterns, such ellipses were found. In Fig. 7 results are shown for natural boundary conditions. The iterative process converged fast in our experiments. Usually after about 200 iterations, there was no apparent change in the images. The parameter λ allows controlling the "smoothness" of the solution. The results in Figures 8 were obtained for $\lambda = 200$. Compare these images with Figure 9 which was obtained for $\lambda = 1000$.

A periodic profile of a face image is shown in Figure 10. The computed ϕ and ψ and the superposition image is shown in Figures 11,12.

The suggested visibility criterion seem to produce good results especially in simple cases such as Fig. 7. In more complicated images (such as the face images) the optimization algorithm seem to converge to a local minimum and the final result depends on the initial conditions. Although in the general case the boundary condition is unknown, experimental results show that this affects only solution pixels near the boundary.

The results of this work suggest another application area for moiré synthsis. If the desired pattern is smooth, the two original images bear little or no resemblance to the desired pattern. The desired pattern is created by the nonlinear superposition from both images. Moiré pattern synthesis may then be used for some sort of visual cryptography. Instead of transmitting the image on an unsecured channel, it is possible to transmit two images which create a moiré pattern of the desired pattern. However, note that for non-smooth images such as the face image areas of discontinuities may disclose the boundary of the face in ψ and ϕ.

A method for visual cryptography for binary images has been proposed in [15] that allows perfect reconstruction but the reconstructed image is half the resolution of the transmitted images. Extending this method for gray-level images will require transmitting two very large images. In moiré synthesis, perfect

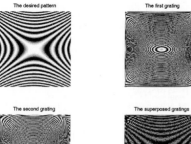

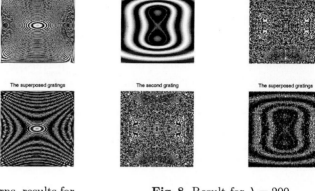

Fig. 7. Hyperbolic patterns, results for natural boundary conditions

Fig. 8. Result for $\lambda = 200$

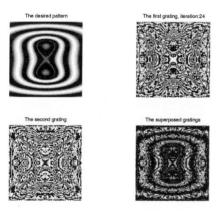

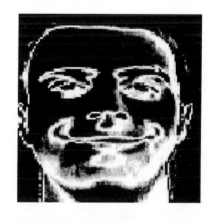

Fig. 9. Result for $\lambda = 1000$

Fig. 10. Periodic profile of a face image

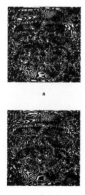

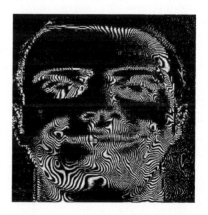

Fig. 11. ψ and ϕ computed for Fig. 10

Fig. 12. The superposition of the images in Fig. 11

reconstruction is not possible. However, as is seen in the previous examples, it is often easy to recognize the pattern from the superposition. Our performance criteria were designed for visibility of the moiré patterns. Other applications, such as true visual cryptography certainly require different performance criteria. The optimization scheme, however, may remain the same.

In our scheme for moiré synthesis the superposition image consists of low frequency and high frequency components. The low frequency components represent the desired pattern and zero order moiré patterns. The high frequency components represent the $(1,1)$ moiré terms which were "pushed" outside the visibility circle and higher order moirés. We can therefore apply low-pass filtering to the superposition image to enhance the desired pattern. If in addition, the periodic profile does not have a DC term, zero order moiré do not exist and hence we expect better reconstruction.

Acknowledgements

We would like to thank Alexander Brook, Ron Kimmel, Avraham Sidi and Marius Ungarish for their helpful advises. This paper was supported in part by the Fund for the Promotion of Research at the Technion.

References

1. Lord Rayleigh. On the manufacture and theory of diffraction-gratings. *Philos. Mag.*, 81:81–93, February 1874. Published also in Indebetouw G. and R. Czarnek, Selected papers on optical moire and applications, SPIE milestone series, Vol. 64.
2. Bryngdahl O. Characteristics of superposed patterns in optics. *J. Opt. Soc. Am.*, 66(2), 1976.
3. I. Amidror. *The theory of the moiré phenomenon.* Kluwer Academic Publishers, Dordecht, 2000.
4. M. Wasserman Oster G. and C. Zwerling. Theoretical interpretations of moiré patterns. *J. Opt. Soc. Am.*, 54(2), 1964.
5. Giger H. Moirés. *Comp. & Math. with Appls*, 12B:329–361, 1986.
6. Bracewell R. *The Fourier transform and its applications.* McGraw-Hill publishing, second edition, 1986.
7. Courant R. and D. Hilbert. *Methods in Mathematical Physics*, volume 1. Interscience Publishers, New York, 1953.
8. Pratt W.K. *Digital Image Processing.* John Wiley & Sons, New York, second edition, 1991.
9. Ulichney R. *Digital halftoning.* MIT Press, Cambridge Mass., 1987.
10. Levine M. *Vision in man and machine.* McGraw-Hill, New York, 1985.
11. Taylor M. Visual discrimination and orientation. *Journal of Applied Optics*, pages 763–765, June 1963.
12. Horn B.K.P. and M.J. Brooks. The variational approach to shape from shading. *Comp. Vision, Graphics Image Processing*, pages 174–203, 1986.
13. Sagan H. *Introduction to the calculus of variations.* Dover Publications, New York, 1969.
14. Strang G. *Introduction to applied mathematics.* Wellesley-Cambridge press, Wellesley, Mass., 1986.
15. A. Shamir Naor M. Visual cryptography. In *EUROCRYPT 1994, Lecture Notes in Computer Science*, volume 950, Springer-Verlag, New York, 1995.

Optimization of Paintbrush Rendering of Images by Dynamic MCMC Methods

Tamás Szirányi[1,3,*] and Zoltán Tóth[2,3]

[1] Analogical Computing Laboratory, Computer. & Automation Research Institue,
Hungarian Academy of Sciences, H-1111 Budapest, Kende u. 13-17, Hungary
sziranyi@sztaki.hu
[2] Distributed System Department, Computer & Automation Institute,
Hungarian Academy of Sciences
sac@samson.aszi.sztaki.hu
[3] University of Veszprém, Department of Image Processing and Neurocomputing,
H-8200 Veszprém, Egyetem u. 10, Hungary

Abstract. We have developed a new stochastic image rendering method for the compression, description and segmentation of images. This paintbrush-like image transformation is based on a random searching to insert brush-strokes into a generated image at decreasing scale of brush-sizes, without predefined models or interaction. We introduced a sequential multiscale image decomposition method, based on simulated rectangular-shaped paintbrush strokes. The resulting images look like good-quality paintings with well-defined contours, at an acceptable distortion compared to the original image. The image can be described with the parameters of the consecutive paintbrush strokes, resulting in a parameter-series that can be used for compression. The painting process can be applied for image representation, segmentation and contour detection. Our original method is based on stochastic exhaustive searching which takes a long time of convergence. In this paper we propose a modified algorithm of speed up of about 2x where the faster convergence is supported by a dynamic Metropolis Hastings rule.

1 Introduction

Images can be interpreted in several ways by decomposition into basic functions: strokes [4, 5], fractals [1], etc. Each of these is natural in some sense: strokes are good representations of letters or shapes, Gabor-functions [8] are natural for human sensation, fractals originate from the self-similarity. When we look at some images or image scenes, we usually search for familiar features. This is exploited in fine arts: small details are sometimes neglected while the main features are enhanced.

Nonlinear partial differential equations [6] can be used for enhancing the main image structure. When compressing the image, anisotropic diffusion, based on the scale-space paradigm, can enhance the basic image features to get visually better quality [10].

---

* This work was partly done during the stay of T. Szirányi at Ariana project, INRIA, 2000

M.A.T. Figueiredo, J. Zerubia, A.K. Jain (Eds.): EMMCVPR 2001, LNCS 2134, pp. 201–215, 2001.
© Springer-Verlag Berlin Heidelberg 2001

Good effects of structured diffusion can be achieved by Gibbs reaction-diffusion method of [14]. A set of about dozen filters is applied to build a potential function for minimization through a stochastic process. Surprisingly good restoring and hiding effects can be demonstrated. This method needs some prior model and it results in partly isotropic morphology.

In our previous paper [11] we introduced a method to follow a painter's process by using simplified artificial strokes. It is not an image-filtering to get a painting-like isotropic transformation. Other image-painting methods of computer graphics deal with model- or edge-controlled methods [e.g. 3,7]. These methods can serve as interesting visual effects (e.g. impressionist style, brush-splines), but they are different from the quality of a 'real-scene' painter (e.g. old-fashion portrait painters or S. Dali). Our first goal is to simulate the painting process to get a picture similar to a 'real-scene' painting where the purpose of the painter is to portray something which looks like to be a real scenery. We deal with a method copying the real visual world into a pleasant form rather than with the artistic interpretation of some special style. Small articles are elaborated with fine brushes, while plain surfaces are painted with greater strokes. On the other hand, the sequential parameters of the consecutive strokes can be applied for image description or some moderate compression as well. We can see that our method enhances the main features, which can easily be followed by eye. The strokes guide our sight.

However, this stochastic stroke-searching and -rendering are exhaustive processes. Any new trial (a new stroke with the color in question) will be accepted if it reduces the distortion. Positioning of a stroke is a random proposal (to avoid ramble-generated "structures"), while the accept/reject decision of the proposed stroke is controlled by the given stage only, namely it is a Markov Chain process.

By selecting an appropriate Monte Carlo Markov Chain (MCMC) process, the exhaustive searching can be replaced with a random decision based on density-approximation of the distribution of the distortion error of strokes. The problem is with the target density: it should be a dynamic definition to avoid the return to the exhaustive search or to fall into the first local minima.

2   The Basic Concepts of the Paintbrush Algorithm [11]

Here we would like to take the human behavior and sensation when looking at and reproducing the visual word into considerations. When looking at an image, there is a very usual way of understanding the visual information:

- Looking at the main outline of the image,
- Looking for the objects,
- Finding small details,
- Relaxed scanning (wandering) on the image.

When interpreting the image content in a visual form, such as representational painting, the re-creation of the image can proceed a similar way:

- Outlining the main areas,
- Elaborating objects,
- Refining the small details.

In both cases (understanding and reproducing) there is a well-defined scale-space line. First the large details, then the finer details are proceeded. In this aspect the representational painting is similar to the anisotropic diffusion that is based on the scale-space theory [6] based on PDEs. However, there is a very important difference between the two scale-space approaches, namely:

Anisotropic diffusion enhances the main edges but smoothes the others, while the present paintbrush transformation has sharp edges at any stage. We get sharp details even in the case of small or low-contrast areas. In the latter sense representational painting gives better segmentation than the anisotropic diffusion. The effect is similar to that of Markov Random Field segmentation [2]. However, MRF has the drawback that the possible number of "colors" is limited to achieve good segmentation in a finite time.

The other important viewpoint is the question of the finest details of an image. When the image contains too many fine details (e.g. sharp photo), our sight may be disturbed by the unnecessary small details. If the image is compressed previously by a function-set of e.g. Cosine or Wavelet functions, then the image results in annoying artifacts in the range of fine details. We can remove the annoying fine information contents at the cost of smoothing the sharp segment-contours. On the contrary, we see a practical effect when we are looking at an image from a distance:

- In case of artwork painting, the visual effect could be perfect, giving high contrast to represent the objects;
- Getting closer to the painting, we can see sharp edges (paintbrush-strokes), but there is a point where there are no more fine details behind it.
- We can relax when looking at the image, since there are no details, which are quivering when scanning through.

When defining what we expect from a new process that follows the main features of representational painting, we can define the main concepts of the new algorithm:

1. It should have sharp edges at any level of image-construction;
2. There are no fine details below a limit;
3. There are sharp edges at the finest level as well;
4. From a given distance the image must give the same visual scenery as the original.

In the following space we can see that the above constraints can be fulfilled by a method, which follows the generation of painting by using different sizes of paintbrush strokes.

3   Our Previous Algorithm

Main steps of the original algorithm of [11] to generate paintbrush strokes follow:
1)   *Starting with the rawest brush-size;*

2) *or Selecting the next, smaller brush-size (δ);*
- If the finest scale is over then, Goto 14;

3) $C_{\varphi\delta}$: *Convolving the I input image by brush-distributions depending on orientation φ and brush-size δ. At δ brush-size we have at least 8 $C_{\varphi\delta}$ maps due to the φ orientations. This map-series is necessary to estimate the brush-color anywhere in the image without further brush-stroke tuning.*

4) *D: Difference image between the original I and the present iterated stage X;*

5) *A: Absolute or square values of the D difference image to get a distortion-map;*

6) *If the error-summation over A converges too slowly*
- then Goto 2;

7) *E: Convolving the A error image by a smoothing due to the diameter of the δ brush-size;*

8) *Calculating histogram of the distortion-map E, defining a threshold value where the probability of higher errors is ε;*

9) *Randomly choose a x,y position in the image and a φ brush-orientation;*

10) *If the distortion value of E at the pixel position of x,y is in the upper region of the distortion-histogram with probability ε, then*
- give the color of $C_{\varphi\delta}(x,y)$ to the brush-stroke centered at position (x,y) with the actual φ orientation and δ brush-size;
- or, in case of large strokes, give the color of the majority vote in the brush-area of the original I image to the brush-stroke centered at position (x,y);

11) *Cover the painted image by the pattern of this brush-stroke;*

12) *If the error-summation between the original and present stage image over the area of this stroke is decreasing,*
- then accept the new stroke;
- else reject and restore the previous stage in the stroke-area;

13) If the counter of the brush-strokes is smaller than a limit-number,
- then Goto 9;
- else Goto 4;

14) Ready.

After completing the rendering process, redundant strokes (fully covered by consecutive strokes) are eliminated from the code of the stroke-series. It usually results in a 20-50% decrease of the number of mounted strokes. Presently, the number of the possible φ stroke-orientations is 8.

We can see that our algorithm is stochastic, error-controlled and multiscale. In our present experiments brush-strokes are simple rectangles (see Figure 1). Since strokes need relatively great convolutions, the $C_{\varphi\delta}$ maps are generated in the Fourier domain. If the process is not random enough (forcing any prior structural constraints when placing a stroke, as considering and modeling 'edgy' places), the result may suffer from structural side-effects, like strong and disturbing contours.

The method has been tested for several parameter sets and test images. Some of the resulted images can be found in Figure 2. The "painted" images seemed to have high quality at the last phase with the finest brush. However, at every stage the edges are sharp and the patterns and textures are appropriate. It is interesting to note that the sharp edges and patterns can be generated without any a priori definitions of contours or textured places.

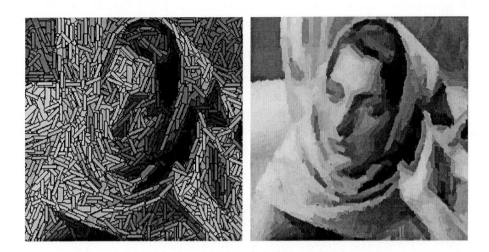

Fig. 1. Painting strokes with border (left) and without border (right) to demonstrate the non-structured random searching of the process (detail of test image "Barbara").

This method demonstrates that a fully random searching process generating brush-strokes can result in a high quality and pleasant-to-see image. This method takes about 10-30 minutes on a Pentium III PC when generating a 512x512 image. However, it can be easily implemented in parallel processor-arrays at high speed, like MRF-based algorithms in [12]. Since the above method is a 'brute-force' algorithm with an exhaustive stochastic searching, any development in the convergence speed and compactness of the generated code of the stroke-series may help in the applications.

4   Generating Series of Strokes Constituting a Markov Chain with Respect to the Metropolis-Hastings [9] Rule

When generating strokes to cover a patch on the image, the process is random: there is a target-density to constrain for the bounding errors and the proposal density depends on the characteristics of the painting process. First, we overview some Metropolis Hastings algorithms that we may use in the sequel.

The paintbrush rendering as originally described in [11] is a brute-force algorithm when considering its goal-function, error-bound and convergence. Applying MH methods, we hope to reach better-defined algorithms, with explicable effects and distributions and well-proven convergence properties.

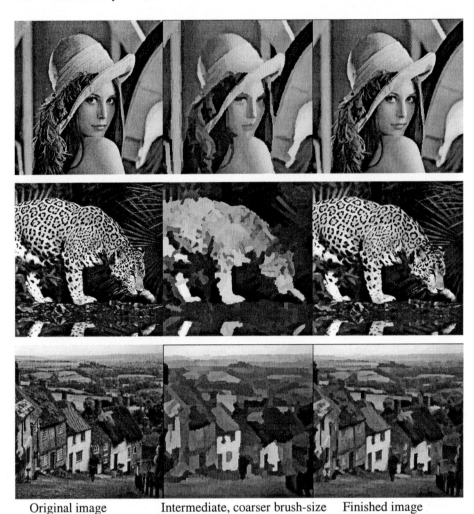

Original image   Intermediate, coarser brush-size   Finished image
                                                          with small brush-size

Fig. 2. Painting stages at different brush-sizes of image "Lena", "Leopard", and "Goldhill" (Number of the scales of brush-strokes was up to 10).

The goal of the painting process is to get a stroke-patched image which differs from the original one by less than a minimum mean-error, the difference being smaller than some minimum for any stroke-position. It can be best described by using an appropriate target density for the similarity-error over the individual strokes.

The individual event $X^{(t)}$ generates a paintbrush stroke at a position (coordinate of its reference point and the tilting angle) $S^{(t)}$ and with color $C^{(t)}$. The distortion error between $X^{(t)}$ and the original image in the area of $X^{(t)}$ is $\mathrm{E}^{(t)} = E\!\left(X^{(t)}\right)$. The position $S^{(t)}$ is randomly generated and may or may not depend on the previous stage and the overall image-parameters, while color $C^{(t)}$ is defined by the mean or majority color behind the proposed stroke in the original (reference) image. The target distribution f is the goal-function of $E(X^{(t)})$: $f = f(E^{(t)})$.

With the above notation, we can generate the series of $X^{(t)}$ s using the following algorithms:

PB-MH Algorithm:

Given $x^{(t)}$, the stroke of the t-th iteration,

1. Generate $Y_t \sim q(y \,|\, x^{(t)})$
2. Take

$$X^{(t+1)} = \begin{cases} Y_t & \text{with probability} & \rho(x^{(t)}, Y_t) \\ x^{(t)} & \text{with probability} & 1 - \rho(x^{(t)}, Y_t) \end{cases} \tag{1}$$

Where $\rho(x, y) = \min\left\{ \dfrac{f(y)\, q(x \,|\, y)}{f(x)\, q(y \,|\, x)}, 1 \right\}$

The algorithm starts with the error-bound of the proposed stroke-approximations as target density f. The conditional density $q(y \,|\, x)$ is a random position-generator of S^{Y_t}, related to the overall controlling error/edge map and the previous $X^{(t)}$ stroke.

Independent PB-MH

Given $x^{(t)}$

1. Generate $Y_t \sim g(y)$ (generated from the error-map and/or edge-map of the input image)
2. Take

$$X^{(t+1)} = \begin{cases} Y_t & \text{with probability} & \min\left\{ \dfrac{f(Y_t)\, g(x^{(t)})}{f(x^{(t)})\, g(Y_t)}, 1 \right\} \\ x^{(t)} & \text{otherwise} \end{cases} \tag{2}$$

Here the proposal density $g(y)$ is a random position-generator of $S^{(t+1)}$, independently of the previous $S^{(t)}$ position. This $g(y)$ might be uniform on the whole image.

Random Walk PB-MH

Given $x^{(t)}$

1. Generate $Y_t \sim g\left(y - x^{(t)}\right)$

2. Take

$$X^{(t+1)} = \begin{cases} Y_t & \text{with probability} \quad \min\left\{\dfrac{f(Y_t)}{f(x^{(t)})}, 1\right\} \\ x^{(t)} & \text{otherwise} \end{cases} \tag{3}$$

Here the proposal density $g\left(y - x^{(t)}\right)$ is a random position-generator of $S^{(t+1)}$, related to the previous $S^{(t)}$ position.

The original exhaustive searching algorithm in [11] operates with the 'Random walk' or 'Independent' proposal positioning, while in the accept/reject method f is a simple threshold on E, ($f(X) = f(E(X))$), where $f\left(x^{(t)}\right)$ and $f(Y_t)$ are considered on the proposed position, and $X^{(t)}$ and $Y^{(t)}$ indicate the whole image at different painted stages. When trying probabilistic accept/reject strategies in the same framework, we cannot get better convergence. As examples, we tested proposals as

$$X^{(t+1)} = \begin{cases} Y_t & \text{with probability} \quad \min\left\{\dfrac{E(x^{(t)})}{E(Y_t)}, 1\right\} \\ x^{(t)} & \text{otherwise} \end{cases} \quad \text{or}$$

$$X^{(t+1)} = \begin{cases} Y_t & \text{with probability} \quad \max\left\{\min\left\{E(x^{(t)}) - E(Y_t), 1\right\}, 0\right\} \\ x^{(t)} & \text{otherwise} \end{cases},$$

but the resulted quality and/or the convergence speed were much poorer than the simple exhaustive searching. We stepped toward a fully stochastic, MCMC-based algorithm.

5   Considering Statistical Tendencies of Densities of Distortion

The above algorithm [11] generates nice painting-like images, but the process needs optimization to get better speed. We can simply apply some quality constraints for $E(x^{(t)}) - E(Y_t) \geq \varepsilon > 0$ to force the acceptance of greater changes, but ε could depend on the image and the current situation, causing a loss of most of the proposals as in Fig 5(left). Practically, choosing $\varepsilon = 0.01$ may improve the compression ratio or convergence speed for several images. However, we should find some more self-calibrated manner for acceptance.

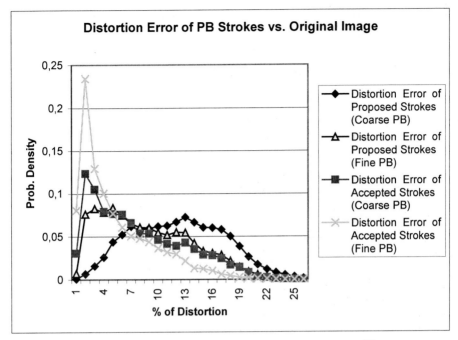

Fig. 3. Probability densities of distortion error of the proposed (Y_t) and accepted $(X^{t+1} = Y_t)$ strokes versus the original image when generating the strokes for 'Barbara' image. First, coarse (20x5), finally, fine (7x2) strokes are generated.

In the following space, $X^{(t)}$ (previous stage) and Y_t (proposed stage) denote state images with events of new strokes at position S^t and $S^{(t+1)}$ on the state image (painted by previous strokes as well).

We define distortion errors against the original image I :

- $E(x^{(t)}) = D\left(X^{(t)}, I\right)$ is the distortion error between the original and the previously painted stage image,
- $E(Y_t) = D\left(Y_t, I\right)$ is the distortion error between the original and the proposed painted stage Y_t,
- $E(x^{(t-1)}) = D\left(X^{(t-1)}, I\right)$ is the distortion error between the original and the last before painted stages.

$D(. , .)$ is defined as the mean square error, normalized by the actual area of the stroke into the [0.0, 1.0] interval.

Figure 3 shows the plot of statistics of the proposed and accepted $D(Y_t, I)$ values. First coarser, later finer strokes are generated, in the meantime the average error rate is decreasing. We can see that the distribution $f\left(D(Y_t, I)\right)$ converges to a Dirac-delta at zero for the accepted ($X^{t+1} = Y_t$) proposals. If we use any of the density functions of Figure 3 for a Metropolis-Hastings approach of eq. (1), the process does not work:

- If we use a long-term statistics of $f(Y_t) = f(D(Y_t, I))_{proposed}$, we get the same or much slower convergence than the exhaustive searching, since it does not fit to the acceptation rule;
- If we use a short-term statistics or the final $f(Y_t) = f(D(Y_t, I))_{accepted}$ (cc. Dirac-delta), the process stops at the beginning or stops at a low quality.

Applying the above statistics anyhow, we have the problem that Metropolis-Hastings MCMC converges relatively slowly, while $f(D(Y_t, I))$ and $f(D(x^{(t)}, I))$ will change considerably. So, the convergence and the basic idea of the process fail during the iterations. The other problem is that we must accept only proposals which decreases the overall error, otherwise the image will be unstructured, as in Fig 5(right).

In our new development of process, the following constraints should be kept:
- Accept error reduction only;
- The previous event and the present proposal of different proposed stroke-position are compared instead of distortion errors in the same place of the proposed stroke;
- The MCMC density-approximation is dynamic, following the changing target density.

Testing several experiments and on the above constraints it is clear that not the $D(.\,,.)$ terms, but their difference is important in the optimization process. Now we define two error differences:

$$Diff(Y_t) = E(x^{(t)}) - E(Y_t)$$
$$Diff(x^{(t)}) = E(x^{(t-1)}) - E(x^{(t)})$$

Figure 4 shows the statistics of the proposed (different cases are nearly the same) and the accepted (two cases) $Diff(Y_t)$ events, as the function of the relative error-rate.

It is clearly demonstrated that density $f(Diff(Y_t)_{accepted})$ is changing considerably through the iterations, while probability of the higher values of the proposed $Diff(Y_t)$ should decrease in time to get better convergence. It means that the stochastic rendering should consider the higher distortion values with a higher probability. Since density $f(Diff(Y_t)_{proposed})$ is nearly a Dirac-delta, containing mostly low $Diff(Y_t)$ values, it can be supposed that the proposed dynamic target density is

- $f(Y_t) = 0$ at $Diff(Y_t) \le 0$, so it is rejected;
- $f(Y_t)$ is progressive for higher $Diff(Y_t)$ values;

- $f(Y_t)$ should be normalized by the variance of the current distribution of $Diff(Y_t)$ values to follow the narrowing of the distribution.

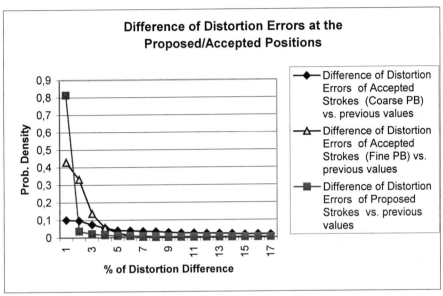

Fig. 4. Probability densities of difference btw distortion errors of the proposed and accepted strokes and the distortion on previous area of the stroke ($Diff(Y_t)$), when generating the strokes for 'Barbara' image. First, coarse (20x5), finally, fine (7x2) strokes are generated.

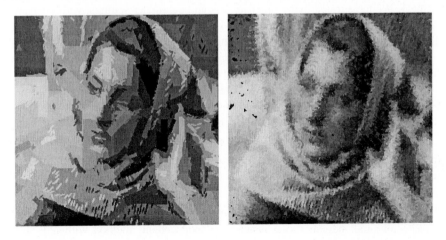

Fig. 5. *Erroneous results of rendering when (left)* Only strokes of high quality increase are accepted, $Diff(Y_t) \geq 0.1$; *(right)* The acceptance of a stroke may increase the overall error-rate. It is nearly the same as a process of fully *random* positioning, proposal and *acceptance*.

On the above considerations, we suppose the next accept/reject rule:

$$X^{(t+1)} = \begin{cases} Y_t & \text{with probability} \quad \rho\left(x^{(t)}, Y_t\right) \\ x^{(t)} & \text{with probability} \quad 1 - \rho\left(x^{(t)}, Y_t\right) \end{cases}$$

Where $\rho(x, y) = \min\left\{\dfrac{f(y)\, q(x\mid y)}{f(x)\, q(y\mid x)}, 1\right\}$ (4)

$$f(y) \sim \begin{cases} 0, & \text{if} \quad Diff(Y_t) < 0 \\ \left(Diff(Y_t)\Big/Var_t\right)^q, & \text{else} \end{cases}$$

$$f(x) \sim \left(Diff(x^{(t)})\Big/Var_t\right)^q$$

Here Var_t is the variance of $Diff(Y_t)$ in a neighborhood time interval around t. Since Var_t is changing slowly by time, it can be eliminated (and neglected) from $\rho(x, y)$ in eq. 4. Although $f(.)$ is the target density, it cannot be measured as a result of long-term statistics, since Var_t causes dynamic windowing effect on the output histogram, as Figure 6 demonstrates it.

Applying eq. 4, we tested it with different exponents q to reach the same image quality in PSNR at the same constraints (starting and stopping conditions, brush-sizes etc.). The results for image Barbara (using 3 different sizes of strokes) can be found in Table 1. We have tested many other images and parameter settings, with very similar conclusions. Tables 2 and 3 demonstrate some results for two 512x512 color images. Tables 4 shows a test of 'Lena' by using 10 different sizes of strokes. Exhaustive search of ε=0.01 also may give good compression result, but at the cost of twice effort, while MCMC at q=2.5 shows a good compromise.

We can see that eq. 4 gives an effective algorithm for image rendering at q=2 ... 3. Convergence speed is much better because of the smaller number of proposing and drawing events, at a considerable gain in the resulted number of paintbrush strokes.

We have also tested the role of the proposal density $q(y\mid x)$. Usually, it is symmetrical, or it is very close to be symmetrical. Step 10 in the algorithm of Section 3 may be asymmetrical, but its outcome is not too important. So, usually, we can consider $q(y\mid x) = q(x\mid y)$.

The proposal method can also be important in some cases. Applying 'Random walk' with small neighborhood instead of 'Independent' method with any sizes of steps, textured images can better converge.

In a recent research we develop the above method to consider MRF-conform neighborhood calculus into the energy term to run a structured MRF-like painting algorithm in a MCMC estimation series.

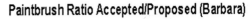

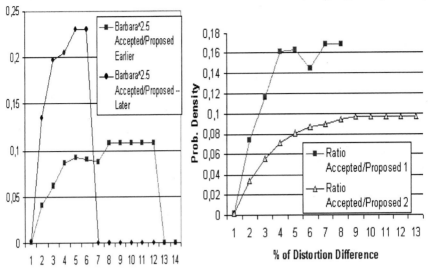

Fig. 6. *Narrowing effect of the distribution of* $Diff(Y_t)$ *and the measured statistics of the conditional probability (left)* Plot of ratio of measured histograms of the accepted and proposed distributions $P(Diff(Y_t)_{accepted})/P(Diff(Y_t)_{proposed})$ in the same size of stroke-series, show-ing the change in the conditional variance; *(right)* The above ratio of histograms for two differ-ent brush-sizes in whole-runs; For less optimized cases the monotonic function becomes a simple thresholding.

Table 1. Painting results for 'Barbara 512x512' at a standard $D(Y_t, I)$=25.5dB PSNR final distortion error rate. Counts are in thousand events.

Method	Number of non-redundant PB strokes # thousand	Number of all drawn strokes $\#((Y_t)_{accepted})$	Number of all proposed strokes $\#\left((Y_t)_{proposed}\right)$
$Diff(Y_t) > 0$	35	61	2645
(exhaustive search)			
q=1	29	40	2380
q=2	26	31	1555
q=3	28	34	1200

6   Conclusions

We have developed a dynamic approximation of target density for image rendering. A Metropolis-Hastings rule is proposed where the target density dynamically fits the process when the characterizing densities are changing through the iterations. This method results in better convergence (lower number of proposed and accepted strokes) and better compression (lower number of non-redundant strokes). The above MCMC-based stochastic search algorithm is quite different from other searching & matching methods, like matching pursuit [8] or effect-oriented paintings [7].

Table 2. Painting results for a 512x512 color image (detail of http://www.sztaki.hu/~sziranyi/ Sz-Barbara.jpg) with room, flowers and a girl at a standard $D(Y_t, I)$=26.5dB PSNR final distortion error rate. Counts are in thousand events.

Method	Number of non-redundant PB strokes # thousand	Number of all drawn strokes $\#((Y_t)_{accepted})$	Number of all pro-posed strokes $\#((Y_t)_{proposed})$
$Diff(Y_t)>0$	32	52	6490
(exhaustive search)			
q=1	26	34	2975
q=2	24	27	1630
q=3	19	22	3445

Table 3. Painting results for a 512x512 color image with a boy and color books, at a standard $D(Y_t, I)$=26.6dB PSNR final distortion error rate. Counts are in thousand events.

Method	Number of non-redundant PB strokes # thousand	Number of all drawn strokes $\#((Y_t)_{accepted})$	Number of all pro-posed strokes $\#((Y_t)_{proposed})$
$Diff(Y_t)>0$	9	16	760
(exhaustive search)			
q =1	7.4	12	860
q =2	7	9.6	560
q =3	7.4	8.7	495

Table 4. Painting results for 'Lena 512x512' at a standard $D(Y_t, I)$=30.45dB PSNR final distortion error rate. Counts are in thousand events.

Method	Number of non-redundant PB strokes # thousand	Number of all drawn strokes $\#((Y_t)_{accepted})$	Number of all pro-posed strokes $\#((Y_t)_{proposed})$
$Diff(Y_t)>0$	28	41	1369
(exhaustive search)			
$Diff(Y_t)>0.01$	11	11	2463
(exhaustive search)			
q =1.5	17	20	2441
q =2.5	14	14	1504

Acknowledgements

Many thanks are due to Josiane Zerubia. This work was supported by the Hungarian Research Fund (OTKA T032307) and by the French Ministry of Education and Research.

References

1. Y. Fisher. (ed.), *Fractal Image Compression*, Springer Verlag (1994)
2. S. Geman, D. Geman, "Stochastic relaxation, Gibbs distributions and the Bayesian restoration of images," *IEEE Tr. PAMI*, Vol. 6, pp. 721-741 (1984)
3. P.E. Haeberli, "Paint by numbers: Abstract image representations", *Computer Graphics*, (Proc. SIGGRAPH' 1990), V.24, pp.207-214, (1990)
4. H. H.S. Ip, H. T. F. Wong, "Generation of Brush Written Characters with fractal Characteristics from True-type Fonts", ICCPOL, *17th Int. Conf. on Computer Processing of Oriental Languages*, pp. 156-161, Hong Kong (1997)
5. H. H S Ip, H. T F Wong, "Calligraphic Character Synthesis using Brush Model", CGI'97, *Computer Graphics International conference*, pp. 13-21, Hasselt-Diepenbeek, Belgium, June 23-27 (1997)
6. T. Lindeberg, B. M. Haar Romeny, "Linear scale-space I-II", Geometry - Driven Diff. In Computer Vision, *Kluwer Academic Publishers,* pp.1-72 (1992)
7. P. Litwinowicz, 'Processing Images and Video for An Impressionist Effect', *Computer Graphics*, (Proc.SIGGRAPH'1997), pp.407-414 (1997)
8. R. Neff, A. Zakhor, "Very low bit-rate video coding based on matching pursuits", *IEEE Tr. CAS VT*, Vol. 7, pp.158-171 (1997)
9. Ch. P. Robert, G. Casella, *"Monte Carlo Statistical Methods"*, *Springer* Text in Statistics (1999)
10. T. Szirányi, I. Kopilovic, B. P. Tóth, "Anisotropic Diffusion as a Preprocessing Step for Efficient Image Compression", *Proc. of the 14th ICPR*, Brisbane, *IAPR&IEEE*, Australia, pp. 1565-1567, August 16-20 (1998)
11. T. Szirányi, Z. Toth, "Random Paintbrush Transformation", *15th ICPR*, Barcelona, IAPR&IEEE, V.3, pp.155-158 (2000)
12. T. Szirányi, J. Zerubia, "Markov Random Field Image Segmentation using Cellular Neural Network", *IEEE CAS I.*, Vol. 44, pp. 86-89 (1997)
13. P. Teo, D. Heeger, "Perceptual Image Distortion", First *IEEE Int.Conf. Image Proc.*, Vol.2, pp.982-986 (1994)
14. S.C. Zhu, D. Mumford, "Prior Learning and Gibbs Reaction-Diffusion",*IEEE Tr. PAMI*, Vol. 19, pp.1236-1250 (1997)

Illumination Invariant Recognition of Color Texture Using Correlation and Covariance Functions

Mohammed Al-Rawi and Yang Jie

Image Processing and Pattern Recognition Institute, Shanghai Jiao Tong University,
Shanghai 200030, P.R. China
rawi707@hotmail.com, jieyang@online.sh.cn

Abstract. In this paper, we derive a complete set of Zernike moment correlation functions used to capture spatial structure of a color texture. The set of moment correlation functions is grouped into moment correlation matrices to be used in illumination invariant recognition of color texture. For any change in the illumination, the moment correlation matrices are related by a linear transformation. Circular and non-circular correlations are discussed and comparisons with a previously suggested color covariance functions have been carried out using about 600 different illuminations and rotations textured images. Using moment correlation matrices in the invariant recognition of color texture, the process can promise in high computation efficiency as well as recognition accuracy. The derived correlation invariants is proposed as a general formalism that can be used directly with other kinds of complex moments, e.g. Fourier Mellin, pseudo Zernike, disc-harmonic coefficients, and wavelet moments, to obtain moment correlation based invariants.

1. Introduction

Early image recognition algorithms were based on computing (geometric) invariant features for gray-level intensity images. The goal was to detect an object or classify a textured image from an image database (gray-level and binary image recognition is still dominant in computer vision and pattern recognition applications). Despite of the increase in dimensionality, the use of colors is unavoidable in recent recognition applications. In fact, using color images may give a better recognition performance than gray-level images due the capability of capturing local and global image features within and between color bands. Moreover, it is not possible to perform illumination invariant recognition without using color properties of an image.

Many techniques had been suggested to investigate the use of multi bands of a color image to achieve geometry, illumination, or illumination-geometry invariant recognition. First, the work of Swain and Ballard [1] in which they showed that color distributions can be used directly for recognition without even paying attention to the spatial structure of the image. Their method, however, fails if the illumination spectral is changed or the spatial structure of the image is high (it is possible for regions with significantly different spatial structure to have similar color distributions). A Color Indexing color constancy algorithm [2] was developed to remove the dependency of color distributions on illumination changes. The algorithm performs well for an object

M.A.T. Figueiredo, J. Zerubia, A.K. Jain (Eds.): EMMCVPR 2001, LNCS 2134, pp. 216–231, 2001.

recognition task but with less success when the image is highly structured as in textures. The other group of color image recognition algorithms deals with computing spatial structure based features, some of the methods are Gabor filters [3], color distributions of spatially filtered images [4], Markov random field models [5] & [6], and spatial covariance functions [7]. Moment invariants of color covariance functions [7] (or as the authors called them color correlation functions but see Rosenfield [8] for the exact terminology which copes with the one we claim in this paper) within and between bands of a color image had been used to recognize three-dimensional textures. The same color covariance functions had been used successfully in a series of illumination recognition experiments of 2-D color texture [9]-[11]. Jain [10] used color covariance functions to recognize multispectral satellite images. In [11], Zernike moment invariants were computed for color covariance functions, the derived Zernike moment invariants, however, were not complete. In this paper a complete set of Zernike moment correlation and covariance matrices is derived. Different color correlations are introduced, circular and non-circular. Experimental results using about 600 different illumination-rotation images are used to compare the proposed model to the previously suggested color covariance functions.

2. Spatial Interaction within and between Color Bands

To be able to recognize the texture of a color image, the interaction within and between its bands is considered in this paper. The spatial covariance family functions forms one of the most reliable schemes used to model the color texture. In this paper we will discuss four different measures of these covariance functions.

2.1 Spatial Covariance Functions

Over the image region defining the texture, each band $I_i(\alpha, \beta)$ is assumed wide-sense stationary and each pair of bands is assumed jointly wide-sense stationary. The set of covariance functions within and between sensor bands ($1 \le i, j \le N$) is defined as

$$C_{ij}(x, \ y) = E\{[I_i(\alpha, \ \beta) - \overline{I}_i][\overline{I}_j(\alpha + x, \beta + y) - \overline{I}_j]\} \tag{1}$$

where $\overline{I}_i$ and $\overline{I}_j$ denote spatial means and E denotes the expected value. For the trichromatic case $N = 3$ we observe the following properties:
- The definition given in (1) will lead to nine covariance functions that include three autocovariance functions and six crosscovariance functions. All the nine spatial covariance functions have the following property $C_{ij}(x, y) = C_{ji}(-x, -y)$ in which only the autocovariance functions are symmetric about the origin. Therefore, we can make use of this symmetry to reduce computations.
- The crosscovariance functions are not symmetric; however, only three should be computed i.e. (C_{12}, C_{13}, C_{23}), the other three (C_{21}, C_{31}, C_{32}) can be obtained

using $C_{ij}(x, y) = C_{ji}(-x, -y)$. It was shown in [7] that it is useful to use only the basic six covariance functions.

- Considering two surfaces S and S' oriented arbitrarily in space where $C_{ij}(\bar{x})$ and $C'_{ij}(\bar{x})$ are the corresponding covariance functions and $\{\bar{x} = [x\ y]^T\}$. From [7], those covariance functions are related by a linear coordinate transform M as $C'_{ij}(\bar{x}) = C_{ij}(M\bar{x})$.

- Values of spatial covariance functions may be negative, zero, or positive.

- If the illumination between the corresponding textures changes, then the relation between their corresponding covariance functions changes. Suppose a textured surface observed at two different orientations in space under different illumination conditions, also suppose that the covariance functions are arranged into a column vector $C_i(\bar{x})$, then we group the covariance functions into a covariance matrix as $C(\bar{x}) = [C_1(\bar{x})\ C_2(\bar{x})\ ...C_6(\bar{x})]$. Following [11], let $C(\bar{x})$ be the covariance matrix of the surface corresponding to the illumination $l(\lambda)$ and $\tilde{C}'(\bar{x})$ be the covariance matrix for the same surface after an orientation change described by M and under illumination $\tilde{l}(\lambda)$, then $C(M\bar{x}) = \tilde{C}'(\bar{x})E$. Where E is a 6×6 matrix with elements that depend on $l(\lambda)$ and $\tilde{l}(\lambda)$. Therefore, for a change in illumination and orientation the covariance matrices are related by a linear transformation E and a linear coordinate transformation M.

The above covariance functions had been used successfully in the recognition of color texture. In all previous works, however, they considered that all crosscovariance functions are symmetric (the fact they were enforced to be symmetric). One reason is the high degree of pixel-to-pixel correlation between different bands belonging to the same image, which leads to a very small symmetric error.

2.2 Spatial Correlation Functions

Here we assume again that over the image region defining the texture, each band $I_i(\alpha, \beta)$ is wide-sense stationary and each pair of bands is assumed jointly wide-sense stationary. We define a set of correlation functions within and between sensor bands $(1 \le i, j \le N)$ as

$$R_{ij}(x, y) = E[I_i(\alpha, \beta)I_j(\alpha + x, \beta + y)],\tag{2}$$

where E denotes the expected value. For the trichromatic case $N = 3$, correlation functions will have the same properties as those given for covariance functions except that correlation functions will always have positive values. Positive values of correlation functions are necessary when used with moments since moments should be computed for nonnegative bounded functions. In the previous work of Kondepudy and Healey [7], they used the absolute value of color covariance functions to eliminate the negative values. This may in turn destroy the color covariance functions and the transform between the original image and its corresponding test image may be non linear or cannot be predicted.

2.3 Circular Correlation and Circular Covariance Functions

It is important to define a third group of correlation functions that capture some circular symmetric properties when the texture region is averaged within and between sensor bands. One way to do this is by averaging or estimating color correlations (or covariances) inside a circular region. We define circular correlations within and between sensor bands as:

$$\hat{R}_{ij} = \begin{cases} E[I_i(\alpha,\beta)I_j(\alpha+x,\beta+y)] & \alpha^2+\beta^2 \leq \Re \\ 0 & \text{elsewhere} \end{cases}, \tag{3}$$

where $\Re$ is the radius of the region to compute the expectation value at. Similarly, circular covariance functions are defined by:

$$\hat{C}_{ij} = \begin{cases} E\{[I_i(\alpha,\beta)-\bar{I}_i][I_j(\alpha+x,\beta+y)-\bar{I}_j] & \alpha^2+\beta^2 \leq \Re \\ 0 & \text{elsewhere} \end{cases}. \tag{4}$$

Circular color correlations and color covariances should give better results due to the ability to capture the same amount of information as an image is rotated by an angle. Experimental results discussed later will show which of the four proposed covariances schemes outperform the others. Figure 1 shows the cloth image photographed with five different illuminations. To consider the effect of different color correlation and color covariance functions, the entire sets of covariance and correlation functions family are used to represent the cloth image under white illumination and are demonstrated in Figs. 2-5.

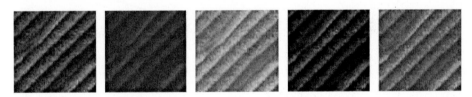

Fig. 1. The image of cloth under five different illuminations. From left to right, used illuminations are; white, red, green, blue, and yellow.

It is our task to show that images shown in Fig. 1, and another 25 cloth images (for each illumination) at different rotation angles belong to the same original class. In Figs. 2-5, we see that the spatial correlation and spatial covariance functions draws a surface that is to be recognized (instead of the original multispectral image). That surface may take the shape of a pyramid like shape or a cone like shape and may be deformed according to the combination of geometry and illumination changes. For this recognition process and how much those shapes are changing, we shall use the method of moment invariants (specifically Zernike moments).

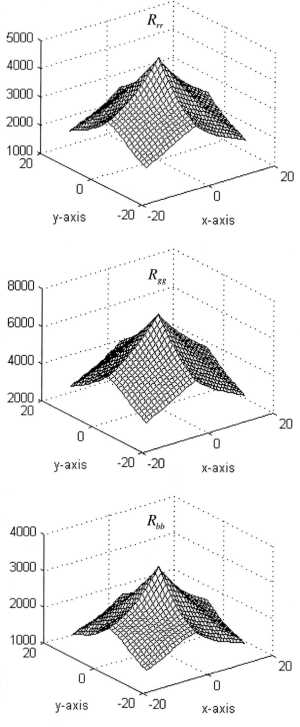

Fig. 2. (a) Correlation functions of cloth image under white illumination.

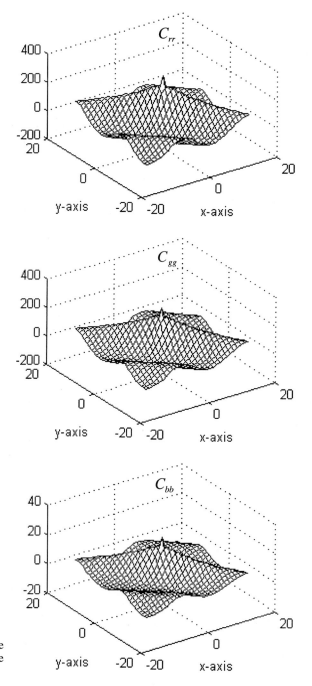

Fig. 3. (a) Covariance functions of cloth image under white illumination.

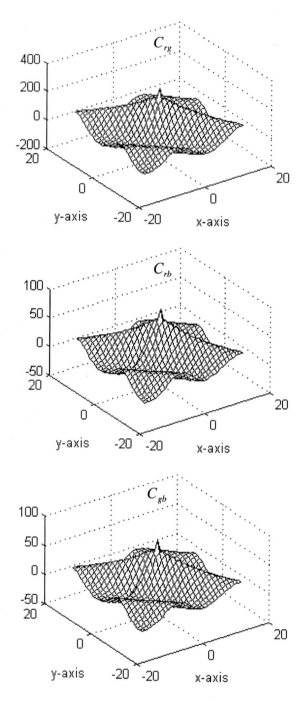

Fig. 3. (b) Covariance functions of cloth image under white illumination.

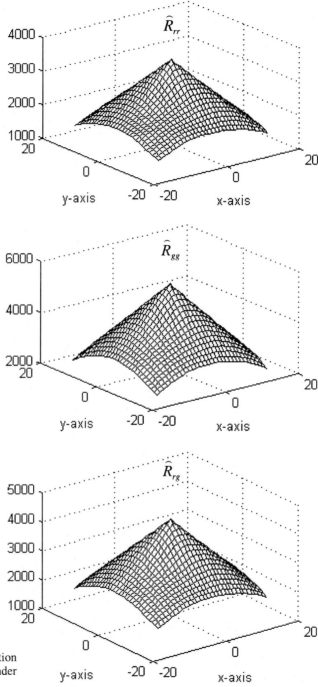

Fig. 4. Circular correlation functions of cloth image under white illumination.

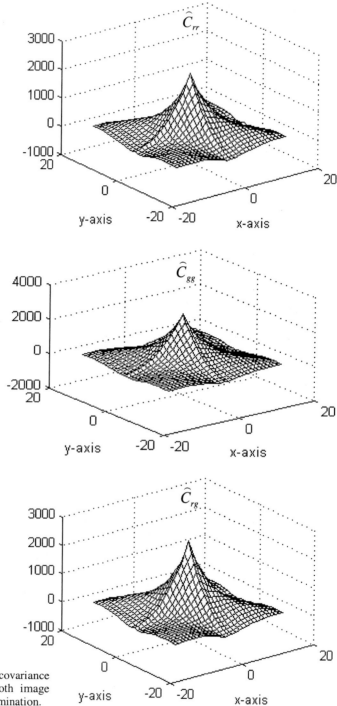

Fig. 5. Circular covariance functions of cloth image under white illumination.

4. Zernike Moments of Correlation and Covariance Functions

Zernike moments [12] may be used to produce one of the most reliable feature set used to achieve invariant pattern recognition, see [13]-[15]. It is our purpose to compute Zernike moments of covariance functions and correlation functions to obtain invariant features that will be used to recognize the color texture. The complex Zernike moments of $f(x, y)$ are defined as:

$$Z_{nl} = \frac{(n+1)}{\pi} \iint dx\, dy\, f(x,y)\, [V_{nl}(r,\theta)]^* = (Z_{n,-l})^*, \tag{5}$$

where the integration is taken inside the unit disk $x^2 + y^2 \leq 1$, $n = 0, 1, 2, ..., \infty$ is the order and l is the repetition which takes on positive and negative integer values subject to the conditions $n - |l|$ is even, and $|l| < n$. Note that, $V_{nl}(r,\theta)$ are the complex Zernike polynomials given as $V_{nl} = R_{nl}(r)\exp(il\theta)$ see [12] for their complete definitions. Zernike moments where l takes negative values can be obtained by making use of the complex conjugate property, which is $Z_{nl} = Z_{n,-l}^*$. In this work, Zernike moments will be used to generate invariants of color correlation and color covariance functions. These invariants are of great importance since they reduce the redundant feature of correlations and covariances. For one specific autocorrelation or crosscorrelation function that correspond to one set of (i, j) value, Zernike moments is computed as

$$Z_{nl}^{ij} = \frac{(n+1)}{\pi} \sum \sum_{x^2+y^2 \leq 1} R_{ij}(x,y)\, [V_{nl}(r,\theta)]^* , \tag{6}$$

and for obtaining Zernike moments of color covariances just use $C_{ij}(x, y)$ instead of $R_{ij}(x, y)$ in the above equation.

4.1 Construction of Zernike Moment Correlation Invariants

Let $R(\bar{x})$ be the correlation matrix of the surface corresponding to the illumination $l(\lambda)$ and let $\tilde{R}'(\bar{x})$ be the correlation matrix for the same surface after an orientation change described by M and under illumination $\tilde{l}(\lambda)$, then

$$R(M\bar{x}) = \tilde{R}'(\bar{x})\, \mathrm{E}, \tag{7}$$

where E is the previously mentioned 6×6 matrix that depends on the illuminations $l(\lambda)$ and $\tilde{l}(\lambda)$. Using the simple representation

$$R_k = \sum_{i=1}^{6} e_{ik} R_i', \tag{8}$$

for $k = 1, 2, ..., 6$. Up to the order n and repetition l, Zernike moments of spatial correlation functions may be computed for both sides of (8) resulting in:

$$Z_{nl}^k = \sum_{i=1}^{6} e_{ik} Z_{nl}^{\prime i} , \qquad (9)$$

where Z_{nl}^k is the moment of $R_k(M\bar{x})$ for $k = 1, 2, \ldots, 6$ and $Z_{nl}^{\prime i}$ is the moment of $R_i'(\bar{x})$. The invariants φ and φ' are constructed as functions to Zernike moments, these invariants may be represented as:

$$\varphi_{uk} = \varphi\left(Z_{nl}^k\right), \qquad (10)$$

$$\varphi_{uk}' = \varphi'\left(\sum_{i=1}^{6} e_{ik} Z_{nl}^{\prime k}\right), \qquad (11)$$

where $u = 1, 2, \ldots$ is the index (or the order) of the invariant and is related (usually) to the order of Zernike moments n. It is desired that

$$\varphi_{uk} = \varphi_{uk}', \qquad (12)$$

will enable us to recognize the desired features independent of illumination and geometry changes. To construct a complete set of Zernike moment invariants (see [12] and [16]) different moment orders may be used to cancel the phase and obtain rotation invariant feature. One way to do this is by taking the magnitude of Zernike moments; the second is using phase cancellation technique. Consider the following combined moment form:

$$\psi_{uk} = Z_{n_1 l_1}^k (Z_{n_2 l_2}^k)^*, \qquad (13)$$

and

$$\psi_{uk}' = \left(\sum_{i=1}^{6} e_{ik} Z_{n_1 l_1}^{\prime i}\right)\left(\sum_{i=1}^{6} e_{ik} Z_{n_1 l_1}^{\prime i}\right)^*, \qquad (14)$$

where $(\cdot)^*$ is the complex conjugate. And for the rules of generating the numerical values of $n_1, l_1, n_2,$ and l_2 that will cancel the phase between the combined moments see [12] and/or [16]. Without loss of generality, lets assume that $(n_1 > n_2)$. The invariants are $\varphi_{uk} = \mathrm{Re}\{\psi_{uk}\}$, thus we can precisely write

$$\varphi_{uk} = \mathrm{Re}\left\{Z_{n_1 l_1}^k (Z_{n_2 l_2}^k)^*\right\}, \qquad (15)$$

and $\varphi_{uk}' = \mathrm{Re}\{\psi_{uk}'\}$ which is obtained by expanding (14), this yields:

$$\varphi_{uk}' = \sum_{i=1}^{6} e_{ik}^2 \,\mathrm{Re}\left\{ Z_{n_1 l_1}^{\prime i} (Z_{n_2 l_2}^{\prime i})^* \right\} + \sum_{i=1}^{5} \sum_{j=i+1}^{6} e_{ik} e_{jk} \,\mathrm{Re}\left\{ Z_{n_1 l_1}^{\prime i} (Z_{n_2 l_2}^{\prime j})^* + Z_{n_1 l_1}^{\prime j} (Z_{n_2 l_2}^{\prime i})^* \right\}. \qquad (16)$$

Wang and Healey [11] computed Zernike moment invariant matrices for the special case $n_1 = n_2$ and some other minor differences. Many in-between invariants were neglected though they belong to the same order or less; therefore, the system of invariants that they were using was not complete. A complete system of invariants can be generated in (16). It is also possible to derive the pseudo Zernike invariants as $P_{uk} = \text{Im}\{\psi_{uk}\}$ and $P'_{uk} = \text{Im}\{\psi'_{uk}\}$ that will be given as

$$P'_{uk} = \sum_{i=1}^{6} e_{ik}^2 \, \text{Im}\left\{ Z_{n_1 l_1}^{\prime i} (Z_{n_2 l_2}^{\prime i})^* \right\} + \sum_{i=1}^{5} \sum_{j=i+1}^{6} e_{ik} e_{jk} \, \text{Im}\left\{ Z_{n_1 l_1}^{\prime i} (Z_{n_2 l_2}^{\prime j})^* + Z_{n_1 l_1}^{\prime jk} (Z_{n_2 l_2}^{\prime i})^* \right\}. \qquad (17)$$

The invariants given in (16) are a general form in which many other invariants can be utilized (depending on other types of moment kernel functions) for instance, pseudo Zernike moments [13], orthogonal Fourier Mellin moments [17], disc-harmonic coefficients moments [18], and wavelet moments [20]. In fact, we are of interest in the invariants given in (16) and it is important to obtain a form that separate e_{ik} elements so that to obtain illumination invariance. For this purpose, we have rearranged (16) to be given as:

$$\varphi'_{uk} = \sum_{m=1}^{21} h_{um} \, g_{mk} , \qquad (18)$$

where

$$g_{um} = \left[\begin{array}{ll} \text{Re}\left\{ Z_{n_1 l_1}^{\prime m} (Z_{n_2 l_2}^{\prime m})^* \right\} & 1 \le m \le 6 \\[2mm] \text{Re}\left\{ Z_{n_1 l_1}^{\prime i_m} (Z_{n_2 l_2}^{\prime j_m})^* + Z_{n_1 l_1}^{\prime j_m} (Z_{n_2 l_2}^{\prime i_m})^* \right\} & 7 \le m \le 21 \end{array} \right. , \qquad (19)$$

and

$$h_{mk} = \left[\begin{array}{ll} e_{mk}^2 & 1 \le m \le 6 \\[2mm] e_{i_m k} \, e_{j_m k} & 7 \le m \le 21 \end{array} \right. , \qquad (20)$$

where the i_m and j_m number set is given by $(i_m, j_m) = \{(1,2),(1,3),(1,4),(1,5),(1,6),$ $(2,3),(2,4),(2,5),(2,6),(3,4),(3,5),(3,6),(4,5),(4,6),(5,6)\}$ for all $m = 7, 8, ..., 21$ respectively, i.e. $(i_7, j_7) = (1,2), ... (i_{21}, j_{21}) = (5,6)$.

It is obvious that (18) takes the form of a matrix multiplication, representing (18) in a matrix form as $\boldsymbol{\varphi'} = \mathbf{GH}$ and from (12) we know that $\boldsymbol{\varphi} = \boldsymbol{\varphi'}$ therefore $\boldsymbol{\varphi} = \mathbf{GH}$. Lets assume using a total of w invariants for which $u = 1, 2...., w$ and in our discussed case $k = 1, 2, ..., 6$, the matrices are

$$\boldsymbol{\varphi} = \begin{vmatrix} \varphi_{11} & \varphi_{12} & \cdots & \varphi_{16} \\ \varphi_{21} & \varphi_{22} & \cdots & \varphi_{26} \\ \vdots & \vdots & \cdots & \vdots \\ \varphi_{w1} & \varphi_{w2} & \cdots & \varphi_{w6} \end{vmatrix} \quad \mathbf{G} = \begin{vmatrix} g_{11} & g_{12} & \cdots & g_{1,21} \\ g_{21} & g_{22} & \cdots & g_{2,21} \\ \vdots & \vdots & \cdots & \vdots \\ g_{w1} & g_{w2} & \cdots & g_{w,21} \end{vmatrix}$$

$$\mathbf{H} = \begin{vmatrix} h_{11} & h_{12} & \cdots & h_{16} \\ h_{21} & h_{22} & \cdots & h_{26} \\ \vdots & \vdots & \cdots & \vdots \\ h_{21,1} & h_{21,2} & \cdots & h_{21,6} \end{vmatrix} \qquad (21)$$

Obviously, $\boldsymbol{\varphi}$ is a $w \times 6$ sized matrix which is the moment invariant matrix (it is translation-rotation invariant), $\mathbf{G}$ is a $w \times 21$ sized matrix, and $\mathbf{H}$ is a 21×6 sized matrix with elements that depend only on $l(\lambda)$ and $\tilde{l}(\lambda)$ which represent the effect of illumination. For texture recognition, $\mathbf{G}$ is represented using an orthonormal bases obtained by a singular value decomposition method [19] as follows

$$\mathbf{G} = \mathbf{U} \Sigma \mathbf{V}, \tag{22}$$

where $\mathbf{U}$ is a $w \times 21$ sized matrix, $\mathbf{U} = [\mathbf{u}_1, \mathbf{u}_2, ..., \mathbf{u}_{21}]$ having columns that are orthonormal eigenvectors of $\mathbf{GG}^T$, Σ is a 21×21 diagonal matrix of singular values $\lambda_1, \lambda_2, ..., \lambda_{21}$, and $\mathbf{V}$ is a 21×21 matrix having columns that are orthonormal eigenvectors of $\mathbf{G}^T \mathbf{G}$. For recognition purpose, the following distance function can be used:

$$D = \sum_{i=1}^{6} \left\| \varphi_i - [(\mathbf{u}_1^T \varphi_i)\mathbf{u}_1 + (\mathbf{u}_2^T \varphi_i)\mathbf{u}_2 + ... + (\mathbf{u}_{21}^T \varphi_i)\mathbf{u}_{21}] \right\|, \tag{23}$$

where $\varphi_1, \varphi_2, ..., \varphi_6$ are the column vectors of $\boldsymbol{\varphi}$. The above distance function characterizes how well the column vectors of $\boldsymbol{\varphi}$ can be approximated as a linear combination of the columns of $\mathbf{U}$. Thus, the smallest value of D for matrices $\boldsymbol{\varphi}$ and $\mathbf{G}$ will correspond to textures related by some combination of rotation and illumination changes. In our work, the matrix $\boldsymbol{\varphi}$ is used to store the feature of the original database under white illumination. The matrix $\mathbf{G}$ is used for the texture under recognition (investigation), i.e., the texture that had undergoes illumination and geometry changes. To clarify the generation of the matrix $\mathbf{G}$ we will give a brief description; first, generate the six color correlation functions using (2), compute Zernike moments for each of the correlation functions using (6), and generate the elements of the $\mathbf{G}$ matrix using the definition given in (19) and by following the rules of generating a complete set of invariants given in [12] and [16].

5. Experimental Results

In this section we intend to test the color covariance model and the developed color correlation model in a texture recognition task. The image database is consisted of 20 textured images as shown in Fig. 6, which contains some homogenous and inhomogeneous textures. For each image class in the database, we generated five image samples under white, red, green, blue, and yellow illuminations using HANSA color filters and the images are photographed with a Sony CCD camera. For each of the five images that have different illuminations, we generated five other rotated images at the rotation angles $30°, 60°, 90°, 120°$ and $150°$ with respect to the original non rotated image.

Thus for each class, we have a total of thirty images photographed at different illuminations and rotations. The whole image database is consisted of 600 images, a total of 20 classes with 30 images per class. For each image in the database, color covariance and color correlation functions are estimated with averages over a finite image region of size 60×60 pixels and for a finite image lag, i.e., $C_{ij}(x, y)$ and/or $R_{ij}(x, y)$ is estimated for $|x| < 16$ and $|y| < 16$. It had been suggested in [8] to normalize color covariance functions against intensity changes by dividing by $C_{rr}(0, 0)$. We will include this normalization scheme in our tests to see whether it is useful or not, $R_{rr}(0,0)$ will be used for normalizing correlation functions.

The test is divided into two stages, the training phase for feature extraction of the original image class and the testing phase that includes feature extraction of the image under investigation that has illumination and geometry changes with respect to the original image class. In the training phase and after computing color covariances and/or color correlations, For comparison purpose, Zernike moment invariant matrices are computed for each image up to the 6_{th}, 8_{th}, 10_{th}, and 12_{th} orders. The training process is performed to each of the 20 color textured images photographed under white illumination and non rotated image, and all the 20 Zernike moment invariant matrices are stored to be used offline. In the testing phase, the unknown textures are extracted from the rest of the 580 images under different illuminations and rotations. The distance function defined in (23) is used as a similarity measure. The recognition performance is measured as the number of correct matches over the total number of images. See Fig. 7 for comparison purpose.

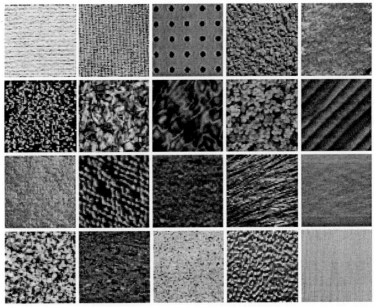

Fig. 6. The original image database used in our experiments, from left to right the first row shows; carpet, carpet back, ceiling tile, coffee grounded and jungle. Second row; algae, ground leaf, wallpaper, leaf, and cloth. Third row; cotton canvas, forest, forest cutting, fur, and water. Fourth row; granite1, granite2, granite3, chrome, and wood.

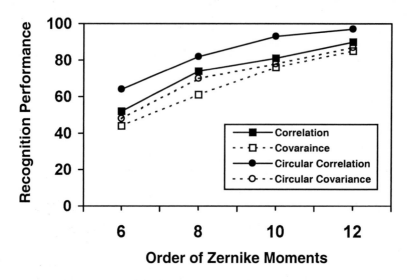

Fig. 7. Performance comparison of using Zernike moment correlation matrices and Zernike moment covariance matrices for the Illumination-rotation invariant recognition of color texture.

The circular correlation functions proposed in this work give the highest recognition performance 97%. On the other hand, the recognition performance value of using the covariance functions proposed by Kondepudy and Healey [7] is 85% and circular covariance functions gives 87%. As we increase the order of Zernike moments, the recognition performance increases for all models. Another test is performed using the normalization shows that using the intensity normalization by dividing each color covariances by $C_{ij}(0, 0)$ and dividing each color correlation by $R_{ij}(0, 0)$ reduces the recognition performance to less than 80%.

6. Conclusions

The spatial correlation functions introduced in this paper is very useful in representing and modeling color texture. Compared to a previous color covariance functions the recognition performance is much higher. We also derived a complete set of Zernike moment invariant correlation and covariance matrices to make correlation functions invariant to rotation changes of textures. The recognition performance is increased as the moment order is increased. The work also investigates four texture modeling functions, ordinary covariance, circular covariance, ordinary correlation, and circular correlation. Using Zernike moments the dimensionality of correlation feature is reduced and it may be useful to use other kinds of moments for the recognition of texture since the derived invariants posses a general form.

References

[1]   M. Swain and D. Ballard, Color indexing, *International Journal of Computer Vision*, vol. 7, pp. 11-32, 1991.

[2]   B. Funt and G. Finalyson, Color constant color indexing, *IEEE Trans. Pattern Anal. Machine Intell.*, vol. 17, pp. 522-528, May 1995.

[3]   A.K. Jain, and F. Farrokhnia, Unsupervised texture segmentation using Gabor filters, *Pattern Recognition*, vol. 24, no. 12, pp. 1167-1186, 1991.

[4]   G. Healey and D. Slater, Computing illumination-invariant descriptors of spatially Filtered Color Image Regions, *IEEE Trans. Image Processing*, vol. 6, no. 7, pp. 1002-1013, July 1997.

[5]   G. Cross, and A.K. Jain, Markov random field texture models, *IEEE Trans. Pattern Anal. Machine Intell.*, vol.5, no. 1, pp. 25-39, 1983.

[6]   D. Panjwani and G. Healey, Selecting neighbors in random field models for color images, *in Proc. IEEE Int. Conf. Image Processing*, Austin, TX, vol. 2, pp. 56-60, 1994.

[7]   R. Kondepudy and G. Healey, Use of invariants for recognition of three-dimensional color texture, *J. Opt. Soc. Amer. A*, vol. 11, pp. 3037-3049, Nov. 1994.

[8]   A. Rosenfield and A.C. Kak, Digital Picture Processing, second Ed., New York, Academic Press, 1982.

[9]   G. Healey and L. Wang, Illumination-invariant recognition of texture in color images, *J. Opt. Soc. Amer. A*, vol.12, pp. 1877-1883. Sept. 1995.

[10] G. Healey and A. Jain, Retrieving multispectral satellite images using physics-based invariant representations, *IEEE Trans. Pattern Anal. Machine Intell.*, vol. 18, pp. 842-848, Aug. 1996.

[11] L. Wang and G. Healey, Using Zernike moments for the illumination and geometry invariant classification of multispectral texture, *IEEE Trans. Image Processing*, vol. 7, no. 2, pp. 196-203, Feb. 1998.

[12] M. R. Teague, Image analysis via the general theory of moments, *J. Opt. Soc. Amer.*, vol. 70, pp. 920-930, Aug. 1980.

[13] C.-H. Teh, and R. T. Chin, On image analysis by moment invariants, *IEEE Trans. Pattern Analysis Machine Intelligence*, vol. 10, no. 4, pp. 496-513, July 1988.

[14] R.R. Bailey, and M. Srinath, Orthogonal moment features for use with parametric and non-parametric classifiers, *IEEE Trans. Pattern Analysis and Machine Intelligence*, vol. 18, no. 4, pp. 389-399, April 1996.

[15] A. Khotanzad, Invariant image recognition by Zernike moments, *IEEE Trans. Pattern Analysis and Machine Intelligence*, vol. 12, no. 5, pp. 489-497, 1990.

[16] A. Wallin and O. Kubler, Complete sets of Zernike moment invariants and the role of Pseudo-invariants, *IEEE T-PAMI*, vol. 17, no. 11, pp. 1106-1110, Nov. 1995.

[17] Y. Sheng and L. Shen, Orthogonal Fourier-Mellin moments for invariant pattern recognition, *J. Opt. Soc. Amer. A*, vol. 11, no. 6, pp. 1748-1757, June 1994.

[18] S.C. Verrall and R. Kakarala, Disk-harmonic coefficients for invariant pattern recognition. *J. Opt. Soc. Amer. A*, vol. 15, no. 2, pp. 389-403, Feb. 1998.

[19] W.H. Press, S.A. Teukolsky, W.T. Vetterling, and B.P. Flannery, Numerical recipes in C: the art of scientific computing, Cambridge university press, second edition, 1992.

[20] D. Shen, H.S. Horace, Discriminative wavelet shape descriptors for recognition of 2D patterns, *Pattern Recognition*, vol.32, pp. 151-165, 1999.

Part III

Clustering, Grouping, and Segmentation

Path Based Pairwise Data Clustering
with Application to Texture Segmentation

Bernd Fischer, Thomas Zöller, and Joachim M. Buhmann

Rheinische Friedrich Wilhelms Universität
Institut für Informatik III, Römerstr. 164
D-53117 Bonn, Germany
{fischerb,zoeller,jb}@cs.uni-bonn.de
http://www-dbv.informatik.uni-bonn.de

Abstract. Most cost function based clustering or partitioning methods measure the compactness of groups of data. In contrast to this picture of a point source in feature space, some data sources are spread out on a low-dimensional manifold which is embedded in a high dimensional data space. This property is adequately captured by the criterion of connectedness which is approximated by graph theoretic partitioning methods.

We propose in this paper a pairwise clustering cost function with a novel dissimilarity measure emphasizing connectedness in feature space rather than compactness. The connectedness criterion considers two objects as similar if there exists a mediating intra cluster path without an edge with large cost. The cost function is optimized in a multi-scale fashion. This new path based clustering concept is applied to segment textured images with strong texture gradients based on dissimilarities between image patches.

1 Introduction

Partitioning a set of objects into groups and thus extracting the hidden structure of the data set is a very important problem which arises in many application areas e.g. pattern recognition, exploratory data analysis and computer vision. Intuitively, a good grouping solution is characterized by a high degree of homogeneity of the respective clusters. Therefore, the notion of *homogeneity* must be given a mathematically precise meaning which strongly depends on the nature of the underlying data.

In this paper we will deal with an important subclass of partitioning methods namely clustering according to pairwise comparisons between objects. Such data is usually called *proximity* or *(dis)similarity* data respectively. This data modality is of particular interest in applications where object (dis)similarities can be reliably estimated even when the objects are not elements of a metric space. There is a rich variety of clustering approaches developed particularly for this data modality in the literature. Most of them fall in the category of agglomerative methods [13]. These methods share as a common trait that they

M.A.T. Figueiredo, J. Zerubia, A.K. Jain (Eds.): EMMCVPR 2001, LNCS 2134, pp. 235–250, 2001.
© Springer-Verlag Berlin Heidelberg 2001

start grouping with a configuration composed of exactly one object per cluster and then they successively merge the two most similar clusters. Agglomerative methods are almost always derived from algorithmic considerations rather than on the basis of an optimization principle which often obscures the underlying modeling assumptions.

A systematic approach to pairwise clustering by objective functions as described in [17] is based on an axiomatization of invariance properties and robustness for data grouping. As a consequence of this axiomatic approach we restrict our discussion to intra cluster criteria. Our second important design decision for pairwise clustering replaces the pairwise object comparison by a path-based dissimilarity measure, thereby emphasizing cluster connectedness. The effective dissimilarity between objects is defined as the largest edge cost on the minimal intra cluster path connecting both objects in feature space. Two objects which are assigned to the same cluster are either similar or there exists a set of mediating objects such that two consecutive objects in this chain are similar.

The distinction between compactness and connectedness principles is also addressed by two other recently proposed clustering methods. Tishby and Slonim [20] introduced a Markovian relaxation dynamics where the Markov transition probability is given by object dissimilarities. Iterating such a relaxation dynamics effectively connects objects by sums over minimal paths. The method, however, does not include the constraint that all considered paths have to be restricted to nodes from the same cluster. The other method which was introduced by Blatt, Wiseman and Domany [2] simulates the dynamics of a locally connected, diluted ferromagnet. The partial order at finite temperature is interpreted as a clustering solution in this model.

2   Pairwise Data Clustering

Notational Prerequisites: The goal of data clustering is formally given by the partitioning of n objects $\mathbf{o}_i$, $1 \leq i \leq n$ into k groups, such that some measure of intra cluster homogeneity is maximized. The memberships of objects to groups can be encoded by a $n \times k$ Matrix $\mathbf{M} \in \{0,1\}^{n \times k}$. In this setting the entry $M_{i\nu}$ is set to 1 if and only if the ith object is assigned to cluster ν which implies the condition $\sum_{\nu=1}^{k} M_{i\nu} = 1, \forall i = 1 \ldots n$. The set of all assignment matrices fulfilling this requirement is denoted in the following by $\mathcal{M}_{n,k}^{\text{part}}$.

The dissimilarity between two objects $\mathbf{o}_i$ and $\mathbf{o}_j$ is represented by D_{ij}. These individual dissimilarity values are collected in a matrix $\mathbf{D} \in \mathbb{R}^{n \times n}$. It is worth noting here that many application domains frequently confront the data analyst with data which violates the triangle inequality. Moreover, the self–dissimilarity of objects often is non vanishing, even negative dissimilarities might occur or a certain percentage of dissimilarities is unknown. For our proposed method, we only require symmetry, i.e. $D_{ij} = D_{ji}$. To distinguish between known and unknown dissimilarities neighborhood sets $\mathcal{N}_1, \ldots, \mathcal{N}_n$ are introduced, i.e., $j \in \mathcal{N}_i$ denotes that the dissimilarity D_{ij} is known.

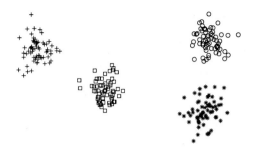

Fig. 1. Prototypical situation for the standard pairwise clustering approach

The Objective Function: With these notational preliminaries, we are now able to address the important modeling step of choosing an appropriate cost function. An axiomatization of objective functions for data clustering based on invariance and robustness criteria is given in [17]. This approach makes explicit the intuitively evident properties that a global shift of the data or a rescaling as well as contamination by noise should not sensitively influence the grouping solution. In accordance with this approach we will focus on the following cost function:

$$\mathcal{H}^{\mathrm{pc}}(\mathbf{M}, \mathbf{D}) = \sum_{\nu=1}^{k} \sum_{i=1}^{n} M_{i\nu} d_{i\nu}, \quad \text{where} \quad d_{i\nu} = \frac{\sum_{j \in \mathcal{N}_i} M_{j\nu} D_{ij}}{\sum_{j \in \mathcal{N}_i} M_{j\nu}}. \tag{1}$$

$\mathcal{H}^{\mathrm{pc}}$ sums up individual contributions $d_{i\nu}$ for each object $\mathbf{o}_i$ and each group $\mathcal{C}_\nu$ where $d_{i\nu}$ stands for the average dissimilarity between $\mathbf{o}_i$ and objects belonging to cluster $\mathcal{C}_\nu$. $\mathcal{H}^{\mathrm{pc}}$ thus favors intra–cluster compactness. It is the use of this normalization that removes the sensitive dependency of the minimum of $\mathcal{H}^{\mathrm{pc}}$ to constant shifts of the dissimilarity values and makes it insensitive to different cluster sizes.

Optimization: The optimization of objective functions like $\mathcal{H}^{\mathrm{pc}}$ is computationally difficult since combinatorial optimization problems of this kind exhibit numerous local minima. Furthermore, most of the data partitioning problems are proven to be $\mathcal{NP}$–hard. For robust optimization, stochastic optimization techniques like *Simulated Annealing* (SA) [11] or *Deterministic Annealing* (DA) ([19, 7]) have shown to perform satisfactorily on many pattern recognition and computer vision applications. Effectively these annealing methods fall in the class of homotopy methods with smoothing controlled by a temperature parameter. In the zero temperature limit the comparatively fast local optimization algorithm known as ICM is obtained [1].

Drawbacks of the Approach: So far we have discussed a very powerful approach to the pairwise data clustering problem. It is theoretically well founded, and showed to be applicable in a wide range of data analysis problems ranging from texture segmentation [8] and document clustering [17] to structuring of

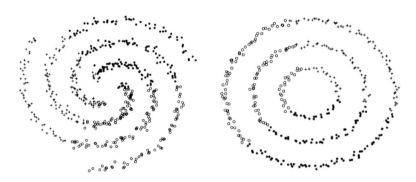

Fig. 2. Data sets on which the naive intra cluster compactness criterion fails

genome data bases [7]. An ideal situation for the cluster compactness criterion is depicted in figure 1 for a toy data set. All objects have been assigned to clusters in an intuitively correct manner.

However there exist situations, where the exclusive focus on compactness fails to capture essential properties of the data. Two prototypical examples are given in figure 2. It is clear that the human data analyst expects that the ring like structures or the spiral arms are detected as clusters. It is the novel contribution of this paper to propose a way of formalizing this goal by determining effective inter object dissimilarities while keeping the well approved clustering objective function.

3   Path Based Clustering

In order to motivate our novel modification of the basic pairwise clustering method we will often try to appeal to readers geometric intuition despite the fact that the objects do not necessarily reside in a metric space.

Modeling: As demonstrated before the pairwise clustering approach according to $\mathcal{H}^{pc}$ is not well suited for the detection of elongated structures in the object domain. This objective function sums all intra-cluster dissimilarities whereby similar objects will be grouped together regardless of their topological relations. This is a good solution as long as the data of one group can be interpreted as a scatter around a single centroid (see figure 1). But if the data is a scatter of a curve (c.f. figure 2) or a surface pairwise clustering as defined by $\mathcal{H}^{pc}$ will fail. In this case the effective dissimilarity of two objects should be mediated by peer objects along that curve, no matter how large the extend of that structure may be.

Assume that the objects o_i and o_j belong to the same manifold. Then with high probability there exists a path from o_i to o_j over other objects of this manifold such that the dissimilarities of two consecutive objects are small. The reason for this is that the density of objects coming from one source is expected to be comparatively high. On the other hand if o_i and o_j belong to different, non-intersecting manifolds then all paths from o_i to o_j have with high probability at least one pair of consecutive objects with high dissimilarity.

As clusters are defined by their coherence one is only interested in paths through the object domain which traverse regions of high density. The part of a path where the density is lowest should thus determine the overall costs of this path. In other words the maximum dissimilarity along a path determines its cost. In order to formalize our ideas about mediating the dissimilarity of any two objects by peers in the same cluster we define the effective dissimilarity D_{ij}^{eff} between objects o_i and o_j to be the length of the minimal connecting path.

$$D_{ij}^{\text{eff}}(\mathbf{M}, \mathbf{D}) = \min_{\mathbf{p} \in \mathcal{P}_{ij}(\mathbf{M})} \left\{ \max_{h \in \{1,\ldots,|\mathbf{p}|-1\}} \left\{ D_{\mathbf{p}[h]\mathbf{p}[h+1]} \right\} \right\}, \text{ where} \tag{2}$$

$$\mathcal{P}_{ij}(\mathbf{M}) = \left\{ \mathbf{p} \in \{1,\ldots,n\}^l \,\middle|\, \exists \nu : \prod_{h=1}^{l} M_{p[h]\nu} = 1 \wedge l \le n \wedge p[1] = i \wedge p[l] = j \right\}$$

is the set of all paths from o_i to o_j through cluster ν if o_i and o_j belong to cluster ν. If both objects belong to different clusters $\mathcal{P}_{ij}(\mathbf{M})$ is the empty set and the effective dissimilarity is not defined.

With the new definition of the effective dissimilarity we are able to define the objective function for path based clustering. It has the same functional form as for pairwise clustering.

$$\mathcal{H}^{\text{pb}}(\mathbf{M}, \mathbf{D}) = \sum_{\nu=1}^{k} \sum_{i=1}^{n} M_{i\nu} d_{i\nu}, \quad \text{where} \quad d_{i\nu} = \frac{\sum_{j=1}^{n} M_{j\nu} D_{ij}^{\text{eff}}(\mathbf{M}, \mathbf{D})}{\sum_{j=1}^{n} M_{j\nu}}. \tag{3}$$

Thereby the desirable properties of shift and scale invariance of the pairwise clustering cost function are conserved:

$$\forall c, D_0 \in \mathbb{R} : \operatorname*{argmin}_{\mathbf{M} \in \mathcal{M}} \mathcal{H}^{\text{pb}}(\mathbf{M}, \mathbf{D}) = \operatorname*{argmin}_{\mathbf{M} \in \mathcal{M}} \mathcal{H}^{\text{pb}}(\mathbf{M}, c\mathbf{D} + D_0), \tag{4}$$

since $\forall c, D_0 \in \mathbb{R}$ holds $\mathcal{H}^{\text{pb}}(\mathbf{M}, c\mathbf{D} + D_0) = c\mathcal{H}^{\text{pb}}(\mathbf{M}, \mathbf{D}) + ND_0$.

Optimization by Iterated Conditional Mode (ICM): Finding the minimum of $\mathcal{H}^{\text{pb}}(\mathbf{M}, \mathbf{D})$ has a high computational complexity. There are many different methods known to avoid a complete search in the assignment configuration space ($|\mathcal{M}| = k^n$). A very effective and simple method is called iterated conditional mode [1]. ICM assigns an object to a cluster under the condition that all other assignments are kept fix. In algorithm 1 the function $s_{\pi[i]}(\mathbf{M}, e_\nu)$ changes the $\pi[i]$-th row of the assignment matrix $\mathbf{M}$ by replacing it with the μth unit vector. This so called single site update is iterated over all objects in a random manner. A complete cycle of visiting all sites is called a sweep. As a common site visitation schedule an arbitrary permutation π of all objects is generated before each sweep in order to avoid local minima due to a fixed visitation order. The algorithm repeats the sweeps until convergence is reached, i.e. no assignment is changed. During each update step the objects are assigned to clusters such that

---

Algorithm 1 Iterated conditional mode (ICM) for Path Based Clustering

---

Require: dissimilarity matrix $\mathbf{D}$
  number of objects n
  number of clusters k
Ensure: $\operatorname{argmin}_{\mathbf{M} \in \mathcal{M}} \mathcal{H}^{\mathbf{pb}}(\mathbf{M}, \mathbf{D})$ with high probability
  choose $\mathbf{M}$ randomly
  repeat
    $\pi = perm(\{1, \ldots, n\})$
    for all $i \in \{1, \ldots, n\}$ **do**
      $\nu^* = \operatorname{argmin}_{\nu \in \{1, \ldots, k\}} \mathcal{H}^{\mathbf{pb}}(s_{\pi[i]}(\mathbf{M}, e_\nu), \mathbf{D})$
      where $s_{\pi[i]}(\mathbf{M}, e_\nu)$ assigns object $\pi[i]$ to cluster ν
      $\mathbf{M} = s_{\pi[i]}(\mathbf{M}, e_{\nu^*})$
    end for
  until converged
  return $\mathbf{M}$

---

the costs of the resulting configuration are minimal. Therefore it is guaranteed that the costs, or energy respectively, decreases in each sweep and ICM will terminate after a finite number of cycles.

Critical for the running time is the update step. Here the recalculations of the dissimilarity matrix dominate the complexity due to the fact that this computational effort is necessary during each assignment update. Basically what has to be solved is an `ALL-PAIRS-SHORTEST-PATH` problem for each group of objects. For a full graph the algorithm of Floyd has a running time of $\mathcal{O}(n^3)$ [3]. If object o_i is updated, the ICM algorithm tries to find the minimum of the local costs by hypothetically assigning the given object to the various groups. Therefore, the effective dissimilarity to each cluster has to be determined once with object o_i inside and once with o_i outside the cluster. Thus $2k$ different effective dissimilarity matrices are needed. In the next paragraph an efficient implementation of this update step is presented.

Efficient Implementation of Update Step: One observes that the instances of the `ALL-PAIRS-SHORTEST-PATH` problems in two consecutive update steps are almost the same. They differ only in one single object: that object, which is to be updated. So it makes sense to check if one effective dissimilarity matrix can be used as a starting point for the calculation of an effective dissimilarity matrices in the next update step. Fortunately, those k dissimilarity matrices which correspond to the current configuration are used again in the next step. What about the other k matrices?

For $k - 1$ of them a possible new configuration is given by adding object o_i, whereas for one cluster the new costs without o_i have to be computed. Consider the first case: object o_i is to be inserted in a certain group. For reasons of computational efficiency a complete recalculation of the effective dissimilarity matrix of that cluster is to be avoided. A closer look at Floyds algorithm leads the way: Its first step is given by the initialization of the matrix with the direct distances between the objects which in our case is given by the input dissimilarity

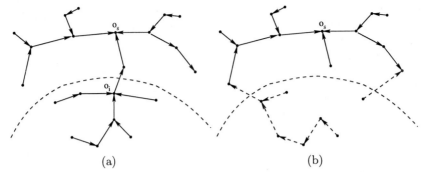

(a)   (b)

Fig. 3. The graphs show the predecessor graph of object o_s before (a) and after (b) object o_i is removed from the cluster. For those objects where the path to o_s does not lead over o_i the effective dissimilarity may not change

matrix. The goal is to get the shortest path distance between each pair of objects. For any object Floyds algorithm tries to put it on a path between each pair of objects. If now o_i is put into a new cluster only the last iteration of the Floyd algorithm has to be performed in which the current object is put on each of the existing paths between entity pairs. This step has a running time of $\mathcal{O}(n^2)$. In order to do so one has to get effective dissimilarities between o_i and all other objects in the considered cluster. Because of the symmetry of the original input dissimilarity matrix the effective dissimilarities are again symmetric. For that reason it is sufficient to solve one SINGLE-SOURCE-SHORTEST-PATH problem in order to arrive at the effective dissimilarities between o_i and all other objects. This can be solved with the Dijkstra's algorithm in a running time of $\mathcal{O}(n^2 \log n)$ [3]. So far we can compute the update step with an overall running time of $\mathcal{O}(n^2 \log n)$.

It remains to describe the necessary recalculations in the case where o_i is to be removed from the cluster it has been assigned to in the previous configuration. Again this goal has to be reached with the least possible computational effort. However in this situation the asymptotic running time of $\mathcal{O}(n^3)$ for a complete recalculation of dissimilarities for the whole group of objects can not be decreased. Nevertheless there is a good heuristic for lowering the running time. If there exists a shortest path from o_s to o_t which does not lead over o_i, the effective dissimilarity D_{st} will not change if o_i is removed from the cluster. One can obtain a predecessor matrix for all objects in a given cluster in the same running time as it takes to compute the effective dissimilarities. For each object we can thus determine the shortest path tree to all other objects in a running time of $\mathcal{O}(n)$. If we have the shortest path tree from o_s then only those dissimilarities between o_s and another object o_t have to be updated where t is an index out of the set of all objects in the subtree with root o_i (see figure 3). The total running time for an assignment update step is thus $\mathcal{O}(n^3)$.

Multi-scale Optimization: As can be seen from the previous section the proposed optimization scheme is computationally highly demanding. An improvement in performance as well as solution quality is reached by using multi-scale techniques. The idea of multi-scale optimization is to lower the complexity by decreasing the number of considered entities in the object space. For example in image processing one can compute the given optimization tasks on a pyramid of different resolution levels of the image. At the first stage of such a procedure one solves the given computational problem on the subsampled image with lowest resolution, maps the result to the next finer resolution level and starts the optimization again. The expectation is that the result from the coarser level provides a reasonable starting point for the next finer level in the sense that convergence to a good solution can be reached within a few iterations. The probability of obtaining the global minimum is raised even if a local optimization scheme is used and the running time will dramatically decrease. A general overview of multi-scale optimization and its mathematically rigorous description is given in [15]. In order to pursue this approach a proper initialization of the coarse levels is needed. To this end three kinds of mappings have to be defined:

First of all, a function I^ℓ is needed, which maps the objects from the finer level ℓ to the next coarser one (level $\ell+1$). The multi-scale operator I^ℓ is defined as a function

$$I^\ell : \mathbb{O}^\ell \to \mathbb{O}^{\ell+1}, \tag{5}$$

where $\mathbb{O}^\ell$ is the set of objects on the ℓth resolution level and $\mathbb{O}^0$ is the set of objects on the finest level. So far this is just a formal definition. There is indeed a large design freedom in choosing the concrete form of this mapping. In the general case subsuming highly similar objects is reasonable. For our most prominent application task texture segmentation however we can use the natural topology of square neighborhoods of image sites in order to determine the fine to coarse mapping.

Second, the input dissimilarity matrix for the coarser level has to be defined in such a way that the basic modeling assumptions which underly the objective function are not violated. If the objects which map to one single entity in the coarser level belong to different clusters, the newly formed super–object in the coarser level should belong to one of these. Otherwise two completely different groups will get closer in the coarser level and the structure of the data is lost.

For that reason a mapping between each object in the coarse level and a representative object in the next finer level has to be defined as the third ingredient of the multi-scale approach. The function R^ℓ will denote the representative object in level ℓ for each object in level $\ell+1$.

$$R^\ell : \mathbb{O}^{\ell+1} \to \mathbb{O}^\ell \quad \text{with} \quad R^\ell(o_I) \in \{o_i | I^\ell(o_i) = o_I\} \tag{6}$$

One possibility of defining such a representative is to choose the object nearest to the center of mass of the set. We are now able to define the input dissimilarity matrix $\mathbf{D}^{\ell+1}$ on the $(\ell+1)^{\text{th}}$ level.

$$\mathbf{D}^{\ell+1}(I, J) = \mathbf{D}^\ell(R^\ell(o_I), R^\ell(o_J)) \tag{7}$$

Having assembled all the necessary parts which constitute the resolution pyramid, the optimization can proceed as described in the beginning of this

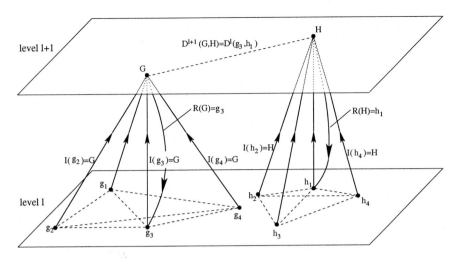

Fig. 4. Illustration of the multi-scale coarsening operators: I is mapping the objects on the finer level to the corresponding super–object in the coarser level, R is back-projecting to the representative in the finer level in order to enable the computation of the coarse level dissimilarity matrix

section. The intermediate coarse to fine mappings of computational results is achieved in a straightforward manner. A pictorial description of the multi-scale pyramid construction is given in figure 4.

4   Texture Segmentation by Pairwise Data Clustering

In order to pose the segmentation of images according to texture content as a pairwise data clustering problem, we follow the approach of Hofmann et al. [8]. A suitable image representation for texture segmentation is given by a multi-scale family of Gabor filters

$$G(\mathbf{x}, \sigma, \mathbf{k}) = \frac{1}{\sqrt{2\pi\sigma^2}} \exp\left(-\frac{\mathbf{x}^t\mathbf{x}}{2\sigma^2} + i\mathbf{k}^t\mathbf{x},\right) \tag{8}$$

which are known to have good discriminatory power for a wide range of textures [8] [10]. In good agreement with psychophysical experiments [4] these Gabor filters extract feature information in the spatial correlation of the texture. The moduli of a bank of such filters at three different scales with octave spacing and four orientations are used as the representation of the input image. Thus the resulting twelve dimensional vector of modulus values $I(\mathbf{x})$ for each image location $\mathbf{x}$ comprises our basic texture features.

By its very nature, texture is a non local property. Although $I(\mathbf{x})$ contains information about spatial relations of pixels in the neighborhood of $\mathbf{x}$, it may not suffice to grasp the complete characterization of the prevalent texture. Therefore the image is covered with a regular grid of image sites. Suppose a suitable binning

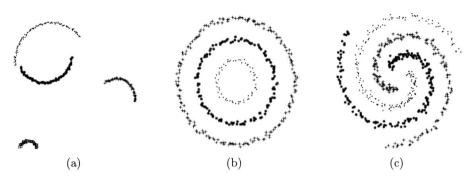

Fig. 5. Results of the novel path based clustering criterion on three toy data sets: a) arcs b) circular structure c) spiral arms

$t^* = 0 < t_1 < \ldots < t_L$ is given. For each site $i, i = 1 \ldots N$ the empirical feature distribution $f_i^{(r)}$ is computed for all Gabor channels r in order to arrive at a texture description for these spatially extend image patches. The dissimilarity between textures at location i and j is then computed independently for each of the channels by a χ^2 statistic.

$$D_{ij}^{(r)} = \chi^2 = \sum_{k=1}^{L} \frac{(f_i^{(r)}(t_k) - \hat{f}^{(r)}(t_k))^2}{\hat{f}^{(r)}(t_k)},$$
$$\text{where } \hat{f}^{(r)}(t_k) = [f_i^{(r)}(t_k) + f_j^{(r)}(t_k)]/2. \tag{9}$$

In order to combine the different values $D_{ij}^{(r)}$ into one dissimilarity value for each pair of objects the L_1–norm is used: $D_{ij} = \sum_r D_{ij}^{(r)}$. As a comparative study shows, this norm outperforms all norms in the L_p family [18].

5   Results

Artificial Data Sets: In section 2 some drawbacks of the formerly developed clustering method were addressed. As the novel path based approach was especially designed to cure such deficits, we first demonstrate its performance on some artificially generated data sets which would pose challenging problems for the conventional method. In figure 5 the results for three different toy data sets are depicted. Evidently the elongated structures apparent in these data sets are grouped in an intuitively appealing manner by our new algorithm.

Recently another interesting paradigm for pairwise data clustering has been proposed by Fred [5]. In this agglomerative procedure clusters are combined if the dissimilarity increment between neighboring objects is sufficiently small according to some smoothness requirement. Our and Fred's results are depicted in figure 6. In contrast to the approach in [5] the outer ring like structure of this data set does not constitute a cluster in the sense of our objective function and we have, therefore, inferred a solution with seven groups. Apart from this deviation, our method is able to match the competitors performance.

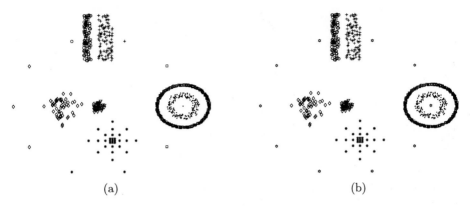

Fig. 6. Comparison between path based pairwise clustering (a) and the most competitive agglomerative procedure (b)

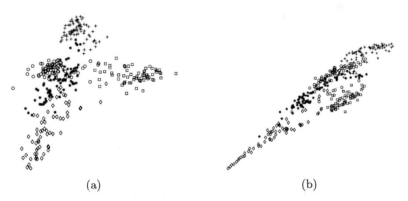

Fig. 7. Multidimensional scaling visualization of texture histograms illustrating the texture drift phenomenon: a) frontal b) tilted view on five textures

Texture Segmentation: A core application domain for pairwise data clustering techniques is the unsupervised segmentation of textured images. In order to obtain test images with known ground truth a set of mixtures of five textures each, so called Mondrians, has been constructed on the basis of micro textures from the Brodatz album.

Before we come to discuss our results a word about the motivation for path based clustering for texture segmentation is in order. Textures in real world images often exhibit a gradient or drift of the describing features due to perspective distortions. This lack of translational and rotational invariance has been recognized early by Gibson [6]. To our knowledge, Lee et al. [14] were the first to address this problem as an important factor in designing models for texture segmentation. The issue is illustrated by figure 7. Here the texture histograms have been treated as vectors. In order to visualize their structural properties the

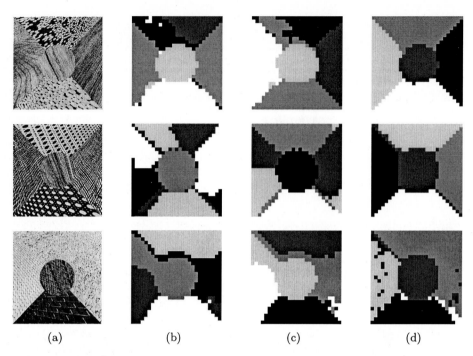

(a)   (b)   (c)   (d)

Fig. 8. Segmentation results for texture Mondrians a) input image b) ACM c) PWC d) Path Based PWC

dimensionality reduction technique *multi–dimensional scaling* (MDS) has been applied to construct a low dimensional embedding of the given vectors while faithfully preserving the inter vector distances. Figure 7 has been generated by using a deterministic annealing implementation of MDS as described in [12]. The left figure shows the case of a frontal view on five exemplary textures whereas the right one depicts the histogram embedding of the same textures when tilting the viewing angle. Clearly, the distorted textures form elongated structures in the feature space, whereas the non-inclined ones are characterized by compact groups.

In order to give an impression of the performance of the novel path based clustering approach three typical grouping solutions on mixtures of tilted Brodatz textures are shown in figure 8. For comparison the results of the conventional pairwise clustering approach (PWC) and another recently proposed and highly competitive histogram clustering method known as *Asymmetric Clustering Model* (ACM) [16] are also shown. All of these results were reached by multi-scale techniques. In this context it is interesting to shed some light on the different topologies in the object and spatial domain. Whereas the novel clustering algorithm presumes a certain topological structure in the object realm, namely that of elongated data sources, the spatial relations of two–dimensional images yield another interesting starting point in terms of the multi-scale coars-

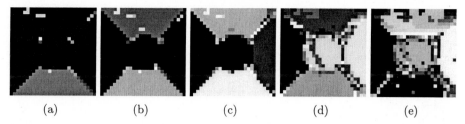

(a)   (b)   (c)   (d)   (e)

Fig. 9. Segmentation results for the texture Mondrian from example 8(a) with Minimum Spanning Tree Clustering using a) 15 cluster b) 26 c) 42 d) 145 and e) 210 cluster

ening strategy. Evidently spatially neighboring sites on the image grid are likely to belong to the same texture category. Therefore combining four by four regions of image sites can be used for defining the multi-scale pyramid in the case of texture segmentation.

As can be seen in figure 8, path based pairwise data clustering clearly outperforms its competitors on this testbed. The results show that the other algorithms tend to split perceptually homogenous regions due to the fact that they cannot handle texture gradients properly. Moreover the image regions in which an edge between adjacent textures occurs are notoriously difficult to handle. The mixed statistics of such image parts do not pose so much of a difficulty for our novel algorithm because often there are links in terms of mediating paths to textures on either side of the edge. Thus the region of concern will then be adjoined to one of these instead of being considered as a group in its own right. However in some cases (c.f. the second row in figure 8) even the novel method fails to achieve the expected results. Thus the problem of mixed statistics can not be considered completely resolved. Another interesting example is given by the last row of figure 8. Here the same texture has been used twice, once in the upper part and once on the right side of the Mondrian. Our method groups these two regions together thereby recognizing the textural similarity whereas the competing approaches separate this texture in different segments.

Path Based Clustering is related, but not identical to the agglomerative minimum spanning tree clustering algorithm (MST) (c.f. [9]). If outliers are present far away from all clusters, MST will put them in single clusters, whereas PBC assigns them to the nearest cluster. Figure 9 shows some results of MST applied to texture segmentation. The agglomerative algorithm has been stopped at different levels. The result with 26 clusters, for instance, contains only 3 groups with more than 3 elements. The result with 145 clusters is the first to distinguish the 5 different texture segments. However this solution suffers from a large amount of noise near the texture boundaries.

Another interesting insight in our novel approach is given by looking at the frequencies with which an edge between objects is lying on an optimal path between any two other objects. Such a visualization for the first and last example of figure 8 is given in figure 10. Here the objects are given by the image sites

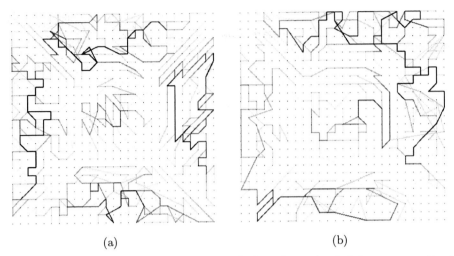

(a)   (b)

Fig. 10. Visualization of frequencies with which a given edge is lying on an optimal path between some objects. a) example one, b) example three of figure 8

lying on a homogeneous grid. The darker the depicted edge, the more often this particular link has appeared on an optimal path. In the case of well separated groups (example 1 of figure 8) the visible edges are all in the interior of the five segments. On the other hand there is a number of frequently used edges forming a chain which traverses the border between Mondrian segments in the case of the merged textures (example three in figure 8).

Apart from artificially created scenarios the ultimate test of a texture segmentation method are real-world images. In this case texture drift occurs as a natural consequence of perspective distortion. Here some results on photographic images taken from the COREL photo gallery are shown in figure 11. Again the path based approach to pairwise data grouping performs best. Furthermore the problem of the competing algorithms with image regions on texture edges becomes apparent again. Our novel method yields satisfactory results not introducing mixed statistics groups.

6   Conclusion

In this contribution a novel algorithm for pairwise data clustering has been proposed. It enhances the conventional approach by redefining inter object dissimilarities on the basis of mediating paths between those entities which belong to the same group or cluster. Moreover an efficient multi-scale optimization scheme for the new clustering approach has been developed. The ability of path based pairwise data clustering to generate high quality grouping solutions has been demonstrated on artificially created data sets as well as for real world applications.

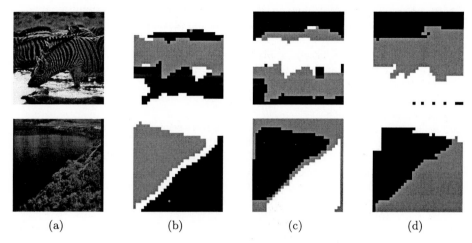

        (a)   (b)   (c)   (d)

Fig. 11. Segmentation results for real world images: a) input image b) ACM c) PWC d) Path Based PWC

However we consider the new grouping criterion to be work in progress. First of all, the current technique for reducing the number of actually considered dissimilarity values is given by simple regular subsampling. Better alternatives in the sense of Gibbs sampling or methods based on the histogram of dissimilarities should be developed. Furthermore, better stochastic optimization methods for our novel clustering approach like simulated annealing have to be formulated and embedded in the multi-scale framework.

Acknowledgement

The authors are grateful to A. Fred for providing the data set in fig. 6.

References

1. J. Besag. On the statistical analysis of dirty pictures. *Journal of the Royal Statistical Society, Series B*, 48:25–37, 1986.
2. M. Blatt, M. Wiesman, and E. Domany. Data clustering using a model granular magnet. *Neural Computation*, 9:1805–1842, 1997.
3. T. H. Cormen, C. E. Leiserson, and R. L. Rivest. *Introduction to Algorithms*. MIT Press, 1989.
4. I. Fogel and D. Sagi. Gabor filters as texture discriminators. *Biological Cybernetics*, 61:103–113, 1989.
5. A. L. N. Fred and J. M. N. Leitão. Clustering under a hypothesis of smooth dissimilarity increment. In *Proceedings of the 15th International Conference on Pattern Recognition*, volume 2, pages 190–194. IEEE Computer Society, 2000.
6. J. J. Gibson. *The Ethological Approach to Visual Perception*. Houghton Mifflin, 1979.

7. T. Hofmann and J. M. Buhmann. Pairwise data clustering by deterministic anneal-ing. *IEEE Transactions on Pattern Analysis and Machine Intelligence*, 19(1):1–14, 1997.

8. T. Hofmann, J. Puzicha, and J. M. Buhmann. Unsupervised texture segmentation in a deterministic annealing framework. *IEEE Transactions on Pattern Analysis and Machine Intelligence*, 20(8):803–818, 1998.

9. A. Jain and R. Dubes. *Algorithms for Clustering Data*. Prentice Hall, Englewood Cliffs, NJ 07632, 1988.

10. A. Jain and F. Farrokhnia. Unsupervised texture segmentation using gabor filters. *Pattern Recognition*, 24(12):1167–1186, 1991.

11. S. Kirkpatrick, C. Gelatt, and M. Vecchi. Optimization by simulated annealing. *Science*, 220(4598):671–680, 1983.

12. H. Klock and J. M. Buhmann. Data visualization by multidimensional scaling: A deterministic annealing approach. *Pattern Recognition*, 33(4):651–669, 1999. partially published in EMMCVPR '97.

13. G. Lance and W. Williams. A general theory of classification sorting strategies: Ii. clustering systems. *Computer Journal*, 10:271 – 277, 1969.

14. T. L. Lee, D. Mumford, and A. Yuille. Texture segmentation by minimizing vector–valued energy functionals : The coupled–membrane model. In *Proceedings of the European Conference on Computer Vision (ECCV'92)*, volume 588 of *LNCS*, pages 165–173. Springer Verlag, 1992.

15. J. Puzicha and J. M. Buhmann. Multiscale annealing for unsupervised image segmentation. *Computer Vision and Image Understanding*, 76(3):213–230, 1999.

16. J. Puzicha, T. Hofmann, and J. M. Buhmann. Histogram clustering for unsuper-vised segmentation and image retrieval. *Pattern Recognition Letters*, 20:899–909, 1999.

17. J. Puzicha, T. Hofmann, and J. M. Buhmann. A theory of proximity based clus-tering: Structure detection by optimization. *Pattern Recognition*, 2000.

18. J. Puzicha, Y. Rubner, C. Tomasi, and J. M. Buhmann. Empirical evaluation of dissimilarity measures for color and texture. In *Proceedings of the International Conference on Computer Vision (ICCV) '99*, pages 1165–1173, 1999.

19. K. Rose, E. Gurewitz, and G. Fox. A deterministic annealing approach to cluster-ing. *Pattern Recognition Letters*, 11:589–594, 1990.

20. N. Tishby and N. Slonim. Data clustering by markovian relaxation and the infor-mation bottleneck method. In *Advances in Neural Information Processing Sytems*, volume 13. NIPS, 2001. to appear.

A Maximum Likelihood Framework
for Grouping and Segmentation

Antonio Robles-Kelly* and Edwin R. Hancock

Department of Computer Science,
University of York, York, Y01 5DD, UK

Abstract. This paper presents an iterative maximum likelihood framework for perceptual grouping. We pose the problem of perceptual grouping as one of pairwise relational clustering. The method is quite generic and can be applied to a number of problems including region segmentation and line-linking. The task is to assign image tokens to clusters in which there is strong relational affinity between token pairs. The parameters of our model are the cluster memberships and the link weights between pairs of tokens. Commencing from a simple probability distribution for these parameters, we show how they may be estimated using an EM-like algorithm. The cluster memberships are estimated using an eigendecomposition method. Once the cluster memberships are to hand, then the updated link-weights are the expected values of their pairwise products. The new method is demonstrated on region segmentation and line-segment grouping problems where it is shown to outperform a non-iterative eigenclustering method.

1 Introduction

Recently, there has been considerable interest in the use of matrix factorisation methods for perceptual grouping. These methods can be viewed as drawing their inspiration from spectral graph theory [4]. The basic idea is to commence from an initial characterisation of the perceptual affinity of different image tokens in terms of a matrix of link-weights. Once this matrix is to hand then its eigenvalues and eigenvectors are located. The eigenmodes represent pairwise relational clusters which can be used to group the raw perceptual entities together. There are several examples of this approach described in the literature. At the level of image segmentation, several authors have used algorithms based on the eigenmodes of an affinity matrix to iteratively segment image data. One of the best known is the normalised cut method of Shi and Malik [16]. Recently, Weiss [17] has shown how this, and other closely related methods, can be improved using a normalised affinity matrix. At higher level, both Sarkar and Boyer [14] and Perona and Freeman [13] have developed matrix factorisation methods for line-segment grouping. These non-iterative methods both use the eigenstructure of a perceptual affinity matrix to find disjoint subgraphs that represent the main arrangements of segmental entities.

---

* Supported by CONACYT, under grant No. 146475/151752.

M.A.T. Figueiredo, J. Zerubia, A.K. Jain (Eds.): EMMCVPR 2001, LNCS 2134, pp. 251–266, 2001.
© Springer-Verlag Berlin Heidelberg 2001

Although elegant by virtue of their use of matrix factorisation to solve the underlying optimization problem, one of the criticisms which can be leveled at these methods is that their foundations are not statistical in nature. The aim in this paper is to overcome this shortcoming by developing a maximum likelihood framework for perceptual grouping. We pose the problem as one of pairwise clustering which is parameterised using two sets of indicator variables. The first of these are cluster membership variables which indicate to which perceptual cluster a segmental entity belongs. The second set of variables are link weights which convey the strength of the perceptual relations between pairs of nodes in the same cluster. We use these parameters to develop a probabilistic model which represents the pairwise clustering of the perceptual entities. We iteratively maximise the likelihood of the configuration of pairwise clusters using an EM-like algorithm. By casting the log-likelihood function into a matrix setting, we are able to estimate the cluster-memberships using matrix factorisation. Once these memberships are to hand, then the link-weights may be estimated.

It is important to stress that although there have been some attempts at using probabilistic methods for grouping elsewhere in the literature [11], our method has a number of unique features which distinguish it from these alternatives. Early work by Dickson [6] has used Bayes nets to develop a hierarchical framework for splitting and merging groups of lines. Cox, Rehg and Hingorani [9] have developed a grouping method which combines evidence from the raw edge attributes delivered by the Canny edge detector. Leite and Hancock [10] have persued similar objectives with the aim of fitting cubic splines to the output of a bank of multiscale derivative of Gaussian filters using the EM algorithm. Castano and Hutchinson [11] have developed a Bayesian framework for combining evidence for different graph-based partitions or groupings of line-segments. The method exploits bilateral symmetries. It is based on a frequentist approach over the set of partitions of the line-segments and is hence free of parameters. Recently, Crevier [5] has developed an evidence combining framework for extracting chains of colinear line-segments. Our work differs from this work in a number of important ways. We use a probabilistic characterisation of the grouping-graph based on a matrix of link weights. The goal of computation is to iteratively recover the maximum likelihood elements of this matrix using the apparatus of the EM algorithm. When posed in this way, the resulting iterative process may also be regarded as the high-level analogue of a number of low-level iterative processes for perceptual grouping. Here several authors have explored the use of iterative relaxation style operators for edgel grouping. This approach was pioneered by Shashua and Ullman [15] and later refined by Guy and Medioni [7] among others. Parent and Zucker have shown how co-circularity can be used to gauge the compatibility of neighbouring edges [12]. Our method differs from these methods by virtue of the fact that it uses a statistical framework rather than a goal directed one dictated by considerations from neurobiology.

The outline of this paper is as follows. Section 2 reviews previous work on how matrix factorisation may be applied to the link-weight matrix to perform perceptual grouping. In Section 3 we develop our maximum likelihood framework and show how the parameters of the model, namely the cluster membership probabilities and the pairwise link-weights can be estimated using an iterative EM-like algorithm. In Section 4 we describe how the method can be applied to image segmentation while Section 5 describes a second application involving motion analysis. Finally, Section 6 concludes the paper by summarising our contributions and offering directions for future research.

2 Grouping by Matrix Factorisation

We pose the problem of perceptual grouping as that of finding the pairwise clusters which exist within a set of image tokens. These objects may be pixels, or segmental entities such as corners, lines, curves or regions. However, in this paper we focus on the two problems of region segmentation and motion analysis. The process of pairwise clustering is somewhat different to the more familiar one of central clustering. Whereas central clustering aims to characterise cluster-membership using the cluster mean and variance, in pairwise clustering it is link-weights between nodes which are used to establish cluster membership. Although less well studied than central clustering, there has recently been renewed interest in pairwise clustering aimed at placing the method on a more principled footing using techniques such as mean-field annealing [8].

To commence, we require some formalism. We are interested in grouping a set of objects which are abstracted using a weighted graph. The problem is characterised by the set of nodes V that represent the objects and the set of weighted edges E between the nodes that represent the state of perceptual grouping. The aim in grouping is to locate the set of edges that parition the node-set V into disjoint and disconnected subsets. If V_ω represents one of these subsets and Ω is the index-set of different partitions, then $V = \bigcup_{\omega \in \Omega} V_\omega$ and $V_{\omega'} \cap V_{\omega''} = \emptyset$ if $\omega' \neq \omega''$. Moreover, since the edges partition the node-set into disconnected subgraphs, then $E \cap (V_{\omega'} \times V_{\omega''}) = \emptyset$ if $\omega' \neq \omega''$. We are interested in perceptual grouping problems which can be characterised using an a $|V| \times |V|$ matrix of link-weights A. The elements of this matrix convey the following meaning in the hard limit

$$A_{ij} = \begin{cases} 1 & \text{if there exists a partition } V_\omega \\ & \text{such that } i \in V_\omega \text{ and } j \in V_\omega \\ 0 & \text{otherwise} \end{cases} \qquad (1)$$

In this paper we are interested in how matrix factorisation methods can be used to locate the set of edges which partition the nodes. One way of viewing this is as the search for the permutation matrix which re-orders the elements of A into non-ovelapping blocks. Howevever, when the elements of the matrix A are not binary in nature, then this is not a straightforward task. However, Sarkar and Boyer [14] have shown how the positive eigenvectors of the matrix of link-weights can be used to assign nodes to perceptual clusters. Using the Rayleigh-Ritz theorem, they observe that the scalar quantity $\underline{x}^t A \underline{x}$, where A is the weighted adjacency matrix, is maximised when $\underline{x}$ is the leading eigenvector of A. Moreover, each of the subdominant eigenvectors corresponds to a disjoint perceptual cluster. We confine our attention to same-sign positive eigenvectors (i.e. those whose corresponding eigenvalues are real and positive, and whose components are either all positive or are all negative in sign). If a component of a positive eigenvector is non-zero, then the corresponding node belongs to the perceptual cluster associated with the associated eigenmodes of the weighted adjacency matrix. The eigenvalues $\lambda_1, \lambda_2....$ of A are the solutions of the equation $|A - \lambda I| = 0$ where I is the $N \times N$ identity matrix. The corresponding eigenvectors $\underline{x}_{\lambda_1}, \underline{x}_{\lambda_2}, \dots$ are found by solving the equation $A\underline{x}_{\lambda_i} = \lambda_i \underline{x}_{\lambda_i}$. Let the set of positive same-sign eigenvectors be represented by $\Omega = \{\omega | \lambda_\omega > 0 \wedge [(\underline{x}_\omega^*(i) > 0 \forall i) \vee \underline{x}_\omega^*(i) < 0 \forall i])\}$. Since the positive eigenvectors are orthogonal, this means that there is only one value of ω for which $\underline{x}_\omega^*(i) \neq 0$. In other words, each node i is associated with a unique cluster. We denote the set of nodes assigned to the cluster with modal index ω as $V_\omega = \{i | \underline{x}_\omega^*(i) \neq 0\}$.

3   Maximum Likelihood Framework

In this paper, we are interested in exploiting the factorisation property of Sarkar and Boyer [14] to develop a maximum likelihood method for updating the link-weight matrix A with the aim of developing a more robust perceptual grouping method. We commence by factorising the likelihood of the observed arrangement of objects over the set of modal clusters of the link-weight matrix. Since the set of modal clusters are disjoint we can write,

$$P(A) = \prod_{\omega \in \Omega} P(\Phi_\omega) \tag{2}$$

where $P(\Phi_\omega)$ is the probability distribution for the set of link-weights belonging to the modal-cluster indexed ω. To model the component probability distributions, we introduce a cluster membership indicator which models the degree of affinity of the object indexed i to the cluster with modal index ω. This is done using the magnitudes of the modal co-efficients and we set

$$s_{iw} = \frac{|\underline{x}_\omega^*(i)|}{\sum_{i \in V_\omega} |\underline{x}_\omega^*(i)|} \tag{3}$$

Using these variables, we develop a model of probability distribution for the link-weights associated with the individual clusters. We commence by assuming that there are putative edges between each pair of nodes (i, j) belonging to the cluster. The set of putative edges is $\Phi_\omega = V_\omega \times V_\omega - \{(i, i) | i \in V\}$. We further assume that the link-weights belonging to each cluster are independent of one another and write

$$P(\Phi_\omega) = \prod_{(i,j) \in \Phi_\omega} P(A_{i,j}) \tag{4}$$

To proceed, we require a model of probability distribution for the link-weights. Here we adopt a model in which the observed link structure of the pairwise clusters arises through a Bernoulli distribution. The parameter of this distribution is the link-probability $A_{i,j}$. The idea behind this model is that any pair of nodes i and j may connect to each with a link. This link is treated as a Bernoulli variable. The probability that this link is the correct is $A_{i,j}$ while the probability that it is in error is $1 - A_{i,j}$. To gauge the correctness of the link, we check whether the nodes i and j belong to the same pairwise cluster. To test for cluster-consistency we make use of the quantity $s_{i\omega}s_{j\omega}$. This is unity if both nodes belong to the same cluster and is zero otherwise. Using this switching property, the Bernoulli distribution becomes

$$p(A_{i,j}) = A_{i,j}^{s_{i\omega}s_{j\omega}}(1 - A_{i,j})^{1 - s_{i\omega}s_{j\omega}} \tag{5}$$

This distribution takes on its largest values when either the link weight A_{ij} is unity and $s_{i\omega} = s_{j\omega} = 1$, or if the link weight $A_{i,j} = 0$ and $s_{i\omega} = s_{j\omega} = 0$.

With these ingredients the log-likelihood function for the observed pattern of link weights is

$$\mathcal{L} = \sum_{\omega \in \Omega} \sum_{(i,j) \in \Phi_\omega} \left\{ s_{i\omega}s_{j\omega} \ln A_{ij} + (1 - s_{i\omega}s_{j\omega})\ln(1 - A_{i,j}) \right\} \tag{6}$$

After some algebra to collect terms, the log-likelihood function simplifies to

$$\mathcal{L} = \sum_{\omega \in \Omega} \sum_{(i,j) \in \Phi_\omega} \left\{ s_{i\omega}s_{j\omega} \ln \frac{A_{ij}}{1 - A_{ij}} + \ln(1 - A_{i,j}) \right\} \tag{7}$$

Posed in this way the structure of the log-likelihood function is reminiscent of that underpinning the expectation-maximisation algorithm. The modes of the link-weight matrix play the role of mixing components. The product of cluster-membership variables $s_{i\omega}s_{j\omega}$ plays the role of an a posteriori measurement probability. Secondly, the link-weights are the parameters which must be estimated. However, there are important differences. The most important of these is that the modal clusters are disjoint. As a result there is no mixing between them.

Based on this observation, we will exploit an EM-like process to update the link-weights and the cluster-membership variables. In the "M" step we will locate maximum likelihood link-weights. In the "E" step we will use the revised link-weight matrix to update the modal clusters. To this end we index the link weights and cluster memberships with iteration number and aim to optimise the quantity

$$Q(A^{(n+1)}|A^{(n)}) = \sum_{\omega \in \Omega} \sum_{(i,j) \in \Phi_\omega} \left\{ s_{i\omega}^{(n)} s_{j\omega}^{(n)} \right.$$
$$\left. \ln \frac{A_{ij}^{(n+1)}}{1 - A_{ij}^{(n+1)}} + \ln(1 - A_{i,j}^{(n+1)}) \right\} \tag{8}$$

The revised link weight parameters are indexed at iteration $n + 1$ while the cluster-memberships are indexed at iteration n.

3.1 Expectation

To update the cluster-membership variables we have used a gradient-based method. We have computed the derivatives of the expected log-likelihood function with respect to the cluster-membership variable

$$\frac{\partial Q(A^{(n+1)}|A^{(n)})}{\partial s_{iw}^{(n+1)}} = \sum_{j \in V_\omega} s_{jw}^{(n)} \ln \frac{A_{ij}^{(n+1)}}{1 - A_{ij}^{(n+1)}} \tag{9}$$

Since the associated saddle-point equations are not tractable in closed form, we use the soft-assign ansatz of Bridle [2] to update the cluster membership assignment variables. This involves exponentiating the partial derivatives of the expected log-likelihood function in the following manner

$$s_{iw}^{(n+1)} = \frac{\exp\left[\frac{\partial Q(A^{(n+1)}|A^{(n)})}{\partial s_{iw}^{(n)}}\right]}{\sum_{i \in V_w} \exp\left[\frac{\partial Q(A^{(n+1)}|A^{(n)})}{\partial s_{iw}^{(n)}}\right]} \tag{10}$$

As a result the update equation for the cluster membership indicator variables is

$$s_{iw}^{(n+1)} = \frac{\exp\left[\sum_{j \in V_\omega} s_{jw}^{(n)} \ln \frac{A_{i,j}^{(n+1)}}{1 - A_{ij}^{(n+1)}}\right]}{\sum_{i \in V_w} \exp\left[\sum_{j \in V_\omega} s_{jw}^{(n)} \ln \frac{A_{i,j}^{(n+1)}}{1 - A_{ij}^{(n+1)}}\right]}$$

$$= \frac{\prod_{j \in V_\omega}\left\{\frac{A_{i,j}^{(n+1)}}{1 - A_{ij}^{(n+1)}}\right\}^{s_{jw}^{(n)}}}{\sum_{i \in V_w} \prod_{j \in V_\omega}\left\{\frac{A_{ij}^{(n+1)}}{1 - A_{ij}^{(n+1)}}\right\}^{s_{jw}^{(n)}}} \tag{11}$$

3.2 Maximisation

Once the revised cluster membership variables are to hand then we can apply the maximisation step of the algorithm to update the link-weight matrix. The updated link-weights are found by computing the derivatives of the expected log-likelihood function

$$\frac{\partial Q(A^{(n+1)}|A^{(n)})}{\partial A_{ij}^{(n+1)}} = \sum_{\omega \in \Omega} \varsigma_{i,j,\omega}^{(n)}\left\{s_{iw}^{(n)} s_{jw}^{(n)}\right.$$

$$\left. \frac{1}{A_{ij}^{(n+1)}(1 - A_{ij}^{(n+1)})} - \frac{1}{1 - A_{ij}^{(n+1)}}\right\} \tag{12}$$

and solving the saddle-point equations

$$\frac{\partial Q(A^{(n+1)}|A^{(n)})}{\partial A_{ij}^{(n+1)}} = 0 \tag{13}$$

As a result the updated link-weights are given by

$$A_{ij}^{(n+1)} = \sum_{\omega \in \Omega} s_{i\omega}^{(n)} s_{j\omega}^{(n)} \tag{14}$$

In other words, the link-weight for the pair of nodes (i, j) is simply the average of the product of individual node cluster memberships over the different perceptual clusters. Since each node is associated with a unique cluster, this means that the updated affinity matrix is composed of non-overlapping blocks. Moreover, the link-weights are are guaranteed to be in the interval $[0, 1]$.

3.3 Modal Structure of the Updated Link-Weight Matrix

Once the updated link-weight matrix is to hand, then we can use the modal analysis of Sarkar and Boyer to refine the set of clusters. The idea is a simple one. For each cluster, we compute an updated link-weight matrix. The leading eigenvector of this matrix provides a measure of the affinity of the different nodes to the cluster.

To proceed, we introduce some matrix notation. We commence by representing the cluster-memberships of the cluster indexed ω using the column vector $\underline{S}_\omega = (s_{1\omega}, ..., s_{|V_\omega|\omega})^T$. We also define a $|V| \times |V|$ weight-matrix W^ω, whose elements are

$$W_{i,j}^\omega = \zeta_{i,j,\omega} \ln \frac{A_{ij}^{(n)}}{1 - A_{ij}^{(n)}} \tag{15}$$

where

$$\zeta_{i,j,\omega} = \begin{cases} 1 \text{ if } s_{i\omega}^{(n)} \neq 0 \text{ and } s_{i\omega}^{(n)} \neq 0 \\ 0 \text{ otherwise} \end{cases} \tag{16}$$

With this notation, the algorithm focuses on the quantity

$$\hat{Q}(A^{(n+1)}|A^{(n)}) = \sum_{\omega \in \Omega} S_\omega^T W^\omega S_\omega \tag{17}$$

In this way the log-likelihood function is decomposed into contributions from the distinct modal clusters. Moreover, each cluster weight matrix W^ω is disjoint. For each such matrix, we will perform a further eigendecomposition to identify the foreground and background modal structure. Recall that Sarkar and Boyer [14] have shown that the scalar quantity $\underline{x}^t A \underline{x}$, where A is the weighted adjacency matrix and $\underline{x}$ is a vector of cluster-membership variables, is maximised when $\underline{x}$ is the leading eigenvector of A. Unfortunately, we can not exploit this property directly. The reasons for this are twofold. First, the utility measure underpinning our maximum likelihood algorithm is a sum of terms of the form $S_\omega^T W^\omega S_\omega$. Second, the elements of W^ω may be negative (since it is computed by taking logarithms) and hence its eigenvalues will not be real. We overcome the first of these problems by applying the Rayleigh-Ritz theorem to each weight matrix W^ω in turn. Each such matrix represents a distinct cluster and its leading eigenvector represents the individual cluster-membership affinities of the nodes. To overcome the second problem we make use of the fact that the directions of the eigenvectors of the matrices A and $\ln A$ are identical. We therefore commence from the matrix $\hat{W}^\omega$ whose elements are

$$\hat{W}_{ij}^\omega = \zeta_{i,j,\omega} \left[\frac{A_{ij}^{(n+1)}}{1 - A_{ij}^{(n+1)}} \right] \tag{18}$$

We use the components of the leading eigenvector $\underline{z}_\omega$ of $\hat{W}^\omega$ to perform "modal sharpening" on the cluster memberships. They are re-assigned according to the following formula

$$s_{i\omega}^{(n+1)} = \frac{|\underline{z}_\omega(i)|}{\sum_{i=1}^{|V_\omega|} |\underline{z}_\omega(i)|} \tag{19}$$

Before proceeding, it is worth pausing to consider the relationship between this modal analysis and the updated cluster membership variables. Using the update formula obtained for the cluster-membership variables given in Equation (11), it is a straightforward matter to show that the log-likelhood function is given by

$$\mathcal{L} = \sum_{\omega \in \Omega} \sum_{(i,j) \in \Phi_\omega} \left\{ T_{ij}^{(n+1)} \right.$$

$$\frac{\exp\left[\sum_{k \in V_\omega} T_{ik}^{(n+1)} s_{k\omega}^{(n)} \right] \exp\left[\sum_{k \in V_\omega} T_{kj}^{(n+1)} s_{k\omega}^{(n)} \right]}{\sum_{i' \in V_\omega} \exp\left[\sum_{k \in V_\omega} T_{i'k}^{(n+1)} s_{k\omega}^{(n)} \right] \sum_{j' \in V_\omega} \exp\left[\sum_{k \in V_\omega} T_{j'k}^{(n+1)} s_{k\omega}^{(n)} \right]} \tag{20}$$

$$\left. + \ln(1 - A_{ij}^{(n+1)}) \right\}$$

where

$$T_{ij}^{(n+1)} = \ln\left(\frac{A_{ij}^{(n+1)}}{1 - A_{ij}^{(n+1)}} \right) \tag{21}$$

To cast the log-likelihood function into a matrix setting suppose that $T^{(n+1)}$ is the matrix whose entry with row i and column j is $T_{i,j}^{(n1+)}$. Further, suppose that $\underline{x}_\omega^{(n)}(\lambda_l^{(n+1)}) = \{x_1^{(n)}, x_2^{(n)}, \ldots, x_m^{(n)}\}^T$ is the eigenvector associated with the eigenvalue $\lambda_l^{(n+1)}$ of $T^{(n+1)}$. For this eigenvector, the eigenvalue equation is

$$T^{(n+1)}\underline{x}_\omega = \lambda_l^{(n+1)}\underline{x}_\omega \tag{22}$$

Furthermore, the jth component of the eigenvector satisfies the equation

$$\sum_{k \in V_\omega} s_{k\omega}^{(n)} T_{kj}^{(n+1)} = \lambda_l^{(n+1)} s_{j\omega}^{(n)}, j = 1, 2, \ldots, m \tag{23}$$

If the vector of cluster membership variables $\underline{s}_\omega^{(n)}(\lambda_l^{(n+1)}) = \{s_1^{(n)}, s_2^{(n)}, \ldots, s_m^{(n)}\}^T$ is an eigenvector of $T^{(n+1)}$ then we can write
    Collecting terms together

$$\mathcal{L} = \sum_{\omega \in \Omega} \sum_{(i,j) \in \Phi_\omega} \left\{ T_{ij}^{(n+1)} \frac{\exp\left[\lambda_l^{(n+1)}(s_{i\omega}^{(n)} + s_{j\omega}^{(n)})\right]}{\sum_{i' \in V_\omega} \exp\left[\lambda_l^{(n+1)} s_{i'\omega}^{(n)}\right] \sum_{j' \in V_\omega} \exp\left[\lambda_l^{(n+1)} s_{j'\omega}^{(n)}\right]} \right.$$
$$\left. + \ln(1 - A_{ij}^{(n+1)}) \right\} \tag{24}$$

For the cluster indexed ω, the contribution to the log-likelihood function is clearly maximised when $\lambda_l^{(n+1)}$ is the largest eigenvalue of $T^{(n+1)}$.

3.4   Algorithm Description

To summarise, the iterative steps of the algorithm are as follows:

- (1) Compute the eignenvectors of the current link-weight matrix $A^{(n)}$. Each same-sign eigenvector whose eigenvalue is positive represents a disjoint pairwise cluster. The number of such eigenvectors determines the number of clusters for the current iteration. This number may vary from iteration to iteration.
- (2) Compute the updated cluster-membership variables using the E-step. At this stage modal sharpening amy be performed to improve the cluster-structure if desired. This sharpening process may be iterated to refine the current set of clusters.
- (3) Update the link-weights using the M-step to compute the updated link weight matrix $A^{(n+1)}$.
- Goto step (1).

4   Grey Scale Image Segmentation

The first application of our new pairwise clustering method involves segmenting grey-scale images into regions. To compute the initial affinity matrix, we use the difference in grey-scale values at different pixel sites. Suppose that g_i is the grey-scale value at the pixel indexed i and g_j is the grey-scale value at the pixel indexed j. The corresponding entry in the affinity matrix is

$$A_{i,j}^{(0)} = \exp[-k_g(g_i - g_j)^2] \tag{25}$$

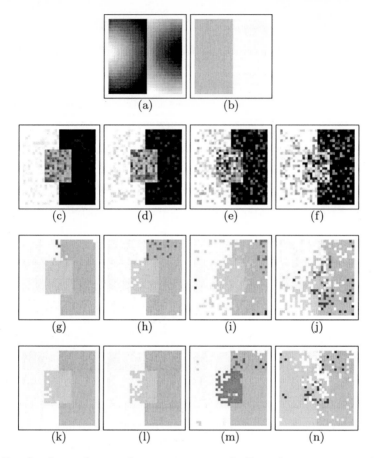

Fig. 1. Results obtained on synthetic images using the Eigendecompositon method and the Softassign.

If we are segmenting an $R \times C$ image of R rows and C columns, then the affinity matrix is of dimensions $RC \times RC$. This initial characterisation of the affinity matrix is similar to that used by Shi and Malik [16] in their normalised-cut method of image segmentation.

By applying the clustering method to this initial affinity matrix we iteratively segment the image into regions. Each eigenmode corresponds to a distinct region.

4.1   Experiments

We have conducted experiments on both synthetic and real images. We commence with some examples on synthetic images aimed at establishing some of the properties of the resulting image segmentation method. In Figure 1 a) and b) we investigate the effect of contrast variations. The left-hand panel shows an image which divided into two rectangular regions. Within each region there is

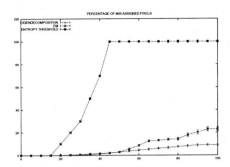

Fig. 2. Number of segmentation errors versus noise standard deviation for non-iterative eigenecomposition (top curve), soft-assign EM (middle curve) and modal sharpening EM (lower curve).

variation in intensity whose distribution is generated using a Lambertian sphere. In the right-hand panel we show the resulting segmentation when the EM-like method is used with modal sharpening. There are two modes, i.e. detected regions. These correspond to the two rectangular regions in the original image. There is no fragmentation due to the spherical intensity variation.

Next we consider the effect of added random noise. In Figure 1 c), d), e) and f) (i.e. the second row) we show a sequence of images in which we have added Gaussian noise of zero mean and known standard deviation to the grey-scale values in an image containing three rectangular regions. The third row (ie 1 g, h, i and j) shows the segmentation result obtained with the EM algorithm when cluster-memberships are updated using the modal refinement process described in Section 3.3. The fourth row (ie 1 k,l,m and n) shows the segmentation obtained using the EM algorithm with cluster membership update using soft-assign. For the different images, standard deviation of the added Gaussian noise is 35%,50%,65% and 95% of the grey-scale difference between the regions. The

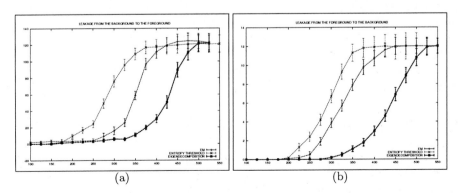

Fig. 3. Comparison between the non-iterative eigendecomposition approach and the two variants of the EM-like algorithm.

final segmentations are obtained with an average of 2.3 iterations per cluster. The final segmentations contain 3,3,4 and 4 clusters respectively. The method begins to fail once the noise exceeds 60%. It is also worth noting that the region boundaries and corners are well reconstructed.

Figure 2 offers a more quantitative evaluation of the segmentation capabilities of the method. Here we compute the fraction of mislabelled pixels in the segmented images as a function of the standard deviation of the added Gaussian noise. The plot shows three performance curves obtained with a) the non-iterative eigendecomposition algorithm, b) the EM-like method with soft-assign and c) the EM-like algorithm with modal sharpening. The non-iterative method fails abruptly at low noise-levels. The two variants of the EM-like algorithm perform much better, with the modal sharpening method offering a useful margin of advantage over the soft-assign method.

We have repeated the experiments described above for a sequence of synthetic images in which the density of distractors increases. For each image in turn we have computed the number of distractors merged with the foreground pattern and the number of foreground line-segments which leak into the background. Figures 3 a and b respectively show the fraction of nodes merged with the foreground and the number of nodes which leak into the background as a function of the number of distractors. The three curves shown in each plot are for the non-iterative eigendecomposition method and for the EM-like algorithm when both soft-assign and modal sharpening are used to update the cluster

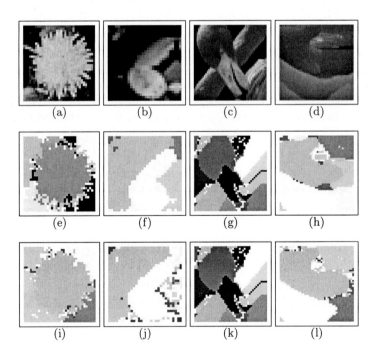

Fig. 4. Segmentations of grey-scale images.

membership weights. In both cases, the shoulder of the response curve for the two variants of the EM-like algorithm occurs at a significantly higher error rate than that for the non-iterative eigen-decomposition method. Of the two alternative methods for updating the cluster membership weights in the EM algorithm, modal sharpening works best.

To conclude this section, in Figure 4 we provide some example segmentations on real-world images. In the ltop row we show the original image, the middle row is the segmentation obtained with EM and modal sharpening, while the bottom row shows the segmentation obtained with EM and soft-assign. On the whole the results are quite promising. The segmentations capture the main region structure of the images. Moreover, they are not unduly disturbed by brightness variations or texture. The modal sharpening method gives the cleanest segmentations. It should be stressed that these results are presented to illustrate the scope offered by our new clustering algorithm and not to make any claims concerning its utility as a tool for image segmentation. To do so would require comparison and sensitivity analysis well beyond the scope of this paper.

One of the interesting properties of our method is that the number of modes or clusters changes with each iteration of the algorithm. This is because we perform a new modal analysis each time the link-weight matrix $A^{(n)}$ is updated. For the segmentation results shown in fig 4, we have investigated how the number of modal clusters varies with iteration number. In Figure 5 we show the number of active clusters as a function of iteration number for each of the real-world images. In each case the number of clusters increase with iteration number. In the best case the number of clusters stabilizes after 2 iterations (figure 4i), and in the worst case after 6 iterations (figure 4l).

5   Motion Segmentation

Our second application involves motion segmentation. To compute motion vectors we have used a single resolution block matching algorithm using spatial/-temporal correlation [3], this kind of block matching algorithms are based on a predictive search that reduces the computational complexity and provides a

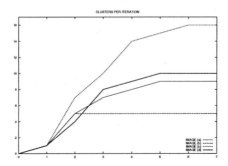

Fig. 5. Number of clusters per iteration for each of the real-world images in fig. 4.

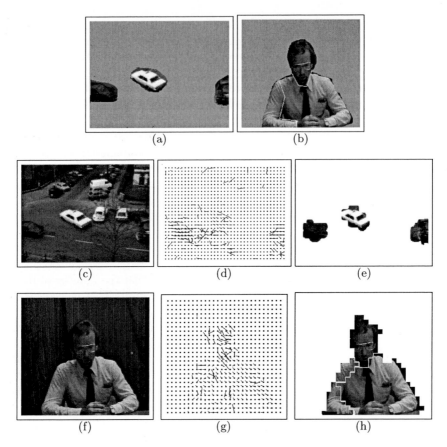

Fig. 6. Results for motion sequences.

reliable performance. The 2D velocity vectors for the extracted motion blocks are characterised using a matrix of pairwise similarity weights. Suppose that $\hat{\mathbf{n}}_i$ and $\hat{\mathbf{n}}_j$ are the unit motion vectors for the blocks indexed i and j. The elements of this weight matrix are given by

$$A_{i,j}^{(0)} = \begin{cases} \frac{1}{2}\left\{1 + \hat{\mathbf{n}}_i.\hat{\mathbf{n}}_j\right\} & \text{if } i \neq j \\ 0 & otherwise \end{cases} \tag{26}$$

5.1   Motion Experiments

We have conducted experiments on motion sequences with known ground truth. In Figures 6a and 6b we show ground truth data for the "Hamburg taxi" and "Trevor White" sequences. The images show the distinct motion components for the two scenes. The corresponding raw images are shown in Figures 6c and 6f.

In both sequences we use 8 × 8 pixel blocks to compute the motion vectors. For the "Hamburg taxi" sequence the motion field is shown in Figure 6d. In Figure 6e we show the pairwise clusters obtained by applying our EM-like algorithm. There are 3 clusters which match closely to the ground truth data shown in Figure 6a. In fact, the three different clusters correspond to distinct moving vehicles in the sequence. Figure 6g shows the corresponding motion field for the "Trevor White" sequence. The motion segmentation is shown in Figure 6h. There are three clusters which correspond to the head, the right arm, and the chest plus left arm. These clusters again match closely to the ground-truth data. It is interesting to note that the results are comparable to those reported in [1] where a 5 dimensional feature vector and a neural network was used. The proposed algorithm converges in an average of four iterations.

Table 1. Error percentage for the two image sequences.

Sequence	Cluster	% of Error
Trevor White	Right arm	8 %
Trevor White	Chest	6 %
Trevor White	Head	12%
Ham. Taxi	Taxi	4 %
Ham. Taxi	Far Left Car	3 %
Ham. Taxi	Far Right Car	10 %

In Table 1 we provide a more quantative analysis of these results. The table lists the fraction of the pixels in each region of the ground truth data which are misasigned by the clustering algorithm. The best results are obtained for the chest-region, the taxi and the far-left car, where the error rate is a few percent. For the far-right car and the head of the Trevor White, the error rates are about 10%. The problems with the far-right cat probably relate to the fact that it is close to the periphery of the image.

6   Conclusions

In this paper, we have presented a new perceptual clustering algorithm which uses an EM-like algorithm to estimate link-weights and cluster membership probabilities. The method is based on an iterative modal decomposition of the link-weight matrix. The modal cluster membership probabilities are modeled using a Bernoulli distribution for the link-weights. We apply the method to the problems of region segmentation and of motion segmentation. The method appears robust to severe levels of background clutter.

References

1. A. G. Bors and I. Pitas. Optical flow estimation and moving object segmentation based on Median RBF network. *IEEE Trans. on Image Processing*, 7(5):693–702, 1998.

2. J. S. Bridle. Training stochastic model recognition algorithms can lead to maximum mutual information estimation of parameters. In *NIPS 2*, pages 211–217, 1990.
3. J. S. Shyn C. H. Hsieh, P. C. Lu and E. H. Lu. Motion estimation algorithm using inter-block correlation. *IEE Electron. Lett.*, 26(5):276–277, 1990.
4. Fan R. K. Chung. *Spectral Graph Theory*. American Mathematical Society, 1997.
5. D. Crevier. A probabilistic method for extracting chains of collinear segments. *Image and Vision Computing*, 76(1):36–53, 1999.
6. W. Dickson. Feature grouping in a hierarchical probabilistic network. *Image and Vision Computing*, 9(1):51–57, 1991.
7. G. Guy and G. Medioni. Inferring global perceptual contours from local features. *International Journal of Computer Vision*, 20(1/2):113–133, 1996.
8. T. Hofmann and M. Buhmann. Pairwise data clustering by deterministic annealing. *IEEE Tansactions on Pattern Analysis and Machine Intelligence*, 19(1):1–14, 1997.
9. J. M. Rehg I. J. Cox and S. Hingorani. A bayesian multiple-hypothesis approach to edge grouping and contour segmentation. *International Journal of Computing and Vision*, 11(1):5–24, 1993.
10. J. A. F. Leite and E. R. Hancock. Iterative curve organisation with the em algorithm. *Pattern Recognition Letters*, 18:143–155, 1997.
11. R. Castan o and S. Hutchinson. A probabilistic approach to perceptual grouping. *Computer Vision and Image Understanding*, 64(3):339–419, 1996.
12. P. Parent and S. Zucker. Trace inference, curvature consistency and curve detection. *IEEE Transactions on Pattern Analysis and Machine Intelligence*, 11(8):823–839, 1989.
13. P. Perona and W. T. Freeman. Factorization approach to grouping. In *Proc. ECCV*, pages 655–670, 1998.
14. S. Sarkar and K. L. Boyer. Quantitative measures of change based on feature organization: Eigenvalues and eigenvectors. *Computer Vision and Image Understanding*, 71(1):110–136, 1998.
15. A. Shashua and S. Ullman. Structural saliency: The detection of globally salient structures using a locally connected network. In *Proc. 2nd Int. Conf. in Comp. Vision*, pages 321–327, 1988.
16. J. Shi and J. Malik. Normalized cuts and image segmentations. In *Proc. IEEE CVPR*, pages 731–737, 1997.
17. Y. Weiss. Segmentation using eigenvectors: A unifying view. In *IEEE International Conference on Computer Vision*, pages 975–982, 1999.

Image Labeling and Grouping
by Minimizing Linear Functionals over Cones

Christian Schellewald, Jens Keuchel, and Christoph Schnörr

Computer Vision, Graphics, and Pattern Recognition Group
Department of Mathematics and Computer Science;
University of Mannheim, D-68131 Mannheim, Germany
{cschelle,jkeuchel,schnoerr}@ti.uni-mannheim.de
Fax: +49 612 181 2744, http://www.cvgpr.uni-mannheim.de

Abstract. We consider energy minimization problems related to image labeling, partitioning, and grouping, which typically show up at mid-level stages of computer vision systems. A common feature of these problems is their intrinsic combinatorial complexity from an optimization point-of-view. Rather than trying to compute the global minimum – a goal we consider as elusive in these cases – we wish to design optimization approaches which exhibit two relevant properties: First, in *each* application a solution with *guaranteed* degree of suboptimality can be computed. Secondly, the computations are based on clearly defined algorithms which do not comprise *any* (hidden) tuning parameters.

In this paper, we focus on the second property and introduce a novel and general optimization technique to the field of computer vision which amounts to compute a suboptimal solution by just solving a *convex* optimization problem. As representative examples, we consider two binary quadratic energy functionals related to image labeling and perceptual grouping. Both problems can be considered as instances of a general quadratic functional in binary variables, which is embedded into a higher–dimensional space such that suboptimal solutions can be computed as minima of linear functionals over cones in that space (semidefinite programs). Extensive numerical results reveal that, on the average, suboptimal solutions can be computed which yield a gap below 5% with respect to the global optimum in case where this is known.

1 Introduction

Many energy-minimization problems in computer vision like image labeling and partitioning, perceptual grouping, graph matching etc., involve discrete decision variables and therefore are intrinsically combinatorial by nature. Accordingly, optimization approaches to efficiently compute good minimizers have a long history in the literature. Important examples include the seminal paper by Geman and Geman [1] on simulated annealing, approaches for suboptimal Markov Random Field (MRF) minimization like the ICM-algorithm [2], the highest-confidence-first heuristic [3], multi-scale approaches [4], and other approximations [5, 6]. A further important class of approaches comprises continuation methods like Leclers partitioning approach [7], the graduated-non-convexity

M.A.T. Figueiredo, J. Zerubia, A.K. Jain (Eds.): EMMCVPR 2001, LNCS 2134, pp. 267–282, 2001.
© Springer-Verlag Berlin Heidelberg 2001

strategy by Blake and Zisserman [8], and various deterministic (approximate) versions of the annealing approach in applications like surface reconstruction [9], perceptual grouping [10], graph matching [11], or clustering [12].

Apart from the simulated annealing approach using annealing schedules which are unpractically slow for real-world applications (but prescribed by theory, see [1]), none of the above-mentioned approaches can guarantee to find the global minimum. And in general, this goal is elusive due to the combinatorial complexity of these minimization problems. Consequently, the important question arises: How good is a minimizer computed relative to the *unknown* global optimum? Can a certain quality of solutions in terms of its suboptimality be guaranteed in *each* application? To the best of our knowledge, none of the approaches above (apart from simulated annealing) seems to be immune against getting trapped in some local minimum and hence does not meet these criteria.

A further problem relates to the *algorithmic properties* of these approaches. Apart from simple greedy strategies [2, 3], most approaches involve some (sometimes hidden) parameters on which the computed local minimum critically depends. A typical example is given by the artificial temperature parameter in deterministic annealing approaches and the corresponding iterative annealing schedule. It is well known [13] that such approaches exhibit complex bifurcation phenomena, the transitions of which (that is, which branch to follow) cannot be controlled by the user. Furthermore, these approaches involve highly nonlinear numerical fixed-point iterations which tend to oscillate in a parallel (synchronous) update mode (see [10, p. 906] and [15]).

These problems can be avoided by going back to the mathematically well-understood class of *convex* optimization problems. Under mild assumptions there exists a global optimum which, in turn, leads to a suboptimal solution of the original problem, along with clear algorithms to compute it. Abstracting from the computational process, we can simply think of a mapping taking the data to this solution. Thus, evidently, no hidden parameter is involved. Concerning global energy-minimization problems in computer vision, this has been exploited for *continuous*-valued functions in [16, 17], for example, to approximate the classical Mumford-Shah functional [18] for image segmentation.

In this paper, however, we focus on more difficult problems by extending this line of research to prototypical energy-minimization problems involving *discrete* decision variables. Our work is based on the seminal paper by Lovász and Schrijver [19] who showed how tight problem relaxations can be obtained by lifting the problem up into some higher-dimensional space and down-projecting to a convex set containing feasible solutions in that space. This idea has been put forward and lead to a remarkable result by Goemans and Williamson [20], who were able to show for a classical combinatorial problem that suboptimal solutions (for the special problem considered) cannot be worse than 14% relative to the unknown global optimum. These two facts – bounds on the suboptimality, and algorithm design based on convex optimization – have motivated our work.

Organisation of the paper. We consider in Section 2 two representatives of the class of quadratic functionals in binary variables. This class of minimization problems is well-known in the context of image labeling, perceptual grouping, MRF-modeling, etc. We derive a problem relaxation leading to a convex optimization problem in Section 3. The corresponding convex programming techniques are sketched in Section 4. In Section 5, we illustrate the properties of our approach by describing ground-truth experiments conducted with one-dimensional signals, for which the global optimum can be easily computed with dynamic programming. Real-world examples are discussed in Section 6, and we conclude our paper by indicating further work in Section 7.

Notation. For a vector $y \in \mathbb{R}^n$, $D(y)$ denotes the diagonal matrix with entries $y_1, \ldots, y_n$. e denotes the vector of one's, $e_i = 1, \forall i$, and $I = D(e)$ the unit matrix. For a matrix X, $D(X)$ denotes the diagonal matrix with the diagonal elements $x_{ii}, \forall i$, of X. $\mathcal{S}^n$ denotes the space of symmetric $n \times n$-matrices $X^t = X$, and $\mathcal{S}^n_+$ denotes the matrices $X \in \mathcal{S}^n$ which are positive semidefinite. For abbreviation, we will also use the symbol $\mathcal{K} = \mathcal{S}^{n+1}_+$. For two matrices $X, Y \in \mathcal{S}^n$, $X \bullet Y = \mathrm{trace}(XY)$ denotes the standard matrix inner product.

2   Problem Statement: Minimizing Binary Quadratic Functionals

In this paper, we consider the problem to minimize functionals of the general form:

$$J(x) = x^t Q x + 2b^t x + const , \quad x \in \{-1, 1\}^n, \ Q \in \mathcal{S}^n, \ b \in \mathbb{R}^n . \qquad (1)$$

In the field of computer vision, such global optimization problems arise in various contexts. In the following sections, we give two examples related to image labeling and perceptual grouping, respectively.

Note that apart from symmetry, no further constraints are imposed on the matrix Q in (1). Hence, the functional J need not to be convex in general. This property along with the integer constraint $x_i \in \{-1, 1\}$, $i = 1, \ldots, n$, makes the minimization problem (1) intrinsically difficult.

In Section 3 we will relax some of these hard constraints so as to arrive at a convex optimization problem which closely approximates the original one.

2.1   Example 1: Binary Image Restoration and Labeling

Consider some scalar-valued feature (grey-value, color feature, texture measure, etc.) $g : \Omega \to \mathbb{R}$ which has been locally computed within the image plane. Suppose that for each pixel position i, feature g is known to originate from either of two prototypical values u_1, u_2. In practice, of course, g is real-valued due to measurement errors and noise. Figure 1 shows an example.

To restore a discrete-valued image function x from the measurements g, we wish to compute x as minimizer of a functional which has the form (1):

$$J(x) = \frac{1}{4} \sum_i \left((u_2 - u_1)x_i + u_1 + u_2 - 2g_i \right)^2 + \frac{\lambda}{2} \sum_{\langle i,j \rangle} (x_i - x_j)^2, \ x_i \in \{-1, 1\}, \ \forall i .$$

$$(2)$$

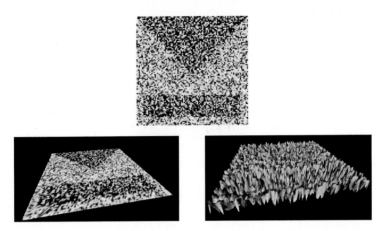

Fig. 1. Top: A binary image, heavily corrupted by (real-valued) noise. **Bottom, left:** The original data textured on a plane. **Bottom, right:** The data as 3D-plot to illustrate the poor signal-to-noise ratio.

Here, the second term sums over all pairwise adjacent variables on the regular image grid.

Functional (2) comprises two terms familiar from many regularization approaches [21]: A data-fitting term and a smoothness term modeling spatial context. However, due to the integer constraint $x_i \in \{-1, 1\}$, the optimization problem considered here is much more difficult than standard regularization problems.

We note further that, depending on the application considered, it might be useful to modify the terms in (2), either to model properties of the imaging device (data-fitting term) or to take into consideration *a priori* known spatial regularities (smoothness term; see, e.g., [22]). These modifications, however, would not increase the difficulty of problem (2) from an optimization point-of-view.

2.2 Example 2: Figure-Ground Discrimination and Perceptual Grouping

Let $g_i, i = 1, \ldots, n$, denote some feature primitive irregularly distributed over the image plane. Suppose that for each pair of primitives g_i, g_j, we can compute some (dis)similarity measure d_{ij} corresponding to some of the well-known "Gestalt laws", or to some specific object properties learned from examples. For instance, g_i might denote an edge-element computed at location i in the image plane, and d_{ij} might denote some measure corresponding to smooth continuation, co-circularity, etc. For an overview over various features and strategies for perceptual grouping we refer to [23].

According to the spatial context modeled by d_{ij}, we wish to separate familiar configurations from the (unknown) background. To this end, following [10], we label each primitive g_i with a decision variable $x_i \in \{-1, 1\}$ ("1" corresponding

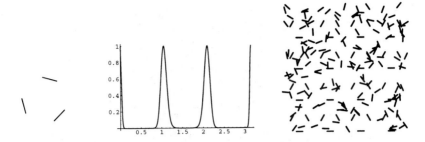

Fig. 2. Left: An "object". **Middle:** The similarity measure for $\Delta\phi_{ij} \in [0, \pi), \beta = 20$, according to the expected relative angles, and allowing for some inaccuracies of a (fictive) preprocessing stage. **Right:** The object was rotated by a fixed arbitrary angle, and translated and scaled copies have been superimposed by noise. Where are these objects?

to figure, "-1" corresponding to background and noise) and wish to minimize a functional of the form (1):

$$J(x) = \sum_{\langle i,j \rangle} (\lambda - d_{ij})x_i x_j + 2 \sum_i (\lambda n - \sum_j d_{ij})x_i, \; x_i \in \{-1, 1\}, \; \forall i . \quad (3)$$

Figure 2 shows a test-problem we use in this paper for illustration. On the left, some "object" is shown which distinguishes itself from background and clutter by the relative angles of edgels. Such edgels typically arise as output of some local edge detector. Accordingly, the difference between the relative angles $\Delta\phi_{ij}$ and the expected ones (due to our knowledge about the object) were chosen as similarity measure d_{ij} with respect to primitives i and j. In addition, we take into consideration inaccuracies of a (fictive) preprocessing stage by virtue of a parameter β (see Figure 2):

$$d_{ij} = \exp(-\beta \prod_k (\Delta\phi_{ij} - \Delta\phi_{k,\text{expected}})^2) .$$

Clearly, this measure is invariant against translation, rotation and scaling of the object. On the right in Figure 2, an unknown number of translated and scaled copies of the object, which has been rotated in advance by an unknown angle, is shown together with a lot of noisy primitives as "background". Trying to find these objects leads to combinatorial search. By contrast, we are interested in suboptimal minimizers of the functional (3) computed by convex programming.

3   Convex Problem Relaxation

Recall that both problems (2) and (3) (and many others) are special cases of problem (1).

In order to relax problem (1), we first drop the constant and homogenize the objective function as follows:

$$x^t Q x + 2 b^t x = \begin{pmatrix} x \\ 1 \end{pmatrix}^t L \begin{pmatrix} x \\ 1 \end{pmatrix}, \quad L = \begin{pmatrix} Q & b \\ b^t & 0 \end{pmatrix}. \tag{4}$$

With slight abuse of notation, we denote the vector $(x \; 1)^t$ again by x.

Next we introduce the Lagrangian with respect to problem (1):

$$x^t L x - \sum_i y_i (x_i^2 - 1) = x^t (L - D(y)) x + e^t y$$

and the corresponding minimax-problem:

$$\sup_y \inf_x x^t (L - D(y)) x + e^t y .$$

Since x is unconstrained now, the inner minimization is finite-valued only if $L - D(y) \in \mathcal{S}_+^{n+1} = \mathcal{K}$ (for notation, see section 1). Hence we arrive at the relaxed problem:

$$\sup_y e^t y , \quad L - D(y) \in \mathcal{K} . \tag{5}$$

The important point here is that problem (5) is a *convex* optimization problem! The set $\mathcal{K}$ is a cone (i.e. a special convex set) and self-dual, that is it coincides with the dual cone [24]

$$\mathcal{K}^* = \{ Y : X \bullet Y \geq 0, \; X \in \mathcal{K} \} .$$

To obtain the connection to our original problem, we derive the dual problem associated with (5). Choosing a Lagrangian multiplier $X \in \mathcal{K}^* = \mathcal{K}$, similar reasoning as above yields:

$$\sup_y e^t y = \sup_y \inf_{X \in \mathcal{K}} e^t y + X \bullet (L - D(y))$$

$$\leq \inf_{X \in \mathcal{K}} \sup_y e^t y + X \bullet (L - D(y))$$

$$= \inf_{X \in \mathcal{K}} \sup_y L \bullet X - D(y) \bullet (X - I) .$$

The inner maximization of the last equation is finite iff $D(X) = I$. Hence, we obtain as the problem dual to (5):

$$\inf_{X \in \mathcal{K}} L \bullet X , \quad D(X) = I . \tag{6}$$

which again is convex.

In order to compare the relaxation (6) with the problems (1) and (4), respectively, we rewrite the latter as follows:

$$\inf_{x \in \{-1,1\}^{n+1}} x^t L x = \inf_{x \in \{-1,1\}^{n+1}} L \bullet x x^t .$$

Note that the matrix $xx^t \in \mathcal{K}$ and has rank one. A comparison with the relaxed problem (6) shows that (i) xx^t is replaced by an arbitrary matrix $X \in \mathcal{K}$ (i.e. the rank one condition is dropped), and (ii) that the integer constraint $x_i \in \{-1, 1\}$ is *weakly* imposed by the constraint $D(X) = I$ in (6).

In the following sections, we will examine the relaxed problem (6) with respect to the criteria discussed in Section 1.

4   Algorithm

The primal–dual pair of optimization problems (6) and (5), respectively, belongs to the class of conic programs. The elegant duality theory corresponding to this class of convex optimization problems can be found in [24]. For "well-behaved" instances of this problem class, optimal primal and dual solutions X^*, y^*, S^* exist (S denotes a matrix of slack variables) and are complementary to each other: $X^* \bullet S^* = 0$. Moreover, no duality gap exists between the optimal values of the corresponding objective functions:

$$L \bullet X^* - e^t y^* = S^* \bullet X^* = 0 .$$

To compute X^*, y^* and S^*, a wide range of iterative interior-point algorithms can be used. Typically, a sequence of minimizers X_η, y_η, S_η, parametrized by a parameter η, is computed until the duality gap falls below some threshold ϵ. A remarkable result in [24] asserts that for the family of self-concordant barrier functions, this can always be done in polynomial time, depending on the number of variables n and the value of ϵ.

For our experiments described in the following two sections, we chose the so-called dual-scaling algorithm using public software from a corresponding website [25]. To get back the solution x to (1) from the solution X to (6), we used the randomized-hyperplane technique described in [20].

A more detailed description of the algorithm, along with useful modifications according to the problem class considered, is beyond the scope of this paper and will be reported elsewhere.

5   Performance: Ground-Truth Numerical Experiments

In this section, we investigate the performance of the relaxed problem (6) experimentally. To this end, we report the statistical results for three different ground-truth experiments using one-dimensional random signals.

We chose one-dimensional signals in this section because ground truth (the global optimum) can be easily computed using dynamic programming. Numerical results concerning two-dimensional signals (images) and grouping experiments are reported in section 6.

In what follows, we denote with x^* the global minimizer of (1), and with x the suboptimal solution reconstructed from the solution X to the convex programming problem (5),(6).

5.1   Ground-Truth Experiments: Partitioning of Random Signals

For the first series of experiments, we generated 1000 random signals, each with 256 pixel values equally distributed in the range $[-1, 1]$. Figure 4, top, shows an example.

To investigate the performance of the relaxed problem we compare the global optimum with the results from the relaxed problem. The optimal objective function is bounded as follows:

$$\inf_{X \in \mathcal{K}, D(X)=I} L \bullet X \leq J(x^*) \leq J(x) . \tag{7}$$

The left inequality holds true due to the relaxation of problem (1), as described in Section 3. The right inequality is obvious because x^* is the global minimizer.

To evaluate this relationship numerically, we used the following quantities:

$\overline{J^*}$: the sample mean of the global optimum $J^* = J(x^*)$ of the functional (2) (computed with dynamic programming),

$\overline{\Delta J}$: the sample mean of the gap $\Delta J = J - J^*$ (measured in % of the optimum) with respect to the objective function values of the suboptimal solution $J(x)$ and the optimal solution J^*, and

$\sigma_{\Delta J}$: the sample standard deviation of the gap ΔJ.

The resulting values of these quantities are shown in Figure 3, for different values of the global parameter λ (1000 random signals were generated for *each* value of λ). Figure 3 shows that for reasonable values of λ, the gap $\overline{\Delta J}$ is about 5% of the optimal value of the objective function.

Taking into consideration that these suboptimal solutions can be computed by solving a mathematically much simpler convex optimization problem, the quality of these solutions is surprisingly good!

The purely random signals considered in this section exhibit another property: There are many solutions having similar values of the objective function which however differ considerably with respect to the Hamming distance. Figure 4 illustrates this fact for an arbitrary random signal and a solution pair x, x^* leading to a gap of $\Delta J = 6.4\%$, but differing at 58 pixel-positions ($=22.7\%$).

On the other hand, no spatial context can be exploited for pure random signals. Accordingly, there is no meaningful parameter value of λ which could give a more accurate solution. Therefore, this negative effect should not be taken too serious because it disappears as soon as the input signal exhibits more structure, as is the case for real signals. This will be confirmed in the following sections.

5.2   Ground-Truth Experiments:
Restoration of Noisy Signals Comprising Multiple Scales

In our second series of experiments, we took the synthetic signal x' depicted in Figure 5 which involves transitions at multiple spatial scales, and superimposed Gaussian white noise with standard deviation $\sigma = 1.0$. Figure 7, top, shows an

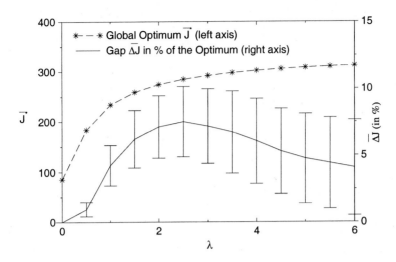

Fig. 3. Sample mean of the optimal value of the objective function $\overline{J^*}$, sample mean of the corresponding gap $\overline{\Delta J}$ with respect to the suboptimal solution, and corresponding standard deviation $\sigma_{\Delta J}$. On the average, the quality of the suboptimal solution is around 5%.

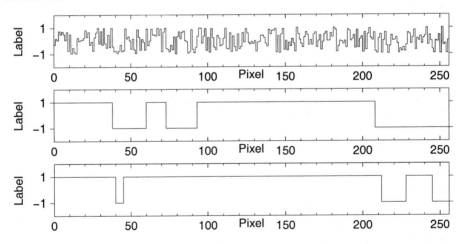

Fig. 4. Top: A purely random input signal. **Middle:** The optimal solution x^*. **Bottom:** The suboptimal solution x. Although the gap $\Delta J = 6.4\%$ only, the Hamming distance between these two solutions is not small. This effect is due to missing structure of the input signal (see text).

example. The goal was to restore the synthetic signal from the noisy input signals. For each value of λ, we repeated this experiment 1000 times using different noise signals.

In addition to the measures introduced in the last section, we computed the following quantities:

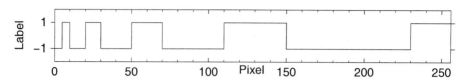

Fig. 5. Signal x' comprising multiple spatial scales.

$\overline{\Delta J'}$: the sample mean of the gap $\Delta J' = |J-J'|$ (measured in % of the optimum) with respect to the objective function values of the suboptimal solution $J(x)$ and the synthetic signal $J' = J(x')$,

$\sigma_{\Delta J'}$: the sample standard deviation of the gap $\Delta J'$.

The statistics of our numerical results are shown in Figure 6. Two observations can be made: First, for values of the scale-parameter $\lambda > 1.5$, the restoration is quite accurate: $\overline{\Delta J'} < 3\%$. Secondly, the fact $\overline{\Delta J} < \overline{\Delta J'}$ indicates that more appropriate criteria should exist for the restoration of signals that are structured like x' (see Fig. 5). The derivation of such functionals is not the objective of this paper. However, we point out that such learning problems can probably be solved within the general class (1). In that case, our optimization framework could be applied, too.

In order not to overload Figure 6, we did not include the measures $\sigma_{\Delta J'}$ and $\sigma_{\Delta J}$. The average values are $\sigma_{\Delta J'} = 3.16\%$ and $\sigma_{\Delta J} = 0.80\%$. These values are significantly smaller than those of the previous experiment, and thus they confirm the statements made at the end of the last section.

5.3 Ground-Truth Experiment: Real 1D-Signal

Before turning to two-dimensional signals in the next section, it is quite illustrative to look at numerical results for a real one-dimensional signal, namely a column of the noisy image depicted in Figure 1. In Figure 8, top, the noisy column of this image is shown.

The following two plots in Figure 1 show the global minimizer x^* computed with dynamic programming, and the suboptimal solution x computed with convex programming, respectively, for an appropriate value of the scale-parameter $\lambda = 2$.

This result demonstrates once more the "tightness" of the convex approximation of the combinatorial optimization problem (1).

6   Numerical Experiments: 2D-Images and Grouping

In the previous section, we showed the performance of the algorithm in the context of one-dimensional signals. We will next discuss the results of applying the algorithm to two-dimensional images. Computing the global optimum for real 2D-signals (images) is no longer possible. To demonstrate the wide range of

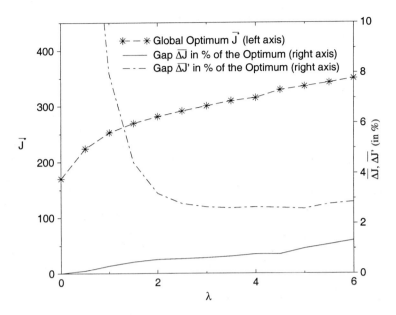

Fig. 6. Average gaps $\overline{\Delta J}$ and $\overline{\Delta J'}$ for noisy versions ($\sigma = 1$) of the signal x' shown in Fig. 5, and for different values of the scale parameter λ. According to the dominating spatial scales in signal x', for $\lambda > 1.5$ the quality of the restoration is remarkably good (below 4%).

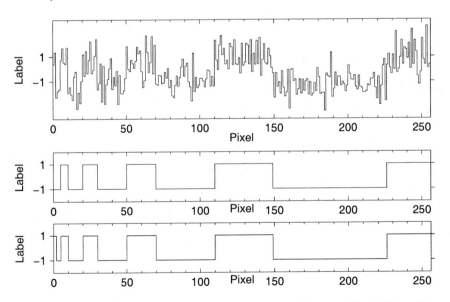

Fig. 7. A representative example illustrating the statistics shown in Fig. 6. **Top:** Noisy input signal. **Middle:** Optimal Solution x^*. **Bottom:** Suboptimal solution x.

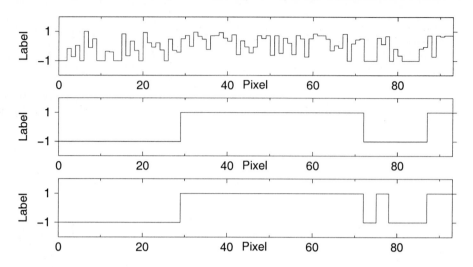

Fig. 8. Top: Column 28 of the very noisy image shown in Fig. 1. **Middle:** Optimal solution x^* computed by dynamic programming. **Bottom:** Suboptimal solution x computed by convex programming.

problems that can in principle be tackled by the general approach (1), we also include results with respect to a grouping problem (see Figure 2).

The results concerning the restoration of the real image shown in Figure 1 are shown in Figure 9. Taking into consideration the quite poor signal-to-noise ratio, the quality of the restoration is encouraging.

Figure 10 shows the same experiment with respect to another image. Note that the desired object to be restored comprises structures at both large and small spatial scales. Again the restoration result using convex programming is surprisingly good.

Next, Figure 11 shows the well known checkerboard experiment. As can be expected, small errors only occur at corners, that is at local structures with a very small spatial structure close to noise.

Finally, the results of the grouping problem (see section 2.2) are depicted in Figure 12. The suboptimal solution computed by convex programming clearly separates structure from background, apart from a small number of edgels. The presence of these extra edgels however is not caused by our optimization approach but is consistent with the chosen similarity measure which fails to label them as dissimilar.

7   Conclusion and Further Work

In this paper, we introduced a novel optimization technique to the field of image processing and computer vision. This technique applies to various energy minimization problems of mid-level vision, the objective function of which typically belongs to the large class of binary quadratic functionals.

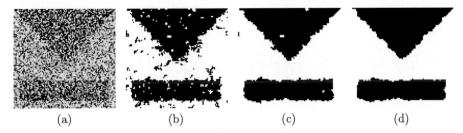

Fig. 9. Arrow and bar real image. **(a)** Noisy original. **(b)**, **(c)**, **(d)**: Suboptimal solutions computed by convex programming for $\lambda = 0.8, 1.5, 3.0$.

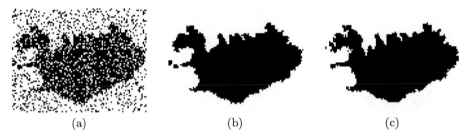

Fig. 10. Iceland image. **(a)** Binary noisy original. **(b)** Suboptimal solution computed by convex programming with $\lambda = 2.0$. **(c)** Original before adding noise.

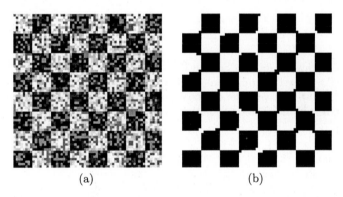

Fig. 11. Checkerboard image. **(a)** Noisy original. **(b)** Suboptimal solution computed by convex programming with $\lambda = 1.5$.

The most important property which distinguishes our approach from related work is its mathematical simplicity: Suboptimal solutions can be computed by just solving a *convex* optimization problem. As a consequence, no additional tuning parameters related to search heuristics, etc. are needed, apart from the parameters of the original model itself, of course.

For two representative functionals related to image labeling and grouping, extensive numerical experiments revealed a surprising quality of suboptimal solutions with an error below 5% on the average. Due to this fact as well as the

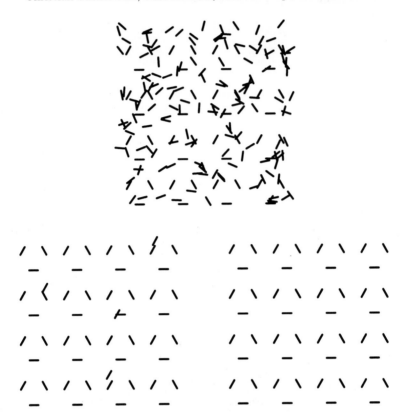

Fig. 12. Top: Input data (see Section 2.2). **Bottom, left:** The suboptimal solution computed with convex optimization ($\lambda = 0.9$). Four false primitives are included which – according to the relative angle measure – cannot be distinguished from object primitives. **Bottom, right:** The true solution.

clear algorithmic properties of our approach, we consider it as an attractive candidate in the context of computational vision.

We will continue our work as follows: First, we will try to prove bounds with respect to the suboptimality of solutions (see Eqn. (7)). Furthermore, we will focus on the algorithmic properties in order to exploit sparsity of specific problems. Finally, other problems in the general class (1) like matching of relational object representations, for example, will be investigated.

Acknowledgements

The authors enjoyed discussing this paper with Daniel Cremers. Programming support by Gregor Schlosser concerning the laborious experiments in Section 5 is gratefully acknowledged. Jens Keuchel has been supported by the German National Science Foundation (DFG) under the grant Sch457/3-1.

References

1. S. Geman and D. Geman. Stochastic relaxation, gibbs distributions, and the bayesian restoration of images. *IEEE Trans. Patt. Anal. Mach. Intell.*, 6(6):721–741, 1984.

2. J.E. Besag. On the analysis of dirty pictures (with discussion). *J. R. Statist. Soc. B*, 48:259–302, 1986.

3. P.B. Chou and C.M. Brown. Multimodal reconstruction and segmentation with markov random fields and hcf optimization. In *Proc. DARPA Image Underst. Workshop*, pages 214–221, Cambridge, Massachussetts, April 6-8 1988.

4. F. Heitz, P. Perez, and P. Bouthemy. Multiscale minimization of global energy functions in some visual recovery problems. *Comp. Vis. Graph. Image Proc.: IU*, 59(1):125–134, 1994.

5. C.-h. Wu and P.C. Doerschuk. Cluster expansions for the deterministic computation of bayesian estimators based on markov random fields. *IEEE Trans. Patt. Anal. Mach. Intell.*, 17(3):275–293, 1995.

6. Y. Boykov, O. Veksler, and R. Zabih. Markov random fields with efficient approximations. In *Proc. IEEE Conf. on Comp. Vision Patt. Recog. (CVPR'98)*, pages 648–655, Santa Barbara, California, 1998.

7. Y.G. Leclerc. Constructing simple stable descriptions for image partitioning. *Int. J. of Comp. Vision*, 3(1):73–102, 1989.

8. A. Blake and A. Zisserman. *Visual Reconstruction*. MIT Press, 1987.

9. D. Geiger and F. Girosi. Parallel and deterministic algorithms from mrf's: Surface reconstruction. *IEEE Trans. Patt. Anal. Mach. Intell.*, 13(5):401–412, 1991.

10. L. Herault and R. Horaud. Figure-ground discrimination: A combinatorial optimization approach. *IEEE Trans. Patt. Anal. Mach. Intell.*, 15(9):899–914, 1993.

11. S. Gold and A. Rangarajan. A graduated assignment algorithm for graph matching. *IEEE Trans. Patt. Anal. Mach. Intell.*, 18(4):377–388, 1996.

12. T. Hofmann and J. Buhmann. Pairwise data clustering by deterministic annealing. *IEEE Trans. Patt. Anal. Mach. Intell.*, 19(1):1–14, 1997.

13. M. Sato and S. Ishii. Bifurcations in mean-field-theory annealing. *Physical Review E*, 53(5):5153–5168, 1996.

14. E. Aarts and J.K. Lenstra, editors. *Local Search in Combinatorial Optimization*, Chichester, 1997. Wiley & Sons.

15. C. Peterson and B. Söderberg. Artificial neural networks. In Aarts and Lenstra [14], chapter 7.

16. C. Schnörr. Unique reconstruction of piecewise smooth images by minimizing strictly convex non-quadratic functionals. *J. of Math. Imag. Vision*, 4:189–198, 1994.

17. C. Schnörr. A study of a convex variational diffusion approach for image segmentation and feature extraction. *J. of Math. Imag. and Vision*, 8(3):271–292, 1998.

18. D. Mumford and J. Shah. Optimal approximations by piecewise smooth functions and associated variational problems. *Comm. Pure Appl. Math.*, 42:577–685, 1989.

19. L. Lovász and A. Schrijver. Cones of matrices and set–functions and 0–1 optimization. *SIAM J. Optimization*, 1(2):166–190, 1991.

20. M.X. Goemans and D.P. Williamson. Improved approximation algorithms for maximum cut and satisfiability problems using semidefinite programming. *J. ACM*, 42:1115–1145, 1995.

21. M. Bertero, T. Poggio, and V. Torre. Ill-posed problems in early vision. *Proc. IEEE*, 76:869–889, 1988.

22. G. Winkler. *Image Analysis, Random Fields and Dynamic Monte Carlo Methods*, volume 27 of *Appl. of Mathematics*. Springer-Verlag, Heidelberg, 1995.

23. S. Sarkar and K.L. Boyer. Perceptual organization in computer vision: A review and a proposal for a classificatory structure. *IEEE Tr. Systems, Man, and Cyb.*, 23(2):382–399, 1993.

24. Y. Nesterov and A. Nemirovskii. *Interior Point Polynomial Methods in Convex Programming*. SIAM, 1994.

25. S.J. Benson, Y. Ye, and X. Zhang. Mixed linear and semidefinite programming for combinatorial and quadratic optimization. *Optimiz. Methods and Software*, 11&12:515–544, 1999.

Grouping with Directed Relationships

Stella X. Yu[1,2] and Jianbo Shi[1]

[1] Robotics Institute
Carnegie Mellon University
[2] Center for the Neural Basis of Cognition
5000 Forbes Ave, Pittsburgh, PA 15213-3890
{stella.yu,jshi}@cs.cmu.edu

Abstract. Grouping is a global partitioning process that integrates local cues distributed over the entire image. We identify four types of pairwise relationships, attraction and repulsion, each of which can be symmetric or asymmetric. We represent these relationships with two directed graphs. We generalize the normalized cuts criteria to partitioning on directed graphs. Our formulation results in Rayleigh quotients on Hermitian matrices, where the real part describes undirected relationships, with positive numbers for attraction, negative numbers for repulsion, and the imaginary part describes directed relationships. Globally optimal solutions can be obtained by eigendecomposition. The eigenvectors characterize the optimal partitioning in the complex phase plane, with phase angle separation determining the partitioning of vertices and the relative phase advance indicating the ordering of partitions. We use directed repulsion relationships to encode relative depth cues and demonstrate that our method leads to simultaneous image segmentation and depth segregation.

1 Introduction

The grouping problem emerges from several practical applications including image segmentation, text analysis and data mining. In its basic form, the problem consists of extracting from a large number of data points, i.e., pixels, words and documents, the overall organization structures that can be used to summarize the data. This allows one to make sense of extremely large sets of data. In human perception, this ability to group objects and detect patterns is called perceptual organization. It has been clearly demonstrated in various perceptual modalities such as vision, audition and somatosensation [6].

To understand the grouping problem, we need to answer two basic questions: 1) what is the right criterion for grouping? 2) how to achieve the criterion computationally? At an abstract level, the criterion for grouping seems to be clear. We would like to partition the data so that elements are well related within groups but decoupled between groups. Furthermore, we prefer grouping mechanisms that provide a clear organization structure of the data. This means to extract big pictures of the data first and then refine them.

M.A.T. Figueiredo, J. Zerubia, A.K. Jain (Eds.): EMMCVPR 2001, LNCS 2134, pp. 283–297, 2001.
© Springer-Verlag Berlin Heidelberg 2001

To achieve this goal, a number of computational approaches have been proposed, such as clustering analysis through agglomerative and divisive algorithms [5], greedy region growing, relaxation labeling [13], Markov random fields (MRF) [4] and variational formulations [2, 7, 9]. While the greedy algorithms are computationally efficient, they can only achieve locally optimal solutions. Since grouping is about finding the global structures of the data, they fall short of this goal. MRF formulations, on the other hand, provide a global cost function incorporating all local clique potentials evaluated on nearby data points. These clique potentials can encode a variety of configuration constraints and probability distributions [18]. One shortcoming of these approaches is a lack of efficient computational solutions.

Recently we have seen a set of computational grouping methods using local pairwise relationships to compute global grouping structures [1, 3, 12, 11, 14–16]. These methods share a similar goal of grouping with MRF approaches, but they have efficient computational solutions. It has been demonstrated that they work successfully in the segmentation of complex natural images [8].

However, these grouping approaches are somewhat handicapped by the very representation that makes them computationally tractable. For example, in graph formulations [16, 15, 3, 11], negative correlations are avoided because negative edge weights are problematic for most graph algorithms. In addition, asymmetric relationships such as those that arise from figure-ground cues in image segmentation and web-document connections in data mining cannot be considered because of the difficulty in formulating a global criterion with efficient solutions.

In this paper, we develop a grouping method in the graph framework that incorporates pairwise negative correlation as well as asymmetric relationships. We propose a representation in which all possible pairwise relationships are characterized in two types of directed graphs, each encoding positive and negative correlations between data points. We generalize the dual grouping formulation of normalized cuts and associations to capture directed grouping constraints. We show that globally optimal solutions can be obtained by solving generalized eigenvectors of Hermitian weight matrices in the complex domain. The real and imaginary parts of Hermitian matrices encode undirected and directed relationships respectively. The phase angle separation defined by the eigenvectors in the complex plane determines the partitioning of data points, and the relative phase advance indicates the ordering of partitions.

The rest of the paper is organized as follows. Section 2 gives a brief review of segmentation with undirected graphs in the normalized cuts formulation. Section 3 expands our grouping method in detail. Section 4 illustrates our ideas and methods on synthetic data. Section 5 concludes the paper.

2   Review on Grouping on One Undirected Graph

The key principles of grouping can often be illustrated in the context of image segmentation. In graph methods for image segmentation, an image is described by an undirected weighted graph $\mathsf{G} = (\mathsf{V}, \mathsf{E}, W)$, where each pixel is a vertex in V and the likelihood of two pixels belonging to one group is described by a weight in W associated with the edge in E between two vertices. The weights are computed from a pairwise similarity function of image attributes such as intensity, color and motion profiles. Such similarity relationships are symmetric and can be considered as mutual attraction between vertices.

After an image is transcribed into a graph, image segmentation becomes a vertex partitioning problem. A good segmentation is the optimal partitioning scheme according to some partitioning energy functions, evaluating how heavily each group is internally connected (associations) and/or how weakly those between-group connections (cuts) are. We are particularly interested in the normalized associations and cuts criteria [15], for they form a duality pair such that the maximization of associations automatically leads to the minimization of cuts and vice versa.

A vertex bipartitioning $(\mathsf{V}_1, \mathsf{V}_2)$ on graph $\mathsf{G} = (\mathsf{V}, \mathsf{E})$ has $\mathsf{V} = \mathsf{V}_1 \cup \mathsf{V}_2$ and $\mathsf{V}_1 \cap \mathsf{V}_2 = \varnothing$. Given weight matrix W and two vertex sets P and Q, let $\mathcal{C}_W(P, Q)$ denote the total W connections from P to Q,

$$\mathcal{C}_W(P, Q) = \sum_{j \in P, k \in Q} W(j, k).$$

In particular, $\mathcal{C}_W(\mathsf{V}_1, \mathsf{V}_2)$ is the total weights cut by the bipartitioning, whereas $\mathcal{C}_W(\mathsf{V}_l, \mathsf{V}_l)$ is the total association among vertices in V_l, $l = 1, 2$. Let $\mathcal{D}_W(P)$ denote the total outdegree of P,

$$\mathcal{D}_W(P) = \mathcal{C}_W(P, \mathsf{V}),$$

which is the total weights connected to all vertices in a set P. Let $\mathcal{S}_W(P, Q)$ denote the connection ratio from P to Q,

$$\mathcal{S}_W(P, Q) = \frac{\mathcal{C}_W(P, Q)}{\mathcal{D}_W(P)}.$$

In particular, $\mathcal{S}_W(\mathsf{V}_l, \mathsf{V}_l)$ is called the *normalized association* of vertex set V_l as it is the association normalized by its degree of connections. Likewise, $\mathcal{S}_W(\mathsf{V}_1, \mathsf{V}_2)$ is called the *normalized cuts* between V_1 and V_2. The sum of these ratios respectively over two partitions are denoted by

$$\epsilon_a = \sum_{l=1}^{2} \mathcal{S}_W(\mathsf{V}_l, \mathsf{V}_l),$$
$$\epsilon_c = \sum_{l=1}^{2} \mathcal{S}_W(\mathsf{V}_l, \mathsf{V} \setminus \mathsf{V}_l).$$

ϵ_a and ϵ_c are called normalized associations and cuts criteria. Since $\forall l, \mathcal{S}_W(\mathsf{V}_l, \mathsf{V}_l) + \mathcal{S}_W(\mathsf{V}_l, \mathsf{V} \setminus \mathsf{V}_l) = 1$, $\epsilon_a + \epsilon_c = 2$, thus ϵ_a and ϵ_c are dual criteria: maximizing ϵ_a is equivalent to minimizing ϵ_c. We seek the optimal solution maximizing ϵ_a such that within-group associations are maximized and between-group cuts are minimized.

The above criteria can be written as Rayleigh quotients of partitioning variables. Let X_l be a membership indicator vector for group l, $l = 1, 2$, where $X_l(j)$

assumes 1 if vertex j belongs to group l and 0 otherwise. Let D_W be the diagonal degree matrix of the weight matrix W, $D_W(j,j) = \sum_k W_{jk}, \forall j$. Let $\mathbf{1}$ denote the all-one vector. Let k denote the degree ratio of V_1: $k = \frac{X_1^T D_W X_1}{\mathbf{1}^T D_W \mathbf{1}}$. We define $y = (1-k) X_1 - k X_2$. Therefore, the optimization problem becomes:

$$\max \epsilon_a = \frac{y^T W y}{y^T D_W y} + 1; \quad \min \epsilon_c = \frac{y^T (D_W - W) y}{y^T D_W y},$$
$$\text{s. t.} \quad y^T D_W \mathbf{1} = 0; \quad y_j \in \{1-k, -k\}, \forall j.$$

When the discreteness constraint is relaxed, the second largest generalized eigenvector of (W, D_W) maximizes ϵ_a subject to the zero-sum constraint $y^T D_W \mathbf{1} = 0$. For eigensystem $M_1 y = \lambda M_2 y$ of a matrix pair (M_1, M_2), let $\lambda(M_1, M_2)$ be the set of distinctive generalized eigenvalues λ and $\Upsilon(M_1, M_2, \lambda)$ be the eigenspace of y. It can be shown that $\forall \lambda \in \lambda(W, D_W), |\lambda| \leq 1$. Let λ_k denote the k-th largest eigenvalue, then $\lambda_1 = 1$ and $1 \in \Upsilon(M_1, M_2, \lambda_1)$. Thus the optimal solution is:

$$\epsilon_a(y_{opt}) = 1 + \lambda_2, \quad y_{opt} \in \Upsilon(W, D_W, \lambda_2).$$

3   Grouping on Two Directed Graphs

The above formulation addresses the grouping problem in a context where we can estimate the *similarity* between a pair of pixels. This set of relationships arises naturally in color, texture and motion segmentation. However, a richer set of pairwise relationships exists in a variety of settings. For example, relative depth cues suggest that two pixels should not belong to the same group; in fact, one of them is more likely to be figure and the other is then the ground. Compared to the similarity measures, this example encapsulates two other distinct attributes in pairwise relationships: repulsion and asymmetry. This leads to a generalization of the above grouping model in two ways. One is to have dual measures of attraction and repulsion, rather than attraction alone; the other is to have directed graph partitioning, rather than symmetric undirected graph partitioning.

3.1   Representation

We generalize the single undirected graph representation for an image to two directed graph representations $G = \{G_A, G_R\}$: $G_A = (V, E_A, A)$, $G_R = (V, E_R, R)$, encoding pairwise attraction and repulsion relationships respectively. Both A and R are *nonnegative* weight matrices. Since G_A and G_R are directed, A and R can be asymmetric. An example is given in Fig. 1.

Whereas directed repulsion can capture the asymmetry between figure and ground, directed attraction can capture the general compatibility between two pixels. For example, a reliable structure at one pixel location might have a higher affinity with a structure at another location, meaning the presence of the former is more likely to attract the latter to the same group, but not the other way around.

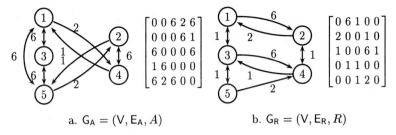

a. $\mathsf{G_A} = (\mathsf{V}, \mathsf{E_A}, A)$ b. $\mathsf{G_R} = (\mathsf{V}, \mathsf{E_R}, R)$

Fig. 1. Two directed graph representation of an image. a. Didrected graph with non-negative asymmetric weights for attraction. b. Directed graph with nonnegative asymmetric weights for repulsion.

3.2 Criteria

To generalize the criteria on nondirectional attraction to directed dual measures of attraction and repulsion, we must address three issues.

1. Attraction vs. repulsion: how do we capture the semantic difference between attraction and repulsion? For attraction A, we desire the association within groups to be as large as possible; whereas for repulsion R, we ask the segregation by between-group repulsion to be as large as possible.
2. Undirected vs. directed: how do we characterize a partitioning that favors between-group relationships in one direction but not the other? There are two aspects of this problem. The first is that we need to evaluate within-group connections regardless of the asymmetry of internal connections. This can be done by partitioning based on its undirected version so that within-group associations are maximized. The second is that we need to reflect our directional bias on between-group connections. The bias favoring weights associated with edges pointing from V_1 to V_2 is introduced by an asymmetric term that appreciate connections in $\mathcal{C}_W(\mathsf{V}_1, \mathsf{V}_2)$ but discourage those in $\mathcal{C}_W(\mathsf{V}_2, \mathsf{V}_1)$. For these two purposes, we decompose $2\,W$ into two terms:

$$2\,W = W_u + W_d, \quad W_u = (W + W^T), \quad W_d = (W - W^T).$$

W_u is an undirected version of graph $\mathsf{G_W}$, where each edge is associated with the sum of the W weights in both directions. The total degree of the connections for an asymmetric W is measured exactly by the outdegree of W_u. W_d is a skew-symmetric matrix representation of W, where each edge is associated with the weight difference of W edges pointing in opposite directions. Their links to W are formally stated below:

$$\mathcal{C}_{W_u}(P,Q) = \mathcal{C}_W(P,Q) + \mathcal{C}_W(Q,P) = \;\;\mathcal{C}_{W_u}(Q,P),$$
$$\mathcal{C}_{W_d}(P,Q) = \mathcal{C}_W(P,Q) - \mathcal{C}_W(Q,P) = -\mathcal{C}_{W_d}(Q,P).$$

This decomposition essentially turns our original graph partitioning on two directed graphs of attraction and repulsion into a simultaneous partitioning on four graphs of nondirectional attraction and repulsion, and directional attraction and repulsion.

3. Integration: how do we integrate the partitioning on such four graphs into one criterion? We couple connection ratios on these graphs through linear combinations. The connection ratios of undirected graphs of A and R are first combined by linear weighting with their total degrees of connections. The connection ratios of directed graphs are defined by the cuts normalized by the geometrical average of the degrees of two vertex sets. The total energy function is then the convex combination of two types of connection ratios for undirected and directed partitioning, with a parameter β determining their relative importance.

With directed relationships, we seek an ordered bipartitioning (V_1, V_2) such that the net directed edge flow from V_1 to V_2 is maximized. The above considerations lead to the following formulation of our criteria.

$$
\epsilon_a(A, R; \beta) = 2\beta \cdot \sum_{l=1}^{2} \frac{\mathcal{S}_{A_u}(V_l, V_l)\mathcal{D}_{A_u}(V_l) + \mathcal{S}_{R_u}(V_l, V \setminus V_l)\mathcal{D}_{R_u}(V_l)}{\mathcal{D}_{A_u}(V_l) + \mathcal{D}_{R_u}(V_l)}
$$
$$
+ 2(1 - \beta) \cdot \frac{\mathcal{C}_{A_d + R_d}(V_1, V_2) - \mathcal{C}_{A_d + R_d}(V_2, V_1)}{\sqrt{[\mathcal{D}_{A_u}(V_1) + \mathcal{D}_{R_u}(V_1)] \cdot [\mathcal{D}_{A_u}(V_2) + \mathcal{D}_{R_u}(V_2)]}},
$$
$$
\epsilon_c(A, R; \beta) = 2\beta \cdot \sum_{l=1}^{2} \frac{\mathcal{S}_{A_u}(V_l, V \setminus V_l)\mathcal{D}_{A_u}(V_l) + \mathcal{S}_{R_u}(V_l, V_l)\mathcal{D}_{R_u}(V_l)}{\mathcal{D}_{A_u}(V_l) + \mathcal{D}_{R_u}(V_l)}
$$
$$
+ 2(1 - \beta) \cdot \frac{\mathcal{C}_{A_d + R_d}(V_2, V_1) - \mathcal{C}_{A_d + R_d}(V_1, V_2)}{\sqrt{[\mathcal{D}_{A_u}(V_1) + \mathcal{D}_{R_u}(V_1)] \cdot [\mathcal{D}_{A_u}(V_2) + \mathcal{D}_{R_u}(V_2)]}}.
$$

Note that the duality between ϵ_a and ϵ_c is maintained as $\epsilon_a + \epsilon_c = 4\beta$.

For undirected graphs, $\mathcal{S}_{A_u}(V_l, V_l)$ is the old normalized association by attraction of set V_l; $\mathcal{S}_{R_u}(V_l, V \setminus V_l)$ is the *normalized dissociation by repulsion* of set V_l. They are summed up using weights from their total degrees of connections: $\mathcal{D}_{A_u}(V_l)$ and $\mathcal{D}_{R_u}(V_l)$.

For directed graphs, only the asymmetry of 'connections matters. We sum up the cross connections regardless of attraction and repulsion: $\mathcal{C}_{A_d + R_d}(V_1, V_2) - \mathcal{C}_{A_d + R_d}(V_2, V_1)$, normalized by the geometrical average of the degrees of the two involved sets. Similar to $\mathcal{S}_W(P, Q)$, this again is a unitless connection ratio.

We write the partitioning energy as functions of (A, R) to reflect the fact that for this pair of directed graphs, we favor both attractive and repulsive edge flow from V_1 to V_2. They can also be decoupled. For example, the ordered partitioning based on $\epsilon_a(A^T, R; \beta)$ favors repulsion flow from V_1 to V_2, but attraction flow from V_2 to V_1.

Finally, we sum up the two terms for undirected and directed relationships by their convex combination, with the parameter β determining their relative importance. When $\beta = 1$, the partitioning ignores the asymmetry in connection weights, while when $\beta = 0$, the partitioning only cares about the asymmetry in graph weights. When $\beta = 0.5$, both graphs are considered equally. The factor 2 is to introduced to make sure that the formula are identical to those in Section 2 for $A = A^T$ and $R = 0$, i.e., $\epsilon_a(A, 0; 0.5) + \epsilon_c(A, 0; 0.5) = 2$.

3.3 Computational Solutions

It turns out that our criteria lead to Rayleigh quotients of Hermitian matrices. Let $i = \sqrt{-1}$. Let $*$ and H denote the conjugate and conjugate transpose operators respectively. We define an equivalent degree matrix D_{eq} and equivalent Hermitian weight matrix W_{eq}, which combines symmetric weight matrix U for an equivalent undirected graph and skew-symmetric weight matrix V for an equivalent directed graph into one matrix:

$$
\begin{aligned}
D_{eq} &= D_{A_u} + D_{R_u}, & U &= 2\beta \cdot (A_u - R_u + D_{R_u}) = & U^T, \\
W_{eq} &= U + i \cdot V = W_{eq}^H, & V &= 2(1-\beta) \cdot (A_d + R_d) = & -V^T.
\end{aligned}
$$

We then have:

$$
\epsilon_a = \sum_{l=1}^{2} \frac{X_l^T U X_l}{X_l^T D_{eq} X_l} + \frac{X_1^T V X_2 - X_2^T V X_1}{\sqrt{X_1^T D_{eq} X_1 \cdot X_2^T D_{eq} X_2}}.
$$

We can see clearly what directed relationships provide in the energy terms. The first term is for undirected graph partitioning, which measures the symmetric connections within groups, while the second term is for directed graph partitioning, which measures the skew-symmetric connections between groups. Such complementary and orthogonal pairings allow us to write the criterion in a quadratic form of one matrix by using complex numbers. Let k denote degree ratio of V_1: $k = \frac{X_1^T D_{eq} X_1}{1^T D_{eq} 1}$. We define a complex vector z, the square of which becomes a real vector we used in the single graph partitioning:

$$
z = \sqrt{1-k}\, X_1 - i \cdot \sqrt{k}\, X_2, \qquad z^2 = (1-k)\, X_1 - k\, X_2.
$$

It can be verified that:

$$
\epsilon_a = 2\frac{z^H W_{eq} z}{z^H D_{eq} z}, \qquad \epsilon_c = 2\frac{z^H (2\beta D_{eq} - W_{eq}) z}{z^H D_{eq} z},
$$

subject to the zero-sum constraint of $(z^2)^T D_{eq} 1 = 0$. Ideally, a good segmentation seeks the solution of the following optimization problem,

$$
z_{opt} = \arg\max_z \frac{z^H W_{eq} z}{z^H D_{eq} z}
$$

$$
\text{s.t.} \quad (z^2)^T D_{eq} 1 = 0, \qquad \forall j, z_j \in \{\sqrt{1-k}, -i\sqrt{k}\}.
$$

The above formulations show that repulsion can be regarded as the extension of attraction measures to negative numbers, whereas directed measures complement undirected measures along an orthogonal dimension. This generalizes graph partitioning on a nonnegative symmetric weight matrix to an arbitrary Hermitian weight matrix.

We find an approximate solution by relaxing the discreteness and zero-sum constraints. W_{eq} being Hermitian guarantees that when z is relaxed to take any complex values, ϵ_a is always a real number. It can be shown that $\forall \lambda \in \lambda(W_{eq}, D_{eq})$, $|\lambda| \leq 3$, and

$$\epsilon_a(z_{opt}) = 2\lambda_1, \qquad z_{opt} \in \Upsilon(W_{eq}, D_{eq}, \lambda_1).$$

As all eigenvalues of an Hermitian matrix are real, the eigenvalues can still be ordered in sizes rather than magnitudes. Because $1 \in \Upsilon(W_{eq}, D_{eq}, \lambda_1)$ when and only when $R = 0$ and $A_d = 0$, the zero-sum constraint $z^2 W_{eq} 1 = 0$ is not, in general, automatically satisfied.

3.4   Phase Plane Embedding of an Ordered Partitioning

In order to understand how an ordered partitioning is encoded in the above model, we need to study the labeling vector z. We illustrate the ideas in the language of figure-ground segregation. If we consider R encoding relative depths with $R_d(j, k) > 0$ for j in front of k, the ordered partitioning based on $\epsilon_a(A, R; \beta)$ identifies V_1 as a group in front (figure) and V_2 as a group in the back (ground).

There are two properties of z that are relevant to partitioning: magnitudes and phases. For complex number $c = a + i b$, where a and b are both real, its magnitude is defined to be $|c| = \sqrt{a^2 + b^2}$ and its phase is defined to be the angle of point (a, b) in a 2D plane: $\angle c = \arctan \frac{b}{a}$. As $z = \sqrt{1-k} X_1 - i \sqrt{k} X_2$, where k is the degree ratio of the figure, the ideal solution assigns real number $\sqrt{1-k}$ to figure and assigns imaginary number $-i\sqrt{k}$ to ground. Therefore, the magnitudes of elements in z indicate sizes of partitions: the larger the magnitude of z_j, the smaller the connection ratio of its own group; whereas the relative phases indicate the figure-ground relationships: $\angle z_j - \angle z_k = 0°$ means that j and k are in the same group, $90°$ (phase advance) for j in front of k, $-90°$ (phase lag) for j behind k. This interpretation remains valid when z is scaled by any complex number c. Therefore, the crucial partitioning information is captured in the phase angles of z rather than the magnitudes as they can become not indicative at all when the connection ratios of two partitions are the same.

When the elements of z are squared, we get $z^2 = (1-k) X_1 - k X_2$. Two groups become antiphase $(180°)$ in z^2 labels. Though the same partitioning remains, the figure-ground information could be lost in cz for constant scaling on z. This fact is most obvious when $A_d + R_d = 0$, where both z and z^* correspond to the same partitioning energy ϵ_a. This pair of solutions suggests two possibilities: V_1 is figure or ground. In other words, the ordering of partitions is created by directed graphs. When we do not care about the direction, z^2 contains the necessary information for partitioning. Indeed, we can show that

$$\epsilon_a = \frac{z^2 W_{eq} z^2}{z^2 D_{eq} z^2} + \frac{1^T W_{eq} 1}{1^T D_{eq} 1}, \qquad \text{if } W_{eq} = 2\beta(A_u - R_u + D_{R_u}).$$

Note that W_{eq} now becomes a real symmetric matrix.

The phase-plane partitioning remains valid in the relaxed solution space. Let $W = D_{eq}^{-\frac{1}{2}} W_{eq} D_{eq}^{-\frac{1}{2}}$, the eigenvectors of which are equivalent (related by $D_{eq}^{\frac{1}{2}}$)

to those of (W_{eq}, D_{eq}). Let U and V denote the real and imaginary parts of W: $W = U + iV$, where U is symmetric and V is skew-symmetric. We consider U_{jk} (the net effect of attraction A and repulsion R) repulsion if it is negative, otherwise as attraction. For any vector z, we have:

$$z^H W z = \sum_{j,k} |z_j| \cdot |z_k| \cdot \left(U_{jk} \cos(\angle z_j - \angle z_k) + V_{jk} \sin(\angle z_j - \angle z_k) \right)$$

$$= 2 \sum_{j<k} |z_j| \cdot |z_k| \cdot |W_{jk}| \cdot \cos(\angle z_j - \angle z_k - \angle W_{jk}) + \sum_j |z_j|^2 \cdot U_{jj}.$$

We see that $z^H W z$ is maximized when $\angle z_j - \angle z_k$ matches $\angle W_{jk}$. Therefore, attraction encourages a phase difference of $0°$, whereas repulsion encourages a phase difference of $180°$, and still directed edge flow encourages a phase difference of $90°$. The optimal solution results from a trade-off between these three processes. If $V_{jk} > 0$ means that j is figural, then the optimal solution tends to have $\angle z_j > \angle z_k$ (phase advance less than $90°$) if U_{jk} is attraction, but phase advance more than $90°$ if it is repulsion. Hence, when there is pairwise repulsion, the relaxed solution in the continuous domain has no longer the ideal bimodal vertex valuation and as a result the zero-sum constraint cannot be satisfied. Nevertheless, phase advance still indicates figure-to-ground relationships.

3.5   Algorithm

The complete algorithm is summarized below. Given attraction measure A and repulsion R, we try to find an ordered partitioning (V_1, V_2) to maximize $\epsilon_a(A, R; \beta)$.

Step 1: $A_u = A + A^T$, $A_d = A - A^T$; $R_u = R + R^T$, $R_d = R - R^T$.
Step 2: $D_{eq} = D_{A_u} + D_{R_u}$.
Step 3: $W_{eq} = 2\beta \cdot (A_u - R_u + D_{R_u}) + i \cdot 2(1 - \beta) \cdot (A_d + R_d)$.
Step 4: Compute the eigenvectors of (W_{eq}, D_{eq}).
Step 5: Find a discrete solution by partitioning eigenvectors in the phase plane.

4   Results

We first illustrate our ideas and methods using the simple example in Fig. 1. The two directed graphs are decomposed into a symmetric part and a skew-symmetric part (Fig. 2).

This example has clear division of figure as $\{1, 3, 5\}$ and ground as $\{2, 4\}$ because: within-group connections are stronger for nondirectional attraction A_u; between-group connections are stronger for nondirectional repulsion R_u; there are only between-group connections pointing from figure to ground for both directional attraction A_d and directional repulsion R_d.

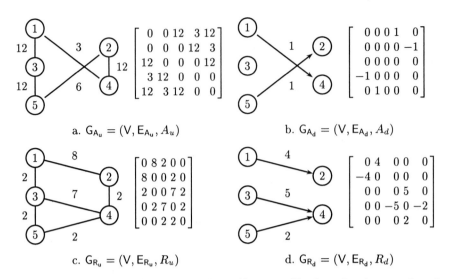

a. $G_{A_u} = (V, E_{A_u}, A_u)$

b. $G_{A_d} = (V, E_{A_d}, A_d)$

c. $G_{R_u} = (V, E_{R_u}, R_u)$

d. $G_{R_d} = (V, E_{R_d}, R_d)$

Fig. 2. Decomposition of directed graphs in Fig. 1. a. Nondirectional attraction A_u. b. Directional attraction A_d. c. Nondirectional repulsion R_u. d. Directional repulsion R_d.

The equivalent degree matrix and weight matrix for $\beta = 0.5$ are:

$$D_{eq} = \begin{bmatrix} 37 & 0 & 0 & 0 & 0 \\ 0 & 25 & 0 & 0 & 0 \\ 0 & 0 & 35 & 0 & 0 \\ 0 & 0 & 0 & 26 & 0 \\ 0 & 0 & 0 & 0 & 31 \end{bmatrix}, \quad W_{eq} = \begin{bmatrix} 10 & -8 & 10 & 3 & 12 \\ -8 & 10 & 0 & 10 & 3 \\ 10 & 0 & 11 & -7 & 10 \\ 3 & 10 & -7 & 11 & -2 \\ 12 & 3 & 10 & -2 & 4 \end{bmatrix} + i \cdot \begin{bmatrix} 0 & 4 & 0 & 1 & 0 \\ -4 & 0 & 0 & 0 & -1 \\ 0 & 0 & 0 & 5 & 0 \\ -1 & 0 & -5 & 0 & -2 \\ 0 & 1 & 0 & 2 & 0 \end{bmatrix}.$$

We expect that the first eigenvector of (W_{eq}, D_{eq}) on $\{1, 3, 5\}$ has phase advance with respect to $\{2, 4\}$. This is verified in Fig. 3.

Fig. 4a shows that how attraction and repulsion complement each other and their interaction gives a better segmentation. We use spatial proximity for attraction. Since the intensity similarity is not considered, we cannot possibly segment this image with attraction alone. Repulsion is determined by relative depths suggested by the T-junction at the center. The repulsion strength falls off exponentially along the direction perpendicular to the T-arms. We can see that repulsion pushes two regions apart at the boundary, while attraction carries this force further to the interior of each region thanks to its transitivity (Fig.4b). Real image segmentation with T-junctions can be found in [17].

Since nondirectional repulsion is a continuation of attraction measures into negative numbers, we calculate the affinity between two d−dimensional features using a Mexican hat function of their difference. It is implemented as the difference of two Gaussian functions:

$$h(X; \Sigma_1, \Sigma_2) = g(X; 0, \Sigma_1) - g(X; 0, \Sigma_2),$$
$$g(X; \mu, \Sigma) = \frac{1}{(2\pi)^{\frac{d}{2}} |\Sigma|^{\frac{1}{2}}} \exp^{-\frac{1}{2}(X-\mu)^T \Sigma^{-1}(X-\mu)},$$

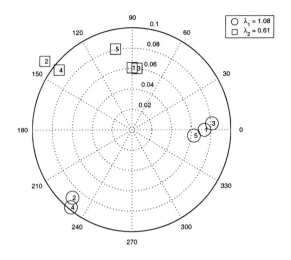

Fig. 3. Partitioning of eigenvectors in the phase-plane. Here we plot the first two eigenvectors of (W_{eq}, D_{eq}) for the example in Fig. 1. The points of the first (second) eigenvector are marked in circles (squares). Both of their phases suggest partitioning the five vertices into $\{1, 3, 5\}$ and $\{2, 4\}$ but with opposite orderings. The first chooses $\{1, 3, 5\}$ as figure for it advances $\{2, 4\}$ by about $120°$, while the second chooses it as ground for it lags $\{2, 4\}$ by about $60°$. The first scheme has a much larger partitioning energy as indicated by the eigenvalues.

where Σ's are $d \times d$ covariance matrices. The evaluation signals pairwise attraction if positive, repulsion if negative and neutral if zero. Assuming $\Sigma_2 = \gamma^2 \Sigma_1$, we can calculate two critical radii, r_0, where affinity changes from attraction to repulsion and r_-, where affinity is maximum repulsion:

$$r_0(\gamma, d) = \sqrt{\frac{2d \ln(\gamma)}{1 - \gamma^{-2}}}, \qquad r_-(\gamma, d) = \sqrt{2 + d} \cdot r_0(\gamma, d).$$

The case of $d = 1$ is illustrated in Fig. 5. With this simple change from Gaussian functions [15, 8, 11] measuring attraction to Mexican hat functions measuring both attraction and repulsion, we will show that negative weights play a very effective role in graph partitioning.

Fig. 6 shows three objects ordered in depth. We compute pairwise affinity based on proximity and intensity similarity. We see that partitioning with attraction measures finds a dominant group by picking up the object of the highest contrast; with the additional repulsion measures, all objects against a common background are grouped together. If we add in directional repulsion measures based on occlusion cues, the three objects are further segregated in depth.

Unlike attraction, repulsion is not an equivalence relationship as it is not transitive. If object 3 is in front of object 2, which is in front of object 1, object 3 is not necessarily in front of object 1. In fact, the conclusion we can draw from the phase plot in Fig. 6 is that when relative depth cues between object 3 and 1 are

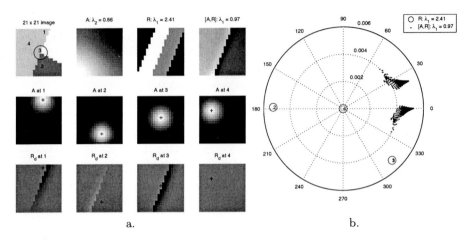

a.   b.

Fig. 4. Interaction of attraction and repulsion. a). The first row shows the image and the segmentation results with attraction A (the second eigenvector), repulsion R, both A and R (the first eigenvectors). The 2nd and 3rd rows are the attraction and repulsion fields at the four locations indicated by the markers in the image. The attraction is determined by proximity, so it is the same for all four locations. The repulsion is determined by the T-junction at the center. Most repulsion is zero, while pixels of lighter(darker) values are in front of (behind) the pixel under scrutiny. Attraction result is not indicative at all since no segmentation cues are encoded in attraction. Repulsion only makes boundaries stand out; while working with the non-informative attraction, the segmentation is carried over to the interiors of regions. b). Figure-ground segregation upon directional repulsion. Here are the phase plots of the first eigenvectors for R and A, R. The numbers in the circles correspond to those in the image shown in a). We rotate the eigenvector for A, R so that the right-lower corner of the image gets phase $0°$. Both cases give the correct direction at boundaries. However, only with A and R together, all image regions are segmented appropriately. The attraction also reduces the figure-to-ground phase advance from $135°$ to $30°$.

missing, object 1 is in front of object 3 instead. When there are multiple objects in an image, the generalized eigenvectors subsequently give multiple hypotheses about their relative depths, as shown in Fig. 7.

These examples illustrate that partitioning with directed relationships can automatically encode border ownerships [10] in the phase plane embedding.

5 Summary

In this paper, we develop a computational method for grouping based on symmetric and asymmetric relationships between pairs of data points. We formulate the problem in a graph partitioning framework using two directed graphs to encode attraction and repulsion measures. In this framework, directed graphs

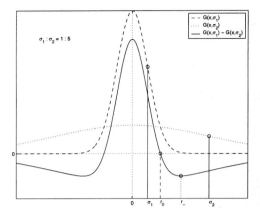

Fig. 5. Calculate pairwise affinity using Mexican hat functions based on difference of Gaussians. When two features are identical, it has maximum attraction; when feature difference is r_0, it is neutral; when feature difference is r_-, it has maximum repulsion.

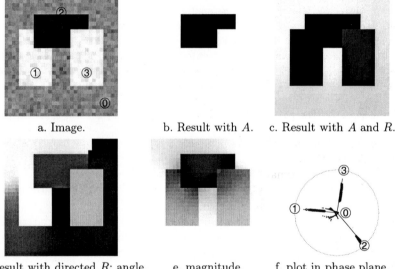

a. Image.   b. Result with A.   c. Result with A and R.

d. Result with directed R: angle,   e. magnitude,   f. plot in phase plane.

Fig. 6. The distinct roles of repulsion in grouping. a) 31×31 image. The background and three objects are marked from 0 to 3. They have average intensity values of 0.6, 0.9, 0.2 and 0.9. Gaussian noise with standard deviation of 0.03 is added to the image. Object 2 has slightly higher contrast against background than objects 1 and 3. Attraction and nondirectional repulsion are measured by Mexican hat functions of pixel distance and intensity difference with σ's of 10 and 0.1 respectively. The neighborhood radius is 3 and $\gamma = 3$. b) Segmentation result with attraction alone. c) Segmentation result with both attraction and repulsion. d), e) and f) show the result when directional repulsion based on relative depth cues at T-junctions are incorporated. With nondirectional repulsion, objects that repel a common ground are bound together in one group. With directional repulsion, objects can be further segregated in depth.

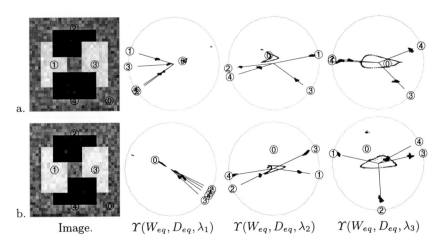

Image. $\Upsilon(W_{eq}, D_{eq}, \lambda_1)$ $\Upsilon(W_{eq}, D_{eq}, \lambda_2)$ $\Upsilon(W_{eq}, D_{eq}, \lambda_3)$

Fig. 7. Depth segregation with multiple objects. Each row shows an image and the phase plots of the first three eigenvectors obtained on cues of proximity, intensity similarity and relative depths. All four objects have the same degree of contrast against the background. The average intensity value of background is 0.5, while that of objects is either 0.2 or 0.8. The same parameters for noise and weight matrices as in Fig. 6 are used. The first row shows four objects ordered in depth layers. The second row shows four objects in a looped depth configuration. Repulsion has no transitivity, so object pair 1 and 3, 2 and 4 tend to be grouped together in the phase plane. The magnitudes indicate the reliability of phase angle estimation. The comparison of the two rows also shows the influence of local depth cues on global depth configuration.

capture the asymmetry of relationships and repulsion complements attraction in measuring dissociation.

We generalize normalized cuts and associations criteria to such a pair of directed graphs. Our formulation leads to Rayleigh quotients of Hermitian matrices, where the imaginary part encodes directed relationships, and the real part encodes undirected relationships with positive numbers for attraction and negative numbers for repulsion. The optimal solutions in the continuous domain can thus be computed by eigendecomposition, with the ordered partitioning embedded in the phases of eigenvectors: the angle separation determines the partitioning, while the relative phase advance indicates the ordering.

We illustrate our method in image segmentation. We show that surface cues and depth cues can be treated equally in one framework and thus segmentation and figure-ground segregation can be obtained in one computational step.

Acknowledgements

This research is supported by (DARPA HumanID) ONR N00014-00-1-0915 and NSF IRI-9817496. Yu has also been supported in part by NSF LIS 9720350 and NSF 9984706.

References

1. A. Amir and M. Lindenbaum. Quantitative analysis of grouping process. In *European Conference on Computer Vision*, pages 371–84, 1996.
2. A. Blake and A. Zisserman. *Visual Reconstruction*. MIT Press, Cambridge, MA, 1987.
3. Y. Gdalyahu, D. Weinshall, and M. Werman. A randomized algorithm for pairwise clustering. In *Neural Information Processing Systems*, pages 424–30, 1998.
4. S. Geman and D. Geman. Stochastic relaxation, Gibbs distributions, and the Bayesian restoration of images. *IEEE Transactions on Pattern Analysis and Machine Intelligence*, 6(6):721–41, 1984.
5. A. K. Jain and R. C. Dubes. *Algorithms for Clustering Data*. Prentice Hall, 1988.
6. K. Koffka. *Principles of Gestalt Psychology*. A Harbinger Book, Harcourt Brace & World Inc., 1935.
7. Y. G. Leclerc. Constructing simple stable descriptions for image partitioning. *International Journal of Computer Vision*, 3:73–102, 1989.
8. J. Malik, S. Belongie, T. Leung, and J. Shi. Contour and texture analysis for image segmentation. *International Journal of Computer Vision*, 2001.
9. D. Mumford and J. Shah. Boundary detection by minimizing functionals. In *IEEE Conference on Computer Vision and Pattern Recognition*, 1985.
10. K. Nakayama, Z. J. He, and S. Shimojo. *Vision. In Invitation to Cognitive Science*, chapter Visual surface representation: a critical link between lower-level and higher level vision, pages 1–70. MIT Press, 1995.
11. P. Perona and W. Freeman. A factorization approach to grouping. In *European Conference on Computer Vision*, pages 655–70, 1998.
12. J. Puzicha, T. Hofmann, and J. Buhmann. Unsupervised texture segmentation in a deterministic annealing framework. *IEEE Transactions on Pattern Analysis and Machine Intelligence*, 20(8):803–18, 1998.
13. A. Rosenfeld, R. A. Hummel, and S. W. Zucker. Scene labeling by relaxation operations. *IEEE Transactions on Systems, Man, and Cybernetics*, 6(6):173–84, 1976.
14. E. Sharon, A. Brandt, and R. Basri. Fast multiscale image segmentation. In *IEEE Conference on Computer Vision and Pattern Recognition*, pages 70–7, 2000.
15. J. Shi and J. Malik. Normalized cuts and image segmentation. In *IEEE Conference on Computer Vision and Pattern Recognition*, pages 731–7, June 1997.
16. Z. Wu and R. Leahy. An optimal graph theoretic approach to data clustering: Theory and its application to image segmentation. *IEEE Transactions on Pattern Analysis and Machine Intelligence*, 11:1101–13, 1993.
17. S. X. Yu and J. Shi. Segmentation with pairwise attraction and repulsion. In *International Conference on Computer Vision*, 2001.
18. S. C. Zhu, Y. N. Wu, and D. Mumford. Filters, random field and maximum entropy: — towards a unified theory for texture modeling. *International Journal of Computer Vision*, 27(2):1–20, 1998.

Segmentations of Spatio-Temporal Images by Spatio-Temporal Markov Random Field Model

Shunsuke Kamijo, Katsushi Ikeuchi, and Masao Sakauchi

Institute of Industrial Science, University of Tokyo.
4-6-1, Komaba Meguro-ku, Tokyo, Japan, 153-8505
{kamijo,ki,sakauchi}@iis.u-tokyo.ac.jp
http://www.sak.iis.u-tokyo.ac.jp/index.html

Abstract. There have been many successful researches on image segmentations that employ Markov Random Field model. However, most of them were interested in two-dimensional MRF, or spatial MRF, and very few researches are interested in three-dimensional MRF model. Generally, 'three-dimensional' have two meaning, that are spatially three-dimensional and spatio-temporal. In this paper, we especially are interested in segmentations of spatio-temporal images which appears to be equivalent to tracking problem of moving objects such as vehicles etc. For that purpose, by extending usual two-dimensional MRF, we defined a dedicated three-dimensional MRF which we defined as Spatio-Temporal MRF model(S-T MRF). This S-T MRF models a tracking problem by determining labels of groups of pixels by referring to their texture and labeling correlations along the temporal axis as well as the x-y image axes. Although vehicles severely occlude each other in general traffic images, segmentation boundaries of vehicle regions will be determined precisely by this S-T MRF optimizing such boundaries through spatio-temporal images. Consequently, it was proved that the algorithm has performed 95% success of tracking in middle-angle image at an intersection and 91% success in low-angle and front-view images at a highway junction.

1   Introduction

Today, one of the most important research efforts in ITS have been the development of systems that automatically monitor the traffic flows. Rather than the current practice of performing a global flow analysis, the automated monitoring systems should be based on local analysis of the behavior of each vehicle out of global flows. The systems should be able to identify each vehicle and track its behavior, and to recognize dangerous situations or events that might result from a chain of such behavior. Tracking in complicated traffics have been often impeded by the occlusion that occurs among vehicles in crowded situations.

Tracking algorithms have a long history in computer vision research. In particular, in ITS areas, vehicle tracking, one of the specialized tracking paradigms, has been extensively investigated. Peterfreund[1] employs the 'Snakes[2]' method to extract contours of vehicles for tracking purposes. Smith[3] and Grimson[4]

M.A.T. Figueiredo, J. Zerubia, A.K. Jain (Eds.): EMMCVPR 2001, LNCS 2134, pp. 298–313, 2001.

employ optical-flow analysis. In particular, Grimson apply clustering and vector quantization to estimated flows. Leuck[5] and Gardner[6] assume 3D models of vehicle shapes, and estimated vehicle images are projected onto a 2D image plane according to appearance angle. Leuck[5] and Gardner[6]'s methods require that many 3D models of vehicles be applied to general traffic images. While these methods are effective in less crowded situations, most of them cannot track vehicles reliably in situations that are complicated by occlusion and clutter.

After some considerations, we have come to the idea that tracking problem against occlusions is equivalent to segmentation of spatio-temporal images. A lot of successful research efforts that had employed Markov Random Field model have been performed by a lot of researchers in the field of Computer Vision. And those researches include image restorations, image segmentations, and image compressions. First of all, the most fundamental work had been done by Geman and Geman[9] which have become the basic research of all on MRF not only for image restorations. And then, Chellapa, Chatterjee, and Bargdzian[10] has applied MRF for image compressions. Here, we are the most interested in image segmentation by MRF models. Methods of merging small segments into large segments can be seen in works of Panjwani and G.Healey[11][12], and these are kinds of unsupervised segmentations. More works for unsupervised segmentations successfully by Manjunath and R.Chellappa[13], R.Hu and M.N.Fahmy[14], F.Cohen and Z.Fan[15], P.Andrey and P.Tarroux[16], S.Barker and P.Rayner[17], and P.Rostaing, J.N.Provost and C.Collet[18]. Although all those researches were successful, those have applied 2D-MRF model to spatial images such as static images. We will then extend 2D-MRF model to Spatio-Temporal MRF model which is able to optimize not only spatial distribution but also temporal axis distribution. An image sequence has correlations at each pixel between consecutive images along a time axis. Our S-T MRF also considers this time-axis correlation. We named the extended MRF the Spatio-Temporal Markov Random Field Model (S-T MRF model).

In order to resolve the segmentation problem of spatio-temporal images, we had developed Spatio-Temporal Markov Random Field model[21], and the algorithm have been applied successfully to traffic event analyses[20]. In this paper, primary idea of Spatio-Temporal MRF model which is define in the previous paper[21] will be briefly described in Section.3. And then, improving the primary model, fine optimizations that enables furthermore precise segmentations of vehicle regions against more severe occlusions are described in Section.4.

2   Basic Ideas of Spatio-Temporal MRF Model

2.1   Connecting Consecutive Images with Motion Vectors

Strictly speaking, S-T MRF should segment spatio-temporal images by each pixel. This means that a cubic clique of twenty-seven pixels should be considered for either labeling or intensity correlations in S-T MRF in substitute for a square clique of nine pixels which is defined in usual 2D-MRF[9].

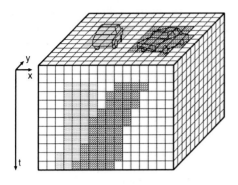

Fig. 1. Segmentation of Spatio-Temporal Images

However, this condition will work only in the case where objects move so slowly as a pixel between the consecutive images and there will be labeling and intensity correlations within such a cubic clique. Since practical moving images cannot be captured in so high frame rates, pixels consisting vehicles move typically in several-ten pixels between the consecutive image frames. Therefore, neighbor pixels within a cubic clique will never have correlations of either intensities or labeling. Consequently, we defined our S-T MRF to divide an image into blocks as a group of pixels and to optimize labeling of such blocks by connecting blocks between consecutive images referring to their motion vectors. Since this algorithm were defined so as to be applicable to gray scaled images, all the experiments has been performed by only using gray scaled images in this paper.

2.2   Initialization of Object-Map

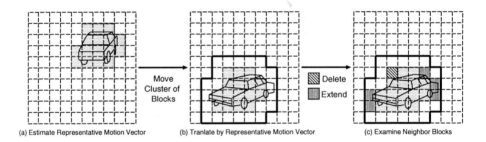

(a) Estimate Representative Motion Vector   (b) Tranlate by Representative Motion Vector   (c) Examine Neighbor Blocks

Fig. 2. Initializing an Object-Map

In preparation for this algorithm, an image which consists of 640x480 pixels is divided into 80x60 blocks where each block consists of 8x8 pixels. Then, one block is considered to be a site in the S-T MRF, and this S-T MRF classifies each block into one of vehicle regions or, equivalently, assigns one vehicle label to each block. Here, only the blocks that have different textures from the background image will be labeled as one of vehicle regions, but the blocks that have similar textures with the background image will never labeled into any vehicle regions. And, such a distribution of classified labels on blocks is referred to as an Object-Map.

Since the S-T MRF converges rapidly to a stable condition when it has a good initial estimation, we use a deductive algorithm to determine an initial label distribution[21]. In this deductive algorithm, a motion vector of each block will be estimated by simple block matching technique, and then a representative motion vector of a cluster will be determined as the most frequent motion vector among all the consisting blocks(Figure.2(a)). In determining the initial state of Object-Map all the blocks of a cluster will be translated in the next Object-Map by referring to this representative motion vector which can be approximately considered as a motion vector of each consisting block(Figure.2(b)). After the translation, if neighbor blocks of the translated blocks have a different texture from the background image, they will be labeled as the cluster. Although a cluster eventually include two or tree vehicles at first, they would be divided after a while by background images.

2.3   Optimization of Object-Map

However, when vehicles are occluding each others, some blocks in the occluded region will be labeled as both of the two vehicles. Such ambiguous labeling will be optimized by Spatio-Temporal MRF model. In the Section.3, the primary idea of this Spatio-Temporal MRF will be described in detail. Since the S-T MRF model in Section.3 approximates a motion vector of each consisting block by representative motion vector of the cluster, and since the S-T MRF model in Section.3 will optimize segmentations by referring to correlations only between the consecutive images, we call this algorithm as 'primary S-T MRF model'.

In Section.4, this primary S-T MRF model will be improved to optimize segmentations globally through spatio-temporal images in order to segment vehicle regions precisely even in the most severe occlusion situations as in low-angle and front-view images.

3   Primary Spatio-Temporal MRF model

3.1   Details of primary S-T MRF model

Some blocks may be classified as having multiple vehicle labels due to occlusion and fragmentation. We can resolve this ambiguity by employing stochastic relaxation with Spatio-Temporal Markov Random Field (MRF) model. Our Spatio-Temporal MRF estimates a current Object-map (a distribution of vehicle labels) according to a previous object map, and previous and current images. Here are the notifications:

- $G(t - 1) = g, G(t) = h$: An image G at time $t - 1$ has a value g, and G at time t has a value h. At each pixel, this condition is described as $G(t - 1; i, j) = g(i, j), G(t; i, j) = h(i, j)$.
- $X(t - 1) = x, X(t) = y$: An object Map X at time $t - 1$ is estimated to have a label distribution as x, and X at time t is estimated to have a label distribution as y. At each block, this condition is described as $X_k(t - 1) = x_k, X_k(t) = y_k$, where k is a block number.

We will determine the most likely $X(t) = y$ so as to have the MAP(Maximum A posteriori Probability) for given $G(t-1) = g, G(t) = h$ and $X(t-1) = x$, previous and current images and a previous object map, and a previous object map $X(t) = y$. A posteriori probability can be described using the Bayesian equation:

$$P(X(t) = y|G(t-1) = g, X(t-1) = x, G(t) = h) =$$
$$\frac{P(G(t-1) = g, X(t-1) = x, G(t) = h|X(t) = y)P(X(t) = y)}{P(G(t-1) = g, X(t-1) = x, G(t) = h)} \quad (1)$$

$P(G(t-1) = g, X(t-1) = x, G(t) = h)$, a probability to have previous and current images and a previous object map, can be considered as a constant. Consequently, maximizing a posteriori probability is equal to maximizing $P(G(t-1) = g, X(t-1) = x, G(t) = h|X(t) = y)P(X(t) = y)$.

$P(X(t) = y)$ is a probability for a block C_k to have $X_k(t-1) = y_k$ (for all ks). Here, y_k is a vehicle label. For each C_k, we can consider its probability as a Boltzmann distribution. Then, $P(X(t) = y)$ is a product of these Boltzmann distributions:

$$P(X(t) = y) = \prod_k exp[-U_N(N_{y_k})]/Z_{Nk} = \prod_k exp[-\frac{1}{2\sigma_{N_y}^2}(N_{y_k} - \mu_{N_y})^2]/Z_{Nk} \quad (2)$$

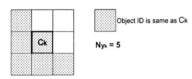

Fig. 3. 8 neighbor blocks

Here, N_{y_k} is the number of neighbor blocks of a block C_k(Figure.3) that belong to the same vehicle as C_k. Namely, the more neighbor blocks that have the same vehicle label, the more likely the block is to have the vehicle label. Currently, we consider eight neighbors as shown in Figure. 3. Thus, $\mu_{N_y} = 8$, because the probability related to block C_k has maximum value when block C_k and all its neighbors have the same vehicle label. Therefore, the energy function $U_N(N_{y_k})$ takes a minimum value at $N_y = 8$ and a maximum value at $N_y = 0$.

We also consider the probability of $G(t-1) = g, G(t) = h, X(t-1) = x$ for a given object map $X(t) = y$ as a Boltzmann function of two independent variables:

$$P(G(t-1) = g, X(t-1) = x, G(t) = h|X(t) = y)$$
$$= \prod_k exp[-U_{pre}(M_{xy_k}, D_{xy_k})]/Z_{DMk}$$
$$= \prod_k exp[-U_M(M_{xy_k})]/Z_{Mk} \cdot \prod_k exp[-U_D(D_{xy_k})]/Z_{Dk}$$
$$= \prod_k exp[-\frac{1}{2\sigma_{M_{xy}}^2}(M_{xy_k} - \mu_{M_{xy}})^2]/Z_{Mk} \cdot \prod_k exp[-\frac{1}{2\sigma_{D_{xy}}^2}(D_{xy_k} - \mu_{D_{xy}})^2]/Z_{Dk} \quad (3)$$

M_{xy_k} is a goodness measure of the previous object map $X(t-1) = x$ under a given current object map $X(t) = y$. Let us assume that a block C_k has a vehicle label O_m in the current object map $X(t)$, and C_k is shifted backward in the

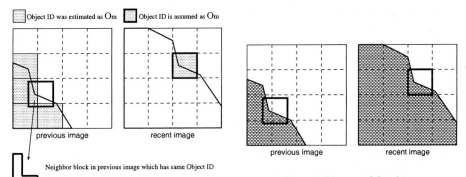

Fig. 4. Neighbor condition between Consecutive Images

Fig. 5. Texture Matching

amount of estimated motion vector, $-\overrightarrow{V_{O_m}} = (-v_{mi}, -v_{mj})$ of the vehicle O_m, in the previous image (Figure.4). Then the degree of overlapping is estimated as M_{xy_k}, the number of overlapping pixels of the blocks with the same vehicle labels. The more pixels that have the same vehicle label, the more likely a block C_k belongs to the vehicle. The maximum number is $\mu_{M_{xy}} = 64$, and the energy function $U_M(M_{xy_k})$ takes a minimum value at $M_{xy_k} = 64$ and a maximum value at $M_{xy_k} = 0$.

For example, when a block is determined to which of vehicle O_1, O_2 it belongs, $U_M(M_{xy_k})$ will be estimated as follows. First, assuming that a block belongs to O_1, the energy function is estimated as $U_M(M_{xy_k}) = U_{M1}$ by referring to $-\overrightarrow{V_{O_1}} = (-v_{1i}, -v_{1j})$. Then assuming that a block belongs to O_2, the energy function is estimated as $U_M(M_{xy_k}) = U_{M2}$ by referring to $-\overrightarrow{V_{O_2}} = (-v_{2i}, -v_{2j})$. As result of these estimations, when U_{M1} is less than U_{M2}, this block more likely belongs to vehicle O_{M1}.

D_{xy_k} represents texture correlation between $G(t-1)$ and $G(t)$. Let us suppose that C_k is shifted backward in the image $G(t-1)$ according to the estimate motion vector $-\overrightarrow{V_{O_m}} = (-v_{mi}, -v_{mj})$. The texture correlation at the block C_k is evaluated as(See Figure.5):

$$D_{xy_k} = \sum_{0 \le di < 8, 0 \le dj < 8} |G(t; i + di, j + dj) - G(t - 1; i + di - v_{mi}, j + dj - v_{mj})| \quad (4)$$

The energy function $U_D(D_{xy_k})$ takes maximum value at $D_{xy_k} = 0$. The smaller D_{xy_k} is, the more likely C_k belong to the vehicle. That is, the smaller $U_D(D_{xy_k})$ is, the more likely C_k belong to the vehicle. For example, when a block is determined to which of vehicle O_1, O_2 it belongs $U_D(D_{xy_k})$ will be estimated as follows. First, assuming that a block belongs to O_1, the energy function is estimated as $U_D(D_{xy_k})) = U_{D1}$ by referring to $\overrightarrow{V_{O_1}} = (v_{1i}, v_{1j})$. Then assuming that a block belongs to O_2, the energy function is estimated as $U_D(D_{xy_k})) = U_{D2}$ by referring to $\overrightarrow{V_{O_2}} = (v_{2i}, v_{2j})$. As result of these estimations, when U_{D1} is less than U_{D2}, this block most likely belongs to vehicle O_{D1}.

Consequently, this optimization problem results in a problem of determining a map $X(t) = y$ which minimizes the following energy function.

$$U(y_k) \equiv U_N(N_{y_k}) + U_{pre}(D_{xy_k}, M_{xy_k}) = U_N(N_{y_k}) + U_D(D_{xy_k}) + U_M(M_{xy_k})$$
$$= a(N_{y_k} - \mu_{N_y})^2 + b(M_{xy_k} - \mu_{M_{xy}})^2 + cD_{xy_k}^2 \qquad (5)$$

$U(y_k)$ is considered to be the energy function for Spatio-Temporal MRF, and $U(y_k)$ will be minimized by the relaxation process.

3.2   Experimental Results

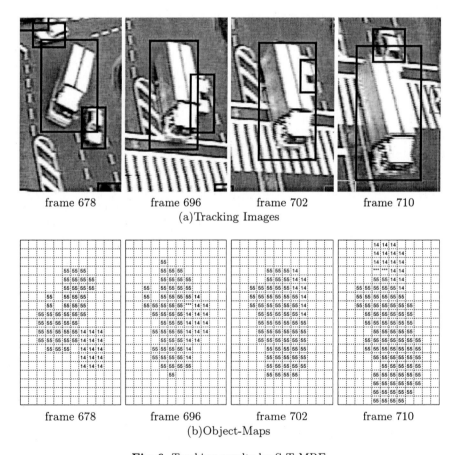

frame 678   frame 696   frame 702   frame 710

(a)Tracking Images

frame 678   frame 696   frame 702   frame 710

(b)Object-Maps

Fig. 6. Tracking results by S-T MRF

Figure.6 shows a sequence of tracking two vehicles that caused an occlusion situation. These images are obtained at the rate of 10 frames/second, and a frame number is attached to each image. Although a car is partly occluded behind a truck, the two vehicles have been successfully segmented.

We applied the tracking algorithm utilizing the Spatio-Temporal MRF model to 25 minute traffic images at the intersection. Three thousand, two hundred and fourteen vehicles traversed the intersection; of these, 541 were occluded. As a result, the method was able to track separated vehicles that did not cause occlusions at over 99% success rate, and the method was able to segment and track 541 occluded vehicles at about 95% success rate.

4 Global Optimization through Accumulated Images

Unfortunately, most of the images captured by cameras on infrastructures are low-angle images, and many of them are front-view images. Therefore, in order to construct traffic monitoring system to be of practical use for various situations, it is necessary to apply this Spatio-Temporal MRF model to those low-angle images and front-view images. However, some characteristics of such images would impede successful tracking as follows: Firstly, more severe occlusions occur in cases of low-angle images than middle-angle images which are used in Section.3. Since occlusion situations would occupy a long period in front-view images, vehicles cannot be divided until they are just under the camera. Secondly, many of vehicles that occlude one another move at almost equal motion vectors in cases of front-view images. These similarities in motion vectors would cause ambiguous boundaries among occluded vehicles.

In order to resolve these problems, it is necessary to apply global optimizations though accumulated images as well as between consecutive images. By observing the principle that tracking problems correspond to segmentation of spatio-temporal images, this improved algorithm will be also applied to middle-angle images as described in Section.3.

4.1 Applying S-T MRF Backward along Temporal Axis

In order to resolve the first problem, it will be effective to apply S-T MRF model backward along temporal axis; we call this procedure 'reversed S-T MRF'. Since the Spatio-Temporal images are symmetrically arranged along temporal axis, this reversed S-T MRF model will be able to divide each vehicle backward to the previous images. In practice, about fifty images along with their corresponding Object-maps are accumulated; the S-T MRF model is applied to such accumulated spatio-temporal images backward to the previous images with re-mapping the Object-maps.

When a cluster is split by background image, S-T MRF model is applied backward along the temporal axis. Since segments of vehicles can be divided individually backward to the previous images against occlusions by this reversed S-T MRF, we will be able to know precise behaviors of such vehicles backward along the temporal axis. Without this process, about half of vehicles will not be divided successfully in low-angle and front-view images until they arrive in just front of the camera.

4.2   Optimization of Motion Vectors

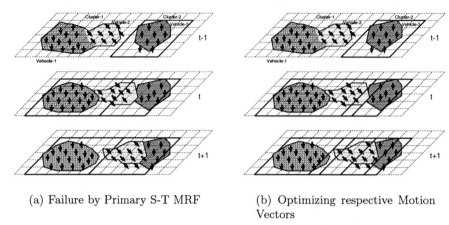

(a) Failure by Primary S-T MRF

(b) Optimizing respective Motion
Vectors

Fig. 7. Optimizations of Motion Vectors

Using the primary algorithm of S-T MRF which was defined in Section.3, blocks belonging to a cluster are re-mapped into the next Object-map by referring to a representative motion vector which was estimated for a cluster. However, when a cluster include two or tree vehicles, this re-mapping method may cause a failure in tracking. For example, as shown at the image frame $t-1$ in Figure.7(a), two vehicles were included in Cluster-1 where Vehicle-1 is occluded behind Vehicle-2, and Cluster-2 was very close to Cluster-1. V-2 then gradually occludes V-3 separating from V-1 at frame $t+1$. Finally, V-2 completely separates from V-1 at frame $t+2$. By only using the primary algorithm of S-T MRF, the algorithm may not be able to recognize that Cluster-1 has include two vehicles.

Such a failure occurs when a representative motion vector of a cluster including V-1 and V-2 is determined to be similar to a representative motion vector of V-1, but to be dissimilar to a representative motion vector of V-2. Therefore, by using only the primary S-T MRF, blocks belonging to V-2 are re-mapped by referring to a representative motion vector of a cluster which is similar to a representative motion vector of V-1. Therefore blocks included in Vehicle-2 will gradually penetrate into Cluster-2. Unfortunately, in low-angle and front-view images, such a kind of failure occurs frequently.

Therefore, we have come to the conclusion that each block should be remapped by referring not to a representative motion vector of a cluster but rather to a motion vector characteristics of each block included in the cluster(Figure.7(b)). Here, we call a group of such a motion vector characteristic of each block as respective motion vectors. By re-mapping each block referring to each respective motion vector, segment boundary of Cluster-1 would extend appropriately according to V-2 moving apart from V-1; V-1 and V-2 will then be divided by background images(Figure.7(b)).

However, since all of the blocks' motion vectors would not be expected to be estimated appropriately only by block matching because of their poor textures, failures would occur in determining appropriate boundaries among clusters. Therefore, in order to optimize such boundaries, it appears to be effective to optimize a motion vector with respect to each block respectively by referring to motion vectors of neighbor blocks. This condition can be defined as the energy function in the following equation(6).

$$P(C_{k_1}, \cdots, C_{k_n}) = \prod_{k_1,\cdots,k_n} exp[-U_{mv}(C_k)]/Z_{mv}; \quad U_{mv}(C_k) = \sum_{B_k} |\overrightarrow{V_{C_k}} - \overrightarrow{V_{B_k}}|^2 \quad (6)$$

Here, V_{C_k} and V_{B_k} represents the estimated motion vector of the block C_k and its neighbor blocks B_k respectively. Summation will be estimated over blocks B_k that have same labels as C_k(see Figure.3). This energy function(6) suggests that neighbor blocks should have similar motion vectors one another.

In this algorithm, each block is re-mapped into the next Object-Map by referring to the motion vector with respect to the block itself instead of the representative motion vector of the cluster. Consequently, in determining a label out of alternative labels, this algorithm minimizes the following energy function;

$$U(y_k(t)) + fU_{mv}(C_k(t-1)) = a(N_{y_k} - \mu_{N_y})^2 + b(M_{xy_k} - \mu_{M_{xy}})^2 + cD_{xy_k}^2$$
$$+ f \sum_{B_k} |\overrightarrow{V_{C_k(t-1)}} - \overrightarrow{V_{B_k(t-1)}}|^2/N_{x_k} \quad (7)$$

Here $U(y_k)$ is defined as function(5) at $T = t$; energy terms of $U_M(M_{xy_k})$ and $U_D(D_{xy_k})$ will be evaluated by referring to respective motion vectors of blocks belonging to the cluster. $U_{mv}(C_k(t-1))$ will be estimated by using motion vectors at $T = t-1$; $C_k(t-1)$ represents the original block of $C_k(t)$, N_{x_k} represents the number of neighbor blocks that have same label as $C_k(t-1)$.

Therefore, motion vectors of blocks at $T = t-1$ and Object-Map at $T = t$ will be optimized simultaneously by considering both similarities in motion vectors among neighbor blocks and in texture correlations between consecutive images.

4.3 Merging Fragmental Segments

In spite of the optimization process in previous subsection, boundaries are sometimes still ambiguous due to similarities in motion vectors and poor textures of the blocks that belong to different vehicles. Such ambiguous boundaries would cause immoderate segmentations of a single vehicle.

For example, consider the case that Vehicle-1 comes close to occlude Vehicle-2, and then the boundary of the vehicles became ambiguous where a segment of Vehicle-1 includes a part of blocks which really belong to Vehicle-2. When Vehicle-1 move apart from Vehicle-2, the segment of Vehicle-1 will be divided into two segments by background images(Figure.8(a)). Although there appears a fragmental segment on Vehicle-2, the segment should be really included into the segment of Vehicle-2. On the other hand, there is a case that such segmentations are correct(Figure.8(b)). That is the case where a cluster including Vehicle-1 and Vehicle-3 came to occlude Vehicle-2, and then Vehicle-1 move apart from

Vehicle-3. In this case, there should be really three segments. Therefore, such immoderate segmentations as in Figure.8(a) could not be found a priori.

Consequently, after the immoderate segmentations by reversed S-T MRF, appropriate segment boundaries should be determined a posteriori by a segment merging process. In order to quantitatively examine whether Vehicle-2 and Vehicle-3 are likely to be merged into a single cluster, we define the following functions:

$$P = exp[-(U_{connect} + U_{mv})] \tag{8}$$

$$U_{connect} = -\alpha N_{connect} + \beta N_{no_{connect}} \tag{9}$$

$$U_{mv} = \gamma \sum_{connected} [\{(v_{xm} - v_{x2})^2 + (v_{ym} - v_{y2})^2\}$$
$$+ \{(v_{xm} - v_{x3})^2 + (v_{ym} - v_{y3})^2\}] \tag{10}$$

Here, $N_{connect}$ means number of frames that segments of Vehicle-2 and Vehicle-3 are connected via blocks differ from a background image. And $N_{no_{connect}}$ means number of frames that segments of Vehicle-2 and Vehicle-3 are not connected as described in frame k in Figure.8(b). (v_{x2}, v_{y2}) and (v_{x3}, v_{y3}) represents motion vectors of Vehicle-2 and Vehicle-3, respectively, and (v_{xm}, v_{ym}) represents motion vectors of a cluster which is a merged segment of Vehicle-2 and Vehicle-3. And summation is estimated only for connected frames.

By using such defined P, likelihood of merging segments of Vehicle-2 and Vehicle-3 into a single segment is written as $P_{merge} = \frac{P}{1+P}$. When the total energy function $U_{connect} + U_{mv} = 0$, P becomes 1 and $\frac{P}{1+P}$ becomes 0.5. That is, when $U_{connect} + U_{mv} = 0$, likelihood and unlikelihood of merging segments are the same. And the lower total energy $U_{connect} + Umv$ becomes, the more the likelihood of merging segments increases. This likelihood function P_{merge} will be estimated between all pairs of segments, and it will then be determined with the probability P_{merge} whether they should be merged into a single segment.

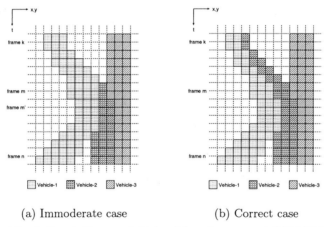

(a) Immoderate case   (b) Correct case

Fig. 8. Spatio-Temporal Object-Maps by reversed S-T MRF

4.4   Experimental Results

In order to verify effectiveness of the global optimization algorithm, we applied this algorithm to forty minute long images of a junction on the Tokyo Metropolitan Expressway. During these forty minute images, 2,381 vehicles have passed this junction. In this experiment, 54 frame images and 54 Object-Maps were accumulated. Since images are captured in a rate of 10 frames/second, 54 frames corresponds to 5.4 seconds. Typically, vehicles run from entrances to under the camera within about 5 seconds. Therefore, applying reversed S-T MRF, most of the vehicles can be tracked from entrances. Parameters were decided by trial and error as: $a = 1/2, b = 1/256, c = 32/1000000, f = 1/4, \mu_{M_{xy}} = 0$.

First of all, Table.1 shows optimization levels that employ primary S-T MRF, reversed S-T MRF, optimization of each motion vector, and segment merging. And each level employs optimization algorithms that are indicated by 'yes'. For example, Level-2 employs primary S-T MRF, reversed S-T MRF, and optimization of each motion vector; however it does not employ segment merging. Here, though only 37.8% out of 2,381 vehicles were tracked successfully by the Level-1 algorithm, the success rate was drastically improved up to 91.2% by the Level-3 algorithm.

	Level-0	Level-1	Level-2	Level-3
Primary S-T MRF	yes	yes	yes	yes
Revered S-T MRF	no	yes	yes	yes
Optimization of each motion vector	no	no	yes	yes
Segment Merging	no	no	no	yes

Table 1. Optimization Levels

Figure.9 shows successful tracking results by applying Level-2 algorithm compared to Level-1. Figure.9(a) shows a tracking result by the Level-1 algorithm which employed reversed S-T MRF and did not employed optimization of each motion vector. Here some vehicles were recognized as a single cluster as indicated by vehicle ID number of 9 and 56. Since boundaries of clusters will be ambiguous without optimization of each motion vector, motion vector of each block would be somehow different from the representative motion vector of the cluster. As a result, such blocks were mis-determined as belonging to a neighbor cluster. Therefore, evaluating Object-Maps of such blocks on ambiguous boundaries referring to their own motion vectors, would enable us to follow such blocks more correctly forward along temporal axis. Then, a cluster including two or more vehicles can be divide correctly in a certain image frame. As a result, such vehicles would be divided into different segments backward to the past frames by applying reversed S-T MRF(Figure.9(b)).

Figure.10 shows successful tracking results to exhibit effectiveness of the segment merging algorithm. Without segment merging, some fragmental segments appeared as shown in Figure.10(a). On the other hand, such fragmental segments are merged by the segment merging algorithm to be correct segments corresponding to vehicles.

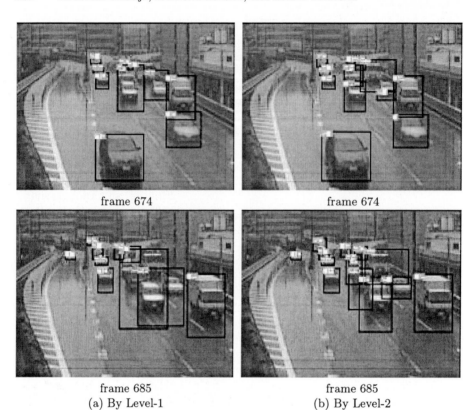

frame 674   frame 674

frame 685   frame 685
(a) By Level-1   (b) By Level-2

Fig. 9. Effects of optimization of each motion vector on Tracking results

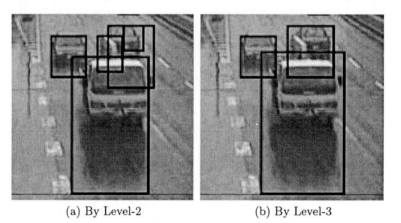

(a) By Level-2   (b) By Level-3

Fig. 10. Effects of Segment Merging on Tracking results

Figure.11 shows dependencies of success rates in tracking results on the algorithm levels. And they were examined by using both of middle-angle images of at the intersection and low-angle images at the expressway junction. In middle-angle images, since most of vehicles were able to recognized vehicle by vehicle, success rate did not decrease even by the use of the Level-1 algorithm. On the other hand in low-angle and front-view images, serious occlusions drastically decreased success rate to less than 40%.

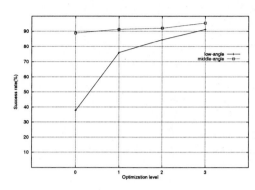

Fig. 11. Success Rates vs. Optimization Levels

Finally, Figure.12 shows dependencies of success rates in tracking results on frame rates. And they also were examined by using both of the middle-angle images and the low-angle images. So far, all of experiments were performed by using images acquired at rate of $10 frames/second$. However, as described in subsection.2.1, one of the essential ideas of the Spatio-Temporal Markov Random Field model is linking images and Object-maps between consecutive frames by motion vectors. Therefore, it is very interesting to examine how the frame rates affect success rates in tracking results. In this experiment, images were captured in the rate of $30 frames/second$. Here in Figure.12, frame rates can be described as $[30/x] frames/second$ by using numbers in x-axis. Therefore, '1' on x-axis corresponds to the rate of $30 frames/second$, and '3' corresponds to $10 frames/second$. In the experiment of Figure.12, Tracking algorithm of Level-3 was used; twenty minute images were examined for this experiment.

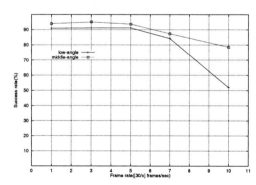

Fig. 12. Success Rates vs. Optimization Frame Rates

As shown in this figure, success rates were decreased steeply at $3 frames/second$ in both kinds of images. It seems that use of block matching algorithm to obtain motion vectors did not work well for low frame rate images as $3 frames/second$ because searching region for matching becomes too broad to find the most likely matched region. In Figure.12, the success rate for middle-angle images does not decrease so steeply as that of low-angle images. However, this should not suggest that middle-angle images are less sensitive to frame rates than low-angle images. At the intersection in middle-angle images, vehicles move more slowly than at the expressway in low-angle images because of crowded traffics, pedestrians, etc.

5   Conclusions

For many years, severe occlusions have been impeded automated analyses and monitoring of traffic images. By some considerations, we have come to a conclusion that such a tracking problem is equivalent to a segmentation problem of spatio-temporal images. For that purpose, we defined Spatio-Temporal Markov Random Field model which optimizes segmentations through spatio-temporal images by referring to texture and labeling correlations along temporal axis as well as x-y axes. In this model, motion vectors of consisting blocks are principal to connect discretized parts of a region along temporal axis into single region.

And then, traffic images at an intersection and highway junction were examined in order to evaluate reliability of this S-T MRF model. As results, 95% of vehicles were tracked successfully in middle-angle images at the intersection, and 91% of vehicles were tracked successfully in low-angle and front-view images at the highway junction. Although severe occlusions occur frequently in low-angle and front-view images, vehicle regions were segmented precisely by global optimizations of S-T MRF model.

Finally, by using such the reliable tracking algorithm, it will be possible to analyze and monitor traffic events in detail and precisely even in complicated situations such at large intersections or highway junctions.

6   Acknowledgment

We would like to express our gratitude for 'Japan Society of Traffic Engineers' who provided us images of the expressway junction.

References

1. Natan Peterfreund, "Robust Tracking of Position and Velocity With Kalman Snakes" IEEE Trans. Pattern Analysis and Machine Intelligence(PAMI), Vol.21 No.6, 1999, pp.564-569.
2. M.Kass,A.Witkin,and D.Terzopoulos, "Snakes: Active contour models" Int'l J.Computer Vision, Vol.1, 1988, pp.321-331.
3. S.M.Smith and J.M.Brady, "ASSET-2:Real-Time Motion Segmentation and Shape Tracking", IEEE Trans. Pattern Analysis and Machine Intelligence(PAMI), Vol.17 No.8, 1995, pp.814-820.
4. C. Stauffer and W.E.L. Grimson, "Adaptive background mixture models for real-time tracking", Proc. of CVPR 1999, Jun 1999, pp246-252.
5. Holger Leuck and Hans-Hellmut Nagel, "Automatic Differentiation Facilitates OF-Integration into Steering-Angle-Based Road Vehicle Tracking", Proc. of Conputer Vision and Pattern Recognition(CVPR) '99, pp.360-365.

6. Warren F.Gardner and Daryl T.Lawton "Interactive Model-Based Vehicle Tracking", IEEE Trans. PAMI, Vol.18 No.11, 1996, pp.1115-1121.
7. N.Metropolis, A.W.Rosenbluth, M.N.Rosenbluth, A.H.Teller and E.Teller, "Equations of State calculations by fast computing machines", J.Chem.Phys., Vol21, pp1087-1091, 1953.
8. S.Kirkpatrick, C.D.Gelatt and M.P.Vecci, "Optimization by Simulated Annealing", Science, 220, pp671-680, 1983.
9. S.Geman and D.Geman, "Stochastic Relaxation, Gibbs Distribution, and the Bayesian Restoration of images", IEEE trans. PAMI, Vol.6, No.6, pp721-741, 1984.
10. R.Chellappa, S.Chatterjee and R.Bargdzian, "Texture Synthesis and Compression Using Gaussian-Markov Random Field Models", IEEE trans. SMC, Vol.15, No.2, 1985.
11. D.K.Panjwani and G.Healey, "Markov random field models for unsupervised segmentation of textured color images", IEEE Trans. PAMI, vol.17, no.10, pp939-954, 1995.
12. D.K.Panjwani and G.Healey, "Selecting neighbors in random field models for color images," Proc. ICIP, vol.II, pp56-60, 1994.
13. B.S.Majunath and R.Chellappa, "Unsupervised Texture Segmentation Using Markov Random Field Models", IEEE Trans. PAMI, vol.13, no.5, pp478-482, May 1991.
14. R.Hu and M.N.Fahmy, "Texture Segmentation based on a Hierarchical Markov Random Field Model", Signal Processing, vol.26, pp.285-305, 1992.
15. F.S.Cohen and Z.Fan, "Maximum Likelihood Unsupervised Texture Image Segmentation", CVGIP: Graphical Models and Image Processing, vol.54, no.3, pp239-251, 1992.
16. P. Andrey, P. Tarroux, "Unsupervised Segmentation of Markov Radom Field Modeled Textured Images Using Selectionist Relaxation", IEEE trans. PAMI, Vol20, No.3, 1998.
17. S.A.Barker and P.J.W.Rayner, "Unsupervised Image Segmentation Using Markov Random Field Models", Proc. EMMCVPR'99(Lecture Notes in CS printed by Springer), pp179-194, May 1997.
18. P.Rostaing, J.N. Provost and C.Collet, "Unsupervised Multispectral Image Segmentation Using Generalized Gaussian Noise Model., Proc. EMMCVPR'99(Lecture Notes in CS printed by Springer), pp142-156, July 1999.
19. Rama Chellappa and Anil Jain, "Markov Random Fields : Theory and Application", Academic Press, 1993.
20. S.Kamijo, Y.Matsushita, K.Ikeuchi, M.Sakauchi, "Traffic Monitoring and Accident Detection at Intersections", IEEE trans. ITS, Vol.1 No.2, June. 2000, pp108-118.
21. S.Kamijo, Y.Matsushita, K.Ikeuchi, M.Sakauchi, "Occlusion Robust Tracking utilizing Spatio-Temporal Markov Random Field Model", International Conference on Pattern Recognition(ICPR), Barcelona, Sep. 2000, Vol.1 pp142-147.

Highlight and Shading Invariant Color Image Segmentation Using Simulated Annealing

Paul Fieguth and Slawo Wesolkowski

Systems Design Engineering
University of Waterloo
Waterloo, Ontario, Canada, N2L-3G1
{swesolko,pfieguth}@uwaterloo.ca
http://ocho.uwaterloo.ca/~pfieguth/

Abstract. Color constancy in color image segmentation is an important research issue. In this paper we develop a framework, based on the Dichromatic Reflection Model for asserting the color highlight and shading invariance, and based on a Markov Random Field approach for segmentation. A given RGB image is transformed into a R'G'B' space to remove any highlight components, and only the vector-angle component, representing color hue but not intensity, is preserved to remove shading effects. Due to the arbitrariness of vector angles for low R'G'B' values, we perform a Monte-Carlo sensitivity analysis to determine pixel-dependent weights for the MRF segmentation. Results are presented and analyzed.

1 Introduction

In recent years the problem of color constancy – the perception of objects in the real world without illumination effects – has been a major research subject in the image science and technology communities. In spite of shading and highlight effects, humans are quite able to perceive object surfaces in a scene, a difficult task for computer systems. An algorithm for color image segmentation, which is invariant to shading and highlight effects, has recently been introduced [23], developed in the context of the Dichromatic Reflection Model of Shafer [12].

In [23] the authors describe a principal component analysis and vector angle clustering-based approach for color image segmentation. In this method, the prototype vector is described as the principal vector (as opposed to principal curve) of the RGB color cluster and the calculation of the distance from this "cluster center" to a pixel in the image is done using the vector angle. The number of clusters is selected and the algorithm chooses the most optimal (in the Mean Squared Error-sense) multi-vector fit to the data [3]. The illumination invariances are well captured by this method, however there are several drawbacks:

1. For small (black) RGB values the algorithm breaks down and produces extremely noisy angles.
2. All colors must fit into a predetermined number of clusters.
3. Border areas composed of composite colors are classified arbitrarily.

M.A.T. Figueiredo, J. Zerubia, A.K. Jain (Eds.): EMMCVPR 2001, LNCS 2134, pp. 314–327, 2001.

Certainly a wide variety of color-segmentation approaches have been proposed. In particular, methods based on color clustering have seen considerable interest, including k-means [15, 21], fuzzy k-means [7], and morphology-based clustering [9]. The most notable drawback of such clustering methods is that they normally do not take any spatial relationships into account, and determine the segmentation strictly on a pixel-by-pixel basis, normally using the Euclidean distance. We will demonstrate for the problems of our interest, specifically the segmentation of images involving illumination effects, some degree of spatial dependence is *crucial* in formulating an adequate approach. The ability for Markov/Gibbs methods to model spatial dependencies will make them a very natural fit to our context.

Ad-hoc local methods have also been proposed for color image segmentation such as [5, 18, 20]. In [5], the authors present a method based on the calculation of principal components of local non-overlapping regions to estimate the region color. The method is also said to be highlight and shading invariant. [18] describes a method based on a region growing technique using the Euclidean distance as a similarity measure which is tested on images of homogenous color. [20] presents another region growing technique in which each region is defined by two values: the color gradient (calculated using the Euclidean distance) between two adjacent pixels and the maximum distance between two colors within this region. The first algorithm suffers from having to quantize the region segmentation information while the last two use the Euclidean distance. All three methods are based on various heuristics.

The focus of the present paper is to formulate a color image processing and segmentation technique in the context of the Dichromatic Reflection Model [12, 19], which is introduced in Section 2. The crucial question is how to measure the *similarity* of two colors. Most previous methods assess the relationship between two multispectral (including color) pixels based on the Euclidean distance [7, 9, 21, 22]. The Euclidean distance is often chosen for its simplicity, mathematical tractability, and is well-suited to feature spaces having an isotropic distribution (for color, a good example is the CIE *Luv* space [11]). However in the case of color images, where each pixel is represented as a RGB vector, the Euclidean distance is a particularly poor measure of color similarity because the RGB space is *an*-isotropic, especially when lighting effects such as specular reflection and shading are present in the image.

In this paper, we propose to use the Dichromatic Reflection Model to transform the RGB image into a different space in which shading and specular reflection are normalized. In this context, highlight and shading invariant color image segmentation means the finding of regions, homogenous in color, irrespective of illumination effects.

Therefore, given the Dichromatic Reflection Model, why can the transformed pixels not be clustered effectively using k-means [10] or other related techniques? The problem is that sufficiently dark shades of any color all look alike (i.e., black), and similarly specular reflections or highlights converge to the same color (the color of the illuminating light, normally white). For example, Figure 1 clearly illustrates highlights (glossy white image patches) and shading (intensity variations on the surface of each fruit, taken under white light illumination. Conse-

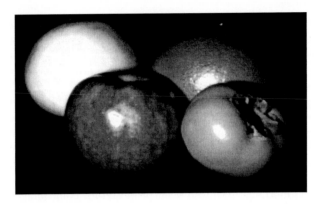

Fig. 1. Original RGB color scene image, showing highlights and shading, captured using white light.

quently, some sort of *spatial* model is *essential* in order to perform segmentation, to assign a highlight pixel to a colored group based on its surrounding context.

We propose to define the spatial context using a Gibbs/Markov approach, as outlined in Section 3. Certainly others have used Markov random fields for image segmentation [1, 6, 24]; however, normally these methods involve Gauss-Markov random fields, where the GMRF defines a spatial texture for the R, G, B components, from which segmentation can proceed as a separate hypothesis-testing procedure applied to the GMRF likelihood [8]. Our approach is quite different: we wish to find the segmented image directly as the result of energy minimization of some appropriately-defined Gibbs random field. Furthermore the regions are not distinguished on the basis of texture, rather on shading and highlight invariant color. That said, textured surfaces where the pixel variations are due to local shading effects (such as the surface of an orange) will be segmented correctly, since the normalized color is similar for all such pixels; whereas textures with intrinsically different colors (such as marble or paisley) are not the focus of our approach.

The formulation of our Gibbs model will be similar to others used for segmentation [4, 6] except for a number of variations due to the peculiarities of our transformed space. We demonstrate the advantages of constructing an energy function for Markov Random Field-driven image segmentation using a measure related to the inner vector product.

This paper first describes the Dichromatic Reflection model and a development of an optimization criterion for segmentation. Next, results on an artificial image and a real scene image are presented and analyzed. Finally, conclusions and directions for future work are given.

2   Color Theory

The Dichromatic Reflection Model [12, 19] will be used in this paper to show highlight and shading invariance properties of the new algorithm. First, the

DRM will be introduced. Next, the highlight invariance property will be briefly explained. Finally, how shading invariance is achieved will be described.

2.1   Preliminaries

The Dichromatic Reflection Model purports to separate light reflected from objects into two different types:

1. specular reflection or highlight characterized visually by a glossy appearance and describing light that is reflected in a mirror-like fashion from a surface;
2. diffuse or body reflection which is the light reflected from a surface in all directions, giving a surface its usual colored appearance.

This model has been described for a variety of materials [16]; the focus here will be on inhomogeneous dielectric materials such as plastics. The presentation of the DRM follows closely that given in [23]. First, light reflected from an object surface o (called the color signal) is described as a function $C^o(\lambda, x)$ of wavelength λ and pixel location x:

$$C^o(\lambda, x) = \text{Body Reflection} + \text{Interface Reflection} \qquad (1)$$
$$= \alpha(x)S^o(\lambda)E(\lambda) + \beta(x)E(\lambda) \qquad (2)$$

where $E(\lambda)$ is the spectral power distribution of a light source, $S^o(\lambda)$ is the spectral-surface reflectance of an object o, $\alpha(x)$ is the shading factor and $\beta(x)$ is a scalar factor for the specular reflection term. The following set of equations can then represent the sensor responses for a camera using R, G, and B coordinates:

$$\begin{bmatrix} R \\ G \\ B \end{bmatrix} = \int C^o(\lambda, x) \begin{bmatrix} R_R(\lambda) \\ R_G(\lambda) \\ R_B(\lambda) \end{bmatrix} d\lambda \qquad (3)$$

where $R_i(\lambda)$, $(i = R, G, B)$ are the spectral sensitivity functions of the camera in the visible spectrum. Substituting (2) into (3), we have

$$\begin{bmatrix} R \\ G \\ B \end{bmatrix} = \alpha(x) \int S^o(\lambda, x)E(\lambda) \begin{bmatrix} R_R(\lambda) \\ R_G(\lambda) \\ R_B(\lambda) \end{bmatrix} d\lambda + \beta(\lambda) \int E(\lambda) \begin{bmatrix} R_R(\lambda) \\ R_G(\lambda) \\ R_B(\lambda) \end{bmatrix} d\lambda \quad (4)$$
$$= \alpha(x)c_b + \beta(x)c_i \qquad (5)$$

where c_b is the body color vector and c_i is the illumination color vector. These color vectors are normalized into a unit vector length.

For the sensor outputs R, G, and B to be white balanced, it is necessary to satisfy the following condition:

$$\int E(\lambda)R_R(\lambda)d\lambda = \int E(\lambda)R_G(\lambda)d\lambda \qquad (6)$$
$$= \int E(\lambda)R_B(\lambda)d\lambda \qquad (7)$$

As long as the illuminant $E(\lambda)$ is a constant white over the visible wavelengths, and the spectral sensitivity functions $R_i(\lambda)$, $(i = R, G, B)$ have the same area, then the above condition obviously holds. However, if the illuminant is not white, a color balancing step [23] is needed where the three sensor outputs are adjusted to be equal to each other. In this paper it will be assumed that the illumination light is white or the image has been white balanced.

2.2   Highlight Invariance

To remove the effects of highlights it is necessary to transform the pixel coordinates according to the following transformation [14, 23]:

$$\begin{bmatrix} R' \\ G' \\ B' \end{bmatrix} = \begin{bmatrix} R \\ G \\ B \end{bmatrix} - AVG \tag{8}$$

where AVG represents the average value of R, G and B. In this transformation, the reflectance variation caused by interface reflection is removed by projecting the observed reflectance in an n-dimensional vector space along the illumination vector onto an $(n\text{-}1)$-dimensional subspace that is perpendicular to the illumination vector [14]. From a practical point of view, a histogram of the RGB pixels making up a homogeneously-colored region containing a highlight patch would show two connected clusters (one for the homogenous color and one for the highlight).

For example, Figure 2 shows such a distribution in the RGB space of pixels from Figure 1. The four clusters appear highly spread-out and are non-linear (do not lie along a straight line in RGB space), because each cluster is composed of both body and specular reflections.

The transformation (8) transforms each set of nonlinear clusters into a single linear cluster representing the body reflection. This is well illustrated in Figure 3, where the original nonlinear clusters now appear as linear groupings. Given that the RGB components are assumed to be white balanced, the application of (5)–(8) eliminates the interface reflection term and reduces to

$$\begin{bmatrix} R' \\ G' \\ B' \end{bmatrix} = \alpha(x) \int S^o(\lambda, x) E(\lambda) \frac{1}{3} \begin{bmatrix} 2R_R(\lambda) - R_G(\lambda) - R_B(\lambda) \\ -R_R(\lambda) + 2R_G(\lambda) - R_B(\lambda) \\ -R_R(\lambda) - R_G(\lambda) + 2R_B(\lambda) \end{bmatrix} d\lambda \tag{9}$$

$$= \alpha(x) \int S^o(\lambda, x) E(\lambda) \begin{bmatrix} R'_R(\lambda) \\ R'_G(\lambda) \\ R'_B(\lambda) \end{bmatrix} d\lambda \tag{10}$$

This formulation is dependent on the shading factor (illumination) and the body reflection (material color), which makes this color representation highlight invariant. Individual elements of the pixel vector in the new representation will be shifted according to the average of the body reflection term. This results in the new space having negative coordinates. Equivalently the spectral sensitivity functions, $R'_R(\lambda)$, $R'_G(\lambda)$, and $R'_B(\lambda)$, in the new system also have negative

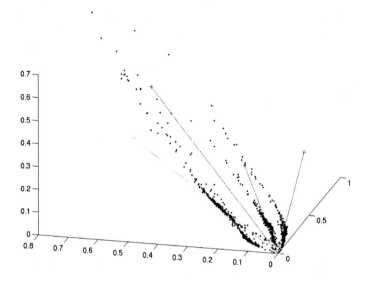

Fig. 2. Distribution of pixels in the RGB space from Figure 1. The straight lines are the principal vectors obtained with the best MSE fit from [23]. Both the red and orange fruits have been clumped into one larger cluster. Whereas three of the four clusters depicted in the image correspond to fruit colors, the fourth represents all of the highlight areas.

values. Three properties were derived from this representation. The first property says that all RGB colors fall into one of six quadrants. The second one says that all gray values (including saturated highlight areas) naturally collapse to the $(0,0,0)$ point. Finally, the third property demonstrates that the same color can only exist in quadrants that have at least one adjacent edge.

2.3   Shading Invariance

Insuring a shading invariance property of the algorithm means that the shading factor shown first in (2) needs to be eliminated from the representation obtained using (10). The simplest way to do this is to normalize the new color vectors to unit length [14]. First, reformulate (10) as

$$c' = \begin{bmatrix} R' \\ G' \\ B' \end{bmatrix} = \alpha(x) \int S^o(\lambda, x) E(\lambda) \begin{bmatrix} R'_R(\lambda) \\ R'_G(\lambda) \\ R'_B(\lambda) \end{bmatrix} d\lambda = \alpha(x) \begin{bmatrix} c^o_R \\ c^o_G \\ c^o_B \end{bmatrix} \quad (11)$$

where c^o_R, c^o_G, c^o_B represent the non-factorable terms of (8). Now normalizing the color vector, c', we obtain:

$$\frac{c'}{|c'|} = \frac{\alpha(x) \begin{bmatrix} c^o_R \\ c^o_G \\ c^o_B \end{bmatrix}}{(\alpha^2(x)[(c^o_R)^2 + (c^o_G)^2 + (c^o_B)^2])^{1/2}} \quad (12)$$

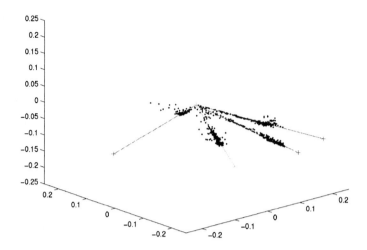

Fig. 3. Distribution of pixels in the R'G'B' space from Figure 1; compare with the RGB distribution in Figure 2. The straight lines are the principal vectors obtained with the best MSE fit from [23]. The alignment of the four cluster prototypes with the four color clusters is clearly seen; each of the four cluster prototypes corresponds to a colored fruit.

$$= \frac{\begin{bmatrix} c_R^o \\ c_G^o \\ c_B^o \end{bmatrix}}{((c_R^o)^2 + (c_G^o)^2 + (c_B^o)^2)^{1/2}} \tag{13}$$

The shading factor has been eliminated and hence this representation is intensity invariant. This operation puts all vectors on the unit hypersphere, except for the null vector (0,0,0) for which this operation is undefined. Since the Euclidean distance between two normalized transformed color vectors does not reflect accurately the perceptual difference between the two vectors, we propose to factor the invariance operation directly into the similarity measure calculation by using one minus the cosine of the vector angle $\theta_{c',d'}$ between two transformed color vectors c', d'; the similarity measure then becomes

$$\Omega(\theta_{c',d'}) = 1 - \frac{<c',d'>}{|c'||d'|} \tag{14}$$

$$= 1 - \frac{\alpha_c(x)\alpha_d(x)(c_R^o d_R^o + c_G^o d_G^o + c_B^o d_B^o)}{(\alpha_c^2(x)(c_R^o c_R^o + c_G^o c_G^o + c_B^o c_B^o))^{1/2}(\alpha_d^2(x)(d_R^o + d_G^o + d_B^o))^{1/2}} \tag{15}$$

$$= 1 - \frac{(c_R^o d_R^o + c_G^o d_G^o + c_B^o d_B^o)}{(c_R^o c_R^o + c_G^o c_G^o + c_B^o c_B^o)^{1/2}(d_R^o + d_G^o + d_B^o)^{1/2}} \tag{16}$$

So if c' and d' are similar in orientation then (16) will be close to zero. Both vectors will be deemed close irrespective of the shading factors $\alpha_c(x)$ and $\alpha_d(x)$ associated with them. Therefore, this method is also shading invariant. In practice, the color vectors R', G', B' are normalized as in (13), which reduces (16) to a simple dot product calculation for each pixel comparison.

2.4 Angle Accuracy

The principal problem with the vector angle formulation derives from the consequences of using (8), which collapses all graylevel values to the origin in the transformed domain, and (13), which performs a vector normalization. Stated more plainly, a collection of noisy, nearly black pixels will be normalized to vastly different transformed locations. This is strictly a reflection of the large degree of sensitivity in the definition of a "hue" for nearly black pixels.

Standard clustering approaches either require such pixels to be rejected (needing an arbitrary rejection threshold) or incorporate them, leading to misleading conclusions. The elegance of the MRF approach to a segmentation algorithm, set up in the next section, is that the penalty term associated with a vector angle can be continuous, rather than discrete admit/reject.

The noise sensitivity of the similarity measure (16) is easily computed, as a preprocessing step, using Monte-Carlo means. In particular, if we model two pixels as noisy

$$c = c_{exact} + \text{noise} \tag{17}$$
$$d = d_{exact} + \text{noise} \tag{18}$$

then the variance $\text{var}(\Omega(\theta_{c'},d'))$ can be efficiently computed; clearly if this variance in angle difference is small then the accuracy of the angle calculation will be deemed high and will be weighted more heavily in the Gibbs energy.

3 Markov Random Fields

The modeling problems in this paper are addressed from the computational viewpoint. There are two primary concerns: how to define an objective function for the optimal solution of the image segmentation problem, and how to find its optimal solution. Given the various uncertainties in the imaging process, it is reasonable to define the desired solution in an optimization sense, such that the "perfect" or "exact" solution to our segmentation problem is interpreted as the optimum solution to the optimization objective.

Some forms of contextual constraints are eventually necessary when trying to interpret visual information. The spatial and visual contexts of the objects in an image scene are necessary for the understanding of the scene; the context of object features at a lower level of representation allow the recognition of the objects; the context of primitives at an even lower level lets the object features be identified; and finally the context of image pixels at the lowest level of abstraction allows for the extraction of those primitives. To create a reliable and effective image analysis system the use of contextual constraints is unavoidable and therefore indispensable.

Gibbs Random Fields (GRFs) [4, 24] provide a natural way of modeling context dependencies between, for example, image pixels of correlated local features

[6]. The practical use of GRF models is largely possible due the improved insights and understanding provided by the Hammersley Clifford theorem [6], which allows Markov random field (MRF) modeling to be reinterpreted as an energy function minimization. The second motivating development is the improved insight and available methods for Gibbs sampling and Simulated Annealing.

The MRF-based segmentation model is defined by the contextual relationships within the local neighborhood structure. Since our goal is the assertion of local constraints, rather than an accurate modeling of spatial textures, as in other GMRF color-segmentation research [8], we shall only be concerned with first order random fields, both simplifying the model and limiting the computational complexity.

Suppose we are given a color image on a pixel lattice $\mathcal{L} = \{i, j\}$. As just discussed in Section 2, each pixel $\{RGB\}_{i,j}$ is transformed to its normalized representation $c'_{i,j}$.

If we precompute the adjacent-pixel vector-angle criteria

$$\psi_{i,j} = \Omega(\theta_{c'_{i,j}, c'_{i+1,j}}) \quad \phi_{i,j} = \Omega(\theta_{c'_{i,j}, c'_{i,j+1}}) \tag{19}$$

then a Gibbs energy E for segmentation can be formulated as follows:

$$E[\{l(i,j)\}] = \sum_{i,j} \alpha \left[\psi_{i,j}^2 \delta_{l(i,j),l(i+1,j)} + \phi_{i,j}^2 \delta_{l(i,j),l(i,j+1)} \right] +$$
$$\beta \left[(1 - \delta_{l(i,j),l(i,j+1)}) + (1 - \delta_{l(i,j),l(i,j+1)}) \right] \tag{20}$$

where each pixel (i, j) is assigned an integer label $0 \le l(i, j) < N$, and where α, β control the relative constraints on the homogeneity of a single region and the degree of region fragmentation, respectively.

The model (20) is intuitive and easily implemented. As mentioned before, it deviates from previous models used for image segmentation in that the inner vector product Ω is used to calculate the minimum energy instead of the Euclidean distance in R, G, B. However it misses one essential point: not all of the vector angles are computed with the same accuracy. Even a small amount of pixel noise on a dark or highlight region results in nearly totally random vector angles, which (20) would choose to separate into single-pixel regions. Given the covariance of the vector angle difference, computed by analytic or Monte-Carlo means as discussed in Section 2.4, we introduce weights

$$w_{i,j} = \frac{1}{\mathrm{var}(\Omega(\theta_{c'_{i,j}, c'_{i+1,j}}))} \quad v_{i,j} = \frac{1}{\mathrm{var}(\Omega(\theta_{c'_{i,j}, c'_{i,j+1}}))} \tag{21}$$

to assert the degree of confidence of the terms in the energy:

$$E[\{l(i,j)\}] = \sum_{i,j} \alpha \left[w_{i,j} \psi_{i,j}^2 \delta_{l(i,j),l(i+1,j)} + v_{i,j} \phi_{i,j}^2 \delta_{l(i,j),l(i,j+1)} \right] +$$
$$\beta \left[(1 - \delta_{l(i,j),l(i,j+1)}) + (1 - \delta_{l(i,j),l(i,j+1)}) \right] \tag{22}$$

Model (22) is a very credible segmentation criterion, representing a considerable advance beyond standard vector-angle methods, and yet (22) is little more complicated than a standard Ising/Potts model [24] and so is well-understood and easily implemented.

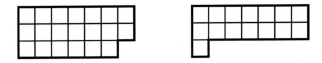

Fig. 4. Boundary length problem: both regions have the same boundary length, although very different volumes.

The primary drawback with (22) is that it is strictly a local, pixel-neighbor model and suffers from the same problems as other region-growing approaches: two vastly differently colored pixels may be grouped into a single region if they are linked by noisy or intermediately-colored pixels. A second undesired effect is that N constrains only the number of region labels, not the number of regions; that is, in regions of noise or color-gradients, (22) can generate a proliferation of small regions. Finally, the label criterion, controlled by β, measures boundary length, rather than region volume (see Figure 4). Therefore, in regions where the vector-angle criterion is vague (that is, in saturated or dark regions), a large number of pixels may have to be flipped to see *any* change in the energy, implying that only the slowest of annealing schedules will successfully converge.

A global model can overcome these drawbacks. If we associate with label l a global transformed color a'_l then each region is forced to be well defined:

$$E[\{l(i,j), a'\}] = \sum_{i,j} \Omega(\theta_{a'_{l(i,j)}, c'_{i,j}})^2 +$$
$$\beta\left[(1 - \delta_{l(i,j),l(i,j+1)}) + (1 - \delta_{l(i,j),l(i,j+1)})\right] \qquad (23)$$

For the purposes of this paper, we propose to fix the region colors $\{a_l\}$; that is, the sampling and annealing takes place only over the label indices $\{l(i,j)\}$ themselves. The $\{a_l\}$ would be found by a preceding step, such as vector quantization [21].

A final modification mirrors that of (22): the degree to which the region color is to be asserted at each pixel should be spatially-varying, now for two reasons:

1. The color-dependent effect of noise, particularly for dark and highlight pixels.
2. We are normally not interested in pixels in regions of high color gradient; at the very least, these pixels should not unduly influence the Gibbs energy by being inconsistent with the region color a.

If we let

$$u_{i,j} = \min\left\{ \frac{1}{\text{var}(\Omega(\theta_{c'_{i,j}, c'_{i+1,j}}))}, \frac{1}{\text{var}_N(\Omega(\theta_{c'_{i,j}, c'_{i+1,j}}))} \right\}, \qquad (24)$$

that is, the variances are the pointwise one, based on a noise model, and a spatial one, computed over a local neighborhood N, then our segmentation model becomes

$$E[\{l(i,j), a_l\}] = \sum_{i,j} u_{i,j}\Omega(\theta_{a'_{l(i,j)}, c'_{i,j}})^2 +$$
$$\beta\left[(1 - \delta_{l(i,j),l(i,j+1)}) + (1 - \delta_{l(i,j),l(i,j+1)})\right] \qquad (25)$$

This gives us a concise and coherent representation of the color image segmentation problem by incorporating both local and global constraints. The global constraints are defined by global color region labels obtained through some vector quantization process such as the one presented in [23]. Local constraints are included by virtue of using pixel level constraints in the MRF model.

Model (25) is a tradeoff between a completely local region growing approach, where many spurious regions can be created, and a global color clustering approach where regions of differing color can be inadvertently merged. Furthermore, the use of vector angle accuracy weights (21) allows the less reliable calculation of vector angle for small R'G'B' values to be appropriately modulated.

4   Results

The Gibbs Sampler [4] will be used to optimize both (22) and (25). To make comparison as straightforward as possible, all MRF results were initialized from a random start, although in practice initializing from an MPC or other segmentation could accelerate convergence. For the global model (25) the label colors a are determined using the algorithm presented in [23].

Results were prepared an artificial image of colored bands, shown in Figure 5 respectively. The artificial image varies in intensity horizontally (i.e., from left to right and a saturated highlight is present near the right border). Some additive uniform uniformly distributed noise was added to this image.

The MPC result on the artificial image is shown in Figure 5(b). The highlight part is clearly a mixture of the three other segmentation classes due to having a nearly null vector representation in the R', G', B' space, and the absence of spatial constraints prevents the ambiguity from being corrected. For the MRF models, the results in Figure 6(a) and Figure 6(b) clearly illustrate the problems of boundary length discussed in Section 3, because of the lack of region-defining constraints such as characteristic region vector, boundary length or area size constraints. It is interesting to note that under careful examination, regions generated on both sides of the border between each color band pair are seldom part of the same class. Figure 6(c) demonstrates the type of result that is obtained using Model (23). As desired, very few highlight parts remain as other highlight areas have been subsumed into their adjacent regions. The remaining few misclassified pixels are due most probably to a too-rapid annealing schedule.

The free parameter β clearly controls the significance of the color-angle dot product in relation to the spatial label contribution in the energy term; clearly in the limit of a small value of β, the MRF result converges to that of MPC. Finally, Figure 6(d) shows the results for the same color bands, but now where the vector angle calculation is weighted in terms of the accuracy to which to the angle can be determined (which is affected by darkness or degree of highlight), as in (25).

5   Conclusions

We have presented a Markov Random Field-based model for shading and highlight invariant color image segmentation. The model's invariance properties have

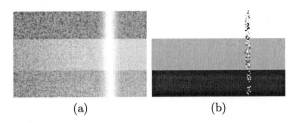

(a)   (b)

Fig. 5. Color band image: (a) Original, (b) MPC segmentation.

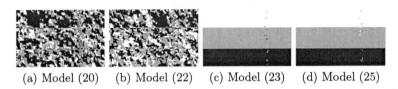

(a) Model (20)   (b) Model (22)   (c) Model (23)   (d) Model (25)

Fig. 6. Color Band image: Results of four proposed MRF models.

been verified using the Dichromatic Reflection Model. Furthermore, the model is based on a vector angle difference measure between color vectors and includes weights to take into account the reliability of calculating angles between various vector pairs.

The MRF model used is a compromise between local-only or global-only color image segmentation methods. It combines the best of both worlds: the ability of the global methods to create well segmented regions and the ability of local methods to adapt to the local variations in pixel values.

There are three immediate considerations for future work. It is not obvious that it is desirable to fix the region colors in models (23), (25). The obvious advantage of doing so is the computational consideration, however the disadvantage is that any error in the vector-quantization step is locked in place and cannot be removed. Instead, the region colors $\{a_l\}$ can be variable, determined as part of the annealing process. Although this requires the Gibbs sampling of continuous values, the effort can remain reasonable if the variables are accurately initialized: $\{a_l\}$ from vector quantization or k-means [10], and the pixel labels $\{l(i,j)\}$ from (22).

Furthermore, the limitation, as illustrated in Figure 4, of using the boundary length as an energy metric for each segmented region, should be revisited. The most obvious choice would be to prefer *larger* regions, where region size is measured by the number of pixels in the region. Although much more robust than boundary length, the number of pixels is a non-local criterion, and is therefore computationally much less convenient.

Finally, parameter estimation to obtain proper convergence of the MRF models is essential. In this paper, parameter estimation was ad-hoc. A formalized parameter estimation technique needs to be applied to fully evaluate the advantages of the MRF models over vector quantization and region growing-based methods when applied to real scene images.

References

1. S. A. Barker, and P. J. W. Rayner, "Unsupervised Image Segmentation Using Markov Random Fields," in M. Pelillo and E. R. Hancock (ed), *Energy Minimization Methods in Computer Vision and Pattern Recognition*, pp. 165-178, Springer-Verlag: 1997.

2. R. Chellappa, and A. Jain, *Markov Random Fields: Theory and Application*. Academic Press, New York, 1993.

3. R. D. Dony, and S. Haykin, "Image segmentation using a mixture of principal components representation," *IEE Proc. VISP*, vol. 144, pp. 73-80, April 1997.

4. S. Geman and D. Geman, "Stochastic Relaxation, Gibbs Distributions, and the Bayesian Restoration of Images," *IEEE Trans-PAMI*, Vol. 6, No. 6, 1984.

5. G.J. Klinker, S.A. Shafer and T. Kanade, "A Physical Approach to Color Image Understanding," *Inter'l J. of Computer Vision*, Vol. 4, No. 1, pp. 7-38, 1990.

6. S. Z. Li, "Modeling Image Analysis Problems Using Markov Random Fields," in C.R. Rao and D.N. Shanbhag (ed), *Stochastic Processes: Modeling and Simulation, Vol. 20 of Handbook of Statistics*. Elsevier Science, 2000, pp. 1-43.

7. Y.W. Lim, and S.U. Lee, "On the color image segmentation algorithm based on the thresholding and fuzzy c-means techniques," *Pattern Recognition*, vol. 23, no. 9, pp. 1235-1252, 1990.

8. D. K. Panjwani, and G. Healey, "Markov Random Field Models for Unsupervised Segmentation of Textured Color Images," *IEEE Trans-PAMI*, Vol. 17, No. 10, 1995.

9. S. H. Park, I. D. Yun, and S.U. Lee, "Color Image Segmentation Based on 3-D Clustering: Morphological Approach," *Pattern Recognition*, vol. 31, no. 8, pp. 1061-1076, 1998.

10. R.J. Schalkoff, *Pattern Recognition: Statistical, Structural and Neural Approaches*. John Wiley & Sons, Inc., New York, 1992.

11. L. Shafarenko, M. Petrou, and J. Kittler, "Automatic watershed segmentation of randomly textured color images," *IEEE Trans. on Image Processing*, vol. 6, pp. 1530-1544, November 1997.

12. S.A. Shafer, "Using color to separate reflection components," TR-136, Computer Sciences Dept., University of Rochester, NY, April 1984.

13. S. Tominaga and B. Wandell, "The standard reflectance model and illuminant estimation", *J. of Optical Society of America A*, Vol. 6, No.4, pp. 576-584, April 1989.

14. S. Tominaga, "Surface Identification Using the Dichromatic Reflection Model," *IEEE Trans. Pattern Analysis and Machine Intelligence*, Vol. 13, No. 7, pp. 658-670, July 1991.

15. S. Tominaga, "Color Classification of Natural Color Images," *Color Research and Application*, Vol. 17, No. 4, pp. 230-239, 1992.

16. S. Tominaga, "Dichromatic Reflection Models for a Variety of Materials," *Color Research and Application*, Vol. 19, No. 4, pp.277 - 285, 1994.

17. S. Tominaga, "Spectral imaging by a multichannel camera," *Journal of Electronic Imaging*, vol. 8, no. 4, pp. 332-342, 1999.

18. A. Tremeau, and N. Borel, "A Region Growing and Merging Algorithm to Color Segmentation," *Pattern Recognition*, vol. 30, no. 7, pp. 1191-1203, 1997.

19. B.A. Wandell. *Foundations of Vision*, Sinauer Associates, Inc. Publishers, Sunderland, MA, 1995.

20. W. Wang, C. Sun, and H. Chao, "Color Image Segmentation and Understanding through Connected Components," *IEEE International Conference on Systems, Man, and Cybernetics*, vol. 2, pp. 1089-1093, October 1997.

21. S. Wesolkowski, M.E. Jernigan, R.D. Dony, "Global Color Image Segmentation Strategies: Euclidean Distance vs. Vector Angle," in Y.-H. Hu, J. Larsen, E. Wilson and S. Douglas (eds.), *Neural Networks for Signal Processing IX*, IEEE Press, Piscataway, NJ, 1999, pp. 419-428.

22. S. Wesolkowski, *Color Image Edge Detection and Segmentation: A Comparison of the Vector Angle and the Euclidean Distance Color Similarity Measures*, Master's thesis, Systems Design Engineering, University of Waterloo, Canada, 1999.

23. S. Wesolkowski, S. Tominaga, and R.D. Dony, "Shading and Highlight Invariant Color Image Segmentation Using the MPC Algorithm," *SPIE Color Imaging: Device-Independent Color, Color Hardcopy, and Graphic Arts VI*, San Jose, USA, January 2001, pp. 229-240.

24. G. Winkler, *Image Analysis, Random Fields and Dynamic Monte Carlo Methods*, Springer-Verlag, Berlin, Germany, 1995.

Edge Based Probabilistic Relaxation
for Sub-pixel Contour Extraction

Toshiro Kubota[1,*], Terry Huntsberger[2], and Jeffrey T. Martin[1]

[1] Department of Computer Science and Engineering
University of South Carolina, Columbia, SC 29205 USA
kubota@cse.sc.edu, j.martin@compaq.com
[2] Jet Propulsion Laboratory, Pasadena, CA 91109
terry@helios.jpl.nasa.gov

Abstract. The paper describes a robust edge and contour extraction technique under two types of degradation: random noise and aliasing. The technique employs unambiguous probabilistic relaxation to distinguish features from noise and refine their spatial locations at sub-pixel accuracy. The most important component in the probabilistic relaxation is a compatibility function. The paper suggests a function with which the optimal orientation of edges can be derived analytically, thus allowing an efficient implementation of the relaxation process. A contour extraction algorithm is designed by combining the relaxation process and a perceptual organization technique. Results on both synthetic and natural images are given and show effectiveness of our approach against noise and aliasing.

Keywords: feature extraction, relaxation labelling, segmentation

1 Introduction

Feature extraction is an essential part of most computer vision problems. Many features such as edges and corners are high frequency components and can be easily obscured by noise. Thus, effective feature extraction processes must incorporate some degree of noise removal capability. Another major obstacle against reliable feature extraction is aliasing due to finite sampling of data. The aliasing obscures the spatial location of features. Researchers are continually working to overcome these problems.

Many feature extraction algorithms proposed in literature often assume that noise has been reduced using some standard smoothing techniques such as Wiener filter, Gaussian smoothing, and non-linear diffusion [1, 9, 20]. A problem with handling noise separately from feature extraction process is that it is difficult to determine the necessary amount of smoothing required to remove noise without removing actual features. Even with an optimal amount of smoothing, some of subtle features would be lost. Another disadvantage associated with

---
* Research partially supported by ONR Grant N00014-97-1-1163

M.A.T. Figueiredo, J. Zerubia, A.K. Jain (Eds.): EMMCVPR 2001, LNCS 2134, pp. 328–343, 2001.
© Springer-Verlag Berlin Heidelberg 2001

smoothing is that it further obscures the spatial location of features. The trade-off between signal to noise ratio (SNR) and localization accuracy is well known, and linear filter based techniques such as Gaussian smoothing have a theoretical limit in its performance in terms of the SNR and localization.

A more reliable approach is to distinguish features from noise by a localized pattern analysis. The underlying assumption is that features form non-random patterns while noise does not. Also prior knowledge of feature patterns can improve the spatial localization of the features. Such pattern analysis is believed to be a part of the human vision processing as evidenced by vernier hyper acuity and contour "pop-out"[4].

Our research goal is to derive a reliable feature extraction and localization system based on simple localized pattern analysis. Such a system is not only for practical interest but also for theoretical one as it can bring some insight on segmentation mechanism of the human vision system. In this paper, we employ probabilistic relaxation or relaxation labeling ([22, 8]) to filter out random noise and extract high frequency features and their spatial locations from low resolution images. The technique searches for a near optimal edge configuration in terms of its location and orientation at the sub-pixel resolution (i.e., we wish to resolve high-resolution edge contours).

The paper suggests a general approach for designing an edge based compatibility function that is a core ingredient for the relaxation process. It then provides a particular realization of the function that allows computationally efficient procedure for performing the relaxation and achieving a near-optimal edge configuration. We then develop a contour extraction technique that combines the result of the relaxation with a perceptual organization technique. The computation is purely local and intrinsically parallel.

The paper is organized as follows. Section 2 provides a brief description of the probabilistic relaxation followed by a detail description of how we designed a compatibility function for recovering edge configuration. Section 3 describes how to perform the relaxation process in a computationally efficient manner. Section 4 provides a contour extraction procedure based on the relaxation and perceptual grouping. Section 5 gives some experimental results of the edge localization and contour extraction processes using both synthetic and natural images. Section 6 provides brief discussion on other related works and some relevant neurological evidence. Finally, Section 7 concludes with a summary.

2   Probabilistic Relaxation

The technique explores global consistency through local iterative interactions or "relaxation". It measures local consistency of an object to its neighbor objects based on a collective sum of a simple pair-wise compatibility measure. The measure captures the prior knowledge of the structural or contextual patterns of interest. At each iteration, the configuration of each object is updated so that it is more consistent to its neighbors. The configuration of an object is represented by the probability distribution of its labels or "states". Through iterative local interaction, the process approaches a more globally consistent configuration. The technique has been studied extensively in both theory and implementation [8, 13, 19, 21], and found many applications in image processing and computer vision. [6, 10]

For any application of the probabilistic relaxation, a compatibility function is necessary. It is often defined as $r_{ij}(\lambda_i, \lambda_j)$, for two objects at i and j having labels λ_i and λ_j, respectively. The function quantifies how likely or how compatible the label λ_i of an object at i is to λ_j of another object at j. We can also associate it with the conditional probability $\Pr(\lambda_i|\lambda_j)$. However, the specification of $r_{ij}(\lambda_i, \lambda_j)$ is less constrained than $\Pr(\lambda_i|\lambda_j)$ as the former is allowed to have negative values and $\sum_{\lambda_i} r_{ij}$ does not have to be 1. When λ_i at site i is compatible (incompatible) with λ_j at site j, the compatibility function should have a large (small or negative) value.

Now a support function is defined based on the compatibility function as

$$S_i(\lambda_i) = \sum_j \sum_{\lambda_j} r_{ij}(\lambda_i, \lambda_j) P_j(\lambda_j), \tag{1}$$

where $P_j(\lambda_j)$ is the probability of having label λ_j at j. In other words, $P_j(\lambda_j)$ is the Probability Density Function (PDF) of λ_j. The support function measures how likely the site i is labelled as λ_i, given the configuration of its neighbors. At last, the total support function is defined as

$$S = \sum_i \sum_{\lambda_i} S_i(\lambda_i) P_i(\lambda_i) = \sum_i \sum_{\lambda_i} \sum_j \sum_{\lambda_j} r_{ij}(\lambda_i, \lambda_j) P_i(\lambda_i) P_j(\lambda_j) \tag{2}$$

The total support function measures the global consistency of the particular configuration. The objective of the probabilistic relaxation is to maximize the total support by iteratively updating P_i $\forall i$.

In its general form, probabilistic relaxation is not computationally amiable. Difficulties associated with the technique are the following:

1. It is difficult to formulate the compatibility function as the function is 4 dimensional (i, j, λ_i and λ_j) in general.
2. It is not simple to update P_i as it has to be projected onto $\{p_i(\lambda_k), k = 1..K | p_i(\lambda_k) \in [0, 1], \sum_k p_i(\lambda_k) = 1\}$ where K is the number of possible labels, and evaluation of the support function is often computationally expensive. [16, 18]

The second difficulty listed above can be alleviated by using unambiguous relaxation [8]. With unambiguous labeling, the only label allowed for an object at i to take is the one that maximizes S_i. By denoting the index of the label that maximizes S_i as $M(i)$ (i.e. $M(i) = \arg\max_k S_i(\lambda_k)$), the PDF becomes $P_i(\lambda_k) = 1$ if $k = M(i)$ and $P_i(\lambda_k) = 0$ if $k \neq M(i)$. Then the support function becomes

$$S_i(\lambda_{M(i)}) = \sum_j r_{ij}(\lambda_{M(i)}, \lambda_{M(j)}), \tag{3}$$

$$S_i(\lambda_k) = 0, k \neq M(i). \tag{4}$$

The total support function is simplified to

$$S = \sum_i \sum_j r_{ij}(\lambda_{M(i)}, \lambda_{M(j)}). \tag{5}$$

Thus, the unambiguous relaxation alleviates the second difficulty listed above at the expense of flexibility in specifying the PDF. However, we still face a problem of designing the compatibility function. In the next sections, we concentrate on designing the compatibility function for application to edge extraction.

2.1 Compatibility Function

As described above, the compatibility function captures the prior knowledge of the patterns of interest; thus it is heavily dependent on a problem one wants to solve. Here, our interest is to extract edges and their attributes. This section first describes a general approach to design a compatibility function for edges. The approach is based on two assumptions: invariance to an Euclidean transform of the coordinate system and invariance to the global illumination level. Then the section describes a particular realization of the approach for extraction of edges under noisy conditions. This realization results in a computationally efficient procedure for maximizing the support function.

First, we consider that an edge is described by three attributes: the location (x, y), orientation θ, and strength m. It will be represented by a vector, $e(x, y)$ whose orientation and strength are $\angle e = \theta$ and $|e| = m$, respectively. Our framework allows the location and orientation to be treated as a label for the relaxation.

We define a compatibility function for edges as

$$r(e_i, e_j) = f(i_x, i_y, \angle e_i, j_x, j_y, \angle e_j, |e_j|) \tag{6}$$

where i_x and i_y are the x and y coordinates of e_i, respectively, likewise for j_x and j_y with respect to e_j. This is a function of 7 variables. Note that the function is not dependent on $|e_i|$ as we do not treat the edge strength as a label.

To simplify the design process, we assume that the compatibility function is invariant to both translation and rotation of the coordinate system. Then, we design a prototype function with $j_x = j_y = 0$ and $\angle e_j = 0$. Later, this prototype function is translated to (j_x, j_y) and rotated by $\angle e_j$ to obtain the general form of $r(e_i, e_j)$. Then the prototype function can be expressed as

$$r_{ij}(e_i, e_j) = f(i_x, i_y, \angle e_i, |e_j|). \tag{7}$$

For convenience, we use a polar coordinate in describing (i_x, i_y). Thus

$$r_{ij}(e_i, e_j) = f(d_i, \alpha_i, \angle e_i, |e_j|). \tag{8}$$

where $d_i = \sqrt{i_x^2 + i_y^2}$ and $\alpha_i = \arctan(i_y, i_x)$.

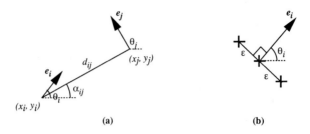

Fig. 1. Geometrical Notations. (a) used in describing the compatibility function. (b) used in describing the support function maximization procedure.

In most image capturing environments, the image irradiance is proportional to the scene radiance. Therefore the edge strength is also proportional to the radiance [25]. Our goal is to obtain a consistent edge configuration based on the structure of objects, as much as possible, without being influenced by the level of illumination. Thus, we impose a constraint that the order of support should be invariant to the constant scaling of the scene illumination. To be more precise mathematically, the ratio of total supports for two different configurations remains constant with respect to the change in the global illumination level.

It can be shown that the above constraint can be satisfied if the compatibility function is proportional to the edge strength. Thus, the prototype compatibility function is

$$r_{ij}(e_i, e_j) = |e_j| f(d_i, \alpha_i, \angle e_i). \tag{9}$$

Note that this is not the only choice for achieving the invariance to the global illumination level. Obviously, making the compatibility function totally independent of the edge strength is another option. However, we found that the scaling of the compatibility measure by the edge strength is important as strong surface discontinuities can strongly influence the neighboring configuration.

The next design step is to decompose f into a product of two terms: r_{loc}, which measures the compatibility of the edge location to e_j, and r_{or}, which measures the compatibility of $\angle e_i$ to e_j given d_i and α_i. The functions r_{loc} and r_{or} will be called compatibility factors. With this decomposition, f is written as

$$f(d_i, \alpha_i, \angle e_j) = r_{loc}(d_i, \alpha_i | e_j) r_{or}(\angle e_i | d_i, \alpha_i, e_j). \tag{10}$$

Note that we used | notation as conditional probability to make the meaning of each factor more clear. One can make an analogy of the decomposition with the product rule of probability. This decomposition can be applied to any function f and does not impose any new constraints on f. However, the design process becomes more tractable by breaking the compatibility relationship into two factors.

Our formulation of the compatibility factors is described next. The design is heavily based on our intuition and other alternatives are possible.

Compatibility Factor r_{loc}. We arrive at our definition of r_{loc} empirically. Colinearity of the Gestalt rules suggest that α_i is most compatible with e_j when it is equal to $\angle e_j$ or $\angle e_j + \pi$ [11]. The degree of the compatibility decreases as α_i deviates from the values. We use $\sin^2(\alpha_i)$ to quantify the deviation. We also assume that the compatibility decreases as the distance between two sites increases. Using the ideas above as guidelines, we suggest the following function for r_{loc} with distributions that are Gaussian in d_i and exponential in $\sin^2(\alpha_i)$.

$$r_{loc}(d_i, \alpha_i) = e^{-\beta \sin^2(\alpha_i) - d_i^2 / 2\sigma^2} \tag{11}$$

where σ^2 and β are parameters for the Gaussian and exponential distributions, respectively.

Compatibility Factor: r_{or}. For r_{or}, we use $cos(\angle e_i - \phi_i(d_i, \alpha_i, e_j))$. where ϕ_i specifies the most compatible $\angle e_i$ to e_j. The function returns 1 when $e_i = \phi_i$ and -1 when $e_i = \phi_i \pm \pi$. It is monotonic between the two extrema.

We found empirically that ϕ_i can be specified further. We collected natural images of various types, measured correlation of gradient angles at different offsets, and obtained PDFs of $\angle \nabla I(x, y) - \angle \nabla I(x + o_x, y + o_y)$ for a distribution of offsets (o_x, o_y). Note that I represents image data and ∇ is the gradient operator. We found that the PDFs are strongly peaked at 0. Figure 2 shows PDFs of $\angle \nabla I(x, y) - \angle \nabla I(x + o_x, y + o_y)$ at two different offsets: $(o_x, o_y) = (2, 0)$ and $(2, 2)$. The results suggest that the most compatible $\angle e_i$ to e_j is $\angle e_j$. Thus, we set $\phi_i = \angle e_j$.

With the compatibility factors so designed, the prototype compatibility function is

$$r(e_i, e_j) = |e_j| e^{-\beta \sin^2(\alpha_i) - d_i^2 / 2\sigma^2} \cos(\angle e_i), \tag{12}$$

and for a general case (i.e. non-prototype condition) e_j,

$$r(e_i, e_j) = |e_j| e^{-\beta \sin^2(\alpha_{ij} - \angle e_j) - d_{ij}^2 / 2\sigma^2} \cos(\angle e_i - \angle e_j), \tag{13}$$

d_{ij} is the distance between (i_x, i_y) and (j_x, j_y), and α_{ij} is the slope of the line connecting (i_x, i_y) and (j_x, j_y). See Figure 1(a).

The use of this compatibility factor results in a computationally efficient procedure for maximizing the total support defined in (5). The next section discusses the maximization process.

3 Relaxation Procedure

3.1 Maximizing Support Function

Computational effort is a major consideration for maximizing the total support function. To show this, denote the number of possible edge locations by N_l, and the number of possible edge orientation by N_o. For simplicity, if we allow multiple edges to share the same site, the number of possible configurations for

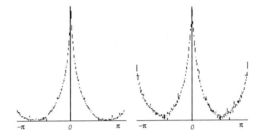

Fig. 2. Correlation of Edge Orientations. The plot shows the PDF of $\angle\nabla I(x,y) - \angle\nabla I(x+o_x, y+o_y)$ at different offsets, (o_x, o_y). Both PDFs show a strong peak at $\angle\nabla I(x,y) - \angle\nabla I(x+o_x, y+o_y) = 0$. (a) $(o_x, o_y) = (2,0)$ (b) $(o_x, o_y) = (2,2)$.

each edge is $N_l N_o$, which can be quite large for moderate cases. For example, with $N_l = 5 \times 5$ and $N_o = 16$, $N_l N_o = 400$. Then, in order to find $M(i)$ which maximizes S_i in (3), a brute force method requires $N_l N_o$ evaluations of S_i. Thus, the total number of evaluation of the compatibility function is $N_n N_l N_o$ where N_n is the number of neighbor sites contributing to the sum in (3).

Maximizing r_{or}. The main reason for using *cos* function in r_{or} to interpolate between the two extrema is to reduce the computational burden and, at the same time, increase the resolution of edge orientation. Assume that we are maximizing S_i in terms of $\angle e_i$. Then by using trigonometry identities, $\cos(a + b) = \cos(a)\cos(b) - \sin(a)\sin(b)$ and $A\sin(\theta) + B\cos(\theta) = \sqrt{A^2 + B^2}\cos(\theta + \phi)$, $\phi = \arctan(A/B)$, the support function can be expressed as

$$S_i(\angle e_i) = \sum_j |e_j| r_{loc} \cos(\angle e_i - \angle e_j) = F_i \cos(\angle e_i - \Theta_i) \qquad (14)$$

where

$$F_i = \sqrt{\left(\sum_j |e_j| r_{loc} \cos(e_j)\right)^2 + \left(\sum_j |e_j| r_{loc} \sin(e_j)\right)^2},$$

$$\Theta_i = \arctan\left(\frac{\sum_j |e_j| r_{loc} \sin(e_j)}{\sum_j |e_j| r_{loc} \cos(e_j)}\right).$$

Therefore $\angle e_j = \Theta_i$ maximizes S_i and Θ_i can be computed with N_n evaluations of r_{loc} instead of $N_o N_n$. Also the domain of $\angle e_i$ becomes continuous without any computational penalty.

Another and more visually intuitive interpretation of the above formula may be to consider a vector f_{ij} whose length and angle are $|e_j| r_{loc}$ and $\angle e_j$, respectively, and a vector F_i whose length and angle are F_i and Θ_i, respectively. Then F_i can be computed as a vector sum of f_{ij}. Thus,

$$F_i = \sum_j f_{ij} \qquad (15)$$

and the $\angle e_j$ that maximizes S_i is $\angle F_i$.

```
Obtain an initial edge configuration with some gradient operator
do {
    for(each edge element i) {
        Compute F_i at the current location and its neighbor sites.
        Move the edge to the location where F_i is the largest
        Set the edge orientation to Θ_i at the new location
    }
} until convergence
```

Fig. 3. Procedure for Maximizing the Total Support.

3.2   Procedure

We propose a local and iterative procedure for obtaining the edge configuration that maximizes S. Because of its local nature, the procedure is not guaranteed to find the global maximum. However, it is computationally efficient, intrinsically parallel and effective in finding a near-optimum solution.

The procedure updates each edge element sequentially. For each e_i, F_i is computed at three different locations: the current edge location and two locations that are ϵ apart from e_i in the direction perpendicular to $\angle e_i$. (Figure 1(b).) The main reasons for this constrained search are the following. If the estimated edge orientation is correct, the shortest path for the edge to reach the contour is along the direction perpendicular to the edge orientation. Thus the maximization process will find the accurate contour location more quickly by moving the edge to the search direction. The search strategy also helps to maintain uniform spacing between edges on the same contour and prevents them from being attracted to those with high edge strength and colliding into a single point.

Figure 3 gives a pseudo code for this procedure. We used Nitzberg-Shiota's gradient operator ([17]) to obtain an initial edge configuration. For each edge element, it requires 3 evaluations of S_i or equivalently F_i. This is a significant reduction from $N_o N_l$.

The edge configuration resulting from this maximization procedure is important for determining object contours in noisy images. Our final goal is to use the resulting edge configuration to obtain high-resolution edge contours.

4   Contour Extraction

It is very useful in many vision applications to extract contours at sub-pixel accuracy. For example, an effective sub-pixel contour extraction process can aid data analysis of low-resolution data, improve visual quality of image expansion, and increase spatial accuracy of matching algorithms.

Using the contour fragments from the edge localization process, we create a boundary contour that is continuous at a high resolution. Furthermore, we want to make the contour in such a way that the grouping result is compatible to our visual perception, and the process is computationally efficient. Many edge grouping techniques have been developed so far. We found it beneficial to develop another one that is tailored to the particular information available to us for both computational and performance reasons. Several steps are necessary to obtain the result.

First, localized edges are resampled on the new finer lattice. Assuming that we are interested in extracting contours at the resolution ρ times higher in both horizontal and vertical directions than the original data, the size of the resulting contour image is $\rho \times \rho$ larger than the original. An edge, $e(x, y)$, is placed at $(round(x\rho), round(y\rho))$ of the new lattice, where $round(x)$ returns the integer closest to x. When multiple edges reside on the same lattice, only the edge with the largest $|e|$ is kept.

Second, edges are grouped into a contour based on proximity and continuation. Since the localization and resampling processes effectively reduce both ambiguity of edge location and the number of spurious edges, a simple perceptual organization technique works well for this task. Also, since edges are distributed very evenly along the contour after the localization process, the search can be restricted to within a small neighborhood. We found that a search distance as small as ρ is often enough for our purpose.

For each edge, our grouping procedure searches in its neighborhood for two edges based on some proximity and continuation criteria. For the first pair, we choose heuristically and empirically the following quantity to measure the continuation of two edges. Denoting e_i as the current edge for the grouping process and e_j as a neighbor edge with which the grouping criteria is being evaluated, the continuation measure, μ_{ij}, is

$$\mu_{ij} = cos^2(\alpha_{ij} - \angle e_i)cos^2(\alpha_{ij} - \angle e_j). \qquad (16)$$

The definition of α_{ij} is the same as before. Thus, the continuation measure ranges between 0 and 1. It is 1 when the orientation of each edge is either the same with α_{ij} or different by π. It is 0 when one of the edge is perpendicular to α_{ij}. The measure varies smoothly between the extrema.

For the second pair, we also take the smoothness of a contour formed by the first pair and e_j into consideration. Then the continuation measure for the second pair, $\hat{\mu}_{ij}$, is the product of the smoothness measure and μ_{ij}.

$$\hat{\mu}_{ij} = sin^2(0.5 * (\alpha_{i1} - \alpha_{ij}))\mu_{ij} \qquad (17)$$

where α_{i1} is the slope of the line connecting the first pair. Again, the measure ranges between 0 and 1. It is 1 when three edges are colinear and point the direction of the line connecting them. It is 0 when either $\mu_{ij} = 0$ or $\alpha_{i1} = \alpha_{ij}$.

The proximity measure is incorporated into the order of the search. We first start the search in the neighborhood whose chessboard distance is 1 from the current lattice site (i.e. $max(|i_x - j_x|, |i_y - j_y|) = 1$). If the maximum of the continuation measure in this neighborhood is above some threshold ζ, then the site associated with the maximum is selected and the search stops. When no sites have continuation measure above ζ, the search continues in the neighborhood at distance 2 then 3 and so on until the distance reaches over pre-defined maximum, D. Advantages of this strategy are, first, that the number of search to find a match is smaller than having the fixed search area and, second, that the formulation of a 'goodness' measure is simplified as only the continuation measure needs to be considered. The disadvantage is that the search can miss the 'best' match when a decent match is detected before.

Note that the grouping process is not symmetric, i.e. e_i selecting e_j as a grouping pair does not guarantee e_j selecting e_i. This asymmetric property is used to form T-junctions.

The next step is to interpolate a pair of edges to form a contour. Typically, the distance between a pair of grouped edges is small, and we found a simple first-order polynomial interpolation is visually acceptable for 4×4 expansion used in our experiments. For higher expansion rates, higher order polynomials may be required. One alternative is to use an *Essentially Non-Oscillatory* interpolation scheme for better preservation of corners and junctions [24]. Another possibility is to use the F_i field so that the curve traces the ridge of the field. These alternatives will give smoother interpolation but are more computationally demanding.

For every grouped pair of edges, an 8-digital straight segment is drawn and lattice sites on the segment including both starting and ending edge sites are marked. Then a contour is defined as a 8-connected component of marked sites, and the contour length is defined as the number of sites contributing to the contour. For details of digital straight segments and how to draw them, see [15].

Now F_i is computed at every contour point. When F_i is below some threshold η, the point is removed from the contour. After the thresholding, the procedure finally removes contours whose lengths are smaller than some threshold L.

5   Experimental Results

5.1   Edge Localization

At low resolution, our maximization procedure effectively refines edge locations while simultaneously removing spurious edges. Figure 4 shows synthetic test images. One is without noise and the other with additive Gaussian noise. The signal to noise ratio of the noisy image is 1.5 The image size is 64×64 pixels. Throughout the experiments, the following set of parameters is used.

$$\beta = 0, \sigma = 0.5, \epsilon = 0.25.$$

Figure 5 shows initial configuration of each test image. Edges are thick mainly due to 3×3 mask used in the Nitzberg-Shiota operator. Thus there is 3-pixel ambiguity in edge location even for the clean image.

Figure 6 shows the results of the maximization procedure. It is evident from the result of the clean image that the procedure effectively resolved the ambiguity of edge location and provided more accurate locations of the edges. For the noisy image, the procedure combined random noise edges and produced some additional patterns. However, due to the random nature of these edges, the patterns are shorter in length than those formed by actual contour edges. They also tend to contain edges whose S_i is small because of high curvature at the

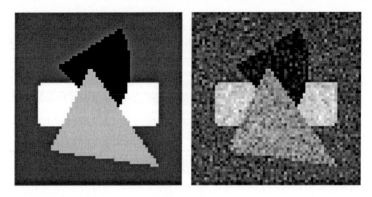

Fig. 4. Synthetic Test Image. The actual size of the images is 64x64 pixels. They are expanded by pixel duplication for viewing.

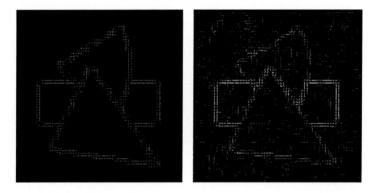

Fig. 5. Initial Edge Configuration. The figure shows the initial edge configuration of test images shown in Figure 4.

locations. By removing edges with S_i smaller than some threshold value, random patterns are broken into even smaller pieces, and the true patterns and random patterns can be separated effectively based on the contour length.

5.2   Contour Extraction

The results of the contour extraction process are shown in Figure 7. Parameter values are given in the figure caption. For the clean image, the complete contour boundaries are extracted with high localization accuracy. For the noisy image, noise edges are effectively removed while most of actual boundaries are extracted. For the clean image, a larger D is used to connect edges at junctions.

This contour extraction process is applied to natural images. Results are given on the right in Figure 8. The process extracted subtle features without being affected by random noise. For example, with the house image, our procedure delineated the outline of the roof more completely than other edge extraction

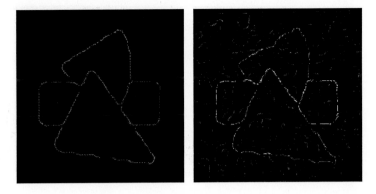

Fig. 6. Localized Edge Configuration. The figure shows the edge configuration of test images shown in Figure 4 after 10 iterations.

techniques we tested. With the seagull image, our procedure extracted the pattern of the feather without picking up relatively strong random patterns in the background.

5.3   Comparison

For comparison, Canny's edge detector ([2]) is applied to the synthetic images. The result is shown in Figure 9. The detector uses Gaussian smoothing followed by a gradient operator for detecting edges. Such a simple linear operator fails to distinguish true boundaries from random noise. As the amount of smoothing is increased, the number of spurious edges decreases and at the same time the real surface boundaries are removed as well.

Overall, the whole process of sub-pixel contour extraction on a 64x64 image expanded to 256x256 with 20 relaxation iterations took 25 seconds on a 300MHz SGI O2. Note that our code is not optimized for ease of maintenance (we implemented it in C++ using vector STL that contains large overheads in both speed and memory usage) and we believe that a significant amount of improvement on the speed can be achieved. The most computationally intensive part of the process is the relaxation, which consumed 90% of computation time.

6   Discussion

As stated in the introduction, our aim of this research is to design a reliable contour extraction system built on simple, localized, and possibly iterative processing. The motivation is to derive a neurologically feasible system from a practical perspective. In the computational vision community, much research on the contour integration problem has been approached from faithful modeling of V1 and V2 neurons with both excitatory and inhibitory connections in a recurrent fashion[14]. It is often cumbersome, however, to build a system purely in

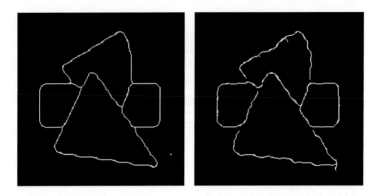

Fig. 7. Result of Contour Detection. Contour detection is applied on 64x64 synthetic images at the 256x256 resolution. The following set of parameters is used. Left: $\zeta = 0.5$, $D = 10$, $\eta = 1.0$, $L = 75$ Right: $\zeta = 0.5$, $D = 4$, $\eta = 1.0$, $L = 75$.

a bottom-up fashion. Our study attempts to bridge two extremes of pure neurological and engineering approaches and give insight in the development of a neuro-morphological contour extraction system that is more faithful to the neurological structures.

In this respect, we found that the probabilistic relaxation is a suitable vehicle to describe a mathematically sound and numerically stable design of a recurrent neural network. With this view and with neural network terminology, the compatibility function provides a weight between two neurons and the projection to the PDF space represents a subsequent non-linear transform. The formulation based on the probabilistic relaxation allows us to concentrate on the algorithmic level of development rather than the network level, which can be laborious.

Another aspect of our development that closely ties with neurophysiological evidence is that the compatibility function derived in Section 2.1 resembles long-range interconnection patterns found in the V1 areas. The long-range interactions are considered to facilitate the contour integration process. *Association field* by Field et al. [4] and the oscillatory intracortical network by Li [14] are models of this neural structures for the contour integration process. Although our formulation is derived empirically and heuristically and is not grounded to any physiological data, it can be replaced with other models without any further changes in its procedure. Our model has only two free parameters, thus it is simpler to implement and adjust than the above models.

Our technique varies from other field based contour integration techniques, in particular works by Elder and Zucker[3], Guy and Medioni [5], Shashua and Ullman[23], and Williams [26]. These techniques use the field representation to measure the *saliency* of features while ours actively reconfigures the edges by the probabilistic relaxation process. our active reconfiguration process tends to increase the saliency of structured patterns more than random ones, resulting in clearer separation of two types of patterns. The mechanism of the reconfiguration process is similar to the recurrent excitation and inhibition of the V1 cells and

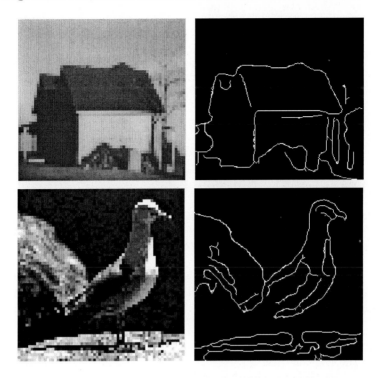

Fig. 8. Result of Contour Detection on Natural Images. Contours are detected at the resolution 4x4 times higher than the original. The left column shows the original images expanded by 4x4 using pixel duplication. The right column shows the corresponding results. Parameters used are $\zeta = 0.1$, $D = 4$, $\eta = 0.5$, $L = 30$ for the house and $\zeta = 0.1$, $D = 4$, $\eta = 0.5$, $L = 50$ for the seagull.

has effects on contour enhancement and texture suppression. [12] Our success in separating patterns reinforces Lee's proposed mechanism.

The research on detecting edges at sub-pixel accuracy under noisy condition dates back to Hueckel's work [7]. Typically, edge locations are estimated in the continuous domain based on theoretical modeling of image formation and edge detection processes. Noise is often handled either by explicit thresholding on the strength of edges or implicit smoothing by interpolation functions. Similarly, our technique employs image formation and edge models that are captured in the compatibility function. However, instead of applying thresholding or smoothing, it delays handling noise until edges are reconfigured based on the relaxation process. The process is effective in isolating noise edges from actual object boundaries as seen in Figure 6, and it becomes easier to separate them by simple heuristical rules as demonstrated in Figure 7.

It is not clear at this point if a localization process similar to the one described here is taking place in the visual cortex. However, as suggested by the visual hyperacuity, some sub-pixel measure of spatial offsets is a part of the cortical

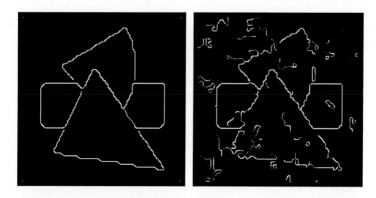

Fig. 9. Result of Canny Edge Detection. Canny edge detection is applied on synthetic images of 4 at the 256x256 resolution. The original 64x64 images are expanded using bi-linear interpolation prior to the edge detection operation.

processing. More study is necessary on both neurological and computational science to reach the conclusion.

7   Conclusion

The paper described a feature extraction process using unambiguous probabilistic relaxation to conduct local pattern analysis of an image. Through local iterative interactions controlled by the relaxation process, globally consistent patterns emerge at sub-pixel accuracy while noise is suppressed to form less consistent patterns. By post-processing the patterns based on the consistency measure derived from the support function, features can be separated from noise. Our formulation of the compatibility function allows efficient relaxation process requiring only 3 evaluations of the support function for each edge per iteration.

We developed a contour extraction procedure on a super-resolution lattice based on the relaxation result and a perceptual organization technique. The effectiveness of the procedure is demonstrated on both synthetic and natural images. Comparison with Canny operator shows superior performance of our technique in terms of noise robustness and localization accuracy.

References

1. L. Albarez, P-L. Lions, and J. M. Morel. Image selective smoothing and edge detection by non-linear diffusion. ii. *SIAM J. Num. Analy.*, 29:845–866, 1992.
2. J. F. Canny. A computational approach to edge-detection. *PAMI*, 8:679–700, 1986.
3. J. H. Elder and S. W. Zucker. Computing contour closure. In *ECCV '96*, 399–412, San Francisco, CA, 1996.
4. D. J. Field, A. Hayes, and R. F. Hess. Contour integration by the human visual system: Evidence for a local "association field". *Vis. Res.*, 33:173–193, 1993.

5. G. Guy and G. Medioni. Inferring global perceptual contours from local features. *IJCV*, 20(1):113–133, 1996.
6. E. R. Hancock and J. Kittler. Edge-labeling using dictionary-based relaxation. *PAMI*, 12(2):165–181, February 1990.
7. M. Hueckel. A local visual operator which recognizes edges and lines. *JACM*, 20(4):634–647, October 1973.
8. R.A. Hummel and S.W. Zucker. On the foundations of relaxation labeling processes. *PAMI*, 5(3):267–287, May 1983.
9. B. Jawerth, P. Lin, and E. Sinzinger. Lattice boltzmann models for anisotropic diffusion of images. *JMIV*, 11(3):231–237, December 1999.
10. J.V. Kittler and J. Illingworth. Relaxation labelling algorithms – a review. *IVC*, 3:206–216, 1985.
11. I. Kovacs. Gestalten of today: Early processing of visual contours and surfaces. *Behav. Brain Research*, 82:1–11, 1996.
12. T.S. Lee, D. Mumford, R. Romero, and V. A. F. Lamme. The role of the primary visual cortex in higher level vision. *Vis. Res.*, 38:2429–2454, 1998.
13. S.Z. Li, H. Wang, K.L. Chan, and M. Petrou. Minimization of mrf energy with relaxation labeling. *JMIV*, 7(2):149–161, March 1997.
14. Zhaoping Li. A neural model of contour integration in the primary visual cortex. *Neural Computation*, 10(4):903–940, 1998.
15. S. Marchand-Maillet and Y. M. Sharaiha. *Binary Digital Image Processing - Discrete Approach*. Academic Press, London, UK, 2000.
16. J.L. Mohammed, R.A. Hummel, and S.W. Zucker. A gradient projection algorithm for relaxation methods. *PAMI*, 5(3):330–332, May 1983.
17. M. Nitzberg and T. Shiota. Nonlinear image filtering with edge and corner enhancement. *PAMI*, 14(8):826–833, August 1992.
18. P. Parent and S.W. Zucker. Radial projection: An efficient update rule for relaxation labeling. *PAMI*, 11(8):886–889, August 1989.
19. M. Pelillo and M. Refice. Learning compatibility coefficients for relaxation labeling processes. *PAMI*, 16(9):933–945, September 1994.
20. P. Perona and J. Malik. Scale-space and edge detection using anisotropic diffusion. *PAMI*, 12(7):629–639, 1990.
21. A. Rangarajan. Self-annealing and self-annihilation: unifying deterministic annealing and relaxation labeling. *PR*, 33(4):635–649, April 2000.
22. A. Rosenfeld, R.A. Hummel, and S.W. Zucker. Scene labeling by relaxation operations. *SMC*, 6(6):420–433, June 1976.
23. A. Shashua and S. Ullman. Structural saliency: the detection of globally salient structures of using a locally connected network. In *ICCV*, 321–327, 1988.
24. K. Siddiqi, B.B. Kimia, and C.W. Shu. Geometric shock capturing eno schemes for subpixel interpolation, computation and curve evolution. *CVGIP*, 59(5):278–301, September 1997.
25. E. Trucco and A. Verri. *Introductory Techniques for 3D Computer Vision*. Prentice-Hall, Upper Saddle River, NJ, 1998.
26. L. Williams and D. W. Jacobs. Local parallel computation of stochastic completion fields. In *CVPR '96*, 161–168, San Francisco, CA, 1996.

Two Variational Models
for Multispectral Image Classification

Christophe Samson[1], Laure Blanc-Féraud[1],
Gilles Aubert[2], and Josiane Zerubia[1]

[1] Ariana*, joint research group I3S (CNRS/UNSA) and INRIA
Inria, 2004 route des Lucioles, BP 93 06902 Sophia Antipolis cedex, France
FirstName.LastName@sophia.inria.fr
http://www.inria.fr/ariana
[2] Laboratoire J.A. Dieudonné, Umr 6621 du Cnrs, Université de Nice Sophia
Antipolis, France
gaubert@math.unice.fr

Abstract. We propose two variational models for supervised classification of multispectral data. Both models take into account contour
and region information by minimizing a functional compound of a data
term (2D surface integral) taking into account the observation data and
knowledge on the classes, and a regularization term (1D length integral)
minimizing the length of the interfaces between regions. This is a free
discontinuity problem and we have proposed two different ways to reach
such a minimum, one using a Γ-convergence approach and the other using a level set approach to model contours and regions.
Both methods have been previously developed in the case of monospectral observations. Multispectral techniques allow to take into account
information of several spectral bands of satellite or aerial sensors. The
goal of this paper is to present the extension of both variational classification methods to multispectral data. We show an application on real
data from SPOT (XS mode) satellite for which we have a ground truth.
Our results are also compared to results obtained by using a hierarchical
stochastic model.

Key-words: classification, multispectral images, Γ-convergence, level-
set methods, active regions, active contours.

1 Introduction

Variational approaches and Partial Differential Equation (PDE) models have
shown to be efficient for a wide variety of image processing problems such as
restoration and edge detection [1, 10, 20–22], or shape segmentation with active
contours [8, 16, 19]. Nevertheless, the notion of classification, which consists of
assigning a label to each site of an image to produce a partition of the image

---

* this work has been conducted in relation with the GdR-PRC ISIS research group
(http://www.isis.enst.fr)

M.A.T. Figueiredo, J. Zerubia, A.K. Jain (Eds.): EMMCVPR 2001, LNCS 2134, pp. 344–356, 2001.
© Springer-Verlag Berlin Heidelberg 2001

into homogeneous labelled areas, has rarely been introduced in a variational formulation (continuous models) mainly because the notion of class has a discrete nature. The classification problem concerns many applications as, for instance, land use management in remote sensing. Many classification models can be found in stochastic approaches (discrete models), with the use of Markov Random Field (MRF) theory as for instance in [4, 7, 12, 17]. Structural approaches such as splitting, merging and region growing models [23], and few other models such as a combination of statistical and deterministic techniques [31, 35] have also been developed for image classification. But, to our knowledge, very few research works have been conducted in the field of classification by the use of variational models. Our goal is to built a functional whose minimum defines a regular classification of the observation, the classes being known (supervised classification). The regularity is obtained by minimizing the length of the discontinuities of the solution, i.e. the length of the region boundaries of the classified image. The classification problem is then a free discontinuity problem in the sense that the main difficulty is to capture information on regions (2D data term) and their contours (1D discontinuities: regularization term). To reach that goal, two methods have been developed for monospectral data [27, 26]. One is based on Γ-convergence results, firstly derived for fluid mechanic problems. The second one uses level set approach to model the regions and contours of each class.

Usually for real multiband applications, as for instance SPOT data in XS mode composed of three images of the same scene with different wave lengths, are used for classification purpose. In this work, we propose an extension of both models to multiband data, taking into account coupled information from these bands.

After setting the classification hypotheses and some notations, we state the properties of the solution we are looking for, and formalize the classification problem through the minimization of a functional. Depending on the variable we use to model a classified image, we obtain two different functionals. The minimum of both functionals being impossible to reach directly (by a gradient descent for example), we propose, as in the monospectral case, approximate functionals to reach the minima. Results are finally given on satellite images and compared with those obtain by using a hierarchical stochastic model, recently proposed in [11].

2   Problem Statement

2.1   Hypothesis and Notation

The considered problem is based on partitioning the image into different areas (i.e. different classes), each area being characterized by a feature. The feature criterion we are interested in is the spatial distribution of the intensity. Of course, other discriminant features than intensity can be used by considering suitable parameters (texture parameters for example). Within this framework, a class is characterized by parameters of the spatial distribution of intensity, i.e. the mean and standard deviation for Gaussian hypothesis (covariance matrix in the multispectral data case). This work takes place in the general framework of supervised classification which means that the number and the parameters of the classes are known. These values are either given by an expert or are pre-computed by a fuzzy Cmeans algorithm with an entropy term (see [18] for instance).

General notation: Ω is an open bounded subset of $\mathbb{R}^2$. Observed data are represented by the function $I : \Omega \to \mathbb{R}$ for the monospectral case and $\boldsymbol{I} : \Omega \to \mathbb{R}^P$, that is $\boldsymbol{I} = [I^1, ..., I^P]^T$ for the multispectral case. P is the number of bands. We assume $\boldsymbol{I} \in L^2(\Omega, \mathbb{R}^P)$.

Classification notation: K is the number of classes. We assume that the number K is the same in each band, each one representing the same scene in different spectral domains. The K classes are characterized by Gaussian parameters as follows:

$$\boldsymbol{\mu}_i = \{\mu_i^p\}_{p=1...P} \quad \text{and} \quad \Sigma_i \quad \text{for} \quad i = 1, ..., K.$$

$\boldsymbol{\mu}_i$ is the mean vector of the ith class, containing the mean for each band p, and Σ_i is the $P \times P$ covariance matrix defined by $\Sigma_i^{mn} = cov(I^m(x), I^n(x))$, x in class i. Σ_i^{pp} is the variance associated to the class i for the band p. This matrix represents a measure of the correlation between bands. A diagonal matrix Σ_i means that for the class i, information in the different bands is totally decorrelated.

2.2 Variational Problem Formulation

As we assume that the repartition of the observed intensity has a Gaussian distribution within each classes, we have chosen to represent each class by its mean (variances will be take into account later in the algorithms). So the label of a class will be its mean in such a way the value of the classes constitutes an approximation of the observed data I (in the L^2 norm sense). Therefore our goal is to find an image $\bar{\boldsymbol{f}}$ such that $\bar{\boldsymbol{f}}(x) = \sum_{i=1}^{K} \chi_{\Omega_i}(x)\boldsymbol{\mu}_i$ where Ω_i is the set of pixels in class i and where the family $(\Omega_i)_{i=1..K}$ forms a partition of Ω. $\bar{\boldsymbol{f}}$ must be close to the observation $\boldsymbol{I}$ in the L^2 norm sense. A third condition is added in order to get a regular solution: $\bar{\boldsymbol{f}}$ should have minimal length discontinuity curves, or equivalently $(\Omega_i)_{i=1..K}$ should have minimal length interfaces.

In order to define a solution in a variational approach, we define a functional which the minimum has the desired properties. The unknown solution can be modelized either by using a function $\boldsymbol{f} : \Omega \to \mathbb{R}^P$ such that at the infimum $\bar{\boldsymbol{f}}$ takes its values in the set $\boldsymbol{\mu}_i, i = 1..K$, or by using sets $(\Omega_i)_{i=1..K}$ such that $\Omega_i = \{x \in \Omega, x \text{ is in class } i\}$, and $(\Omega_i)_{i=1..K}$ form a partition of Ω. In the first approach, the functional is defined as

$$J(\boldsymbol{f}) = \underbrace{\int_{\Omega} \left| \boldsymbol{f}(x) - \boldsymbol{I}(x) \right|_{\mathbb{R}^P}^2 dx}_{\text{data term}} + \underbrace{\mathcal{H}^1(S_f)}_{\text{regularization term}}$$

$$\text{and} \quad \boldsymbol{f}(x) \in \{\boldsymbol{\mu}_1, ..\boldsymbol{\mu}_K\}, \quad \forall x \in \Omega \tag{1}$$

$|.|_{\mathbb{R}^P}$ being a norm in $\mathbb{R}^P$. $\mathcal{H}^1$ denotes the 1D-Hausdorff measure and $S_{\boldsymbol{f}}$ is the set of jumps of $\boldsymbol{f}$ (which identifies to the set of discontinuities of $\boldsymbol{f}$ up to a $\mathcal{H}^1$-negligible set), see [13].

In the second approach, the functional is defined as

$$J(\Omega_1, .., \Omega_K) = \underbrace{\sum_{i=1}^{K} \int_{\Omega_i} [\boldsymbol{I} - \boldsymbol{\mu_i}]^T \Sigma_i^{-1} [\boldsymbol{I} - \boldsymbol{\mu_i}] dx}_{\text{data term}} + \underbrace{\sum_{i=1}^{K} |\Gamma_i|}_{\text{regularization term}}$$

$$\text{and} \quad \{\Omega_i\}_{i=1..K} \text{ is a partition of } \Omega \tag{2}$$

where $\Gamma_i = \partial \Omega_i \cap \Omega$. $|\Gamma_i| = \mathcal{H}^1(\Gamma_i)$ is the one-dimensional measure of Hausdorff of the set Γ_i.

Despite of the fact that the covariance matrix Σ_i is not taken into account in the expression of $J(\boldsymbol{f})$ in (1) (it will be introduce later), both functionals $J(\boldsymbol{f})$ in (1) and $J(\Omega_1, .., \Omega_K)$ in (2) define same constraints on the solution. Minimizing (1) w.r.t $\boldsymbol{f}$ or (2) w.r.t Ω_i is a difficult task since the functionals involve terms of different nature (1D versus 2D terms) and the unknown in (2) are sets and not functions. For each case and for monospectral data, we have developed a method that overcome this difficulty (see [27] and [26]). We present here the methods for multispectral data.

3   Classification with Restoration

Computing a minimum for the functional (1) is difficult due to the presence of 1D regularization term which acts on the discontinuity set of the unknown variable $\boldsymbol{f}$. Based on mathematical results of Γ-convergence for fluid mechanic, we have proposed in [27] to minimize a sequence of functionals. The extension to multispectral data give the following sequence of functionals

$$J_\varepsilon(\boldsymbol{f}) = \underbrace{\int_\Omega \left| \boldsymbol{f}(x) - \boldsymbol{I}(x) \right|^2_{\mathbb{R}^P} dx}_{\text{data term}} + \underbrace{\varepsilon \lambda^2 \int_\Omega \varphi(|\boldsymbol{\nabla} \boldsymbol{f}(x)|_{\mathbb{R}^P}) dx}_{\text{restoration term}} + \underbrace{\frac{\eta^2}{\varepsilon} \int_\Omega W(\boldsymbol{f}(x)) dx}_{\text{classification}},$$

$$\tag{3}$$

and the associated problem consists in finding $\boldsymbol{f}_0$ such as:

$$\boldsymbol{f}_0 = \lim_{\varepsilon \to 0^+} \left[\arg\min_{\boldsymbol{f}} J_\varepsilon(\boldsymbol{f}) \right]. \tag{4}$$

The parameters λ and η are fixed, ε varies. Let us first consider the functional with a fixed ε. The first two terms of (3) are standard for noisy image restoration by anisotropic regularization [10, 21]. Function φ is a smoothing function that will be defined later.

The third term of (3) is a level constraint such that $W : \mathbb{R}^P \to \mathbb{R}^+$ attracts the values of $\boldsymbol{f}(x)$ towards the means $\boldsymbol{\mu_i}$ of classes i, taking into account the

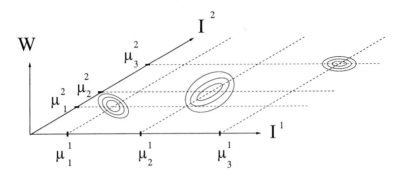

Fig. 1. Vector-valued potential W projected on plane (I^1, I^2) in case of 2 bands and 3 classes.

covariance Σ_i. W has K minima for the values μ_i such that $W(\mu_i) = 0$, $\forall\ i$. W is quadratic in $\mathbb{R}^P$ around each minima (from the Gaussian distribution hypothesis), as illustrated on Figure 1. W is defined by

$$W(f(x)) = \min_{i=1,\dots,K}[f(x) - \mu_i]^T \Sigma_i^{-1}[f(x) - \mu_i] \tag{5}$$

where Σ_i^{-1} is the inverse of the covariance matrix. We can remark that such a W potential is not differentiable at the junction points of the multidimensional parabola. We have not noticed, in the experiences conducted till now, instabilities which could be due to this non differentiability points. However, it should be interesting to construct smoother potential W by building $C^1(\mathbb{R}^P)$ junctions.

Considering a sequence of criteria J_ε when $\varepsilon \to 0$ is inspired from works conducted in the Van der Waals-Cahn-Hilliard theory framework for phase transitions in fluid mechanic [2, 29].

The minimization problem (4) relies upon Γ-convergence arguments [2, 29]. If $\varphi(t) = t^2$, then we can show from [2] that the sequence of functionals (3) Γ-converges to

$$\begin{cases} J_0(f) = \sum_{i=1}^{K} \int_{\Omega_i} |\mu_i - I|_{\mathbb{R}^P}^2 dx + \lambda \sum_{i,j=1}^{K} d(\mu_i, \mu_j)\mathcal{H}^1(\Gamma_{ij}) \\ \qquad \text{if } f \in BV(\Omega), \text{ and } W(f(x)) = 0 \text{ a.e.} \\ J_0(f) = +\infty, \quad \text{otherwise} \end{cases} \tag{6}$$

where Γ_{ij} is the interface between regions Ω_i and Ω_j and $BV(\Omega)$ is the space of functions of bounded variation [13]. The distance d is defined by:

$$d(\mu_i, \mu_j) = \inf_g \left\{ \int_0^1 \sqrt{W(g(s))}|g'(s)|ds;\ g \in C^1([0;1], \mathbb{R}^P) \right.$$

$$\left. \text{and } g > 0,\ g(0) = \mu_i,\ g(1) = \mu_j \right\} \tag{7}$$

From the Γ-convergence theory we know that the sequence of minimizers f_ε of $J_\varepsilon(f)$ converges (up to a subsequence) to a minimizer of J_0. Moreover, f_0 has the form

$$\boldsymbol{f}_0(x) = \sum_{i=1}^{K} \mu_i \chi_{\Omega_i}(x) \tag{8}$$

where χ_{Ω_i} is the characteristic function of Ω_i. So $\boldsymbol{f}_0$ defines a partition of Ω according to the predefined classes, with minimal interfaces with respect to the weighted length (7). Notice that we have not exactly reached the desired minimum of (1) since the regularization term is a weighted distance in $J_0(\boldsymbol{f})$.

From the numerical point of view, when ε varies, the functional turns from a restoration process (the third term in (3) is negligeable) into a classification process.

We have used an edge-preserving regularizing function $\varphi(t) = \frac{t^2}{1+t^2}$ because it numerically gives better results, by preserving high gradients which represent edges [10]. The theoretical justification of the Γ-limit using this function rather the quadratic one is under consideration.

For the numerical minimization of J_ε for a fixed ε, we use the half-quadratic decomposition of functions φ as in [10, 15], in order to avoid nonlinearities in the Euler-Lagrange equations associated to the minimization of (3). By introducing an auxiliary variable $b : \mathbb{R}^2 \to \mathbb{R}$, the minimization of (3) is replaced by the minimization of $J_\varepsilon^*(\boldsymbol{f}, b)$ with respect to $(\boldsymbol{f}, b)$, with:

$$J_\varepsilon^*(\boldsymbol{f}, b) = \int_\Omega \left| \boldsymbol{f}(x) - \boldsymbol{I}(x) \right|_{\mathbb{R}^P}^2 dx + \varepsilon \lambda^2 \int_\Omega \left[b(x)|\boldsymbol{\nabla}\boldsymbol{f}(x)|_{\mathbb{R}^P}^2 + \psi(b(x)) \right] dx$$

$$+ \frac{\eta^2}{\varepsilon} \int_\Omega W(\boldsymbol{f}(x)) dx, \tag{9}$$

where ψ is a convex function with respect to b, defined from φ. Then for each fixed ε value, we solve alternately the Euler-Lagrange equations

$$\begin{cases} b = \psi'^{-1}(-|\boldsymbol{\nabla}\boldsymbol{f}|_{\mathbb{R}^P}^2) \stackrel{[10]}{=} \frac{\varphi'(|\boldsymbol{\nabla}\boldsymbol{f}|_{\mathbb{R}^P})}{2|\boldsymbol{\nabla}\boldsymbol{f}|_{\mathbb{R}^P}} \in \mathbb{R} \text{ with } \boldsymbol{f} \text{ fixed,} \\ \boldsymbol{f} - \lambda^2 \varepsilon \, div(b\boldsymbol{\nabla}\boldsymbol{f}) + \frac{\eta^2}{2\varepsilon} W'(\boldsymbol{f}) = \boldsymbol{I}, \text{ with } b \text{ fixed.} \end{cases} \tag{10}$$

For each ε a solution is computed, which is used to initialize the system (10) for a new value of ε.

Remark on the calculus of $|\boldsymbol{\nabla}\boldsymbol{f}|_{\mathbb{R}^P}$

In order to use inter-band informations for the restoration process, we can replace in equations (10) the divergence term $div(b\boldsymbol{\nabla}\boldsymbol{f})$ by $div(\sqrt{\lambda_+ - \lambda_-}\theta_+)$ where λ_+ and λ_- are respectively the highest and the lowest eigenvalues of the first fundamental form matrix of $\boldsymbol{f}$, and θ_+ is the eigenvector associated to λ_+, that is the direction of the highest slope. This gives an anisotropic smoothing of $\boldsymbol{f}$ along the direction of highest variation. Such smoothing has been first introduced in [33], and also used in [6, 28, 32].

4   Classification by a Dynamical Model

In the second approach, the unknown variables are the sets $\{\Omega_i\}_{i=1..K}$ and the classification problem is stated as a partitioning problem according to the pre-defined classes. Let Ω_i be the region defined as

$$\Omega_i = \{x \in \Omega/x \text{ belongs to the } i^{th} \text{ class}\}. \tag{11}$$

A partitioning of Ω consists of finding a set $\{\Omega_i\}_{i=1...K}$ such that

$$\Omega = \bigcup_{i=1}^{K} \left(\Omega_i \bigcup \Gamma_i\right) \quad \text{and} \quad \Omega_i \bigcap_{i \neq j} \Omega_j = \varnothing. \tag{12}$$

where $\Gamma_i = \partial\Omega_i \cap \Omega$. The interface between Ω_i and Ω_j is denoted by $\Gamma_{ij} = \Gamma_{ji} = \Gamma_i \cap \Gamma_j$, $\forall i \neq j$. We have $\Gamma_i = \bigcup_{j \neq i} \Gamma_{ij}$. $|\Gamma_i| = \mathcal{H}^1(\Gamma_i)$ is the one-dimensional measure of Hausdorff of the set Γ_i satisfying

$$|\Gamma_i| = \sum_{j \neq i} |\Gamma_{ij}| \text{ with } |\varnothing| = 0. \tag{13}$$

We are looking for sets Ω_i such that $\{\Omega_i\}_{i=1...K}$ is a partition of Ω, and such that the Ω_i's define a classification of the observed data $\boldsymbol{I}$, taking into account the gaussian distribution property of the classes (data term). We also impose that the partition is regular in the sense that the sum of the length of interfaces Γ_{ij} is minimum. The functional to minimize is then the one proposed in (2).

In order to change the minimization problem w.r.t the sets Ω_i into a mini-mization problem w.r.t. functions, we have proposed to the use level set method (see [26] for the monospectral data case). Let $\Phi_i : \Omega \rightarrow \mathbb{R}$ be a Lipschitz function associated to the region Ω_i such that $\Phi_i(x) > 0$ if $x \in \Omega_i$, $\Phi_i(x) = 0$ if $x \in \Gamma_i$ and $\Phi_i(x) < 0$ otherwise.

Thus, the region Ω_i is entirely described by the function Φ_i. The resulting model proposed in [26] is inspired from the work of Zhao et al. about multiphase evolution [34], and takes place in the general framework of active contours [8, 9, 16, 19] for region segmentation [24, 35]. For the multispectral data, we propose to minimize

$$F_\alpha(\Phi_1, ..., \Phi_K) = \underbrace{\sum_{i=1}^{K} e_i \int_\Omega H_\alpha(\Phi_i)[\boldsymbol{I} - \mu_i]^T \Sigma_i^{-1}[\boldsymbol{I} - \mu_i]dx}_{\text{mutlispectral data term}}$$

$$+ \underbrace{\sum_{i=1}^{K} \gamma_i \int_\Omega \delta_\alpha(\Phi_i)|\nabla\Phi_i|dx}_{\text{minimization of contour length}} + \underbrace{\frac{\lambda}{2} \int_\Omega \left(\sum_{i=1}^{K} H_\alpha(\Phi_i) - 1\right)^2 dx}_{\text{partition constraint}} \tag{14}$$

where H_α and δ_α are smooth approximations of respectively the Heaviside function H and the Dirac δ distribution. The parameters e_i, γ_i and λ are positive real fixed numbers. The partition constraint is introduced thanks to the third term in (14). As $\alpha \to 0^+$, this term penalizes the formation of vacuum (pixels with no label) and regions overlapping (pixels with more than one label).

By using the coaera formula, we show that [26]

$$\lim_{\alpha \to 0} \int_\Omega \delta_\alpha(\Phi_i(x))|\nabla\Phi_i(x)|dx = |\Gamma_i|.$$

The limiting functional, when $\alpha \to 0$, is:

$$F_0(\Phi_1,...,\Phi_K) = \underbrace{\sum_{i=1}^K e_i \int_{\Omega_i} [I - \mu_i]^T \Sigma_i^{-1}[I - \mu_i]dx}_{\text{data term}} + \underbrace{\sum_{i=1}^K \gamma_i|\Gamma_i|}_{\text{minimization of contour length}}$$

$$+ \underbrace{\frac{\lambda}{2} \int_\Omega \Big(\sum_{i=1}^K H(\Phi_i) - 1\Big)^2 dx}_{\text{partition constraint (cond. A)}} \qquad (15)$$

As $\alpha \to 0^+$, the solution set $\{\Phi_i\}_i$ minimizing $F_\alpha(\Phi_1,...,\Phi_K)$, if it exists, defines a classification compound of homogeneous classes (the so-called Ω_i phases) separated by regularized interfaces, as defined in (2).

Based on numerical results, we have introduced a weighted length term, in order to get improved results. Let $g : \mathbb{R} \to \mathbb{R}^+$ defined by $g(|\nabla I|_\mathbb{R}) = \frac{1}{1+|\nabla I(x)|_\mathbb{R}^2}$, so that it vanishes around high gradients of I. This a standard stopping function used in active contours. This stopping function is introduced in the length term in order to enforce the contours of the classification to be stopped around the high gradients of the data I. The functional we minimize is then

$$F_\alpha(\Phi_1,...,\Phi_K) = \underbrace{\sum_{i=1}^K e_i \int_\Omega H_\alpha(\Phi_i)[I - \mu_i]^T \Sigma_i^{-1}[I - \mu_i]dx}_{\text{mutlispectral data term}}$$

$$+ \underbrace{\sum_{i=1}^K \gamma_i \int_\Omega g(|\nabla I|)\delta_\alpha(\Phi_i)|\nabla\Phi_i|dx}_{\text{minimization of contour weighted length}} + \underbrace{\frac{\lambda}{2} \int_\Omega \Big(\sum_{i=1}^K H_\alpha(\Phi_i) - 1\Big)^2 dx}_{\text{partition constraint}} \qquad (16)$$

To minimize the functional (16), we derive the K Euler -Lagrange equations with respect to the K functions Φ_i. These equations are embedded in a dynamical scheme, where the variable t is the time parameter:

$$\Phi_i^{t+1} = \Phi_i^t - dt\Big\{\delta_\alpha(\Phi_i^t)\Big[e_i[I - \mu_i]^T \Sigma_i^{-1}[I - \mu_i] - \gamma_i g(|\nabla I|)div\Big(\frac{\nabla\Phi_i^t}{|\nabla\Phi_i^t|}\Big)$$

$$-\gamma_i \frac{\nabla g \nabla\Phi_i^t}{|\nabla\Phi_i^t|} + \lambda\Big(\sum_{j=1}^K H_\alpha(\Phi_j^t) - 1\Big)\Big]\Big\} \qquad (17)$$

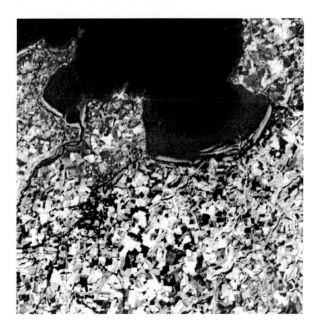

Fig. 2. SPOT Multispectral data (XS3 band) of Lannion bay (August 1997) after histogram equalization.

The K PDEs are coupled through the partition term $\left(\sum_{j=1}^{K} H_\alpha(\Phi_j^t) - 1\right)$. The evolution of each Φ_i is guided by three different forces constraining the solution to be a regular partition of Ω according to the classification of the data. The functions Φ_i are defined as signed distance functions to the zero level set. In order to preserve the constraint $|\nabla\Phi_i| = 1$ (cf. [3, 14]) during the algorithm, the functions Φ_i are regularly updated by using the PDE proposed by Sussman *et al.* [30]: $\frac{\partial \Phi_i}{\partial t} = sign(\Phi_i)(1 - |\nabla\Phi_i|)$.

The parameters are tuned by trial and error according to the dimension and morphology of the regions (for the weights of the length term), and according to the noise (for the weights of the data term). The functions Φ_i are automatically initialized by dividing the image support Ω into N_W windows $W_{n,\,n=1..N_W}$ with a fixed size. In each window, we compute the mean $\boldsymbol{m_n}$ and the standard deviation $\boldsymbol{\sigma_n}$ and we search for the nearest class, that is the k index such that $k = arg\min_j d_B(\mathcal{N}_{(m_p,\sigma_p)}, \mathcal{N}_{(\mu_j,\sigma_j)})$, where d_B is the Bhattacharyya distance [5] which allows to measure the distance between two Gaussian distributions. We do not take into account the correlation between bands for this initialization. Let us remark that the smallest object which could be detected is linked to the size of the initial windows W_n.

5   Results on SPOT Data

We present some results on SPOT data of Lannion Bay in France (see Figure 2) provided from SPOTIMAGE. These data have been used to study and measure

Table 1. For each class: number of **mis** classified pixels and rate of **success** according to the algorithm. Last line is the total of pixels used for the ground truth (GT).

CLASSES

	1 ■ sea water	2 ▦ sand uncovered grounds	3 ■ urban aeras	4 ■ woods heath	5 ▦ grasslands	6 ■ pasturelands	7 ■ vegetables	8 ▦ corn	total
MV	16 (96%)	77 (76%)	119 (63%)	1 (93%)	54 (49%)	182 (4%)	5 (0%)	58 (56%)	512 (65%)
ICM-N0	16 (96%)	73 (77%)	103 (68%)	1 (93%)	50 (53%)	189 (1%)	5 (0%)	61 (54%)	498 (66%)
H-MAP	16 (96%)	76 (76%)	63 (81%)	1 (93%)	41 (61%)	177 (7%)	5 (0%)	54 (59%)	433 (71%)
M1	0 (100%)	79 (75%)	93 (71%)	2 (86%)	52 (51%)	146 (23%)	4 (20%)	44 (67%)	421 (71%)
M2	0 (100%)	105 (67%)	101 (69%)	9 (36%)	41 (61%)	160 (16%)	5 (0%)	19 (86%)	440 (70%)
pix. nb for GT	376	320	323	14	106	190	5	132	1466

how intensive culture changes ground use in this area. A complete study has been made during the PhD thesis of Annabelle Chardin [11] conducted at IRISA in the VISTA research group[1]. She developed a hierchical Markov Random Field model for classification (called H-MAP) and compared her results with those obtained by a Maximum Likelihood (ML) estimator (classification without any restoration) or with those obtained by the restriction of her algorithm at the highest level (called ICM N0). (M1) (resp. (M2)) stands for the first (resp. second) variational model presented in this paper. We also have ground truth given by geographers from COSTEL of Rennes University. The number of classes has been fixed by these experts. They have also chosen small rectangular areas for the estimation of the parameters of the classes and others small rectangular areas for validation with ground truth. The original image is 1480×1024 pixels, and we present results on a portion 400×400 pixels as shown in Figure 2. The classified images are presented on Figure 3 with the corresponding legend presented in Table 1. Numerical results according to ground truth available on small areas of the image are also listed in Table 1.

6   Comments and Conclusion

By visualizing images on Figure 3, we can see that the ML estimator (classification without restoration) results in a noisy image with a lot of small regions which give nonhomogeneous areas. On the contrary, the visually smoothest result is the one given by applying (M2). This is mainly due to the initialization

---

[1] We thank the VISTA research group to have so kindly let these data be available for comparison with our methods.

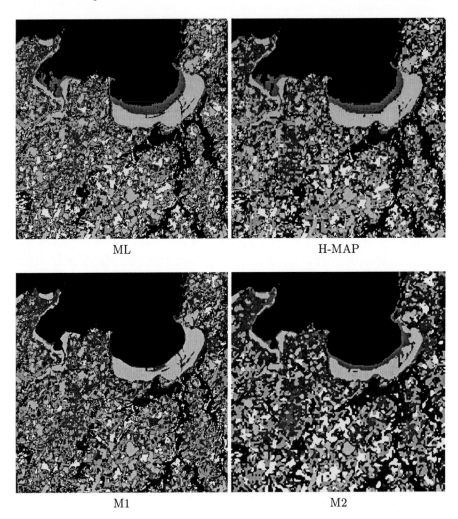

Fig. 3. Results of classification by ML, H-MAP, M1 and M2 (color image).

process where the regions are initialized on windows of 5×5 pixels, limiting the spatial resolution of the model. This is not due to the regularization term (length minimization) because we have some points with high curvature. On (H-MAP) image, we note that contours are mainly horizontal and vertical because of the first order Markov random field (Potts model) used in this approach [11].

Looking at the numerical results in Table 1, the first remark is that classes 4 and 7 are not significant because the number of pixels in the ground truth is too small (14 and 5 respectively). The second remark is that we have mixed classes between classes 5 and 6, which probably explain the bad results obtained for these classes. For the class 3 (urban aeras), we should have taken into account texture parameters rather than grey level values for the classification. It seems that the hierarchical model (H-MAP) is more robust with respect to this bad

modeling. Model (M2) gives smaller performance for class 2 mainly because it is compound of small regions which are not catched at the initialization procedure (5 × 5 pixel windows). This model however gives better results for class 8.
It is difficult to give a general conclusion with respect to the use of these different approaches for classification. Firstly, the number of pixels for the ground truth is too small to analyse results. Notice that the selected areas for estimating the class parameters (different from the previous ones) are sufficient. Secondly, we should also need the evaluation of experts on the final classified images. Thirdly, we should also take into account the computational time for the comparison (for more details see [25]).

References

1. L. Alvarez, P.-L. Lions, and J.-M. Morel. Image selective smoothing and edge detection by nonlinear diffusion. *SIAM J. of Numerical Analysis*, 29(3):845–866, 1992.
2. S. Baldo. Minimal interface criterion for phase transitions in mixtures of Cahn-Hilliard fluids. *Ann. Inst. Henri Poincaré*, 7:67–90, 1990.
3. G. Barles, H. M. Soner, and P.E. Souganidis. Front propagation and phase field theory. *SIAM J. Control and Optimization*, 31:439–479, 1993.
4. M. Berthod, Z. Kato, S. Yu, and J. Zerubia. Bayesian image classification using Markov random fields. *Image and Vision Computing*, 14(4):285–293, 1996.
5. C. Bhattacharyya. A simple method of resolution of a distribution into Gaussian components. *Biometrics*, 23(4):115–135, 1967.
6. P. Blomgren and T.F. Chan. Color TV: Total variation methods for restoration of vector-valued images. *IEEE Trans. on Image Procesing*, 7(3):304–309, March 1998. Special issue on partial differential equations and geometry driven diffusion in image processing and analysis.
7. C.A. Bouman and M. Shapiro. A multiscale random field model for Bayesian image segmentation. *IEEE Trans. on Image Processing*, 3:162–177, March 1994.
8. V. Caselles, F. Catte, T. Coll, and F. Dibos. A geometric model for active contours. *Numerische Mathematik*, 66:1–31, 1993.
9. V. Caselles, R. Kimmel, and G. Sapiro. Geodesic active contours. *International J. of Computer Vision*, 22(1):61–79, 1997.
10. P. Charbonnier, L. Blanc-Féraud, G. Aubert, and M. Barlaud. Deterministic edge-preserving regularization in computed imaging. *IEEE Trans. on Image Processing*, 6(2):298–311, February 1997.
11. A. Chardin. *Modèles énergétiques hiérarchiques pour la résolution des problèmes inverses en analyse d'images*. PhD thesis, Université de Rennes I, France, 2000.
12. X. Descombes, R. Morris, and J. Zerubia. Some improvements to Bayesian image segmentation. Part two : classification. (in french). *Traitement du Signal*, 14(4):383–395, 1997.
13. L. C. Evans and R. F. Gariepy. *Measure theory and fine properties of functions*. CRC Press, 1992.
14. L.C. Evans and J. Spruck. Motion of level sets by mean curvature. part II. *Trans. of the American Mathematical Society*, 330(1):321–332, 1992.
15. D. Geman and G. Reynolds. Constrained restoration and the recovery of discontinuities. *IEEE Trans. on Pattern Analysis and Machine Intelligence*, 14(3):367–383, 1992.

16. M. Kass, A. Witkin, and D. Terzopoulos. Snakes : active contour models. *International J. of Computer Vision*, 1:321–331, 1987.
17. Z. Kato. *Multiresolution Markovian modeling for computer vision. Application to SPOT image segmentation (in French and English)*. PhD thesis, Université de Nice-Sophia Antipolis, France, 1994.
18. A. Lorette, X. Descombes, and J. Zerubia. Texture analysis through a Markovian modelling and fuzzy classification: application to urban area extraction from satellite images. *International Journal of Computer Vision*, 36(3):221–236, 2000.
19. R. Malladi, J.A. Sethian, and B.C. Vemuri. Evolutionary fronts for topology independent shape modeling and recovery. In *Proc. of the 3rd ECCV*, pages 3–13, Stockholm, Sweden, 1994.
20. R. March. Visual reconstruction using variational methods. *Image and Vision Computing*, 10:30–38, 1992.
21. J.-M. Morel and S. Solimini. *Variational methods in image segmentation*. Birkhäuser, 1995.
22. D. Mumford and J. Shah. Boundary detection by minimizing functionals. In *Proc. IEEE Conf. on Computer Vision and Pattern Recognition*, San Francisco, 1985.
23. T. Pavlidis and Y.-T. Liow. Integrating region growing and edge detection. In *Proc. of IEEE CVPR*, 1988.
24. R. Ronfard. Region-based strategies for active contour models. *International J. of Computer Vision*, 13(2):229–251, 1994.
25. C. Samson. *Contribution la classification d'images satellitaires par approche variationnelle et équations aux dérivées partielles*. PhD thesis, Université de Nice-Sophia Antipolis, France, Septembre 2000.
26. C. Samson, L. Blanc-Féraud, G. Aubert, and J. Zerubia. A level set model for image classification. *International Journal of Computer Vision*, 40(3):189–197, December 2000.
27. C. Samson, L. Blanc-Féraud, G. Aubert, and J. Zerubia. A variational model for image classification and restoration. *IEEE Trans. on Pattern Analysis and Machine Intelligence*, 22(5):460–472, May 2000.
28. G. Sapiro and D.L. Ringach. Anisotropic diffusion of multivalued images with applications to color filtering. *IEEE Trans. on Image Procesing*, 5(11):1582–1586, November 1996.
29. P. Sternberg and W.P. Zeimer. Local minimisers of a three-phase partition problem with triple junctions. *Proc. of the Royal Society of Edinburgh*, 124(A):1059–1073, 1994.
30. M. Sussman, P. Smereka, and S. Osher. A level set approach for computing solutions to incompressible two-phase flow. *J. of Computational Physics*, 114:146–159, 1994.
31. P. C. Teo, G. Sapiro, and B. A. Wandell. Creating connected representations of cortical gray matter for functional MRI visualization. *IEEE Trans. on Medical Imaging*, 16(6):852–863, 1997.
32. R. Whitaker and G. Gerig. *Vector-valued diffusion*. in computational imaging and vision: geometry driven diffusion in computer vision, Kluwer, 1994.
33. S. Di Zenzo. A note on the gradient of a multi-image. *CVGIP*, 33:116–125, 1986.
34. H-K. Zhao, T. Chan, B. Merriman, and S. Osher. A variational level set approach to multiphase motion. *J. of Computational Physics*, 127:179–195, 1996.
35. S. C. Zhu and A. Yuille. Integrating region growing and edge detection. *IEEE Trans. on Pattern Analysis and Machine Intelligence*, 18(9):884–900, 1996.

Part IV

Optimization and Graphs

An Experimental Comparison
of Min-cut/Max-flow Algorithms
for Energy Minimization in Vision

Yuri Boykov[1] and Vladimir Kolmogorov[2]

[1] Siemens Corporate Research, Imaging & Visualization, Princeton NJ 08540, USA
yuri@scr.siemens.com
[2] Cornell University, Computer Science, Upson Hall, Ithaca NY 14853, USA
vnk@cs.cornell.edu

Abstract. After [10, 15, 12, 2, 4] minimum cut/maximum flow algorithms on graphs emerged as an increasingly useful tool for exact or approximate energy minimization in low-level vision. The combinatorial optimization literature provides many min-cut/max-flow algorithms with different polynomial time complexity. Their practical efficiency, however, has to date been studied mainly outside the scope of computer vision. The goal of this paper is to provide an experimental comparison of the efficiency of min-cut/max flow algorithms for energy minimization in vision. We compare the running times of several standard algorithms, as well as a new algorithm that we have recently developed. The algorithms we study include both Goldberg-style "push-relabel" methods and algorithms based on Ford-Fulkerson style augmenting paths. We benchmark these algorithms on a number of typical graphs in the contexts of image restoration, stereo, and interactive segmentation. In many cases our new algorithm works several times faster than any of the other methods making near real-time performance possible.

1 Introduction

Greig et. al. [10] were first to discover that powerful min-cut/max-flow algorithms from combinatorial optimization can be used to minimize certain important energy functions in vision. The energies addressed by Greig et. al. and by most later graph based methods (e.g. [15, 12, 2, 11, 4, 1, 18, 13, 16, 17, 3, 14]) can be represented as a posterior energy in MAP-MRF[1] framework:

$$E(L) = \sum_{p \in \mathcal{P}} D_p(L_p) + \sum_{(p,q) \in \mathcal{N}} V_{p,q}(L_p, L_q), \qquad (1)$$

where $L = \{L_p \,|\, p \in \mathcal{P}\}$ is a labeling of image $\mathcal{P}$, $D_p(\cdot)$ is a data penalty function, $V_{p,q}$ is an interaction potential, and $\mathcal{N}$ is a set of all pairs of neighboring pixels. Papers above show that, to date, graph based energy minimization methods provide arguably the most accurate solutions for the specified applications.

---

[1] MAP-MRF stands for Maximum *A Posterior* estimation of a Markov Random Field.

M.A.T. Figueiredo, J. Zerubia, A.K. Jain (Eds.): EMMCVPR 2001, LNCS 2134, pp. 359–374, 2001.

Greig et.al. constructed a two terminal graph such that the minimum cost cut of the graph gives a globally optimal binary labeling L in case of the Potts model of interaction in (1). Previously, exact minimization of energies like (1) was not possible and such energies were approached mainly with iterative algorithms like simulated annealing. In fact, Greig et.al. used their result to show that in practice simulated annealing reaches solutions very far from the global minimum even in very simple image restoration examples.

Unfortunately, the result of Greig et.al. remained unnoticed for almost 10 years mainly because the binary labeling limitation looked too restrictive. In the late 90's new computer vision techniques appeared that used min-cut/max-flow algorithms on graphs. [15] was the first to use these algorithms to compute multi-camera stereo. Later, [12, 2] showed that with the right edge weights on a similar to [15] graph one can minimize the energy in (1) for linear interaction penalties. The exact minimum could be computed when there are more than two labels. The results in [2, 4] showed that iteratively running min-cut/max-flow algorithms on appropriate graphs can be used to find provably good approximate solutions for even more general multi-label case when interaction penalties are *metrics*.

A growing number of publications in vision use graph based energy minimization techniques for applications like image segmentation [12, 18, 13, 3], restoration [10], stereo [15, 2, 11, 14], shape reconstruction [16], object recognition [1], augmented reality [17], and others. The graphs corresponding to these applications are usually huge 2D or 3D grids, and min-cut/max-flow algorithm efficiency is an issue that can not be ignored.

The goal of this paper is to compare experimentally the speed of several min-cut/max-flow algorithms on graphs typical for applications in vision. In Section 2 we provide basic facts about graphs, min-cut and max-flow problems, and some standard combinatorial optimization algorithms for them. Section 3 introduces a new min-cut/max-flow algorithm that we developed while working with graphs in vision. In Section 4 we tested our new algorithm and three standard min-cut/max-flow algorithms: H_PRF and Q_PRF versions of Goldberg-style "push-relabel" method [9, 5], and the Dinic algorithm [7]. We selected several examples in image restoration, stereo, and segmentation where different forms of energy (1) are minimized via graph structures originally described in [10, 12, 2, 4, 14, 3]. Such (or very similar) graphs are used in all computer vision papers known to us that use graph cut algorithms. In many interesting cases our new algorithm was significantly faster than the standard min-cut/max-flow techniques from combinatorial optimization. More detailed conclusions are presented in Section 5.

2   Background on Graphs

In this section we review some basic facts about graphs in the context of energy minimization methods in vision. A graph $\mathcal{G} = \langle \mathcal{V}, \mathcal{E} \rangle$ consists of a set of nodes $\mathcal{V}$ and a set of directed edges $\mathcal{E}$ that connect them. Usually the nodes correspond to pixels, voxels, or other features. A graph normally contains some additional special nodes that are called terminals. In the context of vision, terminals cor-

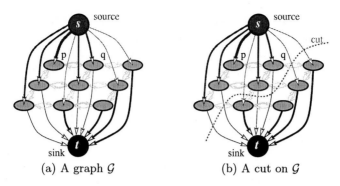

Fig. 1. Example of a graph. Edge costs are reflected by their thickness. This graph construction was first used in Greig et. al. [10].

respond to the set of labels that can be assigned to pixels. We will concentrate on the case of graphs with two terminals. Then the terminals are usually called the *source*, s, and the *sink*, t. In Figure 1(a) we show a simple example of a two terminal graph (due to Greig et. al. [10]) that can be used to minimize the Potts case of energy (1) on a 3×3 image with two labels. There is some variation in the structure of graphs used in other energy minimization methods in vision. However, most of them are based on regular 2D or 3D grid graphs as the one in Figure 1(a). This is a simple consequence of the fact that normal images (or volume data) in vision have grid-like structures.

All edges in the graph are assigned some weight or cost. A cost of a directed edge (p, q) may differ from the cost of the reverse edge (q, p). Normally, there are two types of edges in the graph: n-links and t-links. N-links connect pairs of neighboring pixels or voxels. Thus, they represent a neighborhood system in the image. Cost of n-links corresponds to a penalty for discontinuity between the pixels. These costs are usually derived from the pixel interaction term $V_{p,q}$ in energy (1). T-links connect pixels with terminals (labels). The cost of a t-link connecting a pixel and a terminal corresponds to a penalty for assigning the corresponding label to the pixel. This cost is normally derived from the data term D_p in the energy function (1).

2.1   Min-cut and Max-flow Problems

An s/t cut (or just a *cut*) C on a graph with two terminals is a partitioning of the nodes in the graph into two disjoint subsets $\mathcal{S}$ and $\mathcal{T}$ such that the source s is in $\mathcal{S}$ and the sink t is in $\mathcal{T}$. Figure 1(b) shows one example of a cut. In combinatorial optimization the cost of a cut $C = \{\mathcal{S}, \mathcal{T}\}$ is defined as the sum of the costs of "boundary" edges (p, q) where $p \in \mathcal{S}$ and $q \in \mathcal{T}$. The *minimum cut* problem on a graph is to find a cut that has the minimum cost among all cuts.

One of the fundamental results in combinatorial optimization is that the minimum s/t cut problem can be solved by finding a *maximum flow* from the source s to the sink t. Loosely speaking, maximum flow is the maximum "amount of water" that can be sent from the source to the sink by interpreting graph edges as directed "pipes" with capacities equal to edge weights. The theorem of Ford and Fulkerson [8] states that a maximum flow from s to t saturates a set of edges in the graph dividing the nodes into two disjoint parts $\{S, T\}$ corresponding to a minimum cut. Thus, min-cut and max-flow problems are equivalent. In fact, the maximum flow value is equal to the cost of the minimum cut.

We can also intuitively show how min-cut (or max-flow) on a graph may help with energy minimization over image labelings. Consider an example in Figure 1. The graph corresponds to a 3×3 image. Any s/t cut partitions the nodes into disjoint groups each containing exactly one terminal. Therefore, any cut corresponds to some assignment of pixels (nodes) to labels (terminals). If edge weights are appropriately set based on parameters of an energy, a minimum cost cut will correspond to a labeling with the minimum value of this energy[2].

2.2   Standard Algorithms in Combinatorial Optimization

An important fact in combinatorial optimization is that there are polynomial algorithms for min-cut/max-flow problems on graphs with two terminals. These algorithms can be divided into two main groups: Goldberg-style "push-relabel" methods and algorithms based on Ford-Fulkerson style augmenting paths.

Standard augmenting paths based algorithms, such as Dinic algorithm, work by pushing flow along non-saturated paths from the source to the sink until the maximum flow in the graph G is reached. A typical augmenting path algorithm stores information about the distribution of the current $s \to t$ flow f among the edges of G using a *residual graph* G_f. The topology of G_f is identical to G but capacity of an edge in G_f reflects the residual capacity of the same edge in G given the amount of flow already in the edge. At the initialization there is no flow from the source to the sink (f=0) and edge capacities in the residual graph G_0 are equal to the original capacities in G. At each new iteration the algorithm finds the shortest $s \to t$ path along non-saturated edges of the residual graph. If a path is found then the algorithm *augments* it by pushing the maximum possible flow df that saturates at least one of the edges in the path. The residual capacities of edges in the path are reduced by df while the residual capacities of the reverse edges are increased by df. Each augmentation increases the total flow from the source to the sink $f = f + df$. The maximum flow is reached when any $s \to t$ path crosses at least one saturated edge in the residual graph G_f.

Dinic algorithm uses breadth-first search to find the shortest paths from s to t on the residual graph G_f. After all shortest paths of a fixed length k are saturated, the algorithm starts the breadth-first search for $s \to t$ paths of length $k + 1$ from scratch. Note that the use of shortest paths is an important factor that improves running time complexities for algorithms based on augmenting paths. The worst case running time complexity for Dinic algorithm is $O(mn^2)$ where n is the number of nodes and m is the number of edges in the graph.

---

[2] Different graph based energy minimization methods may use different graph constructions, as well as, different rules for converting graph cuts into image labelings. Details for each method are described in the original publications.

Push-relabel algorithms use quite a different approach. They do not maintain a valid flow during the operation; each node may have a positive "flow excess", and the algorithm tries to push it to neighboring nodes. Push-relabel techniques are harder to describe in just a few sentences and we would rather refer the reader to our favorite text-book on basic graph theory and algorithms [6].

For our experimental tests on graph-based energy minimization methods in vision we selected the following standard algorithms.

DINIC: Algorithm of Dinic [7].
H_PRF: Push-Relabel algorithm [9] with the highest level selection rule.
Q_PRF: Push-Relabel algorithm [9] with the queue based selection rule.

Many previous experimental tests, including the results in [5], show that the last two algorithms work consistently better than a large number of other min-cut/max-flow algorithms of combinatorial optimization. The theoretical worst case complexities for these "push-relabel" algorithms are $O(n^3)$ for Q_PRF and $O(n^2\sqrt{m})$ for H_PRF.

3   New Min-cut/Max-flow Algorithm

In this section we present a new algorithm that we developed while working with graphs that are typical for energy minimization methods in computer vision. The algorithm presented here belongs to the group of algorithms based on augmenting paths. Similarly to DINIC it builds the search tree for finding augmenting paths but it reuses this tree and never starts building it from scratch. The drawback of our approach is that the augmenting paths found are not necessarily shortest augmenting path; thus the time complexity of the shortest augmenting path is no longer valid. The trivial upper bound on the number of augmentations for our algorithm is the cost of the minimum cut $|C|$, which results in the worst case complexity $O(mn^2|C|)$. Theoretically speaking, this is worse than complexities of the standard algorithms discussed in Section 2.2. However, experimental comparison in Section 4 shows that on typical problem instances in vision our algorithm significantly outperforms standard algorithms.

3.1   Algorithm's Overview

We maintain a search tree S with the source as a root where all edges from each parent node to its children are non-saturated. The nodes that are not in S are called "free". The set of free nodes is denoted T. The nodes in the search tree S are divided into "active" and "passive". The active nodes may "grow", that is, they may acquire new children from a set of free nodes. The passive nodes are guaranteed to have no free neighbors connected through non-saturated edges. Thus, the passive nodes can not grow.

The algorithm iteratively repeats the following three stages:

- "growth" stage: the search tree grows until the sink is found

- "augmentation" stage: the path found is augmented, the search tree is broken into a forest.
- "adoption" stage: the forest is transformed back into a tree.

At the growth stage the search tree expands. The active nodes acquire new children from a set of free nodes. The newly acquired nodes become active members of the search tree S. As soon as all neighbors of a given active node are explored the active node becomes passive. The growth stage terminates when the sink is encountered and, thus, a path from the source to the sink is found.

The augmentation stage augments the path found in the growth stage. Since we push through the largest flow possible some edges in the path become saturated. Thus, some of the nodes in the tree become "orphans", that is, the edges linking them to their parents are no longer valid (they are saturated). In fact, the augmentation phase splits the search tree S into a forest. The source is still a root of one of the trees in the forest and the orphans form roots of other trees.

The goal of the adoption stage is to restore a single search tree structure with a root in the source. At this stage we try to find a new valid parent for each orphan. If there is no such parent we remove the orphan from S and make it a free node. We also declare all its former children orphans. The stage terminates when no orphans are left and, thus, the search tree structure of S is restored. Since some orphan nodes in S may become free the adoption stage results in contraction of the set S.

After the adoption stage is completed the algorithm returns to the growth stage. The algorithm terminates when the search tree can not grow (all active nodes checked their neighbors and became passive) while the sink is not found.

3.2   Details of Implementation

Assume that we are given a directed graph $\mathcal{G} = \langle \mathcal{V}, \mathcal{E} \rangle$. As for any augmenting path algorithm, we will maintain a flow f and the residual graph G_f (see Section 2.2). For each node p we will store its parent as $PARENT(p)$. Roots of the forest (the source and the orphans) as well as all free nodes have no parents, t.e. $PARENT(p) = \emptyset$. We will also keep the lists of all active nodes, A, and all orphans, O. The general structure of the algorithm is:

```
initialize: S = A = {s}, T = V − {s}, O = ∅
while true
        grow S to find an augmenting path P from s to t
        if P = ∅ terminate
        augment on P
        adopt orphans
end while
```

The details of the *growth, augmentation,* and *adoption* stages are described below.

Growth Stage: At this stage active nodes acquire new children from a set of free nodes.

```
if t ∈ S return P = PATH_{s→t}
while A ≠ ∅
        pick an active node p ∈ A
        for every non-saturated edge (p, q)
                if q ∈ T add q to the search tree as an active node:
                    S := S ∪ {q},  A := A ∪ {q},  PARENT(q) := p
                if q = t return P = PATH_{s→t}
        end for
        remove p from A
end while
return P = ∅
```

Augmentation Stage: The input for this stage is a path P from s to t. Note that the orphan set is empty in the beginning of the stage, but there will be some orphans in the end since at least one edge in P becomes saturated.

```
find the bottleneck capacity Δ on P
update the residual graph by pushing flow Δ through P
for each edge (p, q) in P that becomes saturated
        set PARENT(q) := ∅
        add q to O
end for
```

Adoption Stage: During this stage all nodes in O are processed until O becomes empty. The node being processed tries to find a new parent in S; in case of success it remains in S but with a new parent, otherwise it is removed from S to the set of free nodes T and all its children are added to O.

```
while O ≠ ∅
        pick a node p ∈ O
        remove p from O
        process p
end while
```

The operation "**process** p" consists of the following steps. First we are trying to find a new parent for p. For each non-saturated edge (q, p) entering p we check whether q is a valid parent. Two conditions should hold for q:

− q should be in S
− the "origin" of q should be the source

Note that it is necessary to check the second condition because some of the nodes in S originate from orphans.

If a new parent q is found, then p remains in S with q as its parent. The active (or passive) status of p in S remains unchanged. If p does not find a valid parent in S then the following three operations are performed:

− p is removed from S (and A) and becomes a free node in T

- for all children q of p we set $PARENT(q) = \emptyset$ and add them to the set of orphans O
- all "potential" parents of p (nodes q in S such that the edge (q, p) is not saturated) are added to the active set A

The last operation is necessary to make sure that no passive node in S connects to a free neighbor through a non-saturated edge. Only active nodes are allowed to have such free neighbors. Suppose that an orphan p becomes free. Without the last operation, the passive neighbors of p in S connected to p via non-saturated edges would remain passive while they should not. At that moment these neighbors did not qualify as valid parents for p because they originated from other orphans and not from the source. After the search tree is fixed one of such neighbors may potentially become a new parent of p.

3.3   Correctness Proof

Let's introduce some invariants which are maintained during the execution of the algorithm.

I1 *S is a forest with roots at either the source or orphans.*
I2 *Edges from a parent to children in the search forest have nonzero residual capacities.*
I3 *There are no orphans during the growth stage.*
I4 *For passive nodes p in S the following property should be true: for all non-saturated edges (p, q) the node q must belong to S.*

These invariants are clearly true at the initialization of the algorithm. It is easy to see these invariants directly follow from the construction of the algorithm.

Let's show that all stages terminate. The growth stage terminates because the number of nodes is finite. The same argument applies to the augmentation stage. Now we prove that the adoption stage is also finite. Note that after a node p in O has been processed it can not become an orphan again during the same adoption stage (it will imply that the adoption stage terminates after processing at most n nodes). Indeed, if p is moved from S to T then this holds since free nodes in T are not involved at the adoption stage. Suppose p found a new parent q and remained in S. The new parent q must originate from the source. Thus, the source is the new origin of p as well. By construction, only descendants of orphans may become orphans during the adoption stage. Therefore, p can not become an orphan again at the same adoption stage.

The algorithm terminates if the number of cycles (augmentations) is finite. Since the algorithm is not a shortest path algorithm the polynomial bound for the number of augmentations does not seem to be valid. We know only a trivial bound given by a minimum cut cost that works if all edge weights are integers.

It remains to show that when the algorithm terminates it generates the maximum flow. In fact, the search tree S and the set of free nodes T at the end of the algorithm give a minimum s/t-cut. Suppose the algorithm has terminated.

It could only have happened in the growth stage when no active nodes were left and $t \notin S$. S and T are disjoint sets such that $S \cup T = \mathcal{V}$, $s \in S$, and $t \in T$. Suppose that the current residual graph contains a non-saturated path from the source to the sink that can be used to increase the flow. Then there is a non-saturated edge (p, q) going from a node $p \in S$ to another node $q \in T$. Since no active nodes are left then p is passive. Hence, the invariant I4 does not hold for p and we get a contradiction.

4   Experimental Tests on Applications in Vision

In this section we experimentally test min-cut/max-flow algorithms for three different applications in computer vision: image restoration (Section 4.1), stereo (Section 4.2), and object segmentation (Section 4.3). We chose formulations where certain appropriate versions of energy (1) can be minimized via graph cuts. The corresponding graph structures were previously described by [10, 12, 2, 4, 14, 3] in detail. These (or very similar) structures are used in all computer vision applications with graph cuts (that we are aware of) to date.

Note that we could not test all known min-cut/max-flow algorithms. We compare our new algorithm presented in Section 3 and standard algorithms of combinatorial optimization introduced in Section 2.2: DINIC, H_PRF, and Q_PRF. Many experimental tests, including the results in [5], show that the last two algorithms work consistently better than a large number of other min-cut/max-flow algorithms of combinatorial optimization. For DINIC, H_PRF, and Q_PRF we took the implementations written by Cherkassky and Goldberg [5] and modified them to our graph representation. Both H_PRF and Q_PRF use global and gap relabeling heuristics. Our algorithm also leaves some choice in implementing certain functions. We found that the order of processing active nodes and orphans may have a significant effect on the running time. We made a tuning and used it in all experiments.

4.1   Image Restoration

Here we consider two examples of energy (1) with the Potts and linear models of interaction. Graph based methods for minimizing Potts energy were used in many different applications including segmentation [13], stereo [2, 4], object recognition [1], shape reconstruction [16], and augmented reality [17]. Linear interaction energy was used for stereo [15] and segmentation [12]. The structures of the corresponding graphs are identical in all applications using the same type of energy. We chose the context of image restoration mainly for its simplicity.

The Potts energy that we use for image restoration is

$$E(I) = \sum_{p \in \mathcal{P}} ||I_p - I_p^o|| + \sum_{(p,q) \in \mathcal{N}} K_{(p,q)} \cdot T(I_p \neq I_q) \qquad (2)$$

where $I = \{I_p \,|p \in \mathcal{P}\}$ is a vector of unknown "true" intensities of pixels on the image $\mathcal{P}$ and $I^o = \{I_p^o \,|p \in \mathcal{P}\}$ are intensities observed in the original image

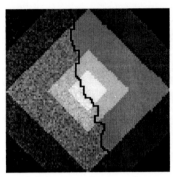
(a) *Diamond* restoration

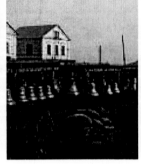
(b) Original *Bell Quad*

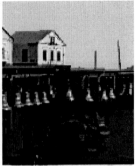
(c) "Restored" *Bell Quad*

method	input		input: *Diamond*			input: *BellQuad*		
	Diamond	*Bell Quad*	$|\mathcal{L}|=27$	$|\mathcal{L}|=54$	$|\mathcal{L}|=108$	$|\mathcal{L}|=32$	$|\mathcal{L}|=64$	$|\mathcal{L}|=128$
DINIC	21	160	24	61	177	24	70	144
H_PRF	10	22	10	22	53	16	50	125
Q_PRF	10	23	7	20	54	9	19	59
Our	6	14	5	16	65	8	27	122

         (d) Potts energy   (e) Linear interactions energy

Fig. 2. Image Restoration Experiments.

corrupted by noise. The Potts interactions are specified by penalties $K_{(p,q)}$ for intensity discontinuities between pairs of neighboring pixels. Function $T(\cdot)$ is 1 if the condition inside parenthesis is true and 0 otherwise. In the case of two labels the Potts energy can be minimized exactly using the graph cut method of Greig et. al. [10]. We consider image restoration with multiple labels where the problem becomes NP hard. We use an iterative graph based method in [4] which is guaranteed to find a solution within a factor of two from the global minimum of the Potts energy. At each iteration [4] computes a minimum cost cut for a certain generalization of the graph introduced in [10].

Our image restoration experiments with the Potts energy are presented in Figure 2(a-c). The sizes of our test images are 100×100 (Diamond) and 112×136 (Bell Quad). The number of allowed labels is 215 and 256, correspondingly. The running times (in seconds, 333MHz Pentium III) for the Potts energy minimization tests are given in Figure 2(d). These running times represent the first cycle of iterations (see [4] for more details).

We also consider image restoration with "linear" interactions energy:

$$E(I) = \sum_{p \in \mathcal{P}} ||I_p - I_p^o|| + \sum_{(p,q) \in \mathcal{N}} A_{(p,q)} \cdot |I_p - I_q| \qquad (3)$$

where constants $A_{(p,q)}$ describe the relative importance of interactions between neighboring pixels p and q. If the set of labels is finite and ordered then this energy can be minimized exactly using either of the two almost identical graph-based methods developed in [12, 2]. In fact, both of them use graphs very similar to the one introduced by [15] in the context of multi-camera stereo. These methods build graphs by consecutively connecting multiple layers of image-grids. Each layer corresponds to one label. The structure of the graphs for linear interactions energy has one important distinction from the graphs that are currently used to minimize other types of energies; the two terminals are connected only to the first and the last layers of the graph. This distinction becomes more pronounced when the number of labels (layers) is large. Note that allocating computer memory for such multi-layered graphs can be problematic even for 2D images.

The table in Figure 2(e) shows how long it took each min-cut/max-flow algorithm to compute the exact minimum of the linear interactions energy above. We used the same *Diamond* and *Bell Quad* images as in the Potts energy tests. In the tests presented in (e) we varied the number of labels (layers) $|\mathcal{L}|$. The experiments show that our algorithm is the fastest when the number of labels is relatively small (less than 50) while Q_PRF wins for larger number of labels. Note that the number of labels affects the structure of the graphs in [15, 12, 2]. In the Potts energy minimization method in [4] the number of labels changes the number of iterations in each cycle but has no effect on the graph structures.

4.2   Stereo with Occlusions

Here we describe our tests on examples in stereo. We consider a recent formulation [14] that takes occlusions into consideration. The problem is formulated as a labeling problem. We want to assign a binary label (0 or 1) to each pair $\langle p, q \rangle$ where p is a pixel in the left image and q is a pixel in the right image that can potentially correspond to p. The set of pairs with the label 1 describes the correspondence between the images.   The energy of configuration f is given by

$$E(f) = \sum_{f_{\langle p,q \rangle}=1} D_{\langle p,q \rangle} + \sum_{p \in \mathcal{P}} C_p \cdot T(p \text{ is occluded in the configuration } f)$$

$$+ \sum_{\{\langle p,q \rangle, \langle p',q' \rangle\} \in \mathcal{N}} K_{\{\langle p,q \rangle, \langle p',q' \rangle\}} \cdot T(f_{\langle p,q \rangle} \neq f_{\langle p',q' \rangle})$$

The first term is the data term, the second is the occlusion penalty, and the third is the smoothness term. $\mathcal{P}$ is the set of pixels in both images, and $\mathcal{N}$ is the neighboring system consisting of tuples of neighboring pairs $\{\langle p, q \rangle, \langle p', q' \rangle\}$ having the same disparity (parallel pairs). [14] gives an approximate algorithm minimizing this energy among all feasible configurations f. In contrast to other energy minimization methods, nodes of the graph constructed in [14] represent *pairs* rather than pixels or voxels.

The tests were done for three stereo examples shown in Figure 3. We used the *Head* pair from the University of Tsukuba, and the well-known *Tree* pair from SRI. To diversify our tests we compared the speed of algorithms on a *Random* pair where the left and the right images did not correspond to each other.

Running times for stereo examples in Figure 3 are shown in seconds (450MHz UltraSPARC II Processor) in the table below. The times are for the first cycle of the algorithm, which is where most of the work is done.

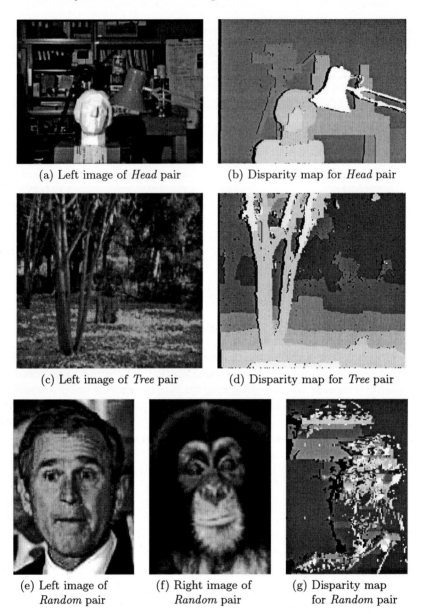

(a) Left image of *Head* pair   (b) Disparity map for *Head* pair

(c) Left image of *Tree* pair   (d) Disparity map for *Tree* pair

(e) Left image of   (f) Right image of   (g) Disparity map
  Random pair   *Random* pair   for *Random* pair

Fig. 3. Stereo Experiments. The sizes of images are 384×288 in (a), 256×233 in (c), and 100×140 in (e,f). The results in (b,d,g) show occluded pixels in black color.

method	input		
	Head pair	*Tree* pair	*Random* pair
DINIC	365.4	39.4	32.6
H_PRF	109.8	20.1	16.0
Q_PRF	56.0	13.4	9.1
Our	17.0	4.0	7.2

4.3   Interactive Object Segmentation

In this section we describe experimental tests that compare min-cut/max-flow algorithms on *Interactive Graph Cuts* segmentation technique in [3]. The method in [3] allows for the segmentation of an object of interest in N-D images/volumes. This technique generalizes the MAP-MRF method of Greig at. al. [10] by incorporating additional hard constraints into the minimization of the Potts energy

$$E(L) = \sum_{p \in \mathcal{P}} D_p(L_p) + \sum_{(p,q) \in \mathcal{N}} K_{(p,q)} \cdot T(L_p \neq L_q)$$

over binary (object/background) labelings of image. The hard constrains come from a user placing some object and background seeds. The technique computes binary segmentation of N-dimensional image with globally optimal regional and boundary properties among all segmentations that satisfy the hard constraints (seeds). The details of the corresponding graph construction are given in [3].

We tested min-cut/max-flow algorithms on 2D and 3D segmentation examples illustrated in Figure 4. We present the original data and the segmentation results corresponding to certain sets of seeds. Note that the user places seeds interactively. New seeds can be added to correct segmentation imperfections. The technique in [3] efficiently recomputes the optimal solution starting at the previous segmentation result.

Figure 4(a-b) shows photo-editing experiment on a picture (200x300 pixels) with a group of people around a bell. Other segmentation examples in (c-h) are for 2D and 3D medical data. The cardiac MR data in (c-d) was tested in both 2D (256x256 pixels) and 3D (256x256x13 voxels) cases. In our 3D experiment the seeds were placed in only one slice in the middle of the volume. This was enough to segment the whole volume "correctly". The tests with lung CT data (e-f) were also made in both 2D (512x512 pixels) and 3D (512x512x5 voxels) cases. In (g-h) we tested the algorithms on 2D liver MR data (512x256 pixels).

The table below compares the running times (in seconds, 600MHz Pentium III processor) of selected min-cut/max-flow algorithms for the segmentation examples described. Note that these times include only the min-cut/max-flow computation[3]. The tests on 3D data are marked by "3D". To diversify our tests we also made a few experiments where inconsistent seeds were placed at random

---

[3] The time it takes the user to place the seeds varies and may depend on image quality, object of interest, and the level of desired details. For the experiments in Figure 4 all seeds were placed within 10 to 40 seconds.

Photo Editing

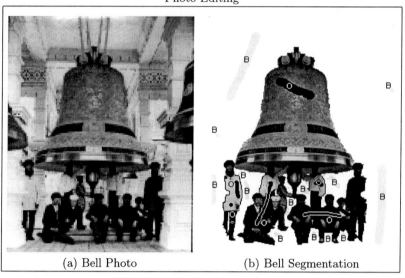

(a) Bell Photo   (b) Bell Segmentation

Medical Data

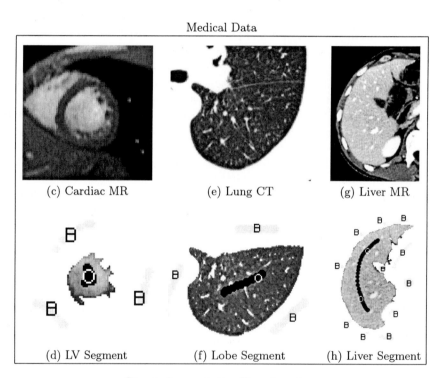

(c) Cardiac MR   (e) Lung CT   (g) Liver MR

(d) LV Segment   (f) Lobe Segment   (h) Liver Segment

Fig. 4. Segmentation Experiments.

places in the image. The corresponding columns in the table are marked as "random". Meaningless segmentations from these tests are not shown in Figure 4.

method	input						
	Liver	Bell	Lung	Heart(3D)	Lung(3D)	Bell(random)	Lung(random)
DINIC	26	7	5	—	—	8	16
H_PRF	3.5	2	2.5	—	—	4	3
Q_PRF	2.5	1	0.5	7	68	1.5	1.5
Our	0.26	0.26	0.16	2	20	1	2.5

Note that 3D segmentation required memory efficient implementations of the graph cut algorithms. We made such implementations only for our new algorithm and for Q_PRF (which outperformed H_PRF and DINIC in most other experiments). H_PRF and DINIC were not tested in 3D segmentation examples.

5   Conclusions

We tested a reasonable sample of typical vision graphs. In most examples our new min-cut/max-flow algorithm worked 2-10 times faster than any of the other methods, including the push-relabel and Dinic algorithms (which are known to outperform other min-cut/max-flow techniques). In some cases the new algorithm made possible near real-time performance of the corresponding applications. One noticeable exception was the energy with linear interactions (3). If the number of labels for (3) was relatively small (< 50) then our algorithm was only marginally the best, while Q_PRF was significantly faster for larger number of labels. We also found that our algorithm's performance was roughly the same as Q_PRF in unrealistic examples with "random" inputs.

Our results also suggest that graphs in vision are a very specific application for min-cut/max-flow algorithms. In fact, Q_PRF outperformed H_PRF in most of our tests despite the fact that H_PRF is generally regarded as the fastest algorithm in combinatorial optimization community. Additional experiments showed that our algorithm was several times slower than H_PRF on standard (outside computer vision) graphs that are used for tests in combinatorial optimization.

Acknowledgements

Olga Veksler (NEC Research, NJ) greatly helped with implementations for Section 4.1. We also thank Professor Ramin Zabih (Cornell, NY) for the discussions that significantly improved our paper. Our research would not be possible without support from Alok Gupta and Gareth Funka-Lea (Siemens Research, NJ).

References

1. Y. Boykov and D. Huttenlocher. A new bayesian framework for object recognition. In *IEEE Conference on Computer Vision and Pattern Recognition*, volume 2, pages 517–523, 1999.

2. Y. Boykov, O. Veksler, and R. Zabih. Markov random fields with efficient approximations. In *IEEE Conference on Computer Vision and Pattern Recognition*, pages 648–655, 1998.
3. Yuri Boykov and Marie-Pierre Jolly. *Interactive graph cuts* for optimal boundary & region segmentation of objects in N-D images. In *International Conference on Computer Vision*, July 2001.
4. Yuri Boykov, Olga Veksler, and Ramin Zabih. Fast approximate energy minimization via graph cuts. In *International Conference on Computer Vision*, volume I, pages 377–384, 1999.
5. B. V. Cherkassky and A. V. Goldberg. On implementing push-relabel method for the maximum flow problem. *Algorithmica*, 19:390–410, 1997.
6. William J. Cook, William H. Cunningham, William R. Pulleyblank, and Alexander Schrijver. *Combinatorial Optimization*. John Wiley & Sons, 1998.
7. E. A. Dinic. Algorithm for solution of a problem of maximum flow in networks with power estimation. *Soviet Math. Dokl.*, 11:1277–1280, 1970.
8. L. Ford and D. Fulkerson. *Flows in Networks*. Princeton University Press, 1962.
9. A. Goldberg and R. Tarjan. A new approach to the maximum flow problem. *Journal of the Association for Computing Machinery*, 35(4):921–940, October 1988.
10. D. Greig, B. Porteous, and A. Seheult. Exact maximum a posteriori estimation for binary images. *Journal of the Royal Statistical Society, Series B*, 51(2):271–279, 1989.
11. H. Ishikawa and D. Geiger. Occlusions, discontinuities, and epipolar lines in stereo. In *5th European Conference on Computer Vision*, pages 232–248, 1998.
12. H. Ishikawa and D. Geiger. Segmentation by grouping junctions. In *IEEE Conference on Computer Vision and Pattern Recognition*, pages 125–131, 1998.
13. Junmo Kim, John W. Fisher III, Andy Tsai, Cindy Wible, Alan S. Willsky, and William M. Wells III. Incorporating spatial priors into an information theoretic approach for fMRI data analysis. In *Medical Image Computing and Computer-Assisted Intervention (MICCAI)*, pages 62–71, 2000.
14. Vladimir Kolmogorov and Ramin Zabih. Computing visual correspondence with occlusions via graph cuts. In *International Conference on Computer Vision*, July 2001.
15. Sebastien Roy and Ingemar Cox. A maximum-flow formulation of the n-camera stereo correspondence problem. In *IEEE Proc. of Int. Conference on Computer Vision*, pages 492–499, 1998.
16. Dan Snow, Paul Viola, and Ramin Zabih. Exact voxel occupancy with graph cuts. In *IEEE Conference on Computer Vision and Pattern Recognition*, volume 1, pages 345–352, 2000.
17. B. Thirion, B. Bascle, V. Ramesh, and N. Navab. Fusion of color, shading and boundary information for factory pipe segmentation. In *IEEE Conference on Computer Vision and Pattern Recognition*, volume 2, pages 349–356, 2000.
18. Olga Veksler. Image segmentation by nested cuts. In *IEEE Conference on Computer Vision and Pattern Recognition*, volume 1, pages 339–344, 2000.

A Discrete/Continuous Minimization Method in Interferometric Image Processing*

José M.B. Dias and José M.N. Leitão

Instituto de Telecomunicações,
Instituto Superior Técnico,
1049-001 Lisboa, Portugal
bioucas@lx.it.pt

Abstract. The 2D absolute phase estimation problem, in interferometric applications, is to infer absolute phase (not simply modulo-2π) from incomplete, noisy, and modulo-2π image observations. This is known to be a hard problem as the observation mechanism is nonlinear. In this paper we adopt the Bayesian approach. The observation density is 2π-periodic and accounts for the observation noise; the *a priori* probability of the absolute phase is modeled by a first order noncausal *Gauss Markov random field* (GMRF) tailored to smooth absolute phase images. We propose an iterative scheme for the computation of the *maximum a posteriori probability* (MAP) estimate. Each iteration embodies a discrete optimization step ($\mathbb{Z}$-step), implemented by network programming techniques, and an *iterative conditional modes* (ICM) step (π-step). Accordingly, we name the algorithm $\mathbb{Z}\pi M$, where letter M stands for maximization. A set of experimental results, comparing the proposed algorithm with other techniques, illustrates the effectiveness of the proposed method.

1 Introduction

In many classes of imaging techniques involving wave propagation, there is need for estimating absolute phase from incomplete, noisy, and modulo-2π observations, as the absolute phase is related with some physical entity of interest. Some relevant examples are [1] synthetic aperture radar, synthetic aperture sonar, magnetic resonance imaging systems, optical interferometry, and diffraction tomography.

In all the applications above referred the observed data relates with the absolute phase in a nonlinear and noisy way; the nonlinearity is sinusoidal and it is closely related with the wave propagation phenomena involved in the acquisition process; noise is introduced both by the acquisition process and by the electronic equipment. Therefore, the absolute phase should be inferred (*unwrapped* in the interfermetric jargon) from noisy and modulo-2π observations (the so-called *principal phase values* or *interferogram*).

---

* This work was supported by the Fundação para a Ciência e Tecnologia, under the project POSI/34071/CPS/2000.

M.A.T. Figueiredo, J. Zerubia, A.K. Jain (Eds.): EMMCVPR 2001, LNCS 2134, pp. 375–390, 2001.

Broadly speaking, absolute phase estimation methods can be classified into four major classes: path following methods, minimum-norm methods, Bayesian and regularization methods, and parametric models. Thesis [2] and paper [3] provide a comprehensive account of these methods.

The mainstream of absolute phase estimation research in interferometry takes a two step approach: in the first step, a filtered interferogram is inferred from noisy images; in the second step, the phase is unwrapped by determining the 2π multiples. Path following and minimum-norm schemes are representative of this approach (see [1] for comprehensive description of these methods). The main drawback of these methods is that the filtering process destroys the modulo-2π information in areas of high phase rate.

In a quite different vein, and recognizing that the absolute phase estimation is an ill-posed problem, papers [4], [5], [6], [7] have adopted the regularization framework to impose smoothness on the solution. The same objective has been pursued in papers [8], [9], [10], [11] by adopting a Bayesian viewpoint. Papers [8], [9] apply a nonlinear recursive filtering technique to determine the absolute phase. Paper [10] considers an InSAR (interferometric synthetic aperture radar) observation model taking into account not only the image absolute phase, but also the *backscattering coefficient* and the *correlation factor* images, which are jointly recovered from InSAR image pairs. Paper [11] proposes a fractal based prior and the simulated annealing scheme to compute the absolute phase image.

Parametric models constrain the absolute phase to belong to a given parametric model. Works [12], [13] have adopted low order polynomials. These approaches yields good results if the low order polynomials represent accurately the absolute phase. However, in practical applications the entire phase function cannot be approximated by a single 2-D polynomial model. To circumvent model mismatches, work [12] proposes a partition of the observed field where each partition element has its own model.

1.1 Proposed Approach

We adopt the Bayesian viewpoint. The likelihood function, which models the observation mechanism given the absolute phase, is 2π-periodic and accounts for the interferometric noise. The *a priori* probability of the absolute phase is modeled by a first order noncausal Gauss Markov random field (GMRF) [14], [15] tailored to smooth fields.

Papers [8], [9], [10] have also followed a Bayesian approach to absolute phase estimation. The prior therein used was a first order causal GMRF. Taking advantage of this prior and using the *reduced order model* (ROM) [16] approximation of the GMRF, the absolute was estimated with a nonlinear recursive filtering technique. Compared with the present approach, the main difference concerns the prior: we use a first order noncausal GMRF prior. In terms of estimation, the noncausal prior has implicit a batch perspective, where the absolute phase estimate at each site is based on the complete observed image. This is in contrast with the recursive filtering technique [8], [9], [10], where the absolute phase estimate of a given site is inferred only from past (in the lexicographic sense) observed data.

To the computation of the MAP estimate, we propose an iterative procedure with two steps per iteration: the first step, termed $\mathbb{Z}$-step, maximizes the posterior density with respect to the field of 2π phase multiples; the second step, termed π-step, maximizes the posterior density with respect to the phase principal values. $\mathbb{Z}$-step is a discrete optimization problem solved by network programming techniques. π-step is a continuous optimization problem solved approximately by the *iterated conditional modes* (ICM) [17] scheme. We term our algorithm $\mathbb{Z}\pi$M, where the letter M stands for maximization.

The paper is organized as follows. Section 2 introduces the observation model, the first order noncausal GMRF prior, and the posteriori density. Section 3 elaborates on the estimation procedure. Namely, we derive solutions for the $\mathbb{Z}$-step and for the π-step. Section 4 presents results.

2   Adopted Models

2.1   Observation Model

The complex envelop of the signal read by the receiver from a given site is given by

$$x = e^{-j\phi} + n, \tag{1}$$

where ϕ is the phase to be estimated and n is complex zero-mean circular Gaussian noise. Model (1), adopted in papers [8] and [9], applies, for example, to laser interferometry [18].

Defining $\sigma_n^2 \equiv E[|n|^2]$, the probability density function[1] of x is (see, e.g., [19, ch. 3])

$$p_{x|\phi}(x|\phi) = \frac{1}{\pi\sigma_n^2} \exp\left\{-\frac{|x - e^{-j\phi}|^2}{\sigma_n^2}\right\}. \tag{2}$$

Developing the quadratic form in (2), one is led to

$$p_{x|\phi}(x|\phi) = ce^{\lambda\cos(\phi - \eta)}, \tag{3}$$

where $c = c(x, \sigma_n)$ and

$$\eta = \arg(x) \tag{4}$$

$$\lambda = \frac{|x|}{\sigma_n^2}. \tag{5}$$

The likelihood function $p_{x|\phi}(x|\phi)$ is 2π-periodic with respect to ϕ with maxima at $\phi = 2\pi k + \eta$, for $k \in \mathbb{Z}$ ($\mathbb{Z}$ denotes the integer set). Thus η is a maximum

---

[1] For compactness, lowercase letters will denote random variables and their values as well.

likelihood estimate of ϕ. The peakiness of the maxima of (3), controlled by parameter λ, is an indication of how trustful data is.

The observation model (1) does not apply to applications exhibiting speckle noise such as synthetic apertura radar and synthetic aperture sonar. We have shown in [10], however, that the observation model of these applications leads to an observation density with the same formal structure given by formula (3). Let $\phi \equiv \{\phi_{ij} \,|\, (i,j) \in Z\}$ and $\mathbf{x} \equiv \{x_{ij} \,|\, (i,j) \in Z\}$ denote the absolute phase and complex amplitude associated to sites $Z \equiv \{(i,j)|\, i,j = 1,\ldots,N\}$ (we assume without lack of generality that images are squared). Assuming that the components of $\mathbf{x}$ are conditionally independent,

$$p_{\mathbf{x}|\phi}(\mathbf{x}|\phi) = \prod_{ij \in Z} p_{x_{ij}|\phi_{ij}}(x_{ij}|\phi_{ij}). \tag{6}$$

The conditional independence assumption is valid if the resolution cells associated to any pair of pixels are disjoint. Usually this is a good approximation, since the *point spread function* of the imaging systems is only slightly larger than the corresponding inter-pixel distance (see [20]).

2.2 Prior Model

Image ϕ is assumed to be smooth. *Gauss-Markov random fields* [14], [15] are both mathematically and computationally suitable for representing local interactions, namely to impose smoothness. We take the *first order* noncausal GMRF

$$p_\phi(\phi) \propto \exp\left\{-\frac{\mu}{2}\sum_{ij \in Z_1}(\Delta\phi_{ij}^h)^2 + (\Delta\phi_{ij}^v)^2\right\}, \tag{7}$$

where $\Delta\phi_{ij}^h \equiv (\phi_{ij} - \phi_{i,j-1})$, $\Delta\phi_{ij}^v \equiv (\phi_{ij} - \phi_{i-1,j})$, $Z_1 \equiv \{(i,j)|\, i,j = 2,\ldots,N\}$, and μ^{-1} means the variance of increments $\Delta\phi_{ij}^h$ and $\Delta\phi_{ij}^v$.

2.3 Posterior Density

Invoking the Bayes rule, we obtain the posterior probability density function of ϕ, given $\mathbf{x}$, as

$$p_{\phi|\mathbf{x}}(\phi|\mathbf{x}) \propto p_{\mathbf{x}|\phi}(\mathbf{x}|\phi)p_\phi(\phi), \tag{8}$$

where the factors not depending on ϕ were discarded. Introducing (6) and (7) into (8), we obtain

$$p_{\phi|\mathbf{x}}(\phi|\mathbf{x}) \propto e^{\displaystyle\sum_{ij \in Z}\lambda_{ij}\cos(\phi_{ij} - \eta_{ij}) - \frac{\mu}{2}\sum_{ij \in Z_1}(\Delta\phi_{ij}^h)^2 + (\Delta\phi_{ij}^v)^2}. \tag{9}$$

The posterior distribution (9) is assumed to contain all information one needs to compute the absolute phase estimate $\widehat{\phi}$.

3   Estimation Procedure

The MAP criterion is adopted for computing $\widehat{\phi}$. Accordingly,

$$\widehat{\phi}_{MAP} = \arg\max_{\phi} p_{\phi|\mathbf{x}}(\phi|\mathbf{x}). \tag{10}$$

Due to the periodic structure of $p_{x|\phi}(x|\phi)$, computing the MAP solution leads to a huge non-convex optimization problem, with unbearable computation burden. Instead of computing the exact estimate $\widehat{\phi}_{MAP}$, we resort to a suboptimal scheme that delivers nearly optimal estimates, with a far less computational load.

Let the absolute phase ϕ_{ij} be uniquely decomposed as

$$\phi_{ij} = \psi_{ij} + 2\pi k_{ij}, \tag{11}$$

where $k_{ij} = \lfloor (\phi_{ij} + \pi)/(2\pi) \rfloor \in \mathbb{Z}$ is the so-called wrap-count component of ϕ_{ij}, and $\psi_{ij} \in [-\pi, \pi[$ is the principal value of ϕ_{ij}. The MAP estimate (10) can be rewritten in terms of $\psi \equiv \{\psi_{ij} \,|\, (i,j) \in Z\}$ and $\mathbf{k} \equiv \{k_{ij} \,|\, (i,j) \in Z\}$ as

$$(\widehat{\psi}_{MAP}, \widehat{\mathbf{k}}_{MAP}) = \arg\max_{\psi, \mathbf{k}} p_{\phi|\mathbf{x}}(\psi + 2\pi\mathbf{k}|\mathbf{x}) \tag{12}$$

$$= \arg\left\{ \max_{\psi} \left\{ \max_{\mathbf{k}} p_{\phi|\mathbf{x}}(\psi + 2\pi\mathbf{k}|\mathbf{x}) \right\} \right\}. \tag{13}$$

Instead of computing (13), we propose a procedure that successively and iteratively maximizes $p_{\phi|\mathbf{x}}(\psi + 2\pi\mathbf{k}|\mathbf{x})$ with respect to $\mathbf{k} \in \mathbb{Z}^{N^2}$ and $\psi \in [-\pi, \pi[^{N^2}$. We term this maximization on the sets $\mathbb{Z}$ and $[-\pi, \pi[$ as the $\mathbb{Z}\pi M$ algorithm; Fig. 1 shows the corresponding pseudo-code.

Initialization: $\widehat{\psi}^{(0)} = \eta$
For $t = 1, 2, \ldots,$

    Unwrapping step:
$$\widehat{\mathbf{k}}^{(t)} = \arg\max_{\mathbf{k}} p_{\phi|\mathbf{x},1}(\psi^{(t-1)} + 2\pi\mathbf{k}|\mathbf{x}) \tag{14}$$

    Smoothing step:
$$\widehat{\psi}^{(t)} = \arg\max_{\psi} p_{\phi|\mathbf{x},1}(\psi + 2\pi\mathbf{k}^{(t)}|\mathbf{x}) \tag{15}$$

    Termination test:
        If $[p_{\phi|\mathbf{x},1}(\widehat{\phi}^{(t)}|\mathbf{x}) - p_{\phi|\mathbf{x},1}(\widehat{\phi}^{(t-1)}|\mathbf{x})] < \xi$
        break loop for

Fig. 1. $\mathbb{Z}\pi M$ Algorithm.

The $\mathbb{Z}\pi M$ algorithm is greedy, since the posterior density $p_{\phi|\mathbf{x}}(\phi|\mathbf{x})$ can not decrease in each step of the each iteration. Thus, the stationary points of the couple (14)-(15) correspond to local maxima of $p_{\phi|\mathbf{x}}(\phi|\mathbf{x})$. Nevertheless, the proposed method yields systematically good results, as we will show in next section.

The unwrapping step (14) finds the maximum of the posterior density $p_{\phi|\mathbf{x}}(\phi|\mathbf{x})$ on a mesh obtained by discretizing each coordinate ϕ_{ij} according to (11). The first estimate $\widehat{\mathbf{k}}^{(1)}$ delivered by the unwrapping step is based on the maximum likelihood estimate $\boldsymbol{\eta} \equiv \{\eta_{ij} \,|\, (i,j) \in Z\}$. Smoothing is implemented by the π-step (15). This is in contrast with the scheme followed by most phase unwrapping algorithms, where the phase is estimated with basis on on a smooth version of $\boldsymbol{\eta}$, under the assumption that the phase ϕ is constant within windows of given size. This assumption leads to strong errors in areas of high phase rate.

3.1 $\mathbb{Z}$-Step

Since the logarithm is strictly increasing and $\cos(\psi_{ij} + 2\pi k_{ij} - \eta_{ij})$ does not depend on k_{ij}, solving the maximization step (14) is equivalent to solve

$$\widehat{\mathbf{k}} = \arg\min_{\mathbf{k}} E(\mathbf{k}|\boldsymbol{\psi}), \tag{16}$$

where the energy $E(\mathbf{k}|\boldsymbol{\psi})$ is given by

$$E(\mathbf{k}|\boldsymbol{\psi}) \equiv \sum_{ij \in Z_1} (\Delta\phi_{ij}^h)^2 + (\Delta\phi_{ij}^v)^2, \tag{17}$$

with

$$\Delta\phi_{ij}^h = [2\pi(k_{ij} - k_{i,j-1}) - \Delta\psi_{ij}^h] \tag{18}$$
$$\Delta\phi_{ij}^v = [2\pi(k_{ij} - k_{i-1,j}) - \Delta\psi_{ij}^v], \tag{19}$$

and $\Delta\psi_{ij}^h = \psi_{i,j-1} - \psi_{ij}$ and $\Delta\psi_{ij}^v = \psi_{i-1,j} - \psi_{ij}$.

A simple but lengthy manipulation of equation (17) allows us to write

$$\widehat{\bar{\mathbf{k}}} = \arg\min_{\bar{\mathbf{k}} \in \mathbb{Z}^{N^2}} (\bar{\mathbf{k}} - \bar{\mathbf{k}}_0)^T \mathbf{A}(\bar{\mathbf{k}} - \bar{\mathbf{k}}_0), \tag{20}$$

where the column vector $\bar{\mathbf{k}}$ is the column by column stacking of matrix $\mathbf{k}$, matrix $\mathbf{A}$ is nonnegative block Toeplitz and symmetric, and vector $\mathbf{k}_0$ depends on $\Delta\psi_{ij}^h$ and $\Delta\psi_{ij}^v$. For nonnegative symmetric matrices $\mathbf{A}$, the integer least square problem (20) is known as the *nearest lattice vector problem* and it is NP-hard [21]. It arises, for example, in highly accurate positioning by Global Positionning System (GPS) [22], [23]. Works [24], [21], [22] propose suboptimal polynomial time algorithms for finding an approximately nearest lattice solution.

In our case, energy $E(\mathbf{k}|\boldsymbol{\psi})$ is a sum of quadratic functions of $(k_{ij} - k_{i-1,j})$ and $(k_{ij} - k_{i,j-1})$. This is a special case of a nearest lattice vector problem, for which we propose a network programming algorithm that finds the exact solution in polynomial time. The algorithm is inspired in the Flyn's minimum discontinuity approach [25], which minimizes the sum of $||\lfloor \Delta\phi_{ij}^h + \pi \rfloor||$ and $||\lfloor \Delta\phi_{ij}^v + \pi \rfloor||$, where $\lfloor x \rfloor$ denotes the hightest integer lower than x. Flyn's objective function is, therefore, quite different from ours. However, both objective functions are the sum of first order click potentials depending only on $\Delta\phi_{ij}^h$, and $\Delta\phi_{ij}^v$. This structural similarity allows us to adapt Flyn's ideas to our problem.

The following lemma assures that if the minimum of $E(\mathbf{k}|\psi)$ is not yet reached, then there exists a binary image $\delta\mathbf{k}$ (i.e., the elements of $\delta\mathbf{k}$ are all 0 or 1) such that $E(\mathbf{k} + \delta\mathbf{k}|\psi) < E(\mathbf{k}|\psi)$.

Lemma 1 *Let $\mathbf{k}_1$ and $\mathbf{k}_2$ be two wrap-count images such that*

$$E(\mathbf{k_2}|\psi) < E(\mathbf{k_1}|\psi). \tag{21}$$

Then, there exists a binary image $\delta\mathbf{k}$ such that

$$E(\mathbf{k_1} + \delta\mathbf{k}|\psi) < E(\mathbf{k_1}|\psi). \tag{22}$$

Proof. See [26].

According to Lemma 1, we can iteratively compute $\mathbf{k}_i = \mathbf{k}_{i-1} + \delta\mathbf{k}$, where $\delta\mathbf{k} \in \{0,1\}^{N^2}$ minimizes $E(\mathbf{k}_{i-1} + \delta\mathbf{k}|\psi)$, until the the minimum energy is reached. Each minimization is a discrete optimization problem that can be exactly solved in polynomial time by using network programming techniques such as maximum flow [27] or minimum cut [28]. We note however that, in the iterative scheme just described, it is not necessary to compute the exact minimizer of $E(\mathbf{k}_{i-1} + \delta\mathbf{k}|\psi)$ with respect to $\delta\mathbf{k}$, but only a binary image $\delta\mathbf{k}$ that decreases $E(\mathbf{k}_{i-1} + \delta\mathbf{k}|\psi)$. Based on this fact we propose an efficient algorithm that iteratively search for improving binary images $\delta\mathbf{k}$.

The following lemma, presented and proofed in the appendix of [25], assures that if there exists an improving binary image $\delta\mathbf{k}$ [i.e., $E(\mathbf{k} + \delta\mathbf{k}|\psi) < E(\mathbf{k}|\psi)$], then there exists another improving binary image $\delta\mathbf{l}$ such that the sets $S_1(\delta\mathbf{l}) \equiv \{(i,j) \in Z \mid \delta l_{ij} = 1\}$ and $S_0(\delta\mathbf{l}) \equiv \{(i,j) \in Z \mid \delta l_{ij} = 0\}$ are both connected in the first order neighborhood sense; i.e., given two sites s_1 and s_n of S_1 (S_0), there exists a sequence of first order neighbors, all in S_1 (S_0), that begins in s_1 and ends in s_n. We call images $\delta\mathbf{l}$ with this property, binary partitions of Z.

Lemma 2 *Suppose that there exits a binary image $\delta\mathbf{k}$ such that*

$$E(\mathbf{k} + \delta\mathbf{k}|\psi) < E(\mathbf{k}|\psi).$$

Then there exists a binary partition of Z, $\delta\mathbf{l}$, such that

$$E(\mathbf{k} + \delta\mathbf{l}|\psi) < E(\mathbf{k}|\psi).$$

Proof. See Lemma 2 in the appendix of [25].

Flyn's central idea is to search for improving binary partitions $\delta\mathbf{l}$ [termed in [25] an elementary operation (EO)]. Once $\delta\mathbf{l}$ is found the wrap-count image $\mathbf{k}$ is updated to $\mathbf{k} + \delta\mathbf{l}$. If no EO is possible then, according to Lemma 2, energy $E(\mathbf{k}|\psi)$

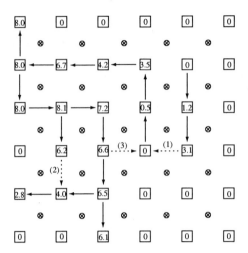

Fig. 2. Auxiliary graph to implement Flyn's algorithm (squared nodes) interleaved with phase sites (circled and crossed nodes). A leftward (rightward) edge indicates an unit increment of the wrap-count below (above) the edge. A downward (upward) edge indicates an unit increment of the wrap-count right (left) to the edge.

can not be decreased by any binary image increment of the actual argument $\mathbf{k}$. Thus, by Lemma 1, $E(\mathbf{k}|\psi)$ has reached its minimum.

To check if a given binary partition $\delta\mathbf{l}$ improves the energy, one has to compute only those click potentials of $E(\mathbf{k}|\psi)$ containing sites on both sets $S_1(\delta\mathbf{l})$ and $S_0(\delta\mathbf{l})$; i.e., one has to compute click potentials of $E(\mathbf{k}|\psi)$ only along loops (this is still true on the boundary of Z by taking zero potentials). The Flyn's algorithm uses graph theory techniques to represent and generate EOs. Figure 2 shows an auxiliary graph, whose nodes are interleaved with the phase sites. The edges sign which wrap-counts are to be incremented: a leftward (rightward) edge indicates an unit increment of the wrap-count below (above) the edge. A downward (upward) edge indicates a unit increment of the wrap-count right (left) to the edge. The algorithm works by creating and extending paths made of directed edges. When a path is extended to form a loop, the algorithm performs an EO, removes the loop from the collection of paths and resumes the path extension.

Assume that the array of auxiliary nodes has indexes in the set $\{(i,j)\,|\,i,j = 1,\ldots,N+1\}$. Define the cost of an edge $\delta V(i,j;i',j')$ between the first order neighbors (i',j') and (i,j) as $E(\mathbf{k}|\psi) - E(\mathbf{k}+\delta\mathbf{k}|\psi)$, where $\delta\mathbf{k}$ is the wrap-count increment induced by the edge. With this definitions and having in attention the structure of $E(\mathbf{k}|\psi)$ [see (17)], we are led to

$$\delta V(i,j;i,j-1) = -4\pi(\pi + \Delta\phi^v_{i,j-1})\bar{h}_{i,j-1}$$
$$\delta V(i,j-1;i,j) = -4\pi(\pi - \Delta\phi^v_{i,j-1})\bar{h}_{i,j-1}$$
$$\delta V(i-1,j;i,j) = -4\pi(\pi + \Delta\phi^h_{i-1,j})\bar{v}_{i-1,j}$$
$$\delta V(i,j;i-1,j) = -4\pi(\pi - \Delta\phi^h_{i-1,j})\bar{v}_{i-1,j}.$$

The values of boundary edges are defined to be zero; i.e., $\delta V(1,j) = \delta V(N+1,j) = \delta V(i,1) = \delta V(i,N+1) = 0$.

Figure 2 represents the state of the graph at a given instant. Assuming that there are no loops, the set of edges defines a given number of trees. The value of each node, $V(i, j)$, is the sum of edge values corresponding to the path between the node and the tree root. In Figure 2 there are two trees. We stress that the node values are real numbers, whereas in the Flyn's algorithm they are integers. The reason is that our energy $E(\mathbf{k}|\boldsymbol{\psi})$ takes values in the non-negative reals while the Flyn's energy takes values on the positive integers.

The basic step of Flyn's algorithm is to revise the set of paths by adding a new edge. An edge from (i, j) to a first order neighbor (i', j'), if not presented, is added if

$$\Delta V \equiv V(i, j) + \delta V(i, j; i', j') - V(i', j') > 0.$$

If $\Delta V \leq 0$ then the new path to (i', j') would have a negative or zero value or would fail to improve an existing path. If the edge is added the set of paths is revised in one of the three possible ways (a minor modification of [25]): 1) edge addition, 2) edge replacement, and 3) edge completion.

The dashed edges in Fig. 2 illustrate graph revision of type 1, 2, and 3. For a more detailed example, see Flyn's paper [25].

The algorithm alternates between type 1 and type 2 revisions until a loop is found, performing then a type 3 revision. If for any attempt of edge addition $\Delta V \leq 0$, then no loop completion is possible and, according to Lemma 2 and Lemma 1, the algorithm terminates.

Flyn's algorithm [25] and Costantini's [29] algorithm are equivalent, as they minimize the L^1 norm. Costantini has shown that L^1 minimization is equivalent to finding the minimum cost flow on a given directed network. Minimum cost flow is a graph problem for which there exists efficient solutions (see, e.g. [30]). We do not implement our $\mathbb{Z}$-step using Costantini's solution because the graph can not be used with L^p norm for $p \neq 1$.

Another alternative to implement the $\mathbb{Z}$-step might be the discrete optimization scheme proposed in [31]. Authors of this paper claim that their approach, based on the maximum flow algorithm applied to a suitable graph, minimizes any energy function in which the smoothness term is convex and involves only pairs of neighboring pixels. However, the graph for a given convex smoothness function is not presented in [31].

3.2   Smoothing Step

The smoothing step (15) amounts to compute $\widehat{\boldsymbol{\psi}}$ given by

$$\widehat{\boldsymbol{\psi}} = \arg \max_{\boldsymbol{\psi} \in [-\pi, \pi]^{N^2}} \sum_{ij \in Z} \lambda_{ij} \cos(\phi_{ij} - \eta_{ij}) - \frac{\mu}{2} \sum_{ij \in Z_1} (\Delta \phi_{ij}^h)^2 + (\Delta \phi_{ij}^v)^2, \quad (23)$$

where $\phi_{ij} = 2\pi k_{ij} + \psi_{ij}$. The function to be maximized in (23) is not convex due to terms $\lambda_{ij} \cos(\phi_{ij} - \eta_{ij})$. Computing $\widehat{\boldsymbol{\psi}}$ is therefore a hard problem. Herein, we adopt the ICM approach [14], which, in spite of being suboptimal, yields good results for the problem at hand.

ICM is a coordinatewise ascent technique where all coordinates are visited according to a given schedule. After some simple algebraic manipulation of the objective function (23), we conclude that its maximum with respect to ψ_{ij} is given by

$$\widehat{\psi}_{ij} = \arg \max_{\psi_{ij} \in [-\pi, \pi[} \left\{ \beta_{ij} \cos(\psi_{ij} - \eta_{ij}) - (\psi_{ij} - \bar{\psi}_{ij})^2 \right\}, \qquad (24)$$

where

$$\beta_{ij} = \frac{\lambda_{ij}}{2\mu} \qquad (25)$$

$$\bar{\psi}_{ij} = \bar{\phi}_{ij} - 2\pi k_{ij} \qquad (26)$$

$$\bar{\phi}_{ij} = \frac{\phi_{i-1,j} + \phi_{i,j-1} + \phi_{i+1,j} + \phi_{i,j+1}}{4}. \qquad (27)$$

There are no closed form solutions for maximization (24), since it involves transcendent and power functions. We compute $\widehat{\psi}_{ij}$ using a simple two-resolution numeric method. First we search $\widehat{\psi}_{ij}$ in the set $\{\pi i/M \,|\, i = -M, \ldots, M-1\}$. Next we refine the search by using the set $\{\pi i_0/M + \pi i/M^2 \,|\, i = -M, \ldots, M-1\}$, where $\pi i_0/M$ is the result of the first search. We have used $M = 20$, which leads to the maximum error of $\pi/(20)^2$.

Phase estimate $\widehat{\psi}_{ij}$ depends in a nonlinear way on data η_{ij} and on the mean weighted phase $\bar{\psi}_{ij}$. The balance between these two components is controlled by parameter β_{ij}. Assuming that $|\bar{\psi}_{ij} - \eta_{ij}| \ll \pi$, then $\cos(\psi_{ij} - \eta_{ij})$ is well approximated by the quadratic form $1 - (\psi_{ij} - \eta_{ij})^2/2$, thus leading to the linear approximation

$$\widehat{\psi}_{ij} \simeq \frac{\beta_{ij}\eta_{ij} + 2\bar{\psi}_{ij}}{\beta_{ij} + 2}. \qquad (28)$$

Reintroducing (28) in the above condition, one gets $|\bar{\psi}_{ij} - \eta_{ij}| \ll 2\pi/(\beta_{ij} + 2)$. If this condition is not met, the solution becomes highly nonlinear on η_{ij} and $\bar{\psi}_{ij}$: as $|\bar{\psi}_{ij} - \eta_{ij}|$ increases, at some point the phase $\widehat{\psi}_{ij}$ becomes thresholded to $\pm\pi$, being therefore independent of the observed data η_{ij}.

Concerning computer complexity the $\mathbb{Z}$-step is, by far, the most demanding one, using a number of floating point operations very close to the Flyn's minimum discontinuity algorithm. Since the proposed scheme needs roughly four $\mathbb{Z}$-steps, is has, approximately 4 times the Flyn's minimum discontinuity algorithm complexity. To our knowledge there is no formula for the Flyn's algorithm complexity (see remarks about complexity in [25]). Nevertheless, we have found, empirically, a complexity of approximately $O(N^3)$ for the $\mathbb{Z}$-step.

4 Experimental Results

The algorithm derived in the previous sections is now applied to synthetic data.

Figure 3 displays the interferogram ($\eta = \{\eta_{ij}\}$ image) generated according to density (2) with noise variance $\sigma_n = 1.05$. The absolute phase image ϕ is

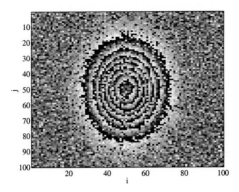

Fig. 3. Interfergram (η-image) of a Gaussian elevation of height 14π rad and standard deviations $\sigma_i = 10$ and $\sigma_j = 15$ pixels. The noise variance is $\sigma_n = 1.05$.

a Gaussian elevation of height 14π rad and standard deviations $\sigma_i = 10$ and $\sigma_j = 15$ pixels. The magnitude of the phase difference $\phi_{i,j+1} - \phi_{ij}$ takes the maximum value of 2.5 and is greater than 2 in many sites. On the other hand a noise variance of $\sigma_n = 1.05$ implies a standard deviation the maximum likelihood estimate η_{ij} of 0.91. This figure is computed with basis on the density of η obtained from the joint density (2). In these conditions, the task of absolute phase estimation is extremely hard, as the interferogram exhibits a large number of inconsistencies; i.e., the observed image η is not consistent with the assumption of absolute phase differences less than π in a large number of sites. In the unwrapping jargon the interferogram is said to have a lot of residues.

The smoothness parameter was set to $\mu = 1/0.8^2$, thus modelling phase images with phase differences (horizontal and vertical) of standard deviation 0.8. This value is too large for most of the true absolute phase image ϕ and too small for sites in the neighborhood of sites ($i = -45, j = 50$) and ($i = 55, j = 50$) (where the magnitude of the phase difference has its largest value). Nevertheless, the $\mathbb{Z}\pi$M algorithm yields good results as it can be read from Fig. 4; Fig. 4(a) shows the phase estimate $\widehat{\phi}^{(1)}$ and Fig. 4(b) shows the phase estimate $\widehat{\phi}^{(10)}$.

Figure 5 plots the logarithm of the posterior density $\ln p_{\phi|\mathbf{x}}(\widehat{\phi}^{(t)}|\mathbf{x})$ and the L^2 norm of the estimation error $\|\widehat{\phi} - \phi\|^2 \equiv N^{-2}\sum_{ij}(\widehat{\phi}_{ij} - \phi_{ij})^2$ as function of the iteration t. The four non-integers ticked between two consecutive integers refer to four consecutive ICM sweeps, implementing the π-step of the $\mathbb{Z}\pi$M algorithm. Notice that the larger increment in $\ln p_{\phi|\mathbf{x}}(\widehat{\phi}^{(t)}|\mathbf{x})$ happens in both steps of the first iteration. For $t \geq 2$ only the $\mathbb{Z}$-step produces noticeable increments in the posterior density. These increments are however possible due to the very small increments produced by the smoothing steep. For $t > 4$ there is practically no improvement in the estimates.

To rank $\mathbb{Z}\pi$M algorithm, we have applied the following phase unwrapping algorithms to the present problem:

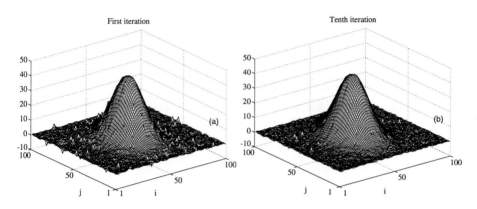

Fig. 4. Phase estimate $\widehat{\phi}^{(t)}$; (a) $t = 1$; (b) $t = 10$.

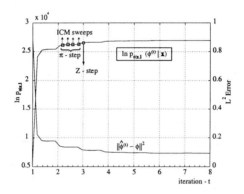

Fig. 5. Evolution of the logarithm of the posterior density $\ln p_{\phi|\mathbf{x}}(\widehat{\phi}^{(t)}|\mathbf{x})$ and of the L^2 norm of the estimation error as function of the iteration t. $\mathbb{Z}$-steps coincide with integers, whereas ICM sweeps implementing π-step are assigned to the non-integer part of t.

- **Path following type:** Golstein's branch cut (GBC) [32]; quality guided (QG) [33], [34]; and mask cut (MC) [35]
- **Minimum norm type:** Flyn's minimum discontinuity (FMD) [25]; weighted least-square (WLS) [36], [37]; and L^0 norm (L0N) (see [1, ch. 5.5])
- **Bayesian type:** recursive nonlinear filters [9] and [10] (NLF).

Path following and minimum norm algorithms were implemented with the code supplied in the book [1], using the following settings: GBC (-dipole yes); QG, MC, (-mode min_var -tsize 3); and WLS (-mode min_var -tsize 3, -thresh yes). We have used the unweighted versions of the FMD and L0N algorithms.

Table 1 displays the L^2 norm of the estimation error $||\widehat{\phi} - \phi||^2$ for each of the classic algorithm referred above. Results on the left column area based on the maximum likelihood estimate of η given by (4), using a 3×3 rectangular window. Results on the right column are based on the interferogram η without

Table 1. L^2 norm of the estimation errors of $\mathbb{Z}\pi$M and other unwrapping algorithms. The left column plots results based of the the maximum likelihood estimate of η using a 3×3 rectangular window; the right column plots results based on the non-smooth η given by (4).

Algorithm	Smooth η	Non-smooth η
	$\|\hat{\phi} - \phi\|^2$	
$\mathbb{Z}\pi$M	–	0.1
GBC	48.0	7.0
QG	10.0	2.2
MC	40.8	28.6
FMD	22.4	3.4
WLS	8.8	3.5
LON	24.1	2.6
NLF	–	40.1

any smoothing. Apart from the proposed $\mathbb{Z}\pi$M scheme, all the algorithms have produced poor results, some of them catastrophic. The reasons depend on the class of algorithms and are are basically the following:

– in the path following and minimum norm methods the noise filtering is the first processing steep and is disconnected from the phase unwrapping process. The noise filtering assumes the phase to be constant within given windows. In data sets as the one at hand, this assumption is catastrophic, even using small windows. On the other hand, if the smoothing steep is not applied, even if algorithm is able to infer most of the 2π multiples, the observation noise is fully present in estimated phase
– the recursive nonlinear approaches [9] and [10] fails basically because they use only the past observed data, in the lexicographic sense, to infer the absolute phase.

5   Concluding Remarks

The paper presented an effective approach to absolute phase estimation in interferometric appliactions. The Bayesian standpoint was adopted. The likelihood function, which models the observation mechanism given the absolute phase, is 2π-periodic and accounts for interferometric noise. The *a priori* probability of the absolute phase is a noncausal first order Gauss Markov random field (GMRF).

We proposed an iterative procedure, with two steps per iteration, for the computation of the *maximum a posteriory probability* MAP estimate. The first step, termed $\mathbb{Z}$-step, maximizes the posterior density with respect to the 2π phase multiples; the second step, termed π-step, maximizes the posterior density with respect to the phase principal values. The $\mathbb{Z}$-step is a discrete optimization problem solved exactly by network programming techniques inspired by Flyn's *minimum discontinuity algorithm* [25]. The π-step is a continuous optimization problem solved approximately by the *iterated conditional modes* (ICM) procedure. We call the proposed algorithm $\mathbb{Z}\pi$M, where the letter M stands for maximization.

The $\mathbb{Z}\pi$M algorithm, resulting from a Bayesian approach, accounts for the observation noise in a model based fashion. More specifically, the observation mechanism takes into account electronic and decorrelation noises. This is a crucial feature that underlies the advantage of the $\mathbb{Z}\pi$M algorithm over path following and minimum-norm schemes, mainly in regions where the phase rate is close to π. In fact, these schemes split the absolute phase estimation problem into two separate steps: in the first step the noise in the interferogram is filtered by applying low-pass filtering; in the second step, termed phase unwrapping, the 2π phase multiples are computed. For high phase rate regions, the application of first step makes it impossible to recover the absolute phase, as the principal values estimates are of poor quality. This is in contrast with the $\mathbb{Z}\pi$M algorithm, where the first step, the $\mathbb{Z}$-step, is an unwrapping applied over the observed interferogram.

To evaluate the performance of the $\mathbb{Z}\pi$M algorithm, a Gaussian shaped surface whit high phase rate, and 0dB of signal to noise ratio was considered. We have compared the computed estimates with those provided by the best path following and minimum-norm schemes, namely the Golstein's branch cut, the quality guided, the Flyn's minimum discontinuity, the weighted least-square, and the L^0 norm. The proposed algorithm yields good results, performing better and in some cases much better than the s technique just referred.

Concerning computer complexity, the $\mathbb{Z}\pi$M algorithm takes, approximately, a number of floating point operations proportional to the 1.5 power of the number of pixels . By far, the $\mathbb{Z}$-step is the most demanding one, using a number of floating point operations very close to the Flyn's minimum discontinuity algorithm. Since the proposed scheme needs roughly four $\mathbb{Z}$-steps, is has, approximately 4 times the Flyn's minimum discontinuity algorithm complexity.

Concerning future developments, we foresee the integration of the principal phase values in the posterior density as a major research direction. If this goal would be attained then the wrapp-count image would be the only unknown of the obtained posterior density and, most important, there would be no need for iterativeness in estimating the wrapp-count image. After obtaining this image, the principal phase values could be obtained using the π-step of the $\mathbb{Z}\pi$M algorithm.

References

1. D. Ghiglia and M. Pritt. *Two-Dimentional Phase Unwrapping. Theory, Algorithms, and Software.* John Wiley & Sons, New York, 1998.
2. J. Strand. *Two-dimensional Phase Unwrapping with Applications.* PhD thesis, Department of Mathematics, Faculty of Mathematics and Natural Sciences, University of Bergen, 1999.
3. J. Strand, T. Taxt, and A. Jain. Two-dimensional phase-unwrapping using a two-dimensional least square method. *IEEE Transactions on Geoscience and Remote Sensing*, 82(3):375–386, March 1999.

4. J. Marroquin and M. Rivera. Quadratic regularization functionals for phase unwrapping. *Journal of the Optical Society of America*, 11(12):2393–2400, 1995.
5. L. Guerriero, G. Nico, G. Pasquariello, and S. Starmaglia. New regularization scheme for phase unwrapping. *Applied Optics*, 37(14):3053–3058, 1998.
6. M. Rivera, J. Marroquin, and R. Rodriguez-Vera. Fast algorithm for integrating inconsistent gradient fields. *Applied Optics*, 36(32):8381–8390, 1995.
7. M. Servin, J. Marroquin, D. Malacara, and F. Cuevas. Phase unwrapping with a regularized phase-tracking system. *Applied Optics*, 37(10):19171–1923, 1998.
8. J. Leitão and M. Figueiredo. Interferometric image reconstruction as a nonlinear Bayesian estimation problem. In *Proceedings of the First IEEE International Conference on Image Processing – ICIP'95*, volume 2, pages 453–456, 1995.
9. J. Leitão and M. Figueiredo. Absolute phase image reconstruction: A stochastic nonlinear filtering approach. *IEEE Transactions on Image Processing*, 7(6):868–882, June 1997.
10. J. Dias and J. Leitão. Simultaneous phase unwrapping and speckle smoothing in SAR images: A stochastic nonlinear filtering approach. In *EUSAR'98 European Conference on Synthetic Aperture Radar*, pages 373–377, Friedrichshafen, May 1998.
11. G. Nico, G. Palubinskas, and M. Datcu. Bayesian approach to phase unwrapping: theoretical study. *IEEE Transactions on Signal processing*, 48(9):2545–2556, Sept. 2000.
12. B. Friedlander and J. Francos. Model based phase unwrapping of 2-d signals. *IEEE Transactions on Signal Processing*, 44(12):2999–3007, 1996.
13. Z. Liang. A model-based for phase unwrapping. *IEEE Transactions on Medical Imaging*, 15(6):893–897, 1996.
14. J. Besag. On the statistical analysis of dirty pictures. *Journal of the Royal Statistical Society B*, 48(3):259–302, 1986.
15. S. Geman and D. Geman. Stochastic relaxation, Gibbs distribution and the Bayesian restoration of images. *IEEE Transactions on Pattern Analysis and Machine Intelligence*, PAMI-6(6):721–741, November 1984.
16. D. Angwin and H. Kaufman. Image restoration using reduced order models. *Signal Processing*, 16:21–28, 89.
17. J. Besag. Spatial interaction and the statistical analysis of lattice systems. *Journal of the Royal Statistical Society B*, 36(2):192–225, 1974.
18. K. Ho. Exact probability-density function for phase-measurement interferometry. *Journal of the Optical Society of America*, 12(9):1984–1989, 1995.
19. K. S. Miller. *Complex Stochastic Processes. An Introduction to Theory and Applications*. Addison–Wesley Publishing Co., London, 1974.
20. E. Rignot and R. Chellappa. Segmentation of polarimetric synthetic aperture radar data. *IEEE Transactions Image Processing*, 1(1):281–300, 1992.
21. M. Grotschel, L. Lovasz, and A. Schrijver. *Beometric Algorithms and Combinatorial Optimization*. Algorithms and Combinatorics. Springer-Verlag, New York, 1988.
22. A Hassibi and S. Boyd. Integer parameter estimation in linear models with applications to gps. *IEEE Transactions on Signal Processing*, 46(11):2938–2952, Nov. 1998.
23. G. Strang and K. Borre. *Linear Algebra, Geodesy, and GPS*. Wellesley-Cambridge Press, New York, 1997.
24. L. Babai. On lovasz lattice reduction and the nearest lattice point problem. *Combinatorica*, 6:1–13, 1986.

25. T. Flynn. Two-dimensional phase unwrapping with minimum weighted disconti-
    nuity. *Journal of the Optical Society of America A*, 14(10):2692–2701, 1997.
26. J. Dias and J. Leitão. Interferometric absolute phase reconstruction in sar/sas: A
    bayesian approach. Thechical report, Instituto Superior Técnico, 2000.
27. D. Greig, B. Porteus, and A. Seheult. Exact maximum a posteriory estimation for
    binary images. *Jounal of Royal Statistics Society B*, 51(2):271–279, 1989.
28. Y. Boykov, O. Veksler, and R. Zabih. A new minimization algorithm for en-
    ergy minimaization with discontinuities. In E. Hancock and M. Pelillo, edi-
    tors, *Energy Minimization Methods in Computer Vision and Pattern Recognition-
    EMMCVPR'99*, pages 205–220, York, 1999. Springer.
29. M. Costantini. A novel phase unwrapping method based on network programing.
    IEEE Transactions on Geoscience and Remote Sensing, 36(3):813–821, May 1998.
30. R. Ahuja, T. Magnanti, and J. Orlin. *Network Flows: Theory, Algorithms and
    Applications*. Prentice Hall, 1993.
31. H. Ishikawa and D. Geiger. Segmentation by grouping junctions. In *Proceedings of
    the IEEE Computer Society Conference on Computer Vision and Pattern Recog-
    nition – CVPR'98*, pages 125–131, 1998.
32. R. Goldstein, H. Zebker, and C. Werner. Satellite radar interferometry: Two-
    dimensional phase unwrapping. In *Symposium on the Ionospheric Effects on Com-
    munication and Related Systems*, volume 23, pages 713–720. Radio Science, 1988.
33. H. Lim, W. Xu, and X. Huang. Two new practical methods for phase unwrapping.
    In *Proc. of the 1995 Internat. Geoscience and Remote Sensing Symposium*, pages
    2044–2046, Lincoln, 1996.
34. W. Xu and I. Cumming. A region growing algorithm for insar phase unwrapping. In
    Proceedings of the 1996 International Geoscience and Remote Sensing Symposium,
    pages 196–198, Firenze, 1995.
35. T. Flynn. Consistent 2-D phase unwrapping guided by a quality map. In *Proceed-
    ings of the 1996 International Geoscience and Remote Sensing Symposium*, pages
    2057–2059, Lincoln, NE, 1996.
36. D. Ghiglia and L. Romero. Robust two-dimensional weighted and unweighted
    phase unwrapping that uses fast transforms and iterative methods. *Journal of the
    Optical Society of America*, 11(1):107–117, 1994.
37. M. Pritt. Phase unwrapping by means of multigrid techniques for interferometric
    SAR. *IEEE Transactions on Geoscience and Remote Sensing*, 34(3):728–738, May
    1996.

Global Energy Minimization: A Transformation Approach

Kar-Ann Toh

Centre for Signal Processing
School of Electrical & Electronic Engineering
Nanyang Technological University, 50 Nanyang Avenue, Singapore 639798
Email: ekatoh@ntu.edu.sg

Abstract. This paper addresses the problem of minimizing an energy function by means of a monotonic transformation. With an observation on global optimality of functions under such a transformation, we show that a simple and effective algorithm can be derived to search within possible regions containing the global optima. Numerical experiments are performed to compare this algorithm with one that does not incorporate transformed information using several benchmark problems. These results are also compared to best known global search algorithms in the literature. In addition, the algorithm is shown to be useful for a class of neural network learning problems, which possess much larger parameter spaces.

1   Introduction

Typically, the overall performance of an application in computer vision, pattern recognition, and many other fields of machine intelligence can be described or approximated by a multivariate function, where the best solution is achieved when the function attains its global extremum. This function to be optimized, the so-called objective function or energy function, is usually formulated to be dependent on a certain number of state variables or parameters. Due to the complexity of physical systems, this objective function is very likely to be nonlinear with respect to its parameters. Depending on the number of parameters and the intrinsic problem nature, the task of locating the global extremum can be extremely difficult. This is due to the unsolvable nature of the general global optimal value problem [17] and the omni-presence of local extrema, whose number may increase exponentially with the size of the parameter vector. Furthermore, in real world applications, there may be flat regions which can mislead gradient-based search methods. Worst still, difficulties may arise when these gradients are different by many orders of magnitude.

As it remains to be the most challenging task to come out with a generic and practical characterization for global optimality, main research effort has been focused on specially structured optimization problems and exhaustive means [6, 7]. While a multitude of ideas have been attempted in devising effective search methods for global solutions via numerical means, the various approaches can

M.A.T. Figueiredo, J. Zerubia, A.K. Jain (Eds.): EMMCVPR 2001, LNCS 2134, pp. 391–406, 2001.

nevertheless be broadly classified as follows: (i) deterministic approaches, (ii) probabilistic/heuristic approaches, and (iii) a mix of deterministic and probabilistic methods. Conceptually, most deterministic methods adopt strategies that are covering-based or grid-search-based, and those that use an ingenious tunneling mechanism or trajectory trace to search through the domain of interest for the global solution [1, 7, 18]. Improvements from such strategies are usually in the form of reducing the computational requirements by narrowing down the search progressively, and discarding regions which are not likely to contain the global optima [6, 7]. For probabilistic methods, various random search methodologies which inherit the 'hill-climbing' capability are employed to locate the global optima (see e.g. [2, 6]). Theoretically, probabilistic methods do not guarantee (this, indeed, is a deterministic requirement) that global optimal solutions are reached within finite search instances, even though asymptotic assurance can usually be achieved. The third class of methods attempts to combine merits of both deterministic and probabilistic methods to achieve efficient means in attaining the global optimal solution.

In this article, the following two issues are addressed: (i) to provide an observation on global optimality of functions under monotonic transformation, and (ii) to illustrate the usefulness of such observation using a deterministic search procedure which is derived from the well-established nonlinear programming literature. We show that it is possible to make use of a structurally known transformation to 'extract' the required structural information from the function of interest. In short, by a notion of "relative structural means for relative structural information", we propose to use the monotonic transformation for characterization of global optimality.

The paper is organized as follows: in next section, we provide notations and definitions related to the subject matter. In section 3, the necessary and sufficient conditions for global optimality based on monotonic transformation are shown. Based on this, regions that contain the global optimal solutions are identified using a level set. In section 4, a global descent algorithm is derived to search within this level set for global optimal solutions. This is followed by section 5 where we compare two settings of our search procedure numerically with one that does not use the proposed transformation. The results in terms of the number of function evaluations and standard CPU time required are also compared with best known global optimization algorithms in the literature. In section 6, we further illustrate the usefulness of the algorithm for neural network applications which represent systems of a larger scale. Finally, some concluding remarks are drawn.

2   Notations And Definitions

Unless otherwise stated, vector and matrix quantities are denoted using bold lowercase characters and bold uppercase characters respectively, to distinguish from scalar quantities. The superscript 'T' on the respective character is used to denote matrix transposition.

2.1   Minimization problem

Let $\mathcal{D}$ be a p-dimensional compact subset of real space $(\mathcal{R}^p)$ and f be a continuous function from $\mathcal{D}$ to $\mathcal{R}$. Since maximization of the function f is equivalent to minimization of $(-f)$, without loss of generality, we define the problem of global optimization to be

$$(\mathcal{P}): \ \arg \min_{\boldsymbol{\theta}} f(\boldsymbol{\theta}), \quad \boldsymbol{\theta} \in \mathcal{D}, \tag{1}$$

assuming existence of at least a solution (see Definition 1, as will be defined next).

2.2   Solution and solution set

In this context, we refer to the solution and solution set of a minimization problem as:

Definition 1 *Let f be a function to be minimized from $\mathcal{D}$ to $\mathcal{R}$ where $\mathcal{D} \subseteq \mathcal{R}^p$ is non-empty and compact. A point $\boldsymbol{\theta} \in \mathcal{D}$ is called a feasible solution to the minimization problem. If $\boldsymbol{\theta}_g^* \in \mathcal{D}$ and $f(\boldsymbol{\theta}) \geqslant f(\boldsymbol{\theta}_g^*)$ for each $\boldsymbol{\theta} \in \mathcal{D}$, then $\boldsymbol{\theta}_g^*$ is called a global optimal solution (global minimum) to the problem. If $\boldsymbol{\theta}^* \in \mathcal{D}$ and if there exists an ε-neighborhood $N_\varepsilon(\boldsymbol{\theta}^*)$ around $\boldsymbol{\theta}^*$ such that $f(\boldsymbol{\theta}) \geqslant f(\boldsymbol{\theta}^*)$ for each $\boldsymbol{\theta} \in \mathcal{D} \cap N_\varepsilon(\boldsymbol{\theta}^*)$, then $\boldsymbol{\theta}^*$ is called a local optimal solution (local minimum). The set which contains both local optimal solutions and global optimal solutions is called a solution set (denoted by Θ^*).*

3   Global Optimality

3.1   Global optimality of functions under monotonic transformation

Denote $\mathcal{R}^+ = (0, \infty)$. Consider a strictly decreasing transformation ϕ on the function to be minimized. Denote by $\phi^\gamma(\cdot)$ a transformation which is raised to some power $\gamma \in \mathcal{R}$. We shall make use of the following observation for our development.

Proposition 1. *Let $f : \mathcal{D} \to \mathcal{R}$ be a continuous function where $\mathcal{D} \subseteq \mathcal{R}^p$ is compact. Let $\phi : \mathcal{R} \to \mathcal{R}^+$ be a strictly decreasing function. Suppose $\boldsymbol{\theta}^* \in \mathcal{D}$. Then $\boldsymbol{\theta}^*$ is a global minimizer of f if and only if*

$$\lim_{\gamma \to \infty} \frac{\phi^\gamma(f(\boldsymbol{\theta}))}{\phi^\gamma(f(\boldsymbol{\theta}^*))} = 0, \quad \forall \boldsymbol{\theta} \in \mathcal{D}, \ f(\boldsymbol{\theta}) \neq f(\boldsymbol{\theta}^*). \tag{2}$$

Proof: This follows from the fact that $\frac{\phi^\gamma(f(\boldsymbol{\theta}))}{\phi^\gamma(f(\boldsymbol{\theta}^*))} > 0$ so that $\lim_{\gamma \to \infty} \frac{\phi^\gamma(f(\boldsymbol{\theta}))}{\phi^\gamma(f(\boldsymbol{\theta}^*))} = 0$ is equivalent to $\frac{\phi(f(\boldsymbol{\theta}))}{\phi(f(\boldsymbol{\theta}^*))} < 1$. ∎

Consider the solution set as defined by Definition 1. Then, using a more structured *convex* transformation ϕ, the following result is a direct consequence of Proposition 1.

Proposition 2. *Let* $f : \mathcal{D} \to \mathcal{R}$ *be a continuous function where* $\mathcal{D} \subseteq \mathcal{R}^p$ *is compact. Let* $\phi : \mathcal{R} \to \mathcal{R}^+$ *be a strictly decreasing and convex function. Denote by* Θ^* *the solution set given by Definition 1. Suppose* $\boldsymbol{\theta}^* \in \Theta^*$. *Then* $\boldsymbol{\theta}^*$ *is a global minimizer of* f *if and only if*

$$\lim_{\gamma \to \infty} \frac{\phi^\gamma(f(\boldsymbol{\theta}))}{\phi^\gamma(f(\boldsymbol{\theta}^*))} = 0, \quad \forall \boldsymbol{\theta} \in \Theta^*, \ f(\boldsymbol{\theta}) \neq f(\boldsymbol{\theta}^*). \tag{3}$$

Remark 1:- Consider $x_0, x_1, x_2 \in \mathcal{R}$ and suppose $x_0 = (1-\alpha)x_1 + \alpha x_2$, $x_1 \neq x_2$, $0 < \alpha \leqslant 1$. Let $\phi(x_2) = \phi(x_1) - \delta$ for some $x_1 < x_2$ and $0 < \delta < \phi(x_1)$. Since $\phi(\cdot)$ is strictly decreasing and convex, it follows that

$$\phi^\gamma(x_0) \leqslant [(1-\alpha)\phi(x_1) + \alpha\phi(x_2)]^\gamma, \quad 0 < \alpha \leqslant 1$$
$$= \left[\phi(x_1)\left(1 - \frac{\alpha\delta}{\phi(x_1)}\right)\right]^\gamma, \tag{4}$$

which implies that

$$\frac{\phi^\gamma(x_0)}{\phi^\gamma(x_1)} \leqslant \left(1 - \frac{\alpha\delta}{\phi(x_1)}\right)^\gamma, \quad 0 < \alpha \leqslant 1. \tag{5}$$

For any arbitrary $\delta \in (0, \phi(x_1))$, we see that the ratio of any transformed points between x_1 and x_2 over the transformed x_1 (i.e. $\phi^\gamma(x_0)/\phi^\gamma(x_1)$) is held under a prescribed curve $(1 - \alpha\delta/\phi(x_1))^\gamma$ for $0 < \alpha \leqslant 1$. The result of such transformation is a structured magnifying effect preserving the relative orders of all extrema. Suppose x_1 is the global minimizer, we see that for any $\gamma > 1$, its neighborhood value x_0 will be held $(1 - \alpha\delta/\phi(x_1))^\gamma$ times below the value of $\phi^\gamma(x_1)$. We shall illustrate this with an example. □

3.2   An illustrative example

Visually, the role of ϕ is to magnify the relative ordering of global minima and local minima, but in a reverse sense. Notice that in the minimization case, a small value of f is mapped to a relatively much higher value of ϕ because ϕ is strictly decreasing and convex. This effect of relative ordering of minima is even more noticeable when ϕ is raised to a high power γ.

Consider the 2-dimensional Rastrigin function [17] for minimization within $[-1, 1]^2$. Let $\phi^\gamma(f) = e^{-\gamma(f - f_L)}$ where $f_L \in \mathcal{R}$ denotes a reference function value. It can be shown that this transformation function is convex and strictly decreasing. In order to maintain similar scalings for the plots, we take $f_L = f_g^*$ (f_g^* is the global minimum value) in this illustration. The 3-D mesh plot for the original Rastrigin function is shown in Fig. 1-(a). Here we see that determining a threshold level directly on f which will differentiate the global minimum from the other local minima is difficult.

The 3-D mesh plots for three versions of the transformed function using $\gamma = 1, 4, 20$ are shown in Fig. 1-(b),(c),(d) respectively. It is clear from Fig. 1 that transformation with a high γ value has made the global minimum 'stands out' from all other local minima. Effectively, the monotonically decreasing convex transformation suppresses local minima to a greater extent than the global minimum, and hence allowing the global minimum to emerge among the omnipresence of local minima.

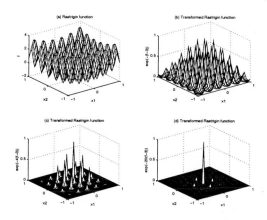

Fig. 1. Rastrigin function f: (a) before transformation, and (b)-(d) after transformation using $\phi^\gamma(f) = e^{-\gamma(f-\hat{f}_L)}$, $\gamma = 1, 4, 20$

3.3   A sufficient condition

Lemma 1. *Let $f : \mathcal{D} \to \mathcal{R}$ be a function to be minimized where f is continuous on the compact set $\mathcal{D}$. Let $\phi : \mathcal{R} \to \mathcal{R}^+$ be a strictly decreasing function. Denote by Θ^* the solution set given by Definition 1. Let $0 < \eta < 1$ and suppose $\theta^* \in \Theta^*$. If there exists $\gamma_o > 1$ such that*

$$\phi^\gamma(f(\boldsymbol{\theta})) \leqslant \eta\phi^\gamma(f(\boldsymbol{\theta}^*)), \quad f(\boldsymbol{\theta}) \neq f(\boldsymbol{\theta}^*) \tag{6}$$

for all $\gamma \geqslant \gamma_o$ and for all $\boldsymbol{\theta} \in \Theta^*$, then $\boldsymbol{\theta}^*$ is a global minimizer of f.

Proof: Let $\boldsymbol{\theta} \in \Theta^*$ where $f(\boldsymbol{\theta}) \neq f(\boldsymbol{\theta}^*)$. By the hypothesis in the lemma, there exists $\gamma_o > 1$ such that $\phi^\gamma(f(\boldsymbol{\theta})) \leqslant \eta\phi^\gamma(f(\boldsymbol{\theta}^*))$ for all $\gamma \geqslant \gamma_o$. Thus $\frac{\phi^\gamma(f(\boldsymbol{\theta}))}{\phi^\gamma(f(\boldsymbol{\theta}^*))} \leqslant \eta < 1$ for $\gamma > \gamma_o$. Passing to limit, we have $\lim_{\gamma\to\infty} \frac{\phi^\gamma(f(\boldsymbol{\theta}))}{\phi^\gamma(f(\boldsymbol{\theta}^*))} = 0$. By Proposition 1, $\boldsymbol{\theta}^*$ is a global minimizer. ∎

Remark 2:- When a structured magnifying effect as shown in section 3.2 is required, Lemma 1 can be adapted according to Proposition 2 for a ϕ which is strictly decreasing and convex.

For the most general problem of global optimization, the global optimal value is unknown. While noting that it is difficult to enumerate the entire solution set to validate (6) for all $\boldsymbol{\theta} \in \Theta^*$ assuming γ_0 exists, we shall observe in what follows, how Lemma 1 can be utilized to solve problem $(\mathcal{P})$. □

Denote the global minimizer by $\boldsymbol{\theta}_g^*$ and let $f_g^* := f(\boldsymbol{\theta}_g^*)$. Suppose we have a γ satisfying Lemma 1. Let

$$\eta\phi^\gamma(f_g^*) < \zeta \leqslant \phi^\gamma(f_g^*), \quad \eta \in (0,1). \tag{7}$$

Then, the problem of locating $\boldsymbol{\theta}_g^*$ in $(\mathcal{P})$ can be narrowed down to a search on

$$(\mathcal{P}') : \quad \arg\min_{\boldsymbol{\theta}} f(\boldsymbol{\theta}) \quad \text{subject to} \quad \boldsymbol{\theta} \in L_\phi(\zeta), \tag{8}$$

where

$$L_\phi(\zeta) = \{\boldsymbol{\theta} \mid \phi^\gamma(f(\boldsymbol{\theta})) \geqslant \zeta, \boldsymbol{\theta} \in \mathcal{D}\} \tag{9}$$

is a level set containing $\boldsymbol{\theta}_g^*$. Here, it is required to locate a $\zeta > 0$ (which satisfies (7)) cutting on $\phi^\gamma(f(\boldsymbol{\theta}))$ so that the global solutions are segregated from all other local solutions. As illustrated, the task of locating such a cutting level ζ in Fig. 1-(d) is easier than that in Fig. 1-(a) since the range of ζ given by (7) is larger than that given by $f^* < \zeta \leqslant f_g^*$ (where f^* denotes the second lowest minimum value of f) on the original function. Moreover, for practical reasons, the right-hand-side of (7) can be relaxed and $(\mathcal{P}')$ can be solved for the best achievable solution closest to qualifying $\phi^\gamma(f(\boldsymbol{\theta})) \geqslant \zeta > \eta\phi^\gamma(f_g^*)$, $\eta \in (0,1)$ and $\boldsymbol{\theta} \in \mathcal{D}$. We shall observe, for the following types of problems, how such cutting level can readily be located for the transformed function.

(i) Minimization of functions with known minimum value or its infimum

There is a class of minimization problems where the global minimum value is known a priori. For instance, the problem of solving $f(\boldsymbol{\theta}) = 0$ can be reformulated as a problem minimizing $(f(\boldsymbol{\theta}))^2$ for $\boldsymbol{\theta}$. This class of problems is, indeed, solvable by the argument using level sets [17]. By our characterization, global optimality is attained at $\phi^\gamma(0)$ where a cutting level at $\zeta \in (\eta\phi^\gamma(0), \phi^\gamma(0)]$, $\eta \in (0,1)$, $\gamma > 1$ can be easily chosen to segregate all other local minima for a sufficiently high γ value that results in a small η value. In short, we can simply choose a ζ that is close to $\phi^\gamma(0)$.

Instead of a known global minimum value, another class of minimization problems may come with knowledge of only an infimum or a lower bound of the global minimum value. This includes approximation problems using least squares type of error criterion where the lowest possible objective function value is approaching zero. Here, zero is a lower bound of the unknown global minimum value. For such cases, a level set can be defined with respect to the required solution quality. For instance, given an approximation problem: $f(\boldsymbol{\theta}) = (g^* - g(\boldsymbol{\theta}))^2$ where the function $g \in \mathcal{R}$ on $\boldsymbol{\theta} \in \mathcal{R}^p$ is to approximate $g^* \in \mathcal{R}$ within a certain error tolerance: $f \leqslant \epsilon = f^* + \varepsilon$, $\varepsilon > 0$, $f^* \in (0, \epsilon)$. In this case, a cutting level constraint can be selected with respect to the error tolerance at $\zeta = \phi^\gamma(\epsilon)$, $\gamma > 1$ when minimizing f.

(ii) Minimization of functions without prior knowledge of global minimum value

For functions with no prior knowledge of the global minimum values or the lower bounds, the following iterative procedure can be adopted to locate a cutting level on the transformed function segregating the global optimal solution from those local ones.

1. **Initialization**: Select a $\gamma > 1$ and initialize a level offset $f_L \in \mathcal{R}$ with respect to an arbitrary estimate $\theta_0 \in \mathcal{D}$, i.e. set $f_L \leqslant f(\theta_0)$. Set initial cutting level for the transformed function as $\zeta_0 = \phi^\gamma(0) + \Delta_0$ for some $\Delta_0 > 0$.

2. **Search**: Locate a local minimizer θ_1 of f satisfying $\phi^\gamma(f(\theta) - f_L) \geqslant \zeta_0$ and $\theta \in \mathcal{D}$. If such a solution exists, set $f_L \leqslant f(\theta_1)$, $\zeta_1 = \phi^\gamma(0) + \Delta_1$ for some $\Delta_1 > 0$ and continue to locate the next local minimizer θ_2 of f satisfying $\phi^\gamma(f(\theta) - f_L) \geqslant \zeta_1$ and $\theta \in \mathcal{D} \cdots$

3. **Termination**: The search terminates until no minimizer θ_{k+1} can be found for the current choice of f_L equal to the local minimum value $f(\theta_k)$ and with smallest possible $\Delta_k > 0$.

While leaving the implementation details to next section, we shall illustrate by an example the fact that the problem of locating such a cutting level becomes 'easier' [1] as the level search proceeds on a transformed function.

3.4   A global level search example

Consider the following univariate function to be minimized:

$$f(x) = x^4 - \cos(20x), \quad -1 \leqslant x \leqslant 1. \tag{10}$$

Note that since the concept applies to multivariate case as well, this example is used without loss of generality. The plot for this function is shown in Fig. 2(a) where we have a unique global optimal solution at $x = 0$. Suppose we do not have prior knowledge of the global minimum value $f_g^* = -1$. We see that even a small difference between two cutting levels on f near the global optimal value can result in minimizers which are far apart. Hence, if a search is performed directly on this function, it is difficult to locate a level such that it just segregates the ultimate minimum from other minima. The situation can be worse if the function is extremely flat near the global solution.

Now, consider the following transformation function where its monotonicity and convexity can be easily verified by checking its first and second derivatives:

$$\phi(f) = \left\{ -\log\left[\frac{1}{1 + e^{-100(f - f_L)}} \right] \right\}^\gamma. \tag{11}$$

---

[1] In the sense of obtaining a clear cutting level on $\phi^\gamma(f(\theta))$ that segregates the global minima from local minima.

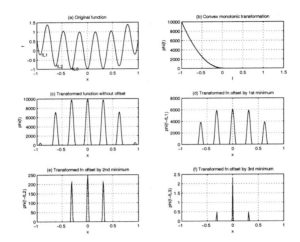

Fig. 2. Level search over the transformed function

The plots for ϕ over f, and ϕ over x, are shown in Fig. 2(b) and (c), respectively, with $f_L = 0$. We note that this particular transformation suppresses function values which are greater than zero.

As we have seen in section 3.2, a high γ eases the task of locating a suitable level to segregate the global minima from local ones (hopefully within a single step). While not expecting to conduct an exhaustive level search for all the local minima in a descending order under most circumstances, we shall walk through a step by step level search, illustrating the convergence. Here, to illustrate only the effect of the level offset, we have set $\gamma = 2$ for all cases in the figure.

The plots for $\phi(f(x))$ over x which are offset at $(f - f_{L1})$ through $(f - f_{L3})$ corresponding to those descending local minima are shown in Fig. 2, (d) through (f) respectively. We see that as the level offset moves downwards, starting from the highest local minimum at f_{L1}, the convex monotonic transformation suppresses f values which are equal to or greater than this local minimum value. At the same time, those minima lower than the current level offset are stretched further apart with their relative ordering preserved. When the level offset reaches the second lowest minimum value (f_{L3}), all other local minima are flattened to almost zero as seen in the transformed function, except the case for $\phi(f - f_{L3}) \approx 0.5$ and the case for a higher value of transformed global minimum. Notice that the transformed function becomes sharper as the level offset approaches the global solution. Existence of a cutting level ζ on the transformed function becomes more obvious as the search proceeds. Hence the convergence in locating such a cutting level.

4   Global Descent Search

Having identified those regions that contain the global optimal solutions in previous section, the well-established constrained search methodologies can be applied to locate the global solutions. Here, we adopt the penalty function method to arrive at a simple and easily reproduceable search utilizing only information from first-order partial derivatives of the objective function. In all subsequent developments, we use $\phi(\cdot) = e^{-(\cdot)}$ as the transformation function.

4.1   Penalty function method

To perform a search within those regions containing the global minima, the unconstrained minimization problem is re-formulated into a constrained one. Here, those regions defined by a cutting level on the transformed function are used as constraints to the minimization problem. In a more formal way, problem $(\mathcal{P})$ in (1) is re-formulated as $(\mathcal{P}')$ given by (8) and (9), and a search is performed on $(\mathcal{P}')$.

Consider the translated minimization problem $\min(f - \xi)$, $\xi \in \mathcal{R}$. Since only translation is involved, the problem of locating $\boldsymbol{\theta}_g^*$ from minimizing f is equivalent to that of minimizing $(f - \xi)$. Suppose $\xi \leqslant f_g^*$, then for $s = (f - \xi)^2$, we can further treat

$$\arg\min_{\boldsymbol{\theta}} \ (f(\boldsymbol{\theta}) - \xi) \equiv \arg\min_{\boldsymbol{\theta}} \ s(\boldsymbol{\theta}). \tag{12}$$

Thus, instead of performing a search directly on f, we can perform a search on s for $\boldsymbol{\theta}_g^*$ when $\xi \leqslant f_g^*$. This dependency on ξ will be removed in subsequent derivation of a search algorithm.

Suppose there are l constraint functions which specify conditions in (9):

$$\mathbf{h}(\boldsymbol{\theta}) = [h_1(\boldsymbol{\theta}), \ h_2(\boldsymbol{\theta}), \ \cdots, \ h_l(\boldsymbol{\theta})]^T \leqslant \mathbf{0}, \tag{13}$$

where $h_1(\boldsymbol{\theta}) = \zeta - e^{-\gamma(f(\boldsymbol{\theta}) - f_L)}$ and $h_2(\boldsymbol{\theta}), ..., h_l(\boldsymbol{\theta})$ are defined by the boundaries given by the domain of interest $\mathcal{D}$ (e.g. $h_2(\boldsymbol{\theta}) = -\theta_1 - 10 \leqslant 0$, $h_3(\boldsymbol{\theta}) = \theta_1 - 20 \leqslant 0$, $h_4(\boldsymbol{\theta}) = -\theta_2 - 5 \leqslant 0$, and so on).

Let

$$\bar{h}_j(\boldsymbol{\theta}) = \max\{0, h_j(\boldsymbol{\theta})\}, j = 1, 2, ..., l \tag{14}$$

and define for $j = 1, 2, ..., l$,

$$\nabla\bar{h}_j(\boldsymbol{\theta}) = \begin{cases} \nabla h_j(\boldsymbol{\theta}) & \text{if } h_j(\boldsymbol{\theta}) \geqslant 0 \\ \mathbf{0} & \text{if } h_j(\boldsymbol{\theta}) < 0 . \end{cases} \tag{15}$$

Then (15) can be packed for $j = 1, 2, ..., l$ as

$$\bar{\mathbf{H}}^T = \nabla\bar{\mathbf{h}}(\boldsymbol{\theta}) = [\nabla\bar{h}_1(\boldsymbol{\theta}), \nabla\bar{h}_2(\boldsymbol{\theta}), \cdots, \nabla\bar{h}_l(\boldsymbol{\theta})] \in \mathcal{R}^{p \times l}. \tag{16}$$

Using a quadratic penalty function [13], the above constrained minimization problem can be written as:

$$(\mathcal{P}_c): \ \ \arg\min_{\boldsymbol{\theta}} q(c, \boldsymbol{\theta}) \tag{17}$$

where

$$q(c, \boldsymbol{\theta}) = s(\boldsymbol{\theta}) + cP(\boldsymbol{\theta}), \tag{18}$$

$$P(\boldsymbol{\theta}) = \psi(\bar{h}_j(\boldsymbol{\theta})) = \bar{\mathbf{h}}^T(\boldsymbol{\theta})\bar{\mathbf{h}}(\boldsymbol{\theta}) = \sum_{j=1}^{l} \left(\bar{h}_j(\boldsymbol{\theta})\right)^2, \tag{19}$$

and $c > 0$ is a large penalty coefficient. $\bar{h}_j(\boldsymbol{\theta})$ is defined in (14).

In [13], it has been shown that as $c \to \infty$, the solution to the minimization problem $(\mathcal{P}_c)$ given by (17) will converge to a solution of the original constrained problem $(\mathcal{P}')$ given by (8). Here, we shall consider the problem of finding the solution of $(\mathcal{P}_c)$ (17)-(19) in the sequel.

Let $\mathbf{F}^T = \nabla f$. For the unconstrained objective function given by $s(\boldsymbol{\theta})$ and the penalty function given by $P(\boldsymbol{\theta})$ in (19), we note that their first- and second-order partial derivatives are written as:

$$\nabla s(\boldsymbol{\theta}) = 2\mathbf{F}^T(f - \xi), \quad \nabla^2 s(\boldsymbol{\theta}) = 2(\mathbf{F}^T\mathbf{F} + (f - \xi)\nabla^2 f) = 2(\mathbf{F}^T\mathbf{F} + \mathbf{R}_s),$$
$$\nabla P(\boldsymbol{\theta}) = 2\bar{\mathbf{H}}^T\bar{\mathbf{h}}, \quad \nabla^2 P(\boldsymbol{\theta}) = 2(\bar{\mathbf{H}}^T\bar{\mathbf{H}} + \mathbf{R}_h).$$

Also, the functional dependency on $\boldsymbol{\theta}$ (and so in the subsequent derivations) are omitted when clarity is not affected. The following descent algorithm is derived to search for the global minima.

4.2   A global descent algorithm

It can now be assumed further that the first partial derivatives of $P(\boldsymbol{\theta})$ are continuous including those points when $\bar{h}_j(\boldsymbol{\theta}) = 0$, $j = 1, 2, ..., l$ following [13]. Taking the quadratic approximation of $q(c, \boldsymbol{\theta})$ (17) about $\boldsymbol{\theta}_o$, we have

$$q(c, \boldsymbol{\theta}) \approx s(\boldsymbol{\theta}_o) + (\boldsymbol{\theta} - \boldsymbol{\theta}_o)^T \nabla s(\boldsymbol{\theta}_o) + \frac{1}{2}(\boldsymbol{\theta} - \boldsymbol{\theta}_o)^T \nabla^2 s(\boldsymbol{\theta}_o)(\boldsymbol{\theta} - \boldsymbol{\theta}_o)$$
$$+ c[P(\boldsymbol{\theta}_o) + (\boldsymbol{\theta} - \boldsymbol{\theta}_o)^T \nabla P(\boldsymbol{\theta}_o) + \frac{1}{2}(\boldsymbol{\theta} - \boldsymbol{\theta}_o)^T \nabla^2 P(\boldsymbol{\theta}_o)(\boldsymbol{\theta} - \boldsymbol{\theta}_o)].$$

The first-order necessary condition for optimality requires that

$$\nabla s(\boldsymbol{\theta}_o) + \nabla^2 s(\boldsymbol{\theta}_o)(\boldsymbol{\theta} - \boldsymbol{\theta}_o) + c[\nabla P(\boldsymbol{\theta}_o) + \nabla^2 P(\boldsymbol{\theta}_o)(\boldsymbol{\theta} - \boldsymbol{\theta}_o)] = 0, \qquad (20)$$

which can also be written as

$$\boldsymbol{\theta} = \boldsymbol{\theta}_o - \left[\nabla^2 s(\boldsymbol{\theta}_o) + c\nabla^2 P(\boldsymbol{\theta}_o)\right]^{-1} (\nabla s(\boldsymbol{\theta}_o) + c\nabla P(\boldsymbol{\theta}_o))$$
$$= \boldsymbol{\theta}_o - \left[\mathbf{F}^T\mathbf{F} + \mathbf{R}_s + c\bar{\mathbf{H}}^T\bar{\mathbf{H}} + c\mathbf{R}_h\right]^{-1} \left(\mathbf{F}^T(f - \xi) + c\bar{\mathbf{H}}^T\bar{\mathbf{h}}\right).$$

If we drop the second-order derivative terms $\mathbf{R}_s$ (which is unknown) and $\mathbf{R}_h$, we can formulate a search algorithm as follows:

$$\boldsymbol{\theta}_{i+1} = \boldsymbol{\theta}_i - \left[\mathbf{F}^T\mathbf{F} + c\bar{\mathbf{H}}^T\bar{\mathbf{H}}\right]^{-1} \left(\mathbf{F}^T(f - \xi) + c\bar{\mathbf{H}}^T\bar{\mathbf{h}}\right). \qquad (21)$$

Since f is always greater than ξ for all $\xi \leqslant f_g^*$, the term $(f - \xi)$ can be replaced by a unit positive term. The required magnitude of search is then taken care of by a *line search* procedure. Hence, no specific knowledge about ξ (and hence f_g^*) is needed. To avoid the search from ill-conditioning when $\mathbf{F}^T\mathbf{F} + c\bar{\mathbf{H}}^T\bar{\mathbf{H}}$ is singular, the above algorithm can be further modified according to Levenberg-Marquardt's method [12, 14] as follows:

$$(\mathcal{A}): \quad \boldsymbol{\theta}_{i+1} = \boldsymbol{\theta}_i - \beta \left[\mathbf{F}^T\mathbf{F} + c\bar{\mathbf{H}}^T\bar{\mathbf{H}} + \alpha\mathbf{I}\right]^{-1} \left(\mathbf{F}^T + c\bar{\mathbf{H}}^T\bar{\mathbf{h}}\right). \qquad (22)$$

where $0 < (\alpha, \beta) \leqslant 1$ and $\mathbf{I}$ corresponds to a $(p \times p)$ identity matrix. In this application, a simple line search sequence is constructed as: $\beta_{k+1} = \beta_k/2$, $k = 0, 1, 2, \dots$.

Remark 3:- Since the local maxima of ϕ are 'flattened' by raising ϕ to high power, the resultant constraint function characterizing the global optimality may be ill-conditioned, i.e. its derivative at regions other than neighborhood of global optima may also be too 'flat' to be useful. Hence, implementation of algorithms utilizing derivatives of the constraint function requires careful selection of γ such that the global optima are segregated and, at the same time, it does not cause ill-conditioning of the constraint function. For the case of $\phi(\cdot) = e^{-(\cdot)}$, introduction of f_L into the transformed functional constraint (i.e. $\phi^\gamma(f(\boldsymbol{\theta}) - f_L) \geqslant \zeta$) can help in achieving a good scaling effect since $e^{-\gamma(f - f_L)} = e^{\gamma f_L} e^{-\gamma f} = \rho e^{-\gamma f}$. Moreover, the penalty constant c provides an additional scaling means for the constrained direction $\bar{\mathbf{H}}^T \bar{\mathbf{H}}$. We shall show in our numerical examples some practical choices of γ, c, f_L and ρ. $\qquad \square$

5   Benchmark Experiments

To illustrate the effectiveness of a search utilizing regions characterized by the proposed monotonic transformation as compared to one that does not use transformation, we conduct numerical experiments on algorithm $(\mathcal{A})$, adopting those level cutting methods according to section 3.3(i) and (ii) (abbreviated as GTL(i) and GTL(ii) respectively), and on an algorithm (GOL) which uses a direct cutting level on the original function to define feasible regions containing the desired solution (i.e. $L_f(\epsilon) = \{\boldsymbol{\theta} | f(\boldsymbol{\theta}) \leqslant \epsilon, \boldsymbol{\theta} \in \mathcal{D}\}$). Several benchmark problems (see Table 1 and [17]) which are considered to be useful for evaluating different aspects of nonlinearity are experimented.

The performance criteria compared include the number of gradient evaluations (equal to the iteration number i in the algorithm) and the number of function evaluations required to arrive at the global minimum within a certain level of accuracy. All examples use those corners defining the domain of interest as initial estimates according to comparative results from the literature. To provide an idea on the physical computing speed, the CPU time taken in standard units (the real time for optimization divided by the real time for 1000 evaluations of Shekel-5 at (4,4,4,4)) for each search processes are also recorded. Noting that the error tolerances as seen in [2] and [1] were set to 1% and 10^{-6} respectively, we think an accuracy of 0.1% with respect to the known global minimum value would be suitable for algorithm termination in these applications.

For GTL(i), since the global minimum function values (f_g^*) are assumed to be known, we set the scaling parameter $\rho = e^{\gamma f_L}$ with $f_L = f_g^*$ throughout all experiments. As for the case of unknown global minimum value, the procedure in section 3.3(ii) is adopted for GTL(ii) starting with $f_L = f(\boldsymbol{\theta}_0) - \delta_{f_L}$ ($\boldsymbol{\theta}_0$ is the initial estimate) and lower this f_L value with level step-size δ_{f_L} whenever $f(\boldsymbol{\theta}_i) \leqslant f_L$ as the search proceeds.

For comparisons to be consistent, similar parameter settings are maintained for all GOL, GTL(i) and GTL(ii) search procedures ($c = 10^8$ and $\alpha = 0.0001$). The cutting level constraint on the non-transformed function for GOL is set according to the desired accuracy ($\epsilon = 0.1\%$ in $L_f(\epsilon)$). Other parameters for GTLs are chosen as: $\gamma = 4$ for both GTL(i) and GTL(ii); $\zeta = 0.9999$ for GTL(i) and $\zeta = 1.04$ for GTL(ii) throughout except for the choices of level step-size δ_{f_L} which are shown in the legends of Table 1. Here, we note that a minimum value of f_L has been set for S5, S7 and S10 at -1.3, -1.4 and -1.3 respectively.

On top of the constraint imposed by global characterization, all search procedures are performed with additional constraints which are defined by the bounding box specifying the domain of interest. To make the global constraint function more dominating, a scaling factor of 100 was used.

5.1   Comparative results

For all functions, as in other comparative reports (e.g.[1]), every corner of the bounding box defining the domain of interest was chosen as initial estimate for the iterative search. The average number of function evaluations for those runs that achieved the desired solutions are summarized in Table 1, together with best known reported results as seen in [1, 2, 9]. The average CPU times for each function in standard units are presented in Table 2. From Table 1, except for GP, BR and H3 problems, significant improvements are seen for GTLs over GOL in terms of convergence of search arriving at desired solutions. While GTL(i) and GTL(ii) searches remained to be simple in design, we note that their speed of convergence in terms of number of function evaluations required and standard CPU time taken are comparable to, if not better than, the fastest global search algorithm reported. Also, we note that the number of function evaluations required for GTL(i) and GTL(ii) is apparently independent of the dimension of problems.

Remark 4:- Main reason for the fast convergence in above applications is that there is no re-start along the search so long as the choice of f_L or δ_{f_L} provides good scaling of the constraint function. This is different from most existing design of global search engines. Effectively, the constrained algorithm when well implemented, shall lead to global optimal solutions with high probability. However, in its present form, we note that the algorithm cannot guarantee to attain the global solutions. Nevertheless, the proposal remains a simple and scientifically reproduceable means to be further explored. We shall leave those issues related to good implementation of the search algorithm for our future work. In the following, we show that this simple search can improve local search in artificial neural network learning problems.   □

6   FNN Application: Parity Patterns Learning

Pattern learning using the artificial Neural Networks represents an important application area in Computer Vision and Pattern Recognition (see e.g. [11]).

Table 1. Best known results in terms of number of function evaluations required by different methods

Method	GP	BR	CA	RA	SH	H3	H6	S5	S7	S10
					Test function					
SDE	5439	2700	10822	−	241215	3416	−	−	−	−
EA	460	430	−	2048	−	−	−	−	−	−
MLSL	148	206	−	−	−	197	487	404	432*	564
IA	−	1354	326	−	7424	−	−	−	−	−
TUN	−	−	1469	−	12160	−	−	−	−	−
TS	486	492	−	540	727	508	2845	−	−	−
ACF	394	20	52	158	−	78	249	−	−	−
TRUST	103	55	31	59	72	58	−	−	−	−
GOL	385	43	166*	**	187*	179	743*	1146*	1011*	775*
GTL(i)	**	57	44	303	239*	213	787	429*	58*	109*
GTL(ii)	222	89	16	49	313	227	63	127	60	71

* Unable to locate the desired solution from some initial points.
** Unable to locate the desired solution from all stated initial points.

Note: SDE is the stochastic method of Aluffi-Pentini et. al.; EA is the evolution algorithms of Yong et. al. or Schneider et. al.; MLSL is the multilevel single-linkage method of Kan and Timmer; IA is the interval arithmetic technique of Ratschek and Rokne; TUN is the tunneling method of Levy and Montalvo; TS is the Taboo search of Cvijovic and TRUST is the method of Barhen et. al. (see [1, 9] for detailed references and results). Choices of δ_{f_L} in GTL(ii) are: GP(2.55), BR(50), CA(10), RA(0.85), SH(0.85), H3(1.15), H6(3.9), S5(0.5), S7(2), S10(0.5).

Table 2. Average CPU time (unit: 1000 S5 evaluations)

Method	GP	BR	CA	RA	SH	H3	H6	S5	S7	S10
					Test function					
EA	−	1.50	−	−	−	−	−	−	−	−
MLSL	−	0.25	−	−	−	0.50	2.00	1.00	1.00*	2.00
GOL	0.86	0.10	0.55*	**	0.28*	0.73	2.56*	3.23*	3.05*	2.48*
GTL(i)	**	0.14	0.10	0.44	0.64*	0.61	2.42	1.08*	0.21*	0.38*
GTL(ii)	0.31	0.14	0.03	0.07	0.75	0.50	0.16	0.39	0.25	0.27

* Unable to locate the desired solution from some initial points.
** Unable to locate the desired solution from all stated initial points.

In this section, we apply the penalty-based algorithm to a class of neural network learning problems which are much more complex than those benchmark problems. Due to the complexity of physical data for approximation and the interconnected nonlinear activation units, the learning problem of artificial neural network represents a highly nonlinear minimization problem with a large number of minimizing parameters (network inter-connection weights) to be solved.

Given a network function $y(\mathbf{x}, \boldsymbol{w}) \in \mathcal{R}$ (see [16] for details) where $\mathbf{x} \in \mathcal{R}^m$ and $\boldsymbol{w} \in \mathcal{R}^p$ represent the m-dimensional network input vector and the p-dimensional network weight vector respectively. A commonly adopted learning objective is to fit a certain target data by minimizing the l_2-error norm given by:

$$s(\boldsymbol{w}) = \sum_{i=1}^{n} \left(y_i^t - y(\mathbf{x}_i, \boldsymbol{w}) \right)^2, \tag{23}$$

where y_i^t, $i = 1, 2..., n$ is the sample target vector with n data elements. It has been shown by several researchers (see e.g. [4, 3, 5]) that multilayer neural networks, under certain conditions, can approximate any nonlinear function to any desired accuracy using different techniques such as Kolmogorov's functional superposition theorem [10], Stone-Weierstrass theorem [see e.g. [15]] and projection pursuit method [8]. Hence, this minimization objective belongs to the class of problems with a known lower bound for global minimum value, when a proper network size is selected.

A strictly two-layer feedforward neural network (FNN) is used to learn several parity functions which are essentially the generalized XOR pattern recognition problem. The output of the network is set to '1' if an odd number of inputs are ones, and '0' otherwise. Since the output changes whenever any single input unit changes, parity problems are considered challenging for evaluating network learning performance. Our aim here is to demonstrate a possible use of the penalty-based algorithm for problems with relatively large number of parameters. As comparable global search results are not available for these examples, we shall compare the global descent algorithm (GTL(i) with $f_L = f_g^* = 0$, $\rho = 10e^{\gamma f_L}$ and $\zeta = 9.9999$; hereon denoted as GTL) with its local *line search* counter-part (LS) in terms of the speed of convergence and percentage of trials reaching the global solution. Also, we shall observe the effect of increasing complexity of the target function on the convergence of the penalty-based algorithm.

The number of hidden-layer neurons (N_j) has been chosen to be the same as the number of input units in each case. Table 3 shows the algorithm settings for the parity problems considered. Here, we note that p is the dimension of the minimizing parameter space. Our largest problem to be solved is $p = 81$. The training error goal (Err, which is the sum of squared error, as shown in the table) was set at 0.025 for all cases. The settings for the penalty-based search parameters were chosen to be similar for most cases as far as nonsingularity of a normalization matrix for the constraint function was maintained.

The experiment was carried out with 100 trials for each parity problem using random initial estimates from $[0, 1]^p$. The results for local search and global search are presented in Table 4 (LS: local line search, GTL: global method). To exclude extreme distributions which can affect the dominant shape of distribution, the statistics (mean, standard deviation) are obtained discarding those with number of iterations exceeding the maximum value indicated. To reflect the physical computation speed with respect to an IBM Pentium (266 MHz) compatible machine, the average CPU time for 10 iterations are also recorded in the table.

Table 3. Settings for parity-3,4,6,8 functions

Fn	N_j	p	α	γ	c	ρ	ζ	Err Goal
P3	3	16	0.0001	4	10	10	9.9999	0.025
P4	4	25	0.0001	4	10	10	9.9999	0.025
P6	6	49	0.0001	4	1000	10	9.9999	0.025
P8	8	81	0.0001	2	1000	10	9.9999	0.025

As seen from Table 4, the GTL algorithm as compared to the local LS method, shows excellent improvement in terms of the number of trials (GOP) attaining the desired error goal for all cases. For the parity-3 and the parity-4 problems, the mean number of iterations is seen to be much lower for GTL algorithm as compared to that of LS algorithm. The slow convergence for the parity-6 problem and the parity-8 problem is a result of high penalty setting that contributes to a much 'flattened' penalized error surface. Due to signifi-

Table 4. Local and global search results for parity-3,4,6,8 functions

LS		CPU	Number of iterations				GOP
Case	Fn	(sec)	min	max	mean	std dev.	(%)
(a)	P3	0.67	9	> 500	66.68	98.57	53
(b)	P4	0.84	12	> 500	70.14	96.28	49
(c)	P6	1.66	22	> 1000	67.89	45.17	36
(d)	P8	7.30	37	> 1000	256.12	234.42	17
GTL		CPU	Number of iterations				GOP
Case	Fn	(sec)	min	max	mean	std dev.	(%)
(e)	P3	0.79	10	> 500	20.81	10.03	99
(f)	P4	1.05	21	145	38.46	20.01	100
(g)	P6	2.31	144	> 1000	399.33	170.29	90
(h)	P8	11.14	147	> 1000	329.24	100.83	72

cant increment in dimension of weight space, the CPU times for GTL algorithm show significant increment for high parity problems as compared to those of LS algorithm.

In this FNN example, we have shown the effectiveness of the transformation based global descent design via minor increase in cost of computational complexity and design effort as compared to many existing global optimization algorithms, though there remains rooms for improvements to guarantee attaining the global optimal solution. The reader is referred to [16] for more application examples.

7 Conclusion And Future Work

Inspired by a visual warping effect, we provided a useful observation on global optimality of functions under monotonic transformation. Based on this observation, a global descent search procedure is designed to minimize the energy functions arising from applications. Comparing to an algorithm that does not use this transformation, we have shown that our approach can improve numerical sensitivity, and hence good numerical convergence, for several penalty-based search applications.

When a suitable level step size is selected, the simple penalty-based constrained search algorithm is shown to be comparable to best known global optimization algorithms in terms of number of function evaluations used, and standard CPU time taken to reach the region of the global optimum on the evaluation of several benchmark problems. The global descent search has also been shown to be applicable to a class of neural network pattern learning problems with significant improvement, on the probability to reach a neighborhood of global optimal solution, over the local line search method.

Several areas which have been identified for our future investigation include: improvement of the constrained minimization search and application to complex computer vision and pattern recognition problems such as support vector machine training and face recognition.

Acknowledgement

The author is thankful to Dr Geok-Choo Tan and Dr Louis Shue for their assistance and comments on various aspects of the paper. The author is also thankful to A/P Wee Ser and Dr Wei-Yun Yau for their kind support.

References

1. Jacob Barhen, Vladimir Protopopescu, and David Reister. TRUST: A deterministic algorithm for global optimization. *Science*, 276:1094–1097, May 1997.
2. Djurdje Cvijović and Jacek Klinowski. Taboo search: An approach to the multiple minima problem. *Science*, 267:664–666, February 1995.
3. G. Cybenko. Approximations by superpositions of a sigmoidal function. *Math. Cont. Signal & Systems*, 2:303–314, 1989.
4. Ken-Ichi Funahashi. On the approximation realization of continuous mappings by neural networks. *Neural Networks*, 2:183–192, 1989.
5. Kurt Hornik, Maxwell Stinchcombe, and Halbert White. Multi-layer feedforward networks are universal approximators. *Neural Networks*, 2(5):359–366, 1989.
6. Reiner Horst and Panos M. Pardalos, editors. *Handbook of Global Optimization*. Kluwer Academics Publishers, 1995.
7. Reiner Horst and Hoang Tuy. *Global Optimization: Deterministic Approaches*. Springer-Verlag, Berlin, 1996.
8. Peter J. Huber. Projection pursuit. *The Annals of Statistics*, 13(2):435–475, 1985.
9. A.H.G Rinnooy Kan and G. T. Timmer. Stochastic global optimization methods part II: Multi level methods. *Mathematical Programming*, 39:57–78, 1987. (North-Holland).
10. Andrei Nikolaevich Kolmogorov. On the representation of continuous functions of many variables by superposition of continuous functions of one variable and addition. *Doklalady Akademii Nauk SSSR*, 114:953–956, 1957. (American Mathematical Society Translation, vol. 28, pp. 55-59, 1963).
11. Steve Lawrence, C. Lee Giles, Ah Chung Tsoi, and Andrew D. Back. Face recognition: A convolutional neural-network approach. *IEEE Tran. Neural Networks*, 8(1):98–113, 1997.
12. Kenneth Levenberg. A method for the solution of certain non-linear problems in least squares. *Quarterly Journal of Applied Mathematics*, 2:164–168, 1944.
13. David G. Luenberger. *Linear and Nonlinear Programming*. Addison-Wesley Publishing Company, Inc., Massachusetts, 1984.
14. Donald W. Marquardt. An algorithm for least-squares estimation of nonlinear parameters. *Journal of the Society for Industrial & Applied Mathematics*, 11(2):431–441, 1963.
15. H. L. Royden. *Real Analysis*. MacMillan Publishing Co., Inc., New York, 2 edition, 1988.
16. K. A. Toh, Juwei Lu, and Wei-Yun Yau. Global feedforward neural networks learning for classification and regression. In *Proceedings of Third International Workshop on Energy Minimization Methods in Computer Vision and Pattern Recognition (EMMCVPR)*. Springer Verlag, Sophia-Antipolis, France, September 2001. (Lecture Notes in Computer Science).
17. Aimo Törn and Antanas Žilinskas. *Global Optimization*. Springer-Verlag, Berlin, 1989. (Lecture Notes in Computer Science).
18. Benjamin W. Wah and Yao-Jen Chang. Traced-based methods for solving non-linear global optimization and satisfiability problems. *J. Global Optimization*, 10(2):107–141, 1997.

Global Feedforward Neural Network Learning for Classification and Regression

Kar-Ann Toh, Juwei Lu, and Wei-Yun Yau

Centre for Signal Processing
School of Electrical & Electronic Engineering
Nanyang Technological University, 50 Nanyang Avenue, Singapore 639798
Email: ekatoh@ntu.edu.sg

Abstract. This paper addresses the issues of global optimality and training of a Feedforward Neural Network (FNN) error funtion incorporating the weight decay regularizer. A network with a single hidden-layer and a single output-unit is considered. Explicit vector and matrix canonical forms for the Jacobian and Hessian of the network are presented. Convexity analysis is then performed utilizing the known canonical structure of the Hessian. Next, global optimality characterization of the FNN error function is attempted utilizing the results of convex characterization and a convex monotonic transformation. Based on this global optimality characterization, an iterative algorithm is proposed for global FNN learning. Numerical experiments with benchmark examples show better convergence of our network learning as compared to many existing methods in the literature. The network is also shown to generalize well for a face recognition problem.

1 Introduction

Backpropagation of error gradients has proven to be useful in layered feedforward neural network learning. However, a large number of iterations is usually needed for adapting the weights. The problem becomes more severe especially when a high level of accuracy is required. It has been an active area of research, between late 1980s and early 1990s, to derive fast training algorithms to circumvent the problem of slow training rate as seen in the error backpropagation algorithm. Among the various methods proposed (see e.g. [6, 14]), significant improvement to the training speed is seen through the application of nonlinear optimization techniques in network training (see e.g. [1, 2, 22]). Very often, this is achieved at the expense of heavier computational requirement.[1] Here, we note that most of them are local methods and training results are very much dependent on the choices of initial estimates.

In light of efficient training algorithm development and network pruning (see [5], page 150-151), exact calculation of the second derivatives (Hessian) and its

---

[1] For example, the complexity of each step in Newton's method is $O(n^3)$ as compared to most first-order methods which are $O(n)$.

M.A.T. Figueiredo, J. Zerubia, A.K. Jain (Eds.): EMMCVPR 2001, LNCS 2134, pp. 407–422, 2001.

multiplied forms were studied [4, 16]. In [4], it was shown that the elements of the Hessian matrix can be evaluated exactly using multiple forward propagation through the network, followed by multiple backward propagation, for a feedforward network without intra-layer connections. In [16], a product form of the Hessian which took about as much computation as a gradient evaluation was presented. The result was then applied to a one pass gradient algorithm, a relaxation gradient algorithm and two stochastic gradient calculation algorithms to train the network. From the review in [7] specifically on the computation of second derivatives of feedforward networks, no explicit expression for the eigenvalues was seen. Here we note that eigenvalues are important for convexity analysis.

In view of the lack of an optimality criterion for global network learning in classification and regression applications, we shall look into the following issues in this paper: (i) characterization of global optimality of a FNN learning objective incorporating the weight decay regularizer, and (ii) derivation of an efficient search algorithm based on results of (i). We shall provide extensive numerical studies to support our claims.

The paper is organized as follows. In section 2, the layered feedforward neural network is introduced. This is followed by explicit Jacobian and Hessian formulations for forthcoming analysis. The FNN learning error function is then regularized using the weight decay method for good generalization capability. Then convexity analysis is performed in section 3 for local solution set characterization. This paves the way for a new approach on global optimality characterization in section 4. In section 5, the analysis results are used to derive a search algorithm to locate the global minima. Several benchmark examples are compared in section 6 in terms of convergence properties. The learning algorithm is also applied to a face recognition problem with good convergence as well as good generalization. Finally, some concluding remarks are drawn.

Unless otherwise stated, vector and matrix quantities are denoted using bold lowercase characters and bold uppercase characters respectively to distinguish from those scalar quantities. The superscript 'T' on the respective character is used to denote matrix transposition. Also, if not otherwise stated, $\| \cdot \|$ is taken to be the l_2-norm.

2   Multilayer Feedforward Neural Network

2.1   Neural feedforward computation

The neural network being considered is the familiar multilayer feedforward network with no recurrent or intra-layer connections. The forward calculation of a strictly 2-layer network with one output-node, i.e. network with one *direct* input-layer, one hidden-layer, and one output-layer consisting a single node (i.e. network with (N_i-N_j-1) structure) can be written as:

$$y(\mathbf{x}, \boldsymbol{w}) = g\left[\sum_{j=0}^{N_j} g\left(\sum_{i=0}^{N_i} w_{ji}^h x_i\right) \cdot w_{kj}^o\right], \quad g(z_0^h) = g(w_{0i}^h x_i) = 1, \; x_0 = 1, \; k = 1 \tag{1}$$

where $\mathbf{x} = \{x_i, i = 1, 2, ..., N_i\}$ denotes the network input vector and $\boldsymbol{w} = \left\{ [w^o_{kj}]_{j=0,...,N_j; k=1}, [w^h_{ji}]_{i=0,...,N_i; j=1,...,N_j} \right\}$ denotes the weight parameters to be adjusted. $g(\cdot)$ is a sigmoidal function given by

$$g(\cdot) = \frac{1}{1 + e^{-(\cdot)}} . \tag{2}$$

The superscripts 'o' and 'h' denote weights that are connected to output-nodes and hidden-nodes respectively.

For n number of data points, input $\mathbf{x}$ becomes a n-tuple vector (i.e. $\mathbf{x} \in \mathcal{R}^{(N_i+1)\times n}$ for N_i number of input-nodes plus a constant bias term) and so is the output $\mathbf{y}$ (i.e. $\mathbf{y} \in \mathcal{R}^n$).

2.2 Explicit Jacobian and Hessian for a two-layer network with single output

Here, we stack the network weights as a parameter vector $\boldsymbol{w} \in \mathcal{R}^p$ ($p = (N_j + 1) + (N_i + 1)N_j$) as follows:

$$\boldsymbol{w} = [w^o_{k,0}, ..., w^o_{k,N_j}, \; w^h_{1,0}, ..., w^h_{1,N_i}, \; \cdots, \; w^h_{N_j,0}, ..., w^h_{N_j,N_i}]^T. \tag{3}$$

Consider a single data point, the first derivative of network output $y(\mathbf{x}, \boldsymbol{w})$ (1) with respect to the weights vector can be written as

$$\mathbf{J}(\boldsymbol{w}) = \nabla^T y(\mathbf{x}, \boldsymbol{w}) = \dot{g}(z^o_k)\mathbf{r}^T, \tag{4}$$

where

$$\mathbf{r} = \left[1, g(z^h_1), ..., g(z^h_{N_j}), \; \dot{g}(z^h_1)w^o_{k,1}\mathbf{u}^T, \; \cdots \; \dot{g}(z^h_{N_j})w^o_{k,N_j}\mathbf{u}^T\right]^T \in \mathcal{R}^p, \tag{5}$$

$$\mathbf{u} = [1, x_1, ..., x_{N_i}]^T \in \mathcal{R}^{N_i+1}, \tag{6}$$

$$\dot{g}(\cdot) = \frac{e^{-(\cdot)}}{(1 + e^{-(\cdot)})^2}, \tag{7}$$

$$z^o_k = \sum_{j=0}^{N_j} g(z^h_j) \cdot w^o_{kj}, \quad g(z^h_0) = 1, \; k = 1, \tag{8}$$

$$z^h_j = \sum_{i=0}^{N_i} w^h_{ji} x_i, \quad g(z^h_0) = g(w^h_{0i} x_i) = 1, \; x_0 = 1, \; j = 1, ..., N_j . \tag{9}$$

The second derivative which is also termed the Hessian for the network function $y(\mathbf{x}, \boldsymbol{w})$ (1) is then

$$\mathbf{Y} = \nabla^2 y(\mathbf{x}, \boldsymbol{w}) = \ddot{g}(z^o_k)\mathbf{P} + \dot{g}(z^o_k)\mathbf{Q}, \tag{10}$$

where

$$\ddot{g}(\cdot) = \frac{\left(e^{-(\cdot)} - 1\right)e^{-(\cdot)}}{(1 + e^{-(\cdot)})^3}, \tag{11}$$

$$\mathbf{P} = \mathbf{r}\mathbf{r}^T, \tag{12}$$

$$\mathbf{Q} = \begin{bmatrix} 0 & \cdots & \cdots & 0 & 0 & \cdots & 0 \\ \vdots & \ddots & & \vdots & \dot{g}(z_1^h)\mathbf{u}^T & & 0 \\ \vdots & & \ddots & \vdots & & \ddots & \\ 0 & \cdots & \cdots & 0 & 0 & & \dot{g}(z_{N_j}^h)\mathbf{u}^T \\ 0\, \dot{g}(z_1^h)\mathbf{u} & & 0 & \ddot{g}(z_1^h)w_{k,1}^o\mathbf{u}\mathbf{u}^T & & 0 & \\ \vdots & \ddots & & & & \ddots & \\ 0 & 0 & \dot{g}(z_{N_j}^h)\mathbf{u} & 0 & & \ddot{g}(z_{N_j}^h)w_{k,N_j}^o\mathbf{u}\mathbf{u}^T \end{bmatrix}. \tag{13}$$

2.3   Learning and generalization

Since the goal of network training is not just to learn the given sample training data, here we adopt the *weight decay* (see e.g. [5, 9]) regularization method to provide some degree of network generalization.

Consider a target learning vector given by $y_i^t, i = 1, ..., n$, the following learning objective for FNN $y(\mathbf{x}_i, \boldsymbol{w})$ is considered:

$$s(\boldsymbol{w}) = s_1(\boldsymbol{w}) + b\,s_2(\boldsymbol{w}), \quad b \geqslant 0 \tag{14}$$

where

$$s_1(\boldsymbol{w}) = \sum_{i=1}^{n} \left(y_i^t - y(\mathbf{x}_i, \boldsymbol{w})\right)^2 = \sum_{i=1}^{n} \epsilon_i^2(\boldsymbol{w}) = \boldsymbol{\epsilon}^T(\boldsymbol{w})\boldsymbol{\epsilon}(\boldsymbol{w}), \tag{15}$$

and

$$s_2(\boldsymbol{w}) = \|w\|_2^2 = \boldsymbol{w}^T\boldsymbol{w}. \tag{16}$$

In what follows, we shall retain s_1 as the minimization objective for regression applications (or by setting $b = 0$ for s in (14)) since only fitting accuracy is required. We shall observe how the learning objective in (14) can influence generalization of FNN learning for classification in a face recognition problem.

3   Convexity Analysis

In this section, we shall analyze the convexity of the more general s such that local optimal solutions can be found. The convexity of s_1 can be directly obtained by setting $b = 0$ from that of s. According to ([17],Theorem 4.5), convexity of a twice continuously differentiable function is conditioned by the positive semidefiniteness of its Hessian matrix.

To determine explicit conditions for our application, consider the l_2-norm training objective given n training data in (14). The Hessian of $s(\boldsymbol{w})$ can be written as

$$\nabla^2 s(\boldsymbol{w}) = 2\left[\mathbf{E}^T(\boldsymbol{w})\mathbf{E}(\boldsymbol{w}) + \mathbf{R}(\boldsymbol{w}) + b\mathbf{I}\right], \tag{17}$$

where $\mathbf{E}(\boldsymbol{w})$ is the Jacobian of $\boldsymbol{\epsilon}(\boldsymbol{w})$ and

$$\mathbf{E}^T(\boldsymbol{w})\mathbf{E}(\boldsymbol{w}) = (-\mathbf{J})^T(\boldsymbol{w})(-\mathbf{J})(\boldsymbol{w}) = \mathbf{J}^T(\boldsymbol{w})\mathbf{J}(\boldsymbol{w}),$$

$$\mathbf{R}(\boldsymbol{w}) = \left[-\sum_{i=1}^{n}\frac{\partial^2 y(\mathbf{x}_i, \boldsymbol{w})}{\partial \boldsymbol{w}\partial \boldsymbol{w}^T}\epsilon_i(\boldsymbol{w})\right] \in \mathcal{R}^{p\times p}. \tag{18}$$

The positive semi-definiteness of $\nabla^2 s(\boldsymbol{w})$ is thus dependent on the matrices $\mathbf{J}^T(\boldsymbol{w})\mathbf{J}(\boldsymbol{w})$, $b\mathbf{I}$ and $\mathbf{R}(\boldsymbol{w})$. By exploring the structure of the above Hessian, we present our convexity result as follows. We shall prove two lemmas before we proceed further:

Lemma 1. *Consider* $\mathbf{v} = [v_1, v_2, ..., v_n]^T \in \mathcal{R}^n$ *for some* $v_i \neq 0, i = 1, 2, ..., n$. *Then, the eigenvalues of* $\mathbf{v}\mathbf{v}^T$ *are given by*

$$\lambda(\mathbf{v}\mathbf{v}^T) = \left\{ \textstyle\sum_{i=1}^n v_i^2, 0, ..., 0 \right\}. \tag{19}$$

Proof: Since $\mathbf{v}\mathbf{v}^T$ is symmetric with rank one, we have one and only one real non-zero eigenvalue which is the trace of $\mathbf{v}\mathbf{v}^T$. This completes the proof. ∎

Lemma 2. *Consider* $\mathbf{v} = [v_1, v_2, ..., v_n]^T$ *for some* $v_i \neq 0, i = 1, 2, ..., n$ *and*

$$\mathbf{A} = \begin{bmatrix} 0 & \cdots & \cdots & 0 & 0 & \cdots & 0 \\ \vdots & \ddots & & \vdots & a_1\mathbf{v}^T & & 0 \\ \vdots & & \ddots & \vdots & & \ddots & \\ 0 & \cdots & \cdots & 0 & 0 & & a_{n-1}\mathbf{v}^T \\ 0 & a_1\mathbf{v} & & 0 & b_1\mathbf{v}\mathbf{v}^T & \cdots & 0 \\ \vdots & & \ddots & \vdots & \vdots & \ddots & \vdots \\ 0 & 0 & & a_{n-1}\mathbf{v} & 0 & \cdots & b_{n-1}\mathbf{v}\mathbf{v}^T \end{bmatrix} \in \mathcal{R}^{n^2 \times n^2}. \tag{20}$$

Then, the eigenvalues of $\mathbf{A}$ *are given by* $\lambda(\mathbf{A}) = \left\{ \lambda_1, ..., \lambda_{2(n-1)}, 0, ..., 0 \right\}$, *where*

$$\lambda_j = \tfrac{1}{2}\left[b_j V \pm \sqrt{(b_j V)^2 + 4(a_j^2 V)} \right], \ j = 1, 2, ..., n-1 \ , \ and \ V = \sum_{i=1}^n v_i^2.$$

Proof: Solve for the eigenvalues block by block will yield the above result. ∎

Now, we are ready to perform convexity analysis for local solution set characterization. The FNN learning problem addressed, in a more precise manner, is stated as:

Problem 1 *The problem of FNN learning is defined by the l_2-norm minimization objective given by (14) where $y(\mathbf{x}_i, \boldsymbol{w})$ is a (N_i-N_j-1) network defined by (1) with sigmoidal activation functions given by (2). The Jacobian of $y(\mathbf{x}_i, \boldsymbol{w})$, $i = 1, 2, ..., n$ is denoted by $\mathbf{J}^T(\boldsymbol{w}) = [\nabla y(\mathbf{x}_1, \boldsymbol{w}), \nabla y(\mathbf{x}_2, \boldsymbol{w}), ..., \nabla y(\mathbf{x}_n, \boldsymbol{w})]$ where each of $\nabla y(\mathbf{x}_i, \boldsymbol{w}), i = 1, 2, ..., n$ is evaluated using (4)-(9).*

First we present a first-order necessary condition for network learning as follows:

Proposition 1. *Given Problem 1. Then, the least squares estimate $\hat{\boldsymbol{w}}$ of $\boldsymbol{w} = [w_1, w_2, ..., w_p]^T$, $p = (N_j + 1) + (N_i + 1)N_j$ in the sense of minimizing $s(\boldsymbol{w})$ of (14) satisfies*

$$\hat{\boldsymbol{w}} - \mathbf{J}^T(\hat{\boldsymbol{w}})[\mathbf{y}^t - \mathbf{y}(\mathbf{x}, \hat{\boldsymbol{w}})] = 0. \tag{21}$$

Proof: Minimizing $s(\boldsymbol{w})$ with respect to $\boldsymbol{w}$ by setting its first derivative to zero yields the normal equation given by (21). $\hat{\boldsymbol{w}}$ is the point satisfying (21). Hence the proof. ∎

The convexity result is presented as follows:

Theorem 1 *Given Problem 1. Then $s(\boldsymbol{w})$ is convex on $\boldsymbol{w} \in \mathcal{W}_c$ if*

$$\sum_{i=1}^{n} \left[\left(\ddot{g}(z_k^o)\lambda_m(\mathbf{P}) \right)_i + \left(\dot{g}(z_k^o)\lambda_m(\mathbf{Q}) \right)_i \right] \epsilon_i \leqslant b, \tag{22}$$

where

$$\lambda_m(\mathbf{P}) = \begin{cases} \sum_{k=1}^{p} r_k^2, \ \epsilon_i \geqslant 0 \\ 0 \qquad \epsilon_i < 0 \end{cases}, \quad i = 1, 2, ..., n, \tag{23}$$

$$[r_1, r_2, ..., r_p] = \left[1, g(z_1^h), ..., g(z_{N_j}^h), \ \dot{g}(z_1^h)w_{k,1}^o \mathbf{u}^T, \ \cdots \ \dot{g}(z_{N_j}^h)w_{k,N_j}^o \mathbf{u}^T \right], \tag{24}$$

$$\lambda_m(\mathbf{Q}) = \begin{cases} \max_j \lambda_j, \ \epsilon_i \geqslant 0 \\ \min_j \lambda_j, \ \epsilon_i < 0 \end{cases}, \quad j = 1, 2, ..., N_j, \tag{25}$$

$$\lambda_j = \frac{1}{2} \left[\ddot{g}\left(z_j^h\right) w_{k,j}^o V \pm \sqrt{\left(\ddot{g}\left(z_j^h\right) w_{k,j}^o V \right)^2 + 4\dot{g}^2\left(z_j^h\right) V} \right], j = 1, ..., N_j, \tag{26}$$

$$V = 1 + \sum_{i=1}^{N_i} x_i^2, \tag{27}$$

with $\dot{g}(\cdot)$, $\ddot{g}(\cdot)$, z_k^o and z_j^h being given by (7) through (9) and (11). Moreover, when the inequality in (22) is strict, strict convexity results.

Proof: For convexity(strict convexity) of $s(\boldsymbol{w})$, we need its Hessian to be positive semidefinite(definite). From (10), (17)-(18), we know that matrices $\mathbf{J}^T\mathbf{J}, \mathbf{R}, \mathbf{I}$ are symmetric. Hence, for the Hessian $[\mathbf{J}^T\mathbf{J} + \mathbf{R} + b\mathbf{I}]$ to be positive semidefinite (definite), it is sufficient to have

$$\lambda_{min}(\mathbf{J}^T\mathbf{J}) + \lambda_{min}(\mathbf{R}) + b \geqslant 0, \tag{28}$$

by Weyl's theorem (see [10], p.181). Substitute $\lambda_{min}(\mathbf{J}^T\mathbf{J}) = 0$, (10), (12) and (13) into above, and apply Weyl's theorem again, we further have

$$b - \sum_{i=1}^{n} \lambda_m \left(\ddot{g}(z_k^o)\mathbf{P} \right)_i \epsilon_i - \sum_{i=1}^{n} \lambda_m \left(\dot{g}(z_k^o)\mathbf{Q} \right)_i \epsilon_i \geqslant 0 \tag{29}$$

where $\lambda_m(\cdot) = \lambda_{max}(\cdot)$ when $\epsilon_i \geqslant 0$ and $\lambda_m(\cdot) = \lambda_{min}(\cdot)$ when $\epsilon_i < 0$. Denote the trace of a matrix $\mathbf{A}$ by $\text{tr}(\mathbf{A})$. According to Lemma 1, we have for $\epsilon_i < 0$

$$\lambda_m \left(\ddot{g}(z_k^o)\mathbf{P} \right)_i = 0, \ i = 1, 2, ..., n, \tag{30}$$

and for $\epsilon_i \geqslant 0$

$$\lambda_m \left(\ddot{g}(z_k^o)\mathbf{P} \right)_i = \left(\ddot{g}(z_k^o)\text{tr}(\mathbf{r}\mathbf{r}^T) \right)_i = \left(\ddot{g}(z_k^o)\sum_{k=1}^{p} r_k^2 \right)_i, \quad i = 1, 2, ..., n, \tag{31}$$

where $\mathbf{r}$ is given in (5). By Lemma 2 with adaptation of $\mathbf{A} \in \mathcal{R}^{n^2 \times n^2}$ to $\mathbf{Q} \in \mathcal{R}^{p \times p}$, $p = (N_j + 1) + (N_i + 1)N_j$, we have $2N_j$ number of non-zero eigenvalues which are identified as in (26) and (27). This completes the proof. ∎

Remark 1:- By exploiting the known canonical structure of the Hessian of the FNN, Theorem 1 presents an explicit convexity condition using eigenvalue characterization. The characterization is general since it can be applied to non-sigmoidal activation functions by replacing g and its derivatives with other activation functions. Here, we note that local optimal solution set can be characterized by Proposition 1 and Theorem 1. These results will be incorporated into global optimality characterization in the following section. □

4 Global Optimality

In this context, we refer to the solution of a minimization problem as:

Definition 1 *Let f be a function to be minimized from $\mathcal{D}$ to $\mathcal{R}$ where $\mathcal{D} \subseteq \mathcal{R}^p$ is non-empty and compact. A point $\boldsymbol{\theta} \in \mathcal{D}$ is called a feasible solution to the minimization problem. If $\boldsymbol{\theta}_g^* \in \mathcal{D}$ and $f(\boldsymbol{\theta}) \geqslant f(\boldsymbol{\theta}_g^*)$ for each $\boldsymbol{\theta} \in \mathcal{D}$, then $\boldsymbol{\theta}_g^*$ is called a global optimal solution (global minimum) to the problem. If $\boldsymbol{\theta}^* \in \mathcal{D}$ and if there exists an ε-neighborhood $N_\varepsilon(\boldsymbol{\theta}^*)$ around $\boldsymbol{\theta}^*$ such that $f(\boldsymbol{\theta}) \geqslant f(\boldsymbol{\theta}^*)$ for each $\boldsymbol{\theta} \in \mathcal{D} \cap N_\varepsilon(\boldsymbol{\theta}^*)$, then $\boldsymbol{\theta}^*$ is called a local optimal solution (local minimum). The set which contains both local optimal solutions and global optimal solutions is called a solution set (denoted by Θ^*).*

4.1 Mathematical construct

Denote $\mathcal{R}^+ = (0, \infty)$. Consider a strictly decreasing transformation ϕ on the function to be minimized. We shall use the following result (see [20] for more details) for global optimality characterization of a FNN error function.

Proposition 2. *Let $f : \mathcal{D} \to \mathcal{R}$ be a continuous function where $\mathcal{D} \subseteq \mathcal{R}^p$ is compact. Let $\phi : \mathcal{R} \to \mathcal{R}^+$ be a strictly decreasing function. Suppose $\boldsymbol{\theta}^* \in \mathcal{D}$. Then $\boldsymbol{\theta}^*$ is a global minimizer of f if and only if*

$$\lim_{\gamma \to \infty} \frac{\phi^\gamma(f(\boldsymbol{\theta}))}{\phi^\gamma(f(\boldsymbol{\theta}^*))} = 0, \quad \forall \boldsymbol{\theta} \in \mathcal{D}, f(\boldsymbol{\theta}) \neq f(\boldsymbol{\theta}^*). \tag{32}$$

Proof: This follows from the fact that $\frac{\phi^\gamma(f(\boldsymbol{\theta}))}{\phi^\gamma(f(\boldsymbol{\theta}^*))} > 0$ so that $\lim_{\gamma \to \infty} \frac{\phi^\gamma(f(\boldsymbol{\theta}))}{\phi^\gamma(f(\boldsymbol{\theta}^*))} = 0$ is equivalent to $\frac{\phi(f(\boldsymbol{\theta}))}{\phi(f(\boldsymbol{\theta}^*))} < 1$. ∎

Consider the solution set given by Definition 1, and using a more structured convex transformation ϕ, the following proposition is a straightforward consequence.

Proposition 3. *Let $f : \mathcal{D} \to \mathcal{R}$ be a continuous function where $\mathcal{D} \subseteq \mathcal{R}^p$ is compact. Let $\phi : \mathcal{R} \to \mathcal{R}^+$ be a strictly decreasing and convex function. Denote by Θ^* the solution set given by Definition 1. Suppose $\boldsymbol{\theta}^* \in \Theta^*$. Then $\boldsymbol{\theta}^*$ is a global minimizer of f if and only if*

$$\lim_{\gamma \to \infty} \frac{\phi^\gamma(f(\boldsymbol{\theta}))}{\phi^\gamma(f(\boldsymbol{\theta}^*))} = 0, \quad \forall \boldsymbol{\theta} \in \Theta^*, \, f(\boldsymbol{\theta}) \neq f(\boldsymbol{\theta}^*). \tag{33}$$

4.2   Global optimality of the modified FNN error function

Consider a feedforward neural network (FNN) with the training objective given by (14). Let $v(\boldsymbol{w})$ be a convex monotonic transformation function given by:

$$v(\boldsymbol{w}) = \phi^\gamma(s(\boldsymbol{w})) = \rho e^{-\gamma s(\boldsymbol{w})}, \quad \boldsymbol{w} \in \mathcal{R}^p, \, \rho > 0, \, \gamma > 1. \tag{34}$$

Notice that $v(\boldsymbol{w}) \in \mathcal{R}^+ = (0, \infty)$ for all finite values of ρ, γ and $s(\boldsymbol{w})$. If a lower bound or the value of global minimum of $s(\boldsymbol{w})$ is known, then we can multiply $s(\boldsymbol{w})$ by $\rho = e^{\gamma s_L}$ for scaling purpose:

$$v(\boldsymbol{w}) = e^{-\gamma(s(\boldsymbol{w}) - s_L)}. \tag{35}$$

This means that the maximum value of $v(\boldsymbol{w})$ can be pivot near to or at 1 while all other local minima can be "flattened" (relative to global minima) using a sufficiently high value of γ. For FNN training adopting a l_2-norm error objective, the ultimate lower bound of $s(\boldsymbol{w})$ is zero. For network with good approximation capability, the global minimum value should be a small value where this zero bound provides a good natural scaling.

Noting that the FNN considered is a continuous function mapping on a compact set of weight space $\boldsymbol{w} \in \mathcal{W}$, characterization of global optimality for the FNN training problem is presented as follows:

Theorem 2 *Consider Problem 1. Denote by $\mathcal{W}^*$ the solution set which satisfies Proposition 1 and strict convexity in Theorem 1. Let $v(s(\boldsymbol{w})) = \rho e^{-\gamma s(\boldsymbol{w})}$, $\rho > 0$. If there exists $\gamma_o > 1$ such that*

$$\frac{v(s(\boldsymbol{w}))}{v(s(\boldsymbol{w}^*))} \leqslant \frac{1}{2}, \quad s(\boldsymbol{w}) \neq s(\boldsymbol{w}^*), \tag{36}$$

for all $\gamma \geqslant \gamma_o$ and for all $\boldsymbol{w} \in \mathcal{W}^*$, then $\boldsymbol{w}^*$ is a global minimizer of $s(\boldsymbol{w})$.

Proof: The solution set $\mathcal{W}^*$ which satisfies Proposition 1 and strict convexity in Theorem 1 defines sufficiency for local optimality of the FNN error function (14). Let $\boldsymbol{w} \in \mathcal{W}^*$ where $s(\boldsymbol{w}) \neq s(\boldsymbol{w}^*)$. By the hypothesis in the theorem, there exists $\gamma_o > 1$ such that (36) holds for all $\gamma \geqslant \gamma_o$. Thus $\frac{v(s(\boldsymbol{w}))}{v(s(\boldsymbol{w}^*))} \leqslant \frac{1}{2} < 1$ for $\gamma > \gamma_o$. Passing to limit, we have $\lim_{\gamma \to \infty} \frac{v(s(\boldsymbol{w}))}{v(s(\boldsymbol{w}^*))} = 0$. By Proposition 3, $\boldsymbol{w}^*$ is a global minimizer. $\blacksquare$

Remark 2:-   Theorem 2 shows that if we can find a $\gamma \geqslant \gamma_o$ such that (36) is satisfied, then a level $\zeta > 0$ can be found to segregate the global minima from all other local minima on the transformed error function v. For FNN training problems adopting a l_2-norm error function s_1, the global optimal value is expected to approach zero if network approximation capability is assumed (i.e. with sufficient layers and neurons). Hence, we can simply choose a cutting level ζ to be slightly less than 1 (since $v(0) = 1$ when $\rho = 1$) on a transformed function v with sufficiently high value of γ. We shall utilize this observation for FNN training in both regression and classification problems.   □

5   Network Training

5.1   Global descent search

In this section, we show that the results of global optimality characterization can be directly applied to network training problem. Here, we treat network training as a nonlinear minimization problem. To achieve global optimality, the minimization is subjected to optimality conditions defined by Theorem 2. Mathematically, the network training can be written as:

$$\min_{\boldsymbol{w}} s(\boldsymbol{w}) \quad \text{subject to} \quad \boldsymbol{w} \in \mathcal{W}_g^*, \tag{37}$$

where $\mathcal{W}_g^*$ defines the solution set containing the global minima according to Theorem 2. Here, the condition given by Proposition 1 is used for iterative search direction design (e.g. Gauss-Newton search). While the convex characterization can be used for verification purpose, the global condition in Theorem 2 is used as a constraint to search for $\boldsymbol{w}$ over a high cutting level on the transformed function:

$$v(s(\boldsymbol{w})) > \zeta \quad or \quad h(\boldsymbol{w}) = \zeta - v(s(\boldsymbol{w})) < 0, \tag{38}$$

where ζ can be chosen to be any value within $(\frac{1}{2}, 1)$.

5.2   Penalty function method

Suppose there are l constraint functions[2] which are put into the following vector form: $\mathbf{h}(\boldsymbol{w}) = [h_1(\boldsymbol{w}), h_2(\boldsymbol{w}), \cdots, h_l(\boldsymbol{w})]^T \leqslant \mathbf{0}$. Let $\bar{h}_j(\boldsymbol{w}) = \max\{0, h_j(\boldsymbol{w})\}$, $j = 1, 2, ..., l$ and define for $j = 1, 2, ..., l$,

$$\nabla \bar{h}_j(\boldsymbol{w}) = \begin{cases} \nabla h_j(\boldsymbol{w}) \text{ if } h_j(\boldsymbol{w}) \geqslant 0 \\ \mathbf{0} \qquad \text{ if } h_j(\boldsymbol{w}) < 0 . \end{cases} \tag{39}$$

Using the more compact matrix notation, (39) can be packed for $j = 1, 2, ..., l$ as $\bar{\mathbf{H}}^T(\boldsymbol{w}) = \nabla \bar{\mathbf{h}}(\boldsymbol{w}) = [\nabla \bar{h}_1(\boldsymbol{w}), \nabla \bar{h}_2(\boldsymbol{w}), \cdots, \nabla \bar{h}_l(\boldsymbol{w})] \in \mathcal{R}^{p \times l}$. By the penalty function method [13], the constrained minimization problem of (37) can be rewritten as:

$$(P_c) : \min q(c, \boldsymbol{w}) = s(\boldsymbol{w}) + cP(\boldsymbol{w}) \tag{40}$$

---

[2] Apart from constraint arising from (36), the boundaries of the domain of interest can also be included as constraints.

where

$$P(\boldsymbol{w}) = \psi(\bar{h}_j(\boldsymbol{w})) = \sum_{j=1}^{l} \left(\bar{h}_j(\boldsymbol{w}) \right)^2, \tag{41}$$

$$\bar{h}_j(\boldsymbol{w}) = \max\{0,\, h_j(\boldsymbol{w})\}, \quad j = 1, 2, ..., l, \tag{42}$$

and $c > 0$ is a large penalty coefficient.

In [13], it has been shown that as $c \to \infty$, the solution to the minimization problem (P_c) given by (40) will converge to a solution of the original constrained problem given by (37). In the sequel, we shall concentrate on finding the solution of (P_c) (40)-(42).

For the unconstrained objective function given by $s(\boldsymbol{w})$ and the penalty function given by $P(\boldsymbol{w})$ in (40), we note that their first- and second-order partial derivatives are written as:

$$\nabla s(\boldsymbol{w}) = -2\mathbf{J}^T\boldsymbol{\epsilon} + 2b\boldsymbol{w}, \qquad \nabla^2 s(\boldsymbol{w}) = 2(\mathbf{J}^T\mathbf{J} + \mathbf{R}_y) + 2b\mathbf{I},$$
$$\nabla P(\boldsymbol{w}) = 2\bar{\mathbf{H}}^T\bar{\mathbf{h}}, \qquad \nabla^2 P(\boldsymbol{w}) = 2(\bar{\mathbf{H}}^T\bar{\mathbf{H}} + \mathbf{R}_h).$$

The functional dependency on $\boldsymbol{w}$ (and so in the subsequent derivations) are omitted when clarity is not affected. The following algorithms are derived to search for the global minima.

5.3   Algorithm

It can be further assumed that the first-order partial derivatives of $P(\boldsymbol{w})$ are continuous including those points where $\bar{h}_j(\boldsymbol{w}) = 0$, $j = 1, 2, ..., l$ following [13]. Hence, by taking the quadratic approximation of $q(\boldsymbol{w})$ (40) about $\boldsymbol{w}_o$ and set the first derivative to zero, we have

$$\boldsymbol{w} = \boldsymbol{w}_o + \left[\mathbf{J}^T\mathbf{J} + \mathbf{R}_y + b\mathbf{I} + c\bar{\mathbf{H}}^T\bar{\mathbf{H}} + \mathbf{R}_h \right]^{-1} \left(\mathbf{J}^T\boldsymbol{\epsilon} - b\boldsymbol{w} - c\bar{\mathbf{H}}^T\bar{\mathbf{h}} \right). \tag{43}$$

If we drop the second-order partial derivatives of network $(\mathbf{R}_y)$ and the second-order partial derivatives of the constraint function $(\mathbf{R}_h)$, we can formulate a search algorithm as follows:

$$\boldsymbol{w}_{i+1} = \boldsymbol{w}_i + \left[\mathbf{J}_i^T\mathbf{J}_i + b\mathbf{I} + c\bar{\mathbf{H}}_i^T\bar{\mathbf{H}}_i \right]^{-1} \left(\mathbf{J}_i^T\boldsymbol{\epsilon}_i - b\boldsymbol{w}_i - c\bar{\mathbf{H}}_i^T\bar{\mathbf{h}}_i \right). \tag{44}$$

By including a weighted parameter norm in the error objective function (14), we note that this has resulted in having a weighted identity matrix $(b\mathbf{I})$ included for the term in (44) which requires matrix inversion. This provides a mechanism to avoid the search from ill-conditioning which is analogous to that of the Levenberg-Marquardt's method.

To further improve numerical properties, the widely distributed eigenvalues of the penalty term can be normalized as shown:

$$\boldsymbol{w}_{i+1} = \boldsymbol{w}_i + \beta \left[\mathbf{J}_i^T\mathbf{J}_i + b\mathbf{I} + c\bar{\mathbf{H}}_i^T\mathbf{A}\bar{\mathbf{H}}_i \right]^{-1} \left(\mathbf{J}_i^T\boldsymbol{\epsilon}_i - b\boldsymbol{w} - c\bar{\mathbf{H}}_i^T\bar{\mathbf{h}}_i \right) \tag{45}$$

where $\mathbf{A} = (\bar{\mathbf{H}}_i\bar{\mathbf{H}}_i^T)^{-1}$. Here, we use the Line Search procedure (with β chosen to minimize the objective function) for iterative search.

In the following, we shall compare the global descent algorithm given by (45) (denoted as LSGO) with its local counter part, the local line search (denoted as LS) obtained from setting $c = 0$ and $bw = 0$ in (45).

6   Numerical Experiments

6.1   Benchmark problems

For the following experiments in this subsection, the FNN learning objective is chosen to be $s_1(w)$ rather than $s(w)$ since only training accuracy for regression is needed. Here the bw term in algorithm (45) is set to zero while the bI term is retained for numerical stability. For all examples, 100 trials using random initial points within the box $[0, 1]^p$ were carried out. Training results in terms of the number of trials reaching a neighborhood of the desired global minimum and the mean number of iterations for these trials are presented.

As the number of iterations required to reach a desired error goal only provides a partial picture of the training algorithm, numerical results on computational aspects are also provided. All the experiments are conducted using an IBM-PC/Pentium compatible machine with 266Hz clock speed. In the following, we tabulate the average CPU time required to run 10 iterations for each algorithm.

For ease of comparison, recent results (mean number of iterations, percentage of trials attaining near global solution) for the XOR problem from [22] are listed: (i) Standard error backpropagation: (332, 91.3%); (ii) Error backpropagation with line minimization: (915.4, 38%); (iii) Davidon-Fletcher-Powell quasi-Newton minimization: (2141.1, 34.1%); (iv) Fletcher-Reeves conjugate gradient minimization: (523, 81.5%); (v) Conjugate gradient minimization with Powell restarts: (79.2, 82.1%). The reader is referred to [22] for more results on $f(x) = \sin(x)\cos(2x)$ fitting problem which requires much more than 600 mean iterations for the above search methods.

As for existing global optimization algorithms, similar statistical comparisons for these examples are not available. We note that the particular training example for XOR given in [8] (TRUST) used about 1000 training iterations to reach the global optimal solution. As for the global algorithm proposed by [19] (GOTA), the convergence speed is reported to be comparable to the backpropagation algorithm for the XOR example.

Example 1: XOR pattern

In this example, 4 samples of the XOR input-output patterns were used for network training. The network chosen was similar to that in [22] where 2 hidden-units were used. The target sum of the squared error was set to be less than 0.025 which was sufficiently closed to the global optimal solution. For both local and global methods, b was chosen to be a fixed value of 0.0001 which was sufficient to provide a stable numerical conditioning. As for other parameters of the global descent algorithm (LSGO), the following settings were used: $\gamma = 4$, $\rho = 1$, $\zeta = 0.9999$, $c = 10$ (γ and ρ appear in $v(\boldsymbol{w})$, ζ is the cutting level on $v(\boldsymbol{w})$ as shown in (38) and c is a penalty constant).

Training results comprising of 100 trials for each of the algorithms are shown in Table 1. The respective statistics (i.e. min: minimum value, max: maximum value, mean: mean value, std dev: standard deviation, and GOP: percentage of trials achieving the desired global error objective within 500 iterations) are also included in Table 1. In order to show the core distribution for trials which took less than 500 iterations, the statistics shown exclude those trials above 500 iterations.

Table 1. Results for the Examples 1,2 and 3

Ex. 1		CPU	Number of iterations				GOP
Case	Algo.	(sec)	min	max	mean	std dev.	(%)
(a)	LS	0.66	5	> 500	13.73	22.46	33
(b)	LSGO	0.77	28	132	39.40	15.76	100
Ex. 2		CPU	Number of iterations				GOP
Case	Algo.	(sec)	min	max	mean	std dev.	(%)
(a)	LS	0.93	21	> 5000	94.70	94.76	50
(b)	LSGO	1.15	29	3191	72.34	26.78	100
Ex. 3		CPU	Number of iterations				GOP
Case	Algo.	(sec)	min	max	mean	std dev.	(%)
(a)	LS	5.50	–	> 500	–	–	0
(b)	LSGO	8.41	49	> 500	73.16	18.85	99

As shown in Table 1, the global descent algorithm (LSGO) have succeeded in locating the approximate global minima within 132 iterations for all the 100 trials using different initial values. This as compared to the local line search algorithm (LS), which scores only 33%, is a remarkable improvement. In terms of computational cost, the global constrained method is found to take slightly higher CPU time than that using unconstrained method.

Example 2: 1-D curve $f(x) = \sin(x)\cos(2x)$

In this example, 20 input-output patterns were uniformly chosen on $0 \leqslant x \leqslant 2\pi$ for network training. Similar to the first example, the sum of the squared error was set to be less than 0.025 which was sufficiently close to the global optimal solution. A single-output network with 10-hidden units was chosen according to [22]. As in previous example, b was set to be 0.0001 throughout. For the global descent algorithm (LSGO), the following settings were chosen: $\gamma = 4$, $\rho = 10$, $\zeta = 9.9999$, $c = 10$. Training results for 100 trials are shown in Table 1, with respective statistics and CPU times. For this example, GOP refers to the percentage of trials achieving the desired error goal within 5000 iterations.

In this example, the global method (LSGO) has achieved a 100% GOP which is much better than the 50% for local method (LS). The largest iteration number for the case in LSGO was found to be 3191. As for the CPU time, the global constrained algorithm takes longer time than its local counterpart in each iteration.

Example 3: 2-D shape

For this example, the network is to learn a two-dimensional *sinc* function. The network size chosen was (2-15-1) and the error goal was set at 0.8 with 289 input-output training sets. Similar to the above examples, b was chosen to be 0.0001 throughout. For the global descent algorithm (LSGO), the following settings were chosen: LSGO: $\gamma = 2$, $\rho = 10$, $\zeta = 9.999999$, $c = 1000$. The training results for 100 trials are shown in Table 1. Here we note that the GOP for this example indicates the percentage of trials reaching the error goal within 500 iterations.

From Table 1, we see that for all 100 trials, the LS method was unable to descent towards the error goal within 500 iterations. In fact, we observed that most of these trials had landed on local minima which are much higher than the error goal. The LSGO had improved the situation with only one trial resulted in SSE slightly greater than the error goal at the end of 500th iteration.

Remark 3:- Despite the remarkable convergence using random initial estimates for all the examples, it is noted that when the initial point was chosen at some of those local minima, the penalty based algorithms converge with extremely slow speed and were unable to locate the global minima within 5000 iterations.   □

6.2   Face recognition

Face recognition represents a difficult classification problem since it has to deal with large amount of variations in face images due to viewpoint, illumination and expression difference even for similar person. As such, many recognition conditions are ill-posed because "the variations between the images of the same face due to illumination and viewing direction are almost always larger than image variation due to change in face identity" [15].

Here we use the ORL Cambridge database [18] for classification. The ORL database contains 40 distinct persons, each having 10 different images taken under different conditions: different times, varying lighting (slightly), facial expression (open/closed eyes, smiling/non-smiling) and facial details (glasses/no-glasses). All the images are taken against a dark homogeneous background and all persons are in up-right, frontal position except for some tolerance in side movement. The face recognition procedure is performed in two stages, namely:

1. *Feature extraction*: the training set and query set are derived in the same way as in [12] where 10 images of each of the 40 persons are randomly partitioned into two sets, resulting in 200 images for training and 200 images for testing with no overlapping between them. Each original image is then projected onto the feature spaces derived from Eigenface [21], Fisherface [3] and D-LDA [23] methods.

2. *Classification*: conventional nearest centre (NC), nearest neighbour (NN) and our proposed FNN method are used for classification. The error rates

are taken only from the averages of test errors obtained from 8 different runs.[3]

The network chosen for this application consists of 40 separate FNN (one network per person), each with (N_i-1-1) structure considering network dilution for good generalization [11]. The number of inputs $N_i = 39$ is set according to the feature dimension obtained from projections using Eigenface, Fisherface and D-LDA. During the training phase, each of the 40 FNN outputs was set to '1' for one corresponding class (person) while the others set to '0'. The global FNN was tested for 5 cases: FNN(a)-(e), each for 500 learning iterations, all using $\gamma = 4$, $\rho = 10$, $\zeta = 9.9999$. Among the 40 individual outputs of the FNNs, the output with the highest value is assigned to the corresponding class. Training and testing error rates were obtained from the number of mis-classified persons divided by 200. The results corresponding to other different FNN settings and various feature extraction methods are shown in Table 2.

Table 2. FNN settings and corresponding error rates

Classification Method	Settings FNN settings			Classification error rate (%)					
				Eigenface		D-LDA		Fisherface	
	w_o	c	b	Train	Test	Train	Test	Train	Test
NC	−	−	−	−	12.25	−	5.56	−	8.12
NN	−	−	−	−	6.50	−	5.38	−	8.81
FNN(a)	$k \times 10^{-4}$	0	10^{-4}	3.69	25.88	34.44	45.31	69.25*	79.25*
FNN(b)	$k \times 10^{-4}$	10^3	10^{-4}	3.56	26.75	34.25	47.06	69.25*	79.38*
FNN(c)	$k \times 10^{-4}$	10^3	0.05	0	5.38	0	5.62	0	12.56
FNN(d)	$\bar{k} \times 10^{-8}$	10^3	0.25	0	5.06	0	5.31	0	7.81
FNN(e)	$R \times 10^{-8}$	10^3	0.05-0.5	0	3.88	0	4.63	0	7.81

* : encounter singularity of matrix for some cases during training.

From Table 2, we see that poor results were obtained for both the conventional FNN (FNN(a): unconstrained minimization on s_1 with $c = 0$) and the global descent FNN for regression (FNN(b): constrained minimization on s_1 with $c = 10^3$). However, remarkable improvement was observed when the weightage b was set at 0.05 as seen in FNN(c). With smaller initial values ($\bar{k}$ indicates $k = 1, ..., p$ offset by its mean) and a higher b, the results were seen to improve further in FNN(d). In FNN(e), we provide our best achievable results from random initial estimates ($R \times 10^{-8}$) and variations of b value. We see that our simple training method can provide good generalization capability as compared to best known network based method that incorporated several ideas: local receptive fields, shared weights, and spatial subsampling [12]. In short, for this case of using half the data set for training, our best FNN provides a good error rate as compared to best known methods reported in [12]: Top-down HMM (13%), Eigenfaces (10.5%), Pseudo 2D-HMM (5%) and SOM+CN (3.8%).

---

[3] Here we note that only 3 runs were tested in [12].

7   Conclusion

In this paper, we propose to train a regularized FNN using a global search method. We have presented explicit vector and matrix canonical forms for the Jacobian and the Hessian of the FNN prior to convexity analysis of the weighted l_2-norm error function. The sufficient conditions for such convex characterization are derived. This permits direct means to analyze the network in aspects of network training and possibly network pruning. Results from the convex characterization are utilized in an attempt to characterize the global optimality of the FNN error function which is suitable for regression and classification applications. By means of convex monotonic transformation, a sufficient condition for the FNN training to attain global optimality is proposed. The theoretical results are applied directly to network training using a simple constrained search. Several numerical examples show remarkable improvement in terms of convergence of our network training as compared to available local methods. The network learning is also shown to possess good generalization property in a face recognition problem. It is our immediate task to generalize these results to a network with multiple outputs. Design of more robust constrained search remains an issue to guarantee global convergence.

Acknowledgement

The authors are thankful to Dr Geok-Choo Tan and Dr Zhongke Wu for their comments and assistance on various aspects of the paper. The authors are also thankful to the anonymous reviewers for providing additional references. Last, but not least, the authors are thankful to A/P Wee Ser for his kind support.

References

1. Etienne Barnard. Optimization for training neural nets. *IEEE Trans. on Neural Networks*, 3(2):232–240, 1992.
2. Roberto Battiti. First- and second-order methods for learning: Between steepest descent and Newton's method. *Neural Computation*, 4:141–166, 1992.
3. P. N. Belhumeur, J. P. Hespanha, and D. J. Kriegman. "Eigenfaces vs. fisherfaces: Recognition using class specific linear projection". *IEEE Transactions on Pattern Analysis and Machine Intelligence*, 19(7):711–720, July 1997.
4. Chris Bishop. Exact calculation of the Hessian matrix for the multilayer perceptron. *Neural Computation*, 4:494–501, 1992.
5. Christopher M. Bishop. *Neural Networks for Pattern Recognition*. Oxford University Press Inc., New York, 1995.
6. Richard P. Brent. Fast training algorithms for multilayer neural networks. *IEEE Trans. on Neural Networks*, 2(3):346–354, 1991.
7. Wray L. Buntine and Andreas S. Weigend. Computing second derivatives in feedforward networks: A review. *IEEE Tran. Neural Networks*, 5(3):480–488, 1994.
8. B. C. Cetin, J. W. Burdick, and J. Barhen. Global descent replaces gradient descent to avoid local minima problem in learning with artificial neural networks. In *IEEE Int. Conf. Neural Networks*, 1993.

9. John Hertz, Anders Krogh, and Richard G. Palmer. *Introduction to the Theory of Neural Computation.* Addison-Wesley Publishing Company, New York, 1991.
10. Roger A. Horn and Charles R. Johnson. *Matrix Analysis.* Cambridge University Press, New York, 1992.
11. Peter Kuhlmann and Klaus-Robert Müller. On the generalisation ability of diluted perceptrons. *J. Phys. A: Math. Gen.,* 27:3759–3774, 1994.
12. Steve Lawrence, C. Lee Giles, Ah Chung Tsoi, and Andrew D. Back. Face recognition: A convolutional neural-network approach. *IEEE Tran. Neural Networks,* 8(1):98–113, 1997.
13. David G. Luenberger. *Linear and Nonlinear Programming.* Addison-Wesley Publishing Company, Inc., Massachusetts, 1984.
14. Martin Fodslette Moller. A scaled conjugate gradient algorithm for fast supervised learning. *Neural Networks,* 6:525–533, 1993.
15. Y. Moses, Y. Adini, and S. Ullman. "Face recognition: The problem of compensating for changes in illumination direction". In *Proceedings of the European Conference on Computer Vision,* volume A, pages 286–296, 1994.
16. Barak A. Pearlmutter. Fast exact multiplication by the Hessian. *Neural Computation,* 4:147–160, 1994.
17. R. Tyrrell Rockafellar. *Convex Analysis.* Princeton University Press, Princeton, New Jersey, 1972.
18. Web site of ORL Cambridge face database:. "http://www.cam-orl.co.uk/facedatabase.html". *AT&T Laboratories Cambridge,* 1994.
19. Zaiyong Tang and Gary J. Koehler. Deterministic global optimal FNN training algorithms. *Neural Networks,* 7(2):301–311, 1994.
20. K. A. Toh. Global energy minimization: A transformation approach. In *Proceedings of Third International Workshop on Energy Minimization Methods in Computer Vision and Pattern Recognition (EMMCVPR).* Springer Verlag, Sophia-Antipolis, France, September 2001. (Lecture Notes in Computer Science).
21. Matthew A. Turk and Alex P. Pentland. "Eigenfaces for recognition". *Journal of Cognitive Neuroscience,* 3(1):71–86, March 1991.
22. P. Patrick van der Smagt. Minimisation methods for training feedforward neural networks. *Neural Networks,* 7(1):1–11, 1994.
23. Jie Yang, Hua Yu, and William Kunz. "An efficient LDA algorithm for face recognition". In *Proceedings of Sixth International Conference on Control, Automation, Robotics and Vision,* Singapore, December 2000.

Matching Free Trees, Maximal Cliques, and Monotone Game Dynamics

Marcello Pelillo

Dipartimento di Informatica
Università Ca' Foscari di Venezia
Via Torino 155, 30172 Venezia Mestre, Italy

Abstract. It is well known that the problem of matching two relational structures can be posed as an equivalent problem of finding a maximal clique in a (derived) association graph. However, it is not clear how to apply this approach to computer vision problems where the graphs are connected and acyclic, i.e. are free trees, since maximal cliques are not constrained to preserve connectedness. Motivated by our recent work on rooted tree matching, in this paper we provide a solution to the problem of matching two free trees by constructing an association graph whose maximal cliques are in one-to-one correspondence with maximal subtree isomorphisms. We then solve the problem using simple payoff-monotonic dynamics from evolutionary game theory. We illustrate the power of the approach by matching articulated and deformed shapes described by shape-axis trees. Experiments on hundreds of larger (random) trees are also presented. The results are impressive: despite the inherent inability of these simple dynamics to escape from local optima, they always returned a globally optimal solution.

1 Introduction

Graph matching is a classic problem in computer vision and pattern recognition, instances of which arise in areas as diverse as object recognition, motion and stereo analysis (see, e.g., [2]). A well-known approach to solving this problem consists of transforming it into the equivalent problem of finding a maximum clique in an auxiliary graph structure, known as the *association graph* [2]. The idea goes back to Ambler *et al.* [1], and has since been successfully employed in a variety of different problems. This framework is attractive because it casts graph matching as a pure graph-theoretic problem, for which a solid theory and powerful algorithms have been developed. Note that, although the maximum clique problem is known to be NP-hard, powerful heuristics exist which efficiently find good approximate solutions [6].

In many computer vision and pattern recognition problems, the graphs at hand have a peculiar structure: they are connected and acyclic, i.e. they are *free trees* [4, 11, 19, 32]. Note that, unlike "rooted" trees, in free trees there is no distinguished node playing the role of the root, and hence no hierarchy is imposed on them. Since in the standard association graph formulation the solutions are not constrained to preserve connectedness, it is not clear how to apply

M.A.T. Figueiredo, J. Zerubia, A.K. Jain (Eds.): EMMCVPR 2001, LNCS 2134, pp. 423–437, 2001.

the framework in these cases, and the extension of association graph techniques to free tree matching problems is therefore of considerable interest.

Motivated by our recent work on rooted tree matching [27], in this paper we propose a solution to this problem by providing a straightforward way of deriving an association graph from two free trees. We prove that in the new formulation there is a one-to-one correspondence between maximal (maximum) cliques in the derived association graph and maximal (maximum) subtree isomorphisms. As an obvious corollary, the computational complexity of finding a maximum clique in such graphs is therefore the same as the subtree isomorphism problem, which is known to be polynomial in the number of nodes [13, 29].

Following [25, 27], we use a recent generalization of the Motzkin-Straus theorem [23] to formulate the maximum clique problem as a quadratic programming problem. To (approximately) solve it we employ *payoff-monotonic dynamics*, a class of simple dynamical systems recently developed and studied in evolutionary game theory [17, 30]. Such continuous solutions to discrete problems are interesting as they can motivate analog and biological implementations.

We illustrate the power of the approach via several examples of matching articulated and deformed shapes described by *shape-axis* trees [19]. We also present experiments on hundreds of much larger (uniformly random) trees. The results are impressive: despite the counter-intuitive maximum clique formulation of the tree matching problem, and the inherent inability of these simple dynamics to escape from local optima, they always found a globally optimal solution.

2   Subtree Isomorphisms and Maximal Cliques

Let $G = (V, E)$ be a graph, where V is the set of nodes and E is the set of (undirected) edges. The *order* of G is the number of nodes in V, while its *size* is the number of edges. Two nodes $u, v \in V$ are said to be *adjacent* (denoted $u \sim v$) if they are connected by an edge. The *adjacency matrix* of G is the the the $n \times n$ symmetric matrix $A_G = (a_{ij})$ defined as

$$a_{ij} = \begin{cases} 1, & \text{if } v_i \sim v_j \\ 0, & \text{otherwise .} \end{cases}$$

The *degree* of a node u, denoted $\deg(u)$, is the number of nodes adjacent to it. A *path* is any sequence of distinct nodes $u_0 u_1 \ldots u_n$ such that for all $i = 1 \ldots n$, $u_{i-1} \sim u_i$; in this case, the *length* of the path is n. If $u_n \sim u_0$ the path is called a *cycle*. A graph is said to be *connected* if any two nodes are joined by a path. The *distance* between two nodes u and v, denoted $d(u, v)$, is the length of the shortest path joining them (by convention $d(u, v) = \infty$, if there is no such path). Given a subset of nodes $C \subseteq V$, the *induced subgraph* $G[C]$ is the graph having C as its node set, and two nodes are adjacent in $G[C]$ if and only if they are adjacent in G. A connected graph with no cycles is called a *free tree*, or simply a *tree*. Trees have a number of interesting properties. One which turns out to be very useful for our characterization is that in a tree any two nodes are connected by a *unique* path.

Let $T_1 = (V_1, E_1)$ and $T_2 = (V_2, E_2)$ be two trees. Any bijection $\phi : H_1 \to H_2$, with $H_1 \subseteq V_1$ and $H_2 \subseteq V_2$, is called a *subtree isomorphism* if it preserves both the adjacency relationships between the nodes and the connectedness of the matched subgraphs. Formally, this means that, given $u, v \in H_1$, we have $u \sim v$ if and only if $\phi(u) \sim \phi(v)$ and, in addition, the induced subgraphs $T_1[H_1]$ and $T_2[H_2]$ are connected. A subtree isomorphism is *maximal* if there is no other subtree isomorphism $\phi' : H_1' \to H_2'$ with H_1 a strict subset of H_1', and *maximum* if H_1 has largest cardinality. The maximal (maximum) subtree isomorphism problem is to find a maximal (maximum) subtree isomorphism between two trees.

The *free tree association graph* (FTAG) of two trees $T_1 = (V_1, E_1)$ and $T_2 = (V_2, E_2)$ is the graph $G = (V, E)$ where

$$V = V_1 \times V_2 \tag{1}$$

and, for any two nodes (u, w) and (v, z) in V, we have

$$(u, w) \sim (v, z) \Leftrightarrow d(u, v) = d(w, z) . \tag{2}$$

Note that this definition of the association graph is stronger than the standard one used for matching arbitrary relational structures [2].

A subset of vertices of G is said to be a *clique* if all its nodes are mutually adjacent. A *maximal* clique is one which is not contained in any larger clique, while a *maximum* clique is a clique having largest cardinality. The maximum clique problem is to find a maximum clique of G.

The following theorem, which is the basis of the work reported here, establishes a one-to-one correspondence between the maximum subtree isomorphism problem and the maximum clique problem

Theorem 1. *Any maximal (maximum) subtree isomorphism between two trees induces a maximal (maximum) clique in the corresponding FTAG, and vice versa.*

Proof (outline). Let $\phi : H_1 \to H_2$ be a maximal subtree isomorphism between trees T_1 and T_2, and let $G = (V, E)$ denote the corresponding FTAG. Let $C_\phi \subseteq V$ be defined as $C_\phi = \{(u, \phi(u)) : u \in H_1\}$. From the definition of a subtree isomorphism it follows that ϕ maps the path between any two nodes $u, v \in H_1$ onto the path joining $\phi(u)$ and $\phi(v)$. This clearly implies that $d(u, v) = d(\phi(u), \phi(v))$ for all $u \in H_1$, and therefore C_ϕ is a clique. Trivially, C_ϕ is a maximal clique because ϕ is maximal, and this proves the first part of the theorem.

Suppose now that $C = \{(u_1, w_1), \cdots, (u_n, w_n)\}$ is a maximal clique of G, and let $H_1 = \{u_1, \cdots, u_n\} \subseteq V_1$ and $H_2 = \{w_1, \cdots, w_n\} \subseteq V_2$. Define $\phi : H_1 \to H_2$ as $\phi(u_i) = w_i$, for all $i = 1 \ldots n$. From the definition of the FTAG and the hypothesis that C is a clique, it is simple to see that ϕ is a one-to-one and onto correspondence between H_1 and H_2, which trivially preserves the adjacency relationships between nodes. The fact that ϕ is a maximal isomorphism is a straightforward consequence of the maximality of C.

To conclude the proof we have to show that the subgraphs that we obtain when we restrict ourselves to H_1 and H_2, i.e. $T_1[H_1]$ and $T_2[H_2]$, are trees, and this is equivalent to showing that they are connected. Suppose by contradiction that this is not the case, and let $u_i, u_j \in H_1$ be two nodes which are not joined by a path in $T_1[H_1]$. Since both u_i and u_j are nodes of T_1, however, there must exist a path $u_i = x_0 x_1 \ldots x_m = u_j$ joining them in T_1. Let $x^* = x_k$, for some $k = 1 \ldots m$, be a node on this path which is not in H_1. Moreover, let $y^* = y_k$ be the k-th node on the path $w_i = y_0 y_1 \ldots y_m = w_j$ which joins w_i and w_j in T_2 (remember that $d(u_i, u_j) = d(w_i, w_j)$, and hence $d(w_i, w_j) = m$). It is easy to show that the set $\{(x^*, y^*)\} \cup C \subseteq V$ is a clique, thereby contradicting the hypothesis that C is a maximal clique. This can be proved by exploiting the obvious fact that if x is a node on the path joining any two nodes u and v, then $d(u, v) = d(u, x) + d(x, v)$.

The "maximum" part of the statement is proved similarly. $\square$

The FTAG is readily derived by using a classical representation for graphs, i.e., the so-called *distance matrix* (see, e.g., [15]) which, for an arbitrary graph $G = (V, E)$ of order n, is the $n \times n$ matrix $D = (d_{ij})$ where $d_{ij} = d(u_i, u_j)$, the distance between nodes u_i and u_j. Efficient, classical algorithms are available for obtaining such a matrix [10]. Note also that the distance matrix of a graph can easily be constructed from its adjacency matrix A_G. In fact, denoting by a_{ij}^n the (i, j)-th entry of the matrix A_G^n, the n-th power of A_G, we have that d_{ij} equals the least n for which $a_{ij}^n > 0$ (there must be such an n since a tree is connected).

3   Continuous Formulation of Maximum Clique

After formulating the free tree matching problem as a maximum clique problem, we now proceed (following [27]) by mapping the latter onto a continuous quadratic programming problem. Let $G = (V, E)$ be an arbitrary graph of order n, and let Δ denote the standard simplex of $\mathbb{R}^n$:

$$\Delta = \{ \mathbf{x} \in \mathbb{R}^n \; : \; \mathbf{e}'\mathbf{x} = 1 \text{ and } x_i \geq 0, \; i = 1 \ldots n \}$$

where $\mathbf{e}$ is the vector whose components equal 1, and a prime denotes transposition. Given a subset of vertices C of G, we will denote by $\mathbf{x}^c$ its *characteristic vector* which is the point in Δ defined as

$$x_i^c = \begin{cases} 1/|C|, & \text{if } i \in C \\ 0, & \text{otherwise} \end{cases}$$

where $|C|$ denotes the cardinality of C.

Now, consider the following quadratic function

$$f_G(\mathbf{x}) = \mathbf{x}' A_G \mathbf{x} + \frac{1}{2}\mathbf{x}'\mathbf{x} \tag{3}$$

where $A_G = (a_{ij})$ is the adjacency matrix of G. The following theorem, recently proved by Bomze [5], expands on the Motzkin-Straus theorem [23], a remarkable result which establishes a connection between the maximum clique problem and certain standard quadratic programs. This has an intriguing computational significance in that it allows us to shift from the discrete to the continuous domain in an elegant manner.

Theorem 2. *Let C be a subset of vertices of a graph G, and let $\mathbf{x}^c$ be its characteristic vector. Then, C is a maximal (maximum) clique of G if and only if $\mathbf{x}^c$ is a local (global) maximizer f_G in Δ. Moreover, all local (and hence global) maximizers of f_G in Δ are strict.*

Unlike the original Motzkin-Straus formulation, which is plagued by the presence of "spurious" solutions [26], the previous result guarantees us that *all* maximizers of f_G on Δ are strict, and are characteristic vectors of maximal/maximum cliques in the graph. In a formal sense, therefore, a one-to-one correspondence exists between maximal cliques and local maximizers of f_G in Δ on the one hand, and maximum cliques and global maximizers on the other hand.

4   Matching Free Trees with Monotone Game Dynamics

Payoff-monotonic dynamics are a wide class of dynamical systems developed and studied in evolutionary game theory, a discipline pioneered by J. Maynard Smith [20] which aims to model the evolution of animal behavior using the principles and tools of noncooperative game theory. In this section we discuss the basic intuition behind these models and present a few theoretical properties that are instrumental for their application to our optimization problem. For a more systematic treatment see [17, 30].

Consider a large, ideally infinite population of individuals belonging to the same species which compete for a particular limited resource, such as food, territory, etc. In evolutionary game theory, this kind of conflict is modeled as a symmetric two-player game, the players being pairs of randomly selected population members. In contrast to traditional application fields of game theory, such as economics or sociology, players here do not behave "rationally," but act instead according to a pre-programmed behavior pattern, or *pure strategy*. Reproduction is assumed to be asexual, which means that, apart from mutation, offspring will inherit the same genetic material, and hence behavioral phenotype, as its parent.

Let $J = \{1, \cdots, n\}$ be the set of available pure strategies and, for all $i \in J$, let $x_i(t)$ be the proportion of population members playing strategy i, at time t. The state of the population at a given instant is the vector $\mathbf{x} = (x_1, \cdots, x_n)'$. Clearly, population states are constrained to lie in the standard simplex Δ. For a given population state $\mathbf{x} \in \Delta$, we shall denote by $\sigma(\mathbf{x})$ the *support* of $\mathbf{x}$, i.e. the set of non-extinct strategies:

$$\sigma(\mathbf{x}) = \{i \in J \ : \ x_i > 0\} \ .$$

Let $A = (a_{ij})$ be the $n \times n$ payoff (or utility) matrix. Specifically, for each pair of strategies $i, j \in J$, a_{ij} represents the payoff of an individual playing strategy i against an opponent playing strategy j. In biological contexts a player's utility can simply be measured in terms of Darwinian fitness or reproductive success, i.e., the player's expected number of offspring. If the population is in state $\mathbf{x}$, the expected payoff earnt by an i-strategist is:

$$\pi_i(\mathbf{x}) = \sum_{j=1}^{n} a_{ij}x_j = (A\mathbf{x})_i \qquad (4)$$

while the mean payoff over the entire population is

$$\pi(\mathbf{x}) = \sum_{i=1}^{n} x_i\pi_i(\mathbf{x}) = \mathbf{x}'A\mathbf{x} . \qquad (5)$$

In evolutionary game theory the assumption is made that the game is played over and over, generation after generation, and that the action of natural selection will result in the evolution of the fittest strategies. If successive generations blend into each other, the evolution of behavioral phenotypes can be described by a set of ordinary differential equations. A general class of evolution equations are given by:

$$\dot{x}_i = x_i g_i(\mathbf{x}) \qquad (6)$$

where a dot signifies derivative with respect to time, and $g = (g_1, \ldots, g_n)$ is a function with open domain containing Δ. Here, the function g_i ($i \in J$) specifies the rate at which pure strategy i replicates. It is usually required that the growth functions g be *regular* [30], which means that it is Lipschitz continuous and that $g(\mathbf{x}) \cdot \mathbf{x} = 0$ for all $\mathbf{x} \in \Delta$. The former condition guarantees us that the system of differential equations (6) has a unique solution through any initial population state. The condition $g(\mathbf{x}) \cdot \mathbf{x} = 0$, instead, ensures that the simplex Δ is invariant under (6), namely any trajectory starting in Δ will remain in Δ.

Payoff-monotonic game dynamics represent a wide class of regular selection dynamics for which useful properties hold. Intuitively, for a payoff-monotonic dynamics the strategies associated to higher payoffs will increase at higher rate. Formally, a regular selection dynamics (6) is said to be payoff-monotonic if:

$$g_i(\mathbf{x}) > g_j(\mathbf{x}) \iff \pi_i(\mathbf{x}) > \pi_j(\mathbf{x}) \qquad (7)$$

for all $\mathbf{x} \in \Delta$.

It is simple to show that all payoff-monotonic dynamics share the same set of stationary points.

Proposition 1. *A point $\mathbf{x} \in \Delta$ is stationary under any payoff-monotonic dynamics if and only if $\pi_i(\mathbf{x}) = \pi(\mathbf{x})$ for all $i \in \sigma(\mathbf{x})$.*

Proof. If $\pi_i(\mathbf{x}) = \pi(\mathbf{x})$ for all $i \in \sigma(\mathbf{x})$, by monotonicity (7), there exists $\mu \in \mathbb{R}$ such that $g_i(\mathbf{x}) = \mu$ for all $i \in \sigma(\mathbf{x})$. But, since g is a regular growth-rate function, $\sum_i x_i g_i(\mathbf{x}) = 0$, and hence $\mu = 0$. Therefore, $\mathbf{x}$ is a stationary point for (6).. On the other hand, if $\mathbf{x}$ is stationary, then $g_i(\mathbf{x}) = 0$ for all $i \in \sigma(\mathbf{x})$. Hence, there exists a $\lambda \in \mathbb{R}$ such that $\pi_i(\mathbf{x}) = \lambda$ for all $i \in \sigma(\mathbf{x})$. But then $\lambda = \sum_i x_i\pi_i(\mathbf{x}) = \pi(\mathbf{x})$. $\qquad\square$

In an unpublished paper [16], Hofbauer shows that the average population payoff is strictly increasing along the trajectories of any payoff-monotonic dynamics. This result generalizes the celebrated fundamental theorem of natural selection [17, 30]. Here, we provide a different proof adapted from [12].

Theorem 3. *If the payoff matrix A is symmetric, then $\pi(\mathbf{x}) = \mathbf{x}'A\mathbf{x}$ is strictly increasing along any non-constant trajectory of any payoff-monotonic dynamics. In other words, $\dot{\pi}(\mathbf{x}(t)) \geq 0$ for all t, with equality if and only if $\mathbf{x} = \mathbf{x}(t)$ is a stationary point.*

Proof. For $\mathbf{x} \in \Delta$, let:

$$\sigma_+(\mathbf{x}) = \{i \in \sigma(\mathbf{x}) \ : \ g_i(\mathbf{x}) \geq 0\}$$

and

$$\sigma_-(\mathbf{x}) = \{i \in \sigma(\mathbf{x}) \ : \ g_i(\mathbf{x}) < 0\} \ .$$

Clearly, $\sigma_+(\mathbf{x}) \cup \sigma_-(\mathbf{x}) = \sigma(\mathbf{x})$. Moreover, let:

$$\overline{\pi}(\mathbf{x}) = \min\{\pi_i(\mathbf{x}) \ : \ i \in \sigma_+(\mathbf{x})\}$$

and

$$\underline{\pi}(\mathbf{x}) = \max\{\pi_i(\mathbf{x}) \ : \ i \in \sigma_-(\mathbf{x})\}$$

Because of payoff-motonicity, note that $\overline{\pi}(\mathbf{x}) \geq \underline{\pi}(\mathbf{x})$. Note also that $\dot{x}_i \geq 0$ if and only if $i \in \sigma_+(\mathbf{x})$.

Because of the symmetry of A, we have:

$$\frac{\dot{\pi}(\mathbf{x})}{2} = \sum_{i \in \sigma(\mathbf{x})} \dot{x}_i \pi_i(\mathbf{x})$$

$$= \sum_{i \in \sigma_+(\mathbf{x})} \dot{x}_i \pi_i(\mathbf{x}) + \sum_{i \in \sigma_-(\mathbf{x})} \dot{x}_i \pi_i(\mathbf{x})$$

$$\geq \overline{\pi}(\mathbf{x}) \sum_{i \in \sigma_+(\mathbf{x})} \dot{x}_i + \underline{\pi}(\mathbf{x}) \sum_{i \in \sigma_-(\mathbf{x})} \dot{x}_i$$

$$= (\overline{\pi}(\mathbf{x}) - \underline{\pi}(\mathbf{x})) \sum_{i \in \sigma_+(\mathbf{x})} \dot{x}_i$$

$$\geq 0$$

where the last equality follows from $\sum \dot{x}_i = 0$. Finally, note that $\dot{\pi}(\mathbf{x}) = 0$ if and only if $\pi_i(\mathbf{x})$ is constant for all $i \in \sigma(\mathbf{x})$ which, from Proposition 1, amounts to saying that $\mathbf{x}$ is stationary. □

A well-known subclass of payoff-monotonic game dynamics is given by:

$$\dot{x}_i = x_i \left(f(\pi_i(\mathbf{x})) - \sum_{j=1}^{n} x_j f(\pi_j(\mathbf{x})) \right) \tag{8}$$

where $f(u)$ is an increasing function of u. These models arise in modeling the evolution of behavior by way of imitation processes, where players are occasionally given the opportunity to change their own strategies [16, 30].

When f is the identity function, i.e., $f(u) = u$, we obtain the standard replicator equations:

$$\dot{x}_i = x_i \left(\pi_i(\mathbf{x}) - \sum_{j=1}^{n} x_j \pi_j(\mathbf{x}) \right) \tag{9}$$

whose basic idea is that the average rate of increase $\dot{x}_i/x_i$ equals the difference between the average fitness of strategy i and the mean fitness over the entire population.

Another popular model arises when $f(u) = e^{\kappa u}$ which yields:

$$\dot{x}_i = x_i \left(e^{\kappa \pi_i(\mathbf{x})} - \sum_{j=1}^{n} x_j e^{\kappa \pi_j(\mathbf{x})} \right) \tag{10}$$

where κ is a positive constant. As κ tends to 0, the orbits of this dynamics approach those of the standard, first-order replicator model (9), slowed down by the factor κ; moreover, for large values of κ the model approximates the so-called "best-reply" dynamics [16, 17]. As it turns out [16], these models behave essentially in the same way as the standard replicator equations (9), the only significant difference being the size of the basins of attraction around stable equilibria. From a computational perspective, exponential replicator dynamics are particularly attractive as they may be considerably faster and even more accurate than the standard, first-order model (see [25] and the results reported below).

In light of their dynamical properties, payoff-monotonic dynamics naturally suggest themselves as simple heuristics for solving the maximal subtree isomorphism problem. Let $T_1 = (V_1, E_1)$ and $T_2 = (V_2, E_2)$ be two free trees, and let A_G denote the adjacency matrix of their FTAG G. By putting

$$A = A_G + \frac{1}{2} I \tag{11}$$

where I is the identity matrix, we know from Theorem 3 that any payoff-monotonic dynamics starting from an arbitrary initial state, will iteratively maximize the function f_G defined in (3) over the simplex and will eventually converge with probability 1 to a strict local maximizer which, by virtue of Theorem 2, will then correspond to the characteristic vector of a maximal clique in the association graph. As stated in Theorem 1, this will in turn induce a maximal subtree isomorphism between T_1 and T_2.

Clearly, in theory there is no guarantee that the converged solution will be a *global* maximizer of f_G, and therefore that it will induce a *maximum* isomorphism between the two original trees. Previous experimental work with standard replicator dynamics [7, 24, 25, 27] and also the results presented in the next section, however, suggest that the basins of attraction of optimal or near-optimal solutions are quite large, and very frequently the algorithm converges to one of them, despite its inherent inability to escape from local optima.

5   Experimental Results

In this section we present experiments of applying payoff-monotonic dynamics to the free tree matching problem. In our simulations, we used the following discrete-time models:

$$x_i(t+1) = \frac{x_i(t)\pi_i(t)}{\sum_{j=1}^n x_j(t)\pi_j(t)} \tag{12}$$

and

$$x_i(t+1) = \frac{x_i(t)e^{\kappa\pi_i(t)}}{\sum_{j=1}^n x_j(t)e^{\kappa\pi_j(t)}} \tag{13}$$

which correspond to well-known discretizations of equations (9) and (10), respectively [9, 14, 17, 30]. Note that model (12) is the standard discrete-time replicator dynamics, which have already proven to be remarkably effective in tackling maximum clique and related problems, and to be competitive to other more elaborated neural network heuristics [5, 7, 8, 24, 25, 27]. Equation (13) has been used in [25] to approximate the graph isomorphism problem. For the latter dynamics the value $\kappa = 10$ was used.

Both the first-order and the exponential processes were started from the simplex barycenter and stopped when either a maximal clique (i.e., a local maximizer of f_G) was found or the distance between two successive points was smaller than a fixed threshold. In the latter case the converged vector was randomly perturbed, and the algorithms restarted from the perturbed point. Because of the one-to-one correspondence between local maximizers and maximal cliques, this situation corresponds to convergence to a saddle point.

5.1   Matching Shape-Axis Trees

Recently, Liu *et al.* [19] introduced a new representation for shape based on the idea of self-similarity. Intuitively, given a closed planar shape, they consider two different parameterizations of its contour, namely one oriented counterclockwise, $\Gamma(s) = \{x(s) : 0 \le s \le 1\}$, and the other clockwise, $\hat{\Gamma}(t) = \{\hat{x}(t) = x(1-t) : 0 \le t \le 1\}$. By minimizing an appropriate cost functional they find a "good" match between Γ and $\hat{\Gamma}$, and then define the shape axis (SA) as the loci of middle points between the matched contour points. From a given SA, it is possible to construct a unique free tree, called the SA-tree, by grouping the discontinuities contained in the SA. In Figure 1 the SA-tree construction process is illustrated, and Figure 2 shows the SA-trees derived from a few example shapes.

The proposed matching algorithms were tested on a selection of 17 shapes (SA-trees) representing six different object classes (horse, human, bird, dog, sheep, and rhino). We matched each shape against each other (and itself) and in *all* the 289 trials both algorithms returned the *maximum* isomorphism, i.e. a maximum clique in the FTAG. Figure 3 shows a few example matches. This is a remarkable fact, considering that replicator dynamics are unable to escape from local solutions. Similar findings on related problems are discussed in [25,

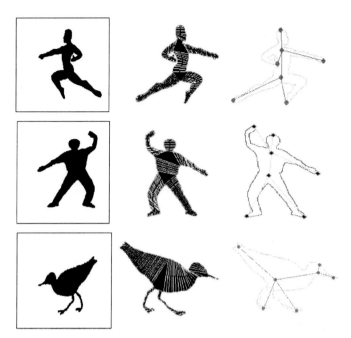

Fig. 1. Illustration of the SA-tree construction. Three shapes (left), their shape-axis model (middle), and the corresponding SA-trees (right).

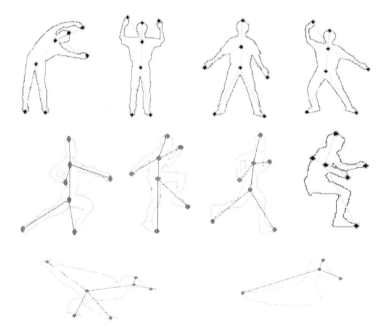

Fig. 2. Examples of SA-trees, under various shape deformations.

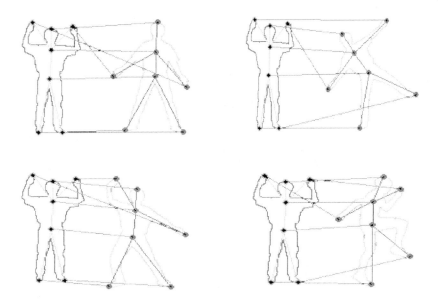

Fig. 3. Some examples of matching SA-trees.

27]. As far as the computational time is concerned, both dynamics took only a few seconds to converge on a 350MHz AMDK6-2 processor, the exponential one being slightly faster than the linear one (but see below for a rather different picture).

5.2   Matching Larger Trees

Encouraged by the results reported above, we proceeded by testing our algorithms over much larger (random) trees. Random structures represent a useful benchmark not only because they are not constrained to any particular application, but also because it is simple to replicate experiments and hence to make comparisons with other algorithms.

In this series of experiments, the following protocol was used. A hundred 100-node free trees were generated uniformly at random using a procedure described by Wilf in [31]. Then, each such tree was subject to a corruption process which consisted of randomly deleting a fraction of its nodes (in fact, the to-be-deleted nodes were constrained to be the terminal ones, otherwise the resulting graph would have been disconnected), thereby obtaining a tree isomorphic to a proper subtree of the original one. Various levels of corruption (i.e., percentage of node deletion) were used, namely 2%, 10%, 20%, 30% and 40%. This means that the order of the pruned trees ranged from 98 to 60. Overall, therefore, 500 pairs of trees were obtained, for each of which the corresponding FTAG was constructed as described in Section 2. To keep the order of the association graph as low as possible, its vertex set was constructed as follows:

$$V = \{(u, w) \in V' \times V'' \; : \; \deg(u) \leq \deg(w)\} \; ,$$

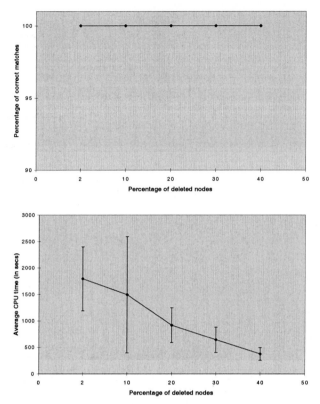

Fig. 4. Results obtained over 100-node random trees with various levels of corruption, using the first-order dynamics (12). Top: Percentage of correct matches. Bottom: Average computational time taken by the replicator equations.

assuming $|V'| \leq |V''|$, the edge set E being defined as in (2). It is straightforward to see that when the first tree is isomorphic to a subtree of the second, Theorem 1 continues to hold. This simple heuristic may significantly reduce the dimensionality of the search space. We also performed some experiments with unpruned FTAG's but no significant difference in performance was noticed apart, of course, heavier memory requirements.

As in the previous series of experiments, both the linear and the exponential dynamics were used, with identical parameters and stopping criterion. After convergence, we calculated the proportion of matched nodes, i.e., the ratio between the cardinality of the clique found and the order of the smaller subtree, and then we averaged. Figure 4(a) shows the results obtained using the linear dynamics (12) as a function of the corruption level. As can be seen, the algorithm was *always* able to find a correct maximum isomorphism, i.e. a maximum clique in the FTAG. Figure 4(b) plots the corresponding (average) CPU time taken by the processes, with corresponding error bars (simulations were performed on the same machine used for the shape-axis experiments).

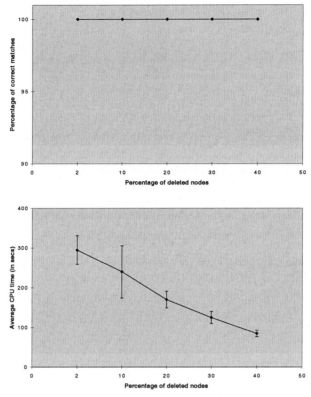

Fig. 5. Results obtained over 100-node random trees with various levels of corruption, using the exponential dynamics (13). Top: Percentage of correct matches. Bottom: Average computational time taken by the replicator equations.

In Figure 5, the results pertaining to the exponential dynamics (13) are shown. In terms of solution's quality the algorithm performed exactly as its linear counterpart, but this time it was dramatically faster. This confirms earlier results reported in [25].

6   Conclusions

We have developed a formal approach for matching connected and acyclic relational structures, i.e. free trees, by constructing an association graph whose maximal cliques are in one-to-one correspondence with maximal subtree isomorphisms. The framework is general and can be applied in a variety of computer vision domains: we have demonstrated its potential for shape matching. The solution is found by using payoff-monotonic dynamical systems, which make them amenable to hardware implementation and offers the advantage of biological plausibility. In particular, these relaxation labeling equations are related to putative neuronal implementations [21, 22]. Extensive experiments on hundreds of uniformly random trees have also been conducted and, as in previous work on graph isomorphism [25] and rooted tree matching [27], the results are impressive. Despite the counter-intuitive maximum clique formulation of the tree matching problem, and the inherent inability of these simple dynamics to escape from local optima, they nevertheless were always able to find a globally optimal solution.

Before concluding, we note that the framework can easily be extended to tackle the problem of matching attributed (free) trees. In this case, the attributes result in weights being placed on the nodes of the association graph, and a conversion of the maximum clique problem to a maximum weight clique problem [27, 8]. Note also that, since the presented approach does not allow for many-to-many correspondences, it cannot be compared as is with edit-distance tree matching algorithms, as the one presented in [18]. However, it is straightforward to formulate many-to-one or many-to-many versions of our framework along the lines suggested in [3, 28] for rooted attributed trees. This will be the subject of future investigations.

Acknowledgments

The author would like to thank M. Zuin for his support in performing the experiments, and T.-L. Liu for kindly providing us with the shape database.

References

1. A. P. Ambler, H. G. Barrow, C. M. Brown, R. M. Burstall, and R. J. Popplestone. A versatile computer-controlled assembly system. In *Proc. 3rd Int. J. Conf. Artif. Intell.*, pages 298–307, Stanford, CA, 1973.

2. D. H. Ballard and C. M. Brown. *Computer Vision*. Prentice-Hall, Englewood Cliffs, NJ, 1982.

3. M. Bartoli, M. Pelillo, K. Siddiqi, and S. W. Zucker. Attributed tree homomorphism using association graphs. In *Proc. ICPR'2000—15th Int. Conf. Pattern Recognition*, volume 2, pages 133–136, Barcelona, Spain, 2000.

4. H. Blum and R. N. Nagel. Shape description using weighted symmetric axis features. *Pattern Recognition*, 10:167–180, 1978.

5. I. M. Bomze. Evolution towards the maximum clique. *J. Global Optim.*, 10:143–164, 1997.

6. I. M. Bomze, M. Budinich, P. M. Pardalos, and M. Pelillo. The maximum clique problem. In D.-Z. Du and P. M. Pardalos, editors, *Handbook of Combinatorial Optimization (Suppl. Vol. A)*, pages 1–74. Kluwer, Boston, MA, 1999.

7. I. M. Bomze, M. Pelillo, and R. Giacomini. Evolutionary approach to the maximum clique problem: Empirical evidence on a larger scale. In I. M. Bomze, T. Csendes, R. Horst, and P. M. Pardalos, editors, *Developments in Global Optimization*, pages 95–108. Kluwer, Dordrecht, The Netherlands, 1997.

8. I. M. Bomze, M. Pelillo, and V. Stix. Approximating the maximum weight clique using replicator dynamics. *IEEE Trans. Neural Networks*, 11(6):1228–1241, 2000.

9. A. Cabrales and J. Sobel. On the limit points of discrete selection dynamics. *J. Econom. Theory*, 57:407–419, 1992.

10. T. H. Cormen, C. E. Leiserson, and R. L. Rivest. *Introduction to Algorithms*. MIT Press, Cambridge, MA, 1991.

11. P. Dimitrov, C. Phillips, and K. Siddiqi. Robust and efficient skeletal graphs. In *Proc. CVPR'2000—IEEE Conf. Comput. Vision Pattern Recognition*, Hilton Head, SC, 2000.

12. D. Fudenberg and D. K. Levine. *The Theory of Learning in Games*. MIT Press, Cambridge, MA, 1998.

13. M. R. Garey and D. S. Johnson. *Computers and Intractability: A Guide to the Theory of NP-Completeness*. W. H. Freeman, San Francisco, CA, 1979.

14. A. Gaunersdorfer and J. Hofbauer. Fictitious play, Shapley polygons, and the replicator equation. *Games Econom. Behav.*, 11:279–303, 1995.

15. F. Harary. *Graph Theory*. Addison-Wesley, Reading, MA, 1969.

16. J. Hofbauer. Imitation dynamics for games. Collegium Budapest, preprint, 1995.

17. J. Hofbauer and K. Sigmund. *Evolutionary Games and Population Dynamics*. Cambridge University Press, Cambridge, UK, 1998.

18. T.-L. Liu and D. Geiger. Approximate tree matching and shape similarity. In *Proc. ICCV'99—7th Int. Conf. Computer Vision*, pages 456–462, Kerkyra, Greece, 1999.

19. T.-L. Liu, D. Geiger, and R. V. Kohn. Representation and self-similarity of shapes. In *Proc. ICCV'98—6th Int. Conf. Computer Vision*, pages 1129–1135, Bombay, India, 1998.

20. J. Maynard Smith. *Evolution and the Theory of Games*. Cambridge University Press, Cambridge, UK, 1982.

21. D. Miller and S. W. Zucker. Efficient simplex-like methods for equilibria of non-symmetric analog networks. *Neural Computation*, 4(2):167–190, 1992.

22. D. Miller and S. W. Zucker. Computing with self-excitatory cliques: A model and an application to hyperacuity-scale computation in visual cortex. *Neural Computation*, 11(1):21–66, 1999.

23. T. S. Motzkin and E. G. Straus. Maxima for graphs and a new proof of a theorem of Turán. *Canad. J. Math.*, 17:533–540, 1965.

24. M. Pelillo. Relaxation labeling networks for the maximum clique problem. *J. Artif. Neural Networks*, 2:313–328, 1995.

25. M. Pelillo. Replicator equations, maximal cliques, and graph isomorphism. *Neural Computation*, 11(8):2023–2045, 1999.

26. M. Pelillo and A. Jagota. Feasible and infeasible maxima in a quadratic program for maximum clique. *J. Artif. Neural Networks*, 2:411–420, 1995.

27. M. Pelillo, K. Siddiqi, and S. W. Zucker. Matching hierarchical structures using association graphs. *IEEE Trans. Pattern Anal. Machince Intell.*, 21(11):1105–1120, 1999.

28. M. Pelillo, K. Siddiqi, and S. W. Zucker. Many-to-many matching of attributed trees using association graphs and game dynamics. In C. Arcelli, L. P. Cordella, and G. Sanniti di Baja, editors, *Visual Form 2001*, pages 583–593. Springer, Berlin, 2001.

29. S. W. Reyner. An analysis of a good algorithm for the subtree problem. *SIAM J. Comput.*, 6:730–732, 1977.

30. J. W. Weibull. *Evolutionary Game Theory*. MIT Press, Cambridge, MA, 1995.

31. H. Wilf. The uniform selection of free trees. *J. Algorithms*, 2:204–207, 1981.

32. S. C. Zhu and A. L. Yuille. FORMS: A flexible object recognition and modeling system. *Int. J. Computer Vision*, 20(3):187–212, 1996.

Efficiently Computing Weighted Tree Edit Distance Using Relaxation Labeling

Andrea Torsello and Edwin R. Hancock

Department of Computer Science University of York
York, YO10 5DD, UK
`atorsell@cs.york.ac.uk`

Abstract. This paper investigates an approach to tree edit distance problem with weighted nodes. We show that any tree obtained with a sequence of cut and relabel operations is a subtree of the transitive closure of the original tree. Furthermore, we show that the necessary condition for any subtree to be a solution can be reduced to a clique problem in a derived structure. Using this idea we transform the tree edit distance problem into a series of maximum weight clique problems and then we use relaxation labeling to find an approximate solution.

1 Introduction

The problem of how to measure the similarity of pictorial information which has been abstracted using graph-structures has been the focus of sustained research activity for over twenty years in the computer vision literature. Moreover, the problem has recently acquired significant topicality with the need to develop ways of retrieving images from large data-bases. Stated succinctly, the problem is one of inexact or error-tolerant graph-matching. Early work on the topic included Barrow and Burstall's idea [1] of locating matches by searching for maximum common subgraphs using the association graph, and the extension of the concept of string edit distance to graph-matching by Fu and his co-workers [6]. The idea behind edit distance [18] is that it is possible to identify a set of basic edit operations on nodes and edges of a structure, and to associate with these operations a cost. The edit-distance is found by searching for the sequence of edit operations that will make the two graphs isomorphic with one-another and which has minimum cost. By making the evaluation of structural modification explicit, edit distance provides a very effective way of measuring the similarity of relational structures. Moreover, the method has considerable potential for error tolerant object recognition and indexing problems.

Unfortunately, the task of calculating edit distance is a computationally hard problem and most early efforts can be regarded as being goal-directed. However, in an important series of recent papers, Bunke has demonstrated the intimate relationship between the size of the maximum common subgraph and the edit distance [4] . In particular, he showed that, under certain assumptions concerning the edit-costs, computing the MCS and the graph edit distance are equivalent. The restriction imposed on the edit-costs is that the deletions and re-insertions

M.A.T. Figueiredo, J. Zerubia, A.K. Jain (Eds.): EMMCVPR 2001, LNCS 2134, pp. 438–453, 2001.

of nodes and edges are not more expensive than the corresponding node or edge relabeling operations. In other words, there is no incentive to use relabeling operations, and as a result the edit operations can be reduced to those of insertion and deletion.

The work reported in this paper builds on a simple observation which follows from Bunke's work. By re-casting the search for the maximum common subgraph as a max clique problem [1], then we can efficiently compute the edit distance. A diverse array of powerful heuristics and theoretical results are available for solving the max clique problem. In particular the Motzkin-Straus theorem [10] allows us to transform the max clique problem into a continuous quadratic programming problem. An important recent development is reported by Pelillo [11] who shows how probabilistic relaxation labeling can be used to find a (local) optimum of this quadratic programming problem.

In this paper we are interested in measuring the similarity of tree structures obtained from a skeletal representation of 2D shape. While trees are a special case of graphs, because of the connectivity and partial order constraints which apply to them, the methods used to compare and match them require significant specific adaptation. For instance, Bartoli et al. [2], use the graph theoretic notion of a path string to transform the tree isomorphism problem into a single max weighted clique problem. This work uses a refinement of the Motzkin Strauss theorem to transform the max weighted clique problem into a quadratic programming problem on the simplex [3], the quadratic problem is then solved using relaxation labeling.

Because of the added connectivity and partial order constraints mentioned above, Bunke's result linking the computation of edit distance to the size of the maximum common subgraph does not translate in a simple way to trees. Furthermore, specific characteristics of trees suggest that posing the tree-matching problem as a variant on graph-matching is not the best approach. In particular, both the tree isomorphism and the subtree isomorphism problems have efficient polynomial time solutions. Moreover, Tai [16] has proposed a generalization of the string edit distance problem from the linear structure of a string to the non-linear structure of a tree. The resulting tree edit distance differs from the general graph edit distance in that edit operations are carried out only on nodes and never directly on edges. The edit operations thus defined are node deletion, node insertion and node relabeling. This simplified set of edit operations is guaranteed to preserve the connectivity of the tree structure. Zhang and Shasha [22] have investigated a special case which involves adding the constraint that the solution must maintain the order of the children of a node. With this order among siblings, they showed that the tree-matching problem is still in P and gave an algorithm to solve it. In subsequent work they showed that the unordered case was indeed an NP hard problem [23]. The NP-completeness, though, can be eliminated again by adding particular constraints to the edit operations. In particular, it can be shown that the problem returns to P when we add the constraint of strict hierarchy, that is when separate subtrees are constrained to be mapped to separate subtrees [21].

In this paper we propose an energy minimization method for efficiently computing the weighted tree edit distance. We follow Pelillo [11] by casting the problem into the Motzkin-Straus framework. To achieve n this goal we use the graph-theoretic notion of tree closure. We show that, given a tree T, then any tree obtained by cutting nodes from T is a subtree of the closure of T. Furthermore, we can eliminate subtrees that can not be obtained from T by solving a series of max-clique problems. In this way we provide a divide and conquer method for finding the maximum edited common subtree by searching for maximal cliques of an association graph formed from the closure of the two trees. With this representation to hand, we follow Bomze et al. [3] and use a variant of the Motzkin Straus theorem to convert the maximum weighted clique problem into a quadratic programming problem which can be solved by relaxation labeling.

2   Exact Tree Matching

In this section we describe a polynomial time algorithm for the subtree isomorphism problem. This allows us to formalize some concepts and give a starting point to extend the approach to the minimum tree edit distance problem.

2.1   Association Graph

The phase space we use to represent the matching of nodes is the directed association graph, a variant of the association graph. The association graph is a structure that is frequently used in graph matching problems. The nodes of the association graph are the Cartesian products of nodes of the graphs to be matched. Hence, each node represents a possible association, or match, of a node in one graph to a node in the other. The edges of the association graph represent the pairwise constraints of the problem: they represent both connectivity on the original graphs and the feasibility of a solution with the linked associations.

Hierarchical graphs have an order relation induced by paths: given two nodes a and b, (a, b) is in this relation if and only if there is a path from a to b. When the directed graph is acyclical, this relation can be shown to be an (irreflexive) order relation. The use of directed arcs in the association graph allows us to make use of this order. We connect nodes with directed arcs in a way that preserves the ordering of the associated graph. The graph obtained can be shown to be ordered still. Specifically, an association graph for the tree isomorphism problem can be shown to be a forest.

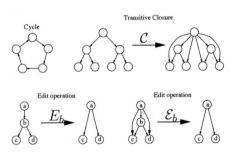

Fig. 1. Terminology on directed graphs

For the exact isomorphism problem (maximum common subgraph) the edges of the association graphs are:

$$(v, v') \rightarrow (u, u') \text{ iff } v \rightarrow u \text{ and } v' \rightarrow u' \tag{1}$$

where v and u are nodes on one graph and v' and u' are nodes on the other.

Proposition 1. *The directed association graph of two directed acyclic graphs (DAGs) G and G' is acyclic.*

Proof. Let us assume that $(u_1, v_1) \rightarrow \cdots \rightarrow (u_n, v_n)$ is a cycle. Then, since an arc $(v, v') \rightarrow (u, u')$ in the association graph exists only if the arcs $v \rightarrow u$ and $v' \rightarrow u'$ exist in G and G' respectively, we have that $u_1 \rightarrow \cdots \rightarrow u_n$ is a cycle in G and $v_1 \rightarrow \cdots \rightarrow v_n$ is a cycle in G' against the hypothesis that they are DAGs.

Proposition 2. *The directed association graph of two trees t and t' is a forest.*

Proof. We already know that the association graph is a DAG, we have to show that for each node (u, u') there is at most one node (v, v') such that $(v, v') \rightarrow (u, u')$. Due to the way the association graph is constructed this means that either u or u' must have at most one incoming edge. But t and t' are trees, so both u and u' have at most one incoming edge, namely the one from the parent.

The directed association graph can be used to reduce a tree matching problem into subproblems: the best match given the association of nodes v and v' can be found examining only descendents of v and v' This gives us a divide and conquer solution to the maximum common subtree problem: use the association graph to divide the problem and transform it into maximum bipartite match subproblems, the subproblems can then be efficiently conquered with known polynomial time algorithms. We then extend the approach to the minimum unlabeled tree edit problem and present an evolutionary method to conquer the subproblems. Finally, we present a method to convert the divide and conquer approach into a multi-population evolutionary approach.

2.2   Maximum Common Subtree

We present a divide and conquer approach to the exact maximum common subtree problem. We call the maximum common subtree rooted at (v, v') a solution to the maximum common subtree problem applied to two subtrees of t and t'. In particular, the solution is on the subtrees of t and t' rooted at v and v' respectively. This solution is further constrained with the condition that v and v' are roots of the matched subtrees.

With the maximum rooted isomorphism problem for each children of (v, v') at hand, the maximum isomorphism rooted at (v, v') can be reduced to a maximum bipartite match problem. The two partitions V and V' of the bipartite match consist of the children of v and v' respectively. The weight of the match between $u \in V$ and $u' \in V'$ is the sum of the matched weights of the maximum isomorphism rooted at (u, u'). In case of a non weighted tree this is the cardinality of the isomorphism. With this structure we have a one-to-one relationship between matches in the bipartite graph and the children of (v, v') in the association graph. The solution of the bipartite matching problem identifies a set of children of (v, v') that satisfy the constraint of matching one node of t to no more than one node of t'. Furthermore, among such sets is the one that guarantees the maximum total weight of the isomorphism rooted at (v, v').

The maximum isomorphism between t and t' is a maximum isomorphism rooted at (v, v'), where either v or v' is the root of t or t' respectively. This reduces the isomorphism problem to $n + m$ rooted isomorphism problems, where n and m are the cardinality of t and t'. Furthermore, since there are nm nodes in the association graph, the problem is reduced to nm maximum bipartite match problems.

3   Inexact Tree Matching

We want to extend the algorithm to provide us with an error-tolerant tree isomorphism. There is a strong connection between the computation of maximum common subtree and the tree edit distance. In [4] Bunke showed that, under certain constraints applied to the edit-cost function, computing the maximum common subgraph problem and the minimum graph edit distance are equivalent to one-another.

This is not directly true for trees, because of the added constraint that a tree must be connected. But, extending the concept to the common edited subtree, we can use common substructures to find the minimum cost edited tree isomorphism. In particular, we want to match weighted trees. These are trees with weight associated to the nodes and with the property that the cost of an edit operation is a function of the weight of the nodes involved.

Following common use, we consider three fundamental operations:

- *node removal:* this operation removes a node and links the children to the parent of said node.
- *node insertion:* the dual of node removal
- *node relabel:* this operation changes the weight of a node.

In our model the cost node removal and insertion is equal to the weight of the node, while the cost of relabeling a node is equal to the difference in the weights. This approach identifies node removal to relabel to 0 weight and is a natural interpretation when the weight represents the "importance" of the node.

Since a node insertion on the data tree is dual to a node removal on the model tree, we can reduce the number of operations to be performed to only node removal, as long as we perform the operations on both trees.

At this point we introduce the concept of *edited isomorphism*. Assuming that we have two trees T_1 and T_2 and a tree T' that can be obtained from both with node removal and relabel operations, T' will induce an isomorphism between nodes in T_1 and T_2 so that places two nodes in correspondence if and only if they get cut down to the same node in T'. We call such isomorphism an edited isomorphism induced by T'. From the definition it is clear that there is a tree T', obtained only with node removal and relabel operations, so that the sum of the edit distance from this tree to T_1 and T_2 is equal to the edit distance between T_1 and T_2, i.e. a median tree. We say that the isomorphism induced by this tree is a *maximum edited isomorphism* because it maximizes $W_m = \sum_{(i,j)} \min(w_i, w_j)$, where i and j are nodes matched by the isomorphism, and w_i and w_j are their weights. In fact, if we W_1 and W_2 be the weights in T_1 and T_2 respectively, the edit distance between T_1 and T' is $W_1 - W_m$, the distance between T_1 and T_2 is $W_1 + W_2 - 2W_m$. Clearly, finding the maximum edited isomorphism is equivalent to solving the tree edit distance problem.

3.1   Editing the Transitive Closure of a Tree

For each node v of t, we can define an edit operation E_v on the tree and an edit operation $\mathcal{E}_v$ on the closure Ct of the tree t (see Figure 1). In both cases the edit operation removes the node v, all the incoming edges, and all the outgoing edges.

We show that the transitive closure operation and the node removal operation commute, that is we have:

Lemma 1. $\mathcal{E}_v(\mathcal{C}(t)) = \mathcal{C}(E_v(t))$

Proof. If a node is in $\mathcal{E}_v(\mathcal{C}(t))$ it is clearly also in $\mathcal{C}(E_v(t))$. What is left is to show is that an edge (a, b) is in $\mathcal{E}_v(\mathcal{C}(t))$ if and only if it is in $\mathcal{C}(E_v(t))$.

If (a, b) is in $\mathcal{C}(E_v(t))$ then neither a nor b is v and there is a path from a to b in $E_v(t)$. Since the edit operation E_v preserves connectedness and the hierarchy, there must be a path from a to b in t as well. This implies that (a, b) is in $\mathcal{C}(t)$. Since neither a nor b is v, the operation $\mathcal{E}_v$ will not delete (a, b). Thus (a, b) is in $\mathcal{E}_v(\mathcal{C}(t))$.

If (a, b) is in $\mathcal{E}_v(\mathcal{C}(t))$, then it is also in $\mathcal{C}(t)$, because $\mathcal{E}_v(\mathcal{C}(t))$ is obtained from $\mathcal{C}(t)$ by simply removing a node and some edges. This implies that there is a path from a to b in t and, as long as neither a nor b are v, there is a path from a to b in $E_v(t)$ as well. Thus (a, b) is in $\mathcal{C}(E_v(t))$. Since (a, b) is in $\mathcal{E}_v(\mathcal{C}(t))$, both a and b must be nodes in $\mathcal{E}_v(\mathcal{C}(t))$ and, thus, neither can be v.

Furthermore, the transitive closure operation clearly commutes with node relabeling as well, since one acts only on weights and the other acts only on node connectivity.

We call a subtree s of Ct *consistent* if for each node v of s there cannot be two children a and b so that (a, b) is in Ct. In other words, given two nodes a and b, siblings in s, s is consistent if and only if there is no path from a to b in t.

We can, now, prove the following:

Theorem 1. *A tree $\hat{t}$ can be obtained from a tree t with an edit sequence composed of only node removal and node relabeling operations if and only if $\hat{t}$ is a consistent subtree of the DAG Ct.*

Proof. Let us assume that there is an edit sequence $\{E_{v_i}\}$ that transforms t into $\hat{t}$, then, by virtue of the above lemma, the dual edit sequence $\{\mathcal{E}_{v_i}\}$ transforms Ct into $C\hat{t}$. By construction we have that $\hat{t}$ is a subtree of $C\hat{t}$ and $C\hat{t}$ is a subgraph of Ct, thus $\hat{t}$ is a subtree of Ct. Furthermore, since the node removal operations respect the hierarchy, $\hat{t}$ is a consistent subtree of Ct.

To prove the converse, assume that $\hat{t}$ is a consistent subtree of Ct. If (a, b) is an edge of $\hat{t}$, then it is an edge on Ct as well, i.e. there is a path from a to b in t and we can define a sequence of edit operations $\{E_{v_i}\}$ that removes any node between a and b in such a path. Showing that the nodes $\{v_i\}$ deleted by the edit sequence cannot be in $\hat{t}$ we show that all the edit operations defined this way are orthogonal. As a result they can be combined to form a single edit sequence that solves the problem.

Let v in $\hat{t}$ be a node in the edited path and let p be the minimum common ancestor of v and a in $\hat{t}$. Furthermore, let w be the only child of p in $\hat{t}$ that is an ancestor of v in $\hat{t}$ and let q be the only child of p in $\hat{t}$ that is an ancestor of a in $\hat{t}$. Since a is an ancestor of v in t, an ancestor of v can be a descendant of a, an ancestor of a, or a itself. This means that w has to be in the edited path. Were it not so, then w had to be a or an ancestor of a against the hypothesis that p is the minimum common ancestor of v and a. Since q is an ancestor of a in t and a is an ancestor of w in t, q is an ancestor of w in t, but q and w are siblings in $\hat{t}$ against the hypothesis that $\hat{t}$ is consistent.

Using this result, we can show that the minimum cost edited tree isomorphism between two trees t and t' is a maximum common consistent subtree of the two DAGs Ct and Ct', provided that the cost of node removal and node matching depends only on the weights.

The minimum cost edited tree isomorphism is a tree that can be obtained from both model tree t and data tree t' with node removal and relabel operations. By virtue of the theorem above, this tree is a consistent subtree of both Ct and Ct'. The tree must be obtained with minimum combined edit cost. Since node removal can be considered as matching to a node with 0 weight, the isomorphism that grants the minimum combined edit cost is the one that gives the maximum combined match, i.e. it must be the maximum common consistent subtree of the two DAGs.

3.2   Cliques and Common Consistent Subtrees

In this section we show that the directed association graph induces a divide and conquer approach to edited tree matching as well. Given two trees t and t' to be matched, we create the directed association graph of the transitive closures Ct and Ct' and we look for a consistent matching tree in the graph. That is we seek a tree in the graph that corresponds to two consistent trees in the transitive closures Ct and Ct'. The maximum such tree corresponds to the maximum common consistent subtree of Ct and Ct'.

In analogy to what we did for the exact matching case, we divide the problem into a maximum common consistent subtree rooted at (v, w), for each node

(v, w) of the association graph. We show that, given the weight of the maximum common consistent subtree rooted at each child of (v, w) in the association graph, then we can transform the rooted maximum common consistent subtree problem into a max weighted clique problem. Solving this problem for each node in the association graph and looking for the maximum weight rooted common consistent subtree, we can find the solution to the minimum cost edited tree isomorphism problem.

Let us assume that we know the weight of the isomorphism for every child of (v, w) in the association graph. We want to find the consistent set of siblings with greatest total weight. Let us construct an undirected graph whose nodes consist of the children of (v, w) in the association graph. We connect two nodes (p, q) and (r, s) if and only if there is no path connecting p and r in t and there is no path connecting q and s in t'. This means that we connect two matches (p, q) and (r, s) if and only if they match nodes that are consistent siblings in each tree. Furthermore, we assign to each association node (a, b) a weight equal to the weight of the maximum common consistent subtree rooted at (a, b). The maximum weight clique of this graph will be the set of consistent siblings with maximum total weight. The weight of the maximum common consistent subtree rooted at (v, w) will be this weight plus the minimum of the weights of v and w, i.e. the maximum weight that can be obtained by the match. Furthermore, the nodes of the clique will be the children of (v, w) in the maximum common consistent subtree.

3.3   Heuristics for the Maximum Weighted Clique

As we have seen, we have transformed an inexact tree matching problem into a series of maximum weighted clique problems. That is, we transformed one NP-complete problem into multiple NP-complete problems. The reason behind this approach lies in the fact that the max clique problem is, on average, a relatively easy problem. Furthermore, since the seminal paper of Barrow and Burstall [1], it is a standard technique for structural matching and a large number of approaches and very powerful heuristics exist to solve it or approximate it.

The approach we will adopt to solve each single instance of the max weight clique problem is an evolutionary one introduced by Bomze, Pelillo and Stix [3]. This approach is based on a continuous formulation of the combinatorial problem and transforms it into a symmetric quadratic programming problem in the simplex Δ. For more detail we refer to the appendix.

Relaxation labeling is a evidence combining process developed in the framework of constraint satisfaction problems. Its goal is to find a classification p that satisfies pairwise constraints and interactions between its elements. The process is determined by the update rule

$$p_i^{t+1}(\lambda) = \frac{p_i^t(\lambda)q_i^t(\lambda)}{\sum_\mu p_i^t(\mu)q_i^t(\mu)}, \tag{2}$$

where the compatibility component is $q_i(\lambda) = \sum_{j=1}^n \sum_{\mu=1}^m r_{ij}(\lambda, \mu)p_j(\mu)$.

In [12] Pelillo showed that the function $A(\mathbf{p}) = \sum_{i\lambda} p_i(\lambda) q_i(\lambda)$ is a Lyapunov function for the process, i.e. $A(\mathbf{p}^{t+1}) \geq A(\mathbf{p}^t)$, with equality if and only if $\mathbf{p}^t$ is stationary.

3.4   Putting It All Together

In the previous sections we proved that the maximum edited tree isomorphism problem can be reduced to nm maximum weight clique problem and we have given an iterative process that is guaranteed to find maximal weight cliques. In this section we will show how to use these ideas to develop a practical algorithm.

A direct way is to use the relaxation labeling dynamics starting from the leaves of the directed association graph and propagate the result upwards in the graph using the weight of the extracted clique to initialize the compatibility matrix of every parent association. For a subproblem rooted at (u, v) the compatibility coefficients can be calculated knowing the weight M of every isomorphism rooted at the descendants of u and v. Specifically, the compatibility coefficients are initialized as $R_{(u,v)} = \gamma \mathbf{e}\mathbf{e}^T - C$, or, equivalently, $r_{(u,v)}(a, a'b, b') = \gamma - c^{(u,v)}_{(a,a')(b,b')}$, where

$$
c^{(u,v)}_{(a,a')(b,b')} = \begin{cases} \dfrac{1}{2M_{(a,a')}} & \text{if } (a, a') = (b, b') \\ c^{(u,v)}_{(a,a')(a,a')} + c^{(u,v)}_{(b,b')(b,b')} & \text{if } (a, a') \text{ and } (b, b') \text{ are consistent} \\ 0 & \text{otherwise.} \end{cases}
$$

This approach imposes a sequentiality to an otherwise highly parallel algorithm. An alternative can be obtained transforming the problem into a single multi-object labeling process. With this approach we set up a labeling problem with one object per node in the association graph, and at each iteration we update the label distribution for each object. We, then, update the compatibility matrices according to the new weight estimate.

This multi-object approach uses the fact that the compatibility matrix for one rooted matching subproblem does not depend upon which nodes are matched below the root, but only on the number of matches. That is, to solve one subproblem we need to know only the weight of the cliques rooted at the children, not the nodes that form the clique.

Gibbons' result [7] guarantees that the weight of the clique is equal to $\frac{1}{\mathbf{x}^T B \mathbf{x}}$, where $\mathbf{x}$ is the characteristic vector of the clique and B is the weight matrix defined in (3). This allows us to generate an estimate of the clique at each iteration: given the current distribution of label probability $\mathbf{p}$ for the subproblem rooted at (u, v), we estimate the number of nodes matched under (u, v) as $\frac{1}{\mathbf{p}^T B \mathbf{p}}$, and thus we assign to (u, v) the weight $M_{(u,v)} = \frac{1}{\mathbf{p}^T B \mathbf{p}} + \min(w_u, w_v)$, that is the weight of the maximum set of consistent descendants plus the the weight that can be obtained matching node u with node v.

We obtain a two step update rule: at each iteration we update the label probability distribution according to equation (2), and then we use the updated distributions to generate new compatibility coefficients according to the rule $r_{u,v}(a, a', b, b') = \gamma - c^{(u,v)}_{(a,a')(b,b')}$, where

$$c_{(a,a')(b,b')}^{(u,v)} = \begin{cases} \frac{1}{2}\mathbf{P}_{a,a'} B^{(a,a')} \mathbf{P}_{a,a'} & \text{if } (a,a') = (b,b') \\ c_{(a,a')(a,a')}^{(u,v)} + c_{(b,b')(b,b')}^{(u,v)} & \text{if } (a,a') \text{ and } (b,b') \text{ are consistent} \\ 0 & \text{otherwise} \end{cases}$$

Another possible variation to the algorithm can be obtained using different initial assignments for the label distribution of each subproblem.

A common approach is to initialize the assignment with a uniform distribution so that we have an initial assignment close to the baricenter of the simplex. A problem with this approach is that the dimension of the basin of attraction of one maximal clique grows with the number of nodes in the clique.

With our problem decomposition the wider cliques are the ones that map nodes at lower levels. As a result the solution will be biased towards matches that are very low on the graph, even if these matches require cutting a lot of nodes and are, thus, less likely to give an optimum solution.

A way around this problem is to choose an initialization that assigns a higher initial likelihood to matches that are higher up on the subtree. In our experiments we decided to initialize the probability of the association (a, b) for the subproblem rooted at (u, v) as $p_{(u,v)}(a, b) = e^{-(d_a+d_b+\epsilon)}$, where d_a is the depth of a with respect to u, d_b is the depth of b with respect to v, and ϵ is a small perturbation. Of course, we then renormalize $\mathbf{P}_{(u,v)}$ to ensure that it is still in the simplex.

4   Experimental Results

We evaluate the new tree-matching method on the problem of shock-tree matching. The idea of characterizing boundary shape using the differential singularities of the reaction equation was first introduced into the computer vision literature by Kimia, Tannenbaum and Zucker [8]. The idea is to evolve the boundary of an object to a canonical skeletal form using the reaction-diffusion equation. The skeleton represents the singularities in the curve evolution, where inward moving boundaries collide. The reaction component of the boundary motion corresponds to morphological erosion of the boundary, while the diffusion component introduces curvature dependent boundary smoothing. In practice, the skeleton can be computed in a number of ways, here we use a variant of the method Siddiqi, Tannenbaum and Zucker, which solves the eikonal equation which underpins the reaction-diffusion analysis using the Hamilton-Jacobi formalism of classical mechanics [14]. Once the skeleton is to hand, the next step is to devise ways of using it to characterize the shape of the original boundary. Here we follow Zucker, Siddiqi, and others, by labeling points on the skeleton using so-called shock-labels [15]. According to this taxonomy of local differential structure, there are different classes associated with behavior of the radius of the osculating circle from the skeleton to the nearest pair of boundary points. The so-called shocks distinguish between the cases where the local osculating circle has maximum radius, minimum radius, constant radius or a radius which is strictly increasing or decreasing. We abstract the skeletons as trees in which the level in the tree is determined by their time of formation [13,15]. The later the time of formation, and hence their proximity to the center of the shape, the higher the shock in the hierarchy. While this temporal notion of relevance can work well with isolated shocks (maxima and minima of the radius function), it fails on monotonically increasing or decreasing shock groups. To give an example, a protrusion that ends on a vertex will always have the earliest time of creation, regardless of its relative relevance to the shape.

We generate two variants of this matching problem. In the first variant we use aq purely symbolic approach: Here the shock trees have uniform weight and we match only the structure. The second variant is weighted: we assign to each shock group a weight proportional to the length of the border that generates the shock; this value proves to be a good measure of skeletal similarity [17].

For our experiments we used a database consisting of 16 shapes. For each shape in the database, we computed the maximum edited isomorphism with the other shapes. In the unweighted version the "goodness" measure of the match is the average fraction of nodes matched,that is, $W(t_1, t_2) = \frac{1}{2} \left(\frac{\#\hat{t}}{\#t_1} + \frac{\#\hat{t}}{\#t_2} \right)$, where $\#t$ indicates the number of nodes in the tree t. Conversely, to calculate the goodness of the weighted match we weights so that the sum over all the nodes of a tree is 1. The way we use the total weight of the maximum common edited isomorphism as a measure for the match. In figure 2 we show the shapes and the goodness measure of their match. The top value of each cell is the result for the unweighted case, the bottom value is represents the weighted match.

To illustrate the usefullness of the set of similarity measures, we have used them as input to a pairwise clustering algorithm [9]. The aim here is see whether the clusters extracted from the weighted or the unweighted tree edit distance correspond more closely to the different perceptual shape categories in the data-base. In the unweighted case the process yielded six clusters (brush (1) + brush (2) + wrench (4); spanner (3) + horse (13) ; pliers (5) + pliers (6) + hammer (9) ;pliers (7) +hammer (8) + horse (12); fish (10) + fish (12); hand (14) + hand (15) + hand (16). Clearly there is merging and leakage between the different shape categories. Clustering on the weighted tree edit distances gives better results yielding seven clusters: brush (1) + brush (2) ; spanner (3) + spanner (4); pliers (5) + pliers (6) + pliers (7); hammer (8) + hammer (9); fish (10) + fish (11); horse (12) + horse (13); hand (14) + hand (15) + hand (16)). These correspond exactly to the shape categories in the data-base.

5   Sensitivity Study

To augment these real world experiments, we have performed a sensitivity analysis. The aim here is to characterise the effects measurement errors resulting from noise or jitter on the weights and the structural errors resulting from node removal.

Node removal tests the capability of the method to cope with structural modification. To do this we remove an increasing fraction of nodes from a randomly generated tree. We then we match the modified tree against its unedited version. Since we remove nodes only from one tree, the edited tree will have an exact match against the unedited version. Hence, we know the optimum value of the

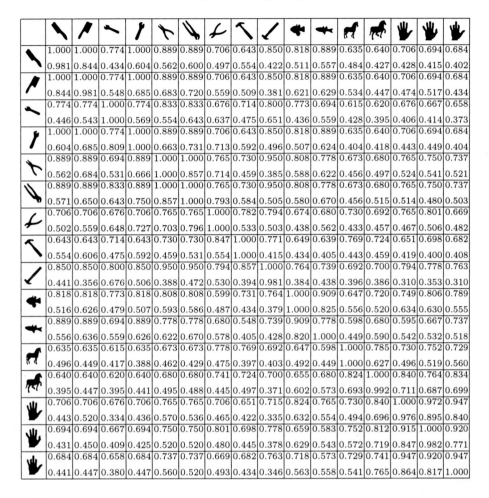

Fig. 2. Matching result for unweighted (top) and weighted (bottom) shock trees

weight that should be attained by the maximum edited isomorphism. This is equalt to the total weight of the edited tree.

By adding measurement errors or jitter to the weights, we test how the method copes with a modification in the weight distribution. The measurement errors are normally distributed with zero mean and controlled variance. Here we match the tree of noisy or jittered weights against its noise-free version. In this case we have no easy way to determine the optimal weight of the isomorphism, but we do expect a smooth drop in total weight with increasing noise variance.

We performed the experiments on trees with 10, 15, 20, 25, and 30 nodes. For each experimental run we used 11 randomly generated trees. The procedure for generating the random trees was as follows: we commence with an empty tree (i.e. one with no nodes) and we iteratively add the required number of nodes. At each iteration nodes are added as children of one of the existing nodes. The

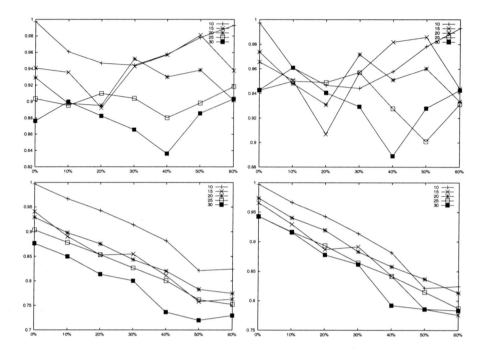

Fig. 3. Sensitivity analysis: top-left node removal, top-right node removal without outliers, bottom-left weight jitter, bottom-right weight jitter without outliers.

parents are randomly selected with uniform probability from among the existing nodes. The weight of the newly added nodes are selected at random from an exponential distribution with mean 1. This procedure will tend to generate trees in which the branch ratio is highest closest to the root. This is quite realistic of real-world situations, since shock trees tend to have the same characteristic.

The fraction of nodes removed was varied from 0% to 60%. In figure 3 top left we show the ratio of the computed weighted edit distance to the optimal value of the maximum isomorphism. Interestingly, for certain trees the relaxation algorithm failed to converge within the allotted number of iterations. Furthermore, the algorithm also failed to converge on the noise corrupted variants of these trees. In other cases, the algorithm exhibited particularly rapid convergence. Again, the variants of these trees also showed rapid algorithm convergence. When the method fails to converge in an allocated number of iterations, we can still give a lower bound to the weight. However, this bound is substantially lower than the average value obtained when the algorithm does converge. The top right-hand graph of figure 3 shows the ratio of weight matched when we eliminate these convergence failures. The main conclusion that can be drawn from these two plots are as follows. First, the effect of increasing structural error is to cause a systematic underestimation of the weighted edit distance. The different curves all exhibit a minimum value of the ratio. The reason for this is that the matching problem becomes trivial as the trees are decimated to extinction,

The bottom row of figure 3 shows the results obtained when we have added measurement errors or jitter to the weights. We noise corrupted weights were obtained with randomly added Gaussian noise with standard deviation ranging from 0 to 0.6. The bottom left-hand graph shows the result of this test. It is clear that the matched weight decreases almost linearly with the noise standard deviation. In these experiments, we encountered similar problems with algorithm non-convergence. Furthermore, the problematic instances were identical. This further supports the observation that the problem strongly depends on the instance. The bottom right-hand plot shows the results of the jitter test with the convergence failures removed.

6   Conclusions

In this paper we have investigated a optimization approach to tree matching. We based the work on to tree edit distance framework. We show that any tree obtained with a sequence of cut operation is a subtree of the transitive closure of the original tree. Furthermore we show that the necessary condition for any subtree to be a solution can be reduced a clique problem in a derived structure. Using this idea we transform the tree edit distance problem into a series of maximum weight cliques problems and then we use relaxation labeling to find an approximate solution.

In a set of experiments we apply this algorithm to match shock graphs, a graph representation of the morphological skeleton. The results of these experiments are very encouraging, showing that the algorithm is able to match similar shapes together. Furthermore we provide some sensitivity analysis of the method.

A   Motzkin-Strauss Heuristic

In 1965, Motzkin and Strauss [10] showed that the (unweighted) maximum clique problem can be reduced to a quadratic programming problem on the n-dimensional simplex $\Delta = \{\mathbf{x} \in \mathbb{R}^n | x_i \geq 0$ for all $i = 1 \ldots n, \sum_i x_i = 1\}$, here x_i are the components of vector $\mathbf{x}$. More precisely, let $G = (V, E)$ be a graph where V is the node set and E is the edge set, and let $C \subseteq V$ be a maximum clique of G, then the vector $\mathbf{x}^* = \{x_i^* = 1/\#C$ if $i \in C$, 0 otherwise$\}$, maximizes in Δ the function $g(\mathbf{x}) = \mathbf{x}^T A \mathbf{x}$, where A is the adjacency matrix of G. Furthermore, given a set $S \subseteq V$, we define the *characteristic* vector $\mathbf{x}^S$

$$
x_i^S = \begin{cases} 1/\#S & \text{if } i \in S \\ 0 & \text{otherwise,} \end{cases}
$$

S is a maximum (maximal) clique if and only if $g(\mathbf{x}^S)$ is a global (local) maximum for the function g.

Gibbons *et al.* [7] generalized this result to the weighted clique case. In their formulation the association graph is substituted with a matrix $B = (b_{ij})_{i,j \in V}$ is related to the weights and connectivity of the graph by the relation

$$b_{ij} = \begin{cases} 1/w_i & \text{if } i = j \\ k_{ij} \geq \frac{b_{ii}+b_{jj}}{2} & \text{if } (i,j) \notin E \\ 0 & \text{otherwise.} \end{cases} \tag{3}$$

Let us consider a weighted graph $G = (V, E, w)$, where V is the set of nodes, E the set of edges, and $w : V \to \mathbb{R}$ a weight function that assigns a weight to each node. Gibbons et $al.$ proved that, given a set $S \subseteq V$ and its $characteristic$ vector $\mathbf{x}^S$ defined as

$$x_i^S = \begin{cases} \frac{w(i)}{\sum_{j \in S} w(j)} & \text{if } i \in S, \\ 0 & \text{otherwise,} \end{cases}$$

S is a maximum (maximal) weight clique if and only if $\mathbf{x}^S$ is a global (local) minimizer for equation $\mathbf{x}^T B \mathbf{x}$. Furthermore, the weight of the clique S is $w(S) = \frac{1}{\mathbf{x}^{S^T} B \mathbf{x}^S}$.

Unfortunately, under this formulation, the minima are not necessarily isolated: when we have more than one clique with the same maximal weight, any convex linear combinations of their characteristic vectors will give the same maximal value. What this implies is that, if we find a minimizer $\mathbf{x}^*$ we can derive the weight of the clique, but we might not be able to tell the nodes that constitute it.

Bomze, Pelillo and Stix [3] introduce a regularization factor to the quadratic programming method that generates an equivalent problem with isolated solutions. The new quadratic program minimizes $\mathbf{x}^T C \mathbf{x}$ in the simplex, where the matrix $C = (c_{ij})_{i,j \in V}$ is defined as

$$c_{ij} = \begin{cases} \frac{1}{2w_i} & \text{if } i = j \\ k_{ij} \geq c_{ii} + c_{jj} & \text{if } (i,j) \notin E, i \neq j \\ 0 & \text{otherwise.} \end{cases} \tag{4}$$

Once again, S is a maximum (maximal) weighted clique if and only if $\mathbf{x}^S$ is a global (local) minimizer for the quadratic program.

To solve the quadratic problem we transform it into the equivalent problem of maximizing $\mathbf{x}^T (\gamma \mathbf{e} \mathbf{e}^T - C) \mathbf{x}$, where $\mathbf{e} = (1, \cdots, 1)^T$ is the vector with every component equal to 1 and γ is a positive scaling constant.

References

1. H. G. Barrow and R. M. Burstall, Subgraph isomorphism, matching relational structures and maximal cliques, $Inf.$ $Proc.$ $Letter$, Vol. 4, pp.83, 84, 1976.
2. M. Bartoli et al., Attributed tree homomorphism using association graphs, In $ICPR$, 2000.
3. I. M. Bomze, M. Pelillo, and V. Stix, Approximating the maximum weight clique using replicator dynamics, $IEEE$ $Trans.$ on $Neural$ $Networks$, Vol. 11, 2000.
4. H. Bunke and A. Kandel, Mean and maximum common subgraph of two graphs, $Pattern$ $Recognition$ $Letters$, Vol. 21, pp. 163-168, 2000.

5. W. J. Christmas and J. Kittler, Structural matching in computer vision using probabilistic relaxation, *PAMI*, Vol. 17, pp. 749-764, 1995.
6. M. A. Eshera and K-S Fu, An image understanding system using attributed symbolic representation and inexact graph-matching, *PAMI*, Vol 8, pp. 604-618, 1986.
7. L. E. Gibbons et al., Continuous characterizations of the maximum clique problem, *Math. Oper. Res.*, Vol. 22, pp. 754-768, 1997
8. B. B. Kimia, A. R. Tannenbaum, and S. W. Zucker, Shapes, shocks, and deforamtions I, *International Journal of Computer Vision*, Vol. 15, pp. 189-224, 1995.
9. B. Luo, et al., Clustering shock trees, submitted 2001.
10. T. S. Motzkin and E. G. Straus, Maxima for graphs and a new proof of a theorem of Turán, *Canadian Journal of Mathematics*, Vol. 17, pp. 533-540, 1965.
11. M. Pelillo, Replicator equations, maximal cliques, and graph isomorphism, *Neural Computation*, Vol. 11, pp.1935-1955, 1999.
12. M. Pelillo, The dynamics of relaxation labeling process, *J. Math. Imaging Vision*, Vol. 7, pp. 309-323, 1997.
13. A. Shokoufandeh, S. J. Dickinson, K. Siddiqi, and S. W. Zucker, Indexing using a spectral encoding of topological structure, In *CVPR*, 1999.
14. K. Siddiqi, S. Bouix, A. Tannenbaum, and S. W. Zucker, The hamilton-jacobi skeleton, In *ICCV*, pp. 828-834, 1999.
15. K. Siddiqi et al., Shock graphs and shape matching, *Int. J. of Comp. Vision*, Vol. 35, pp. 13-32, 1999.
16. K-C Tai, The tree-to-tree correction problem, *J. of the ACM*, Vol. 26, pp. 422-433, 1979.
17. A. Torsello and E.R. Hancock, A skeletal measure of 2D shape similarity, *Int. Workshop on Visual Form*, 2001.
18. W. H. Tsai and K. S. Fu, Error-correcting isomorphism of attributed relational graphs for pattern analysis, *Sys., Man, and Cyber.*, Vol. 9, pp. 757-768, 1979.
19. J. T. L. Wang, K. Zhang, and G. Chirn, The approximate graph matching problem, In *ICPR*, pp. 284-288, 1994.
20. R. C. Wilson and E. R. Hancock, Structural matching by discrete relaxation, *PAMI*, 1997.
21. K. Zhang, A constrained edit distance between unordered labeled trees, *Algorithmica*, Vol. 15, pp. 205-222, 1996.
22. K. Zhang and D. Shasha, Simple fast algorithms for the editing distance between trees and related problems, *SIAM J. of Comp.*, Vol. 18, pp. 1245-1262, 1989.
23. K. Zhang, R. Statman, and D. Shasha, On the editing distance between unorderes labeled trees, *Inf. Proc. Letters*, Vol. 42, pp. 133-139, 1992.

Estimation of Distribution Algorithms: A New Evolutionary Computation Approach for Graph Matching Problems

Endika Bengoetxea[1], Pedro Larrañaga[2],
Isabelle Bloch[3], and Aymeric Perchant[3]

[1] Department of Computer Architecture and Technology,
University of the Basque Country, San Sebastian, Spain
`endika@si.ehu.es`
[2] Department of Computer Science and Artificial Intelligence,
University of the Basque Country, San Sebastian, Spain
`pedro@si.ehu.es`
[3] Department of Signal and Image Processing
Ecole Nationale Supérieure des Télécommunications, CNRS URA 820,
Paris, France
{`Isabelle.Bloch,Aymeric.Perchant`}`@enst.fr`

Abstract. The interest of graph matching techniques in the pattern recognition field is increasing due to the versatility of representing knowledge in the form of graphs. However, the size of the graphs as well as the number of attributes they contain can be too high for optimization algorithms. This happens for instance in image recognition, where structures of an image to be recognized need to be matched with a model defined as a graph.

In order to face this complexity problem, graph matching can be regarded as a combinatorial optimization problem with constraints and it therefore it can be solved with evolutionary computation techniques such as Genetic Algorithms (GAs) and Estimation Distribution Algorithms (EDAs).

This work proposes the use of EDAs, both in the discrete and continuous domains, in order to solve the graph matching problem. As an example, a particular inexact graph matching problem applied to recognition of brain structures is shown. This paper compares the performance of these two paradigms for their use in graph matching.

1   Introduction

Many articles about representation of structural information by graphs in domains such as image interpretation and pattern recognition can be found in the literature [1]. In those, graph matching is used for structural recognition of images: the model (which can be an atlas or a map depending on the application) is represented in the form of a graph, where each node contains information for a particular structure and arcs contain information about relationships between

M.A.T. Figueiredo, J. Zerubia, A.K. Jain (Eds.): EMMCVPR 2001, LNCS 2134, pp. 454–468, 2001.

structures; a data graph is generated from the images to be analyzed and contains similar information. Graph matching techniques are then used to determine which structure in the model corresponds to each of the structures in a given image.

Most existing problems and methods in the graph matching domain assume graph isomorphism, where both graphs being matched have the same number of nodes and links. In some cases this bijective condition between the two graphs is too strong and it is necessary to weaken it and to express the correspondence as an inexact graph matching problem.

When the generation of the data graph from an original image is done without the aid of an expert, it is difficult to segment accurately the image into meaningful entities, that is why over-segmentation techniques need to be applied [1–3]. As a result, the number of nodes in the data graph increases and isomorphism condition between the model and data graphs cannot be assumed. Such problems call for inexact graph matching, and similar examples can be found in other fields.

Several techniques have been applied to inexact graph matching, including combinatorial optimization [4–6], relaxation [7–11], EM algorithm [12, 13], and evolutionary computation techniques such as Genetic Algorithms (GAs) [14, 15].

This work proposes the use of Estimation Distribution Algorithm (EDA) techniques in both the discrete and continuous domains, showing the potential of this new evolutionary computation approach among traditional ones such as GAs.

The outline of this work is as follows: Section 2 is a review of the EDA approach. Section 3 illustrates the inexact graph matching problem and shows how to face it with EDAs. Section 4 describes the experiment carried out and the results obtained. Finally, Section 5 gives the conclusions and suggests further work.

2   Estimation Distribution Algorithms

2.1   Introduction

EDAs [16–18] are non-deterministic, stochastic heuristic search strategies that form part of the evolutionary computation approaches, where number of solutions or individuals are created every generation, evolving once and again until a satisfactory solution is achieved. In brief, the characteristic that most differentiates EDAs from other evolutionary search strategies such as GAs is that the evolution from a generation to the next one is done by estimating the probability distribution of the fittest individuals, and afterwards by sampling the induced model. This avoids the use of crossing or mutation operators, and the number of parameters that EDAs require is reduced considerably.

In EDAs, the individuals are not said to contain genes, but variables which dependencies have to be analyzed. Also, while in other heuristics from evolutionary computation the interrelations between the different variables representing the individuals are kept in mind implicitly (e.g. building block hypothesis), in

---

EDA

    $D_0 \leftarrow$ Generate N individuals (the initial population) randomly

    Repeat for $l = 1, 2, \ldots$ until a stopping criterion is met

        $D_{l-1}^{Se} \leftarrow$ Select $Se \leq N$ individuals from D_{l-1} according to
           a selection method

        $\rho_l(\boldsymbol{x}) = \rho(\boldsymbol{x}|D_{l-1}^{Se}) \leftarrow$ Estimate the probability distribution
           of an individual being among the selected individuals

        $D_l \leftarrow$ Sample N individuals (the new population) from $\rho_l(\boldsymbol{x})$

Fig. 1. Pseudocode for EDA approach.

EDAs the interrelations are expressed explicitly through the joint probability distribution associated with the individuals selected at each iteration. The task of estimating the joint probability distribution associated with the database of the selected individuals from the previous generation constitutes the hardest work to perform, as this requires the adaptation of methods to learn models from data developed in the domain of probabilistic graphical models.

Figure 1 shows the pseudocode of EDA, in which we distinguish four main steps in this approach:

1. At the beginning, the first population D_0 of N individuals is generated, usually by assuming an uniform distribution (either discrete or continuous) on each variable, and evaluating each of the individuals.
2. Secondly, a number Se ($Se \leq N$) of individuals are selected, usually the fittest ones.
3. Thirdly, the n–dimensional probabilistic model that better expresses the interdependencies between the n variables is induced.
4. Next, the new population of N new individuals is obtained by simulating the probability distribution learned in the previous step.

Steps 2, 3 and 4 are repeated until a stopping condition is verified. The most important step of this new paradigm is to find the interdependencies between the variables (step 3). This task will be done using techniques from the field of probabilistic graphical models.

Next, some notation is introduced. Let $\boldsymbol{X} = (X_1, \ldots, X_n)$ be a set of random variables, and let x_i be a value of X_i, the ith component of $\boldsymbol{X}$. Let $\boldsymbol{y} = (x_i)_{X_i \in \boldsymbol{Y}}$ be a value of $\boldsymbol{Y} \subseteq \boldsymbol{X}$. Then, a probabilistic graphical model for $\boldsymbol{X}$ is a graphical factorization of the joint generalized probability density function, $\rho(\boldsymbol{X} = \boldsymbol{x})$ (or simply $\rho(\boldsymbol{x})$). The representation of this model is given by two components: a structure and a set of local generalized probability densities.

With regard to the structure of the model, the structure S for $\boldsymbol{X}$ is a directed acyclic graph (DAG) that describes a set of conditional independences between the variables on $\boldsymbol{X}$. $\boldsymbol{Pa}_i^S$ represents the set of parents –variables from which an arrow is coming out in $S-$ of the variable X_i in the probabilistic graphical model, the structure of which is given by S. The structure S for $\boldsymbol{X}$ assumes that X_i and its non descendants are independent given $\boldsymbol{Pa}_i^S$, $i = 2, \ldots, n$. Therefore, the factorization can be written as follows:

$$\rho(\boldsymbol{x}) = \rho(x_1, \ldots, x_n) = \prod_{i=1}^{n} \rho(x_i \mid \boldsymbol{pa}_i^S). \tag{1}$$

Furthermore, regarding the local generalized probability densities associated with the probabilistic graphical model, these are; precisely the ones appearing in Equation 1.

A representation of the models of the characteristics described above assumes that the local generalized probability densities depend on a finite set of parameters $\boldsymbol{\theta}_S \in \boldsymbol{\Theta}_S$, and as a result the previous equation can be rewritten as follows:

$$\rho(\boldsymbol{x} \mid \boldsymbol{\theta}_S) = \prod_{i=1}^{n} \rho(x_i \mid \boldsymbol{pa}_i^S, \boldsymbol{\theta}_i) \tag{2}$$

where $\boldsymbol{\theta}_S = (\boldsymbol{\theta}_1, \ldots, \boldsymbol{\theta}_n)$.

After having defined both components of the probabilistic graphical model, the model itself will be represented by $M = (S, \boldsymbol{\theta}_S)$.

2.2   EDAs in Discrete Domains

In the particular case where every variable $X_i \in \boldsymbol{X}$ is discrete, the probabilistic graphical model is called *Bayesian network* [19]. If the variable X_i has r_i possible values, $x_i^1, \ldots, x_i^{r_i}$, the local distribution, $p(x_i \mid \boldsymbol{pa}_i^{j,S}, \boldsymbol{\theta}_i)$ is:

$$p(x_i^k \mid \boldsymbol{pa}_i^{j,S}, \boldsymbol{\theta}_i) = \theta_{x_i^k \mid \boldsymbol{pa}_i^j} \equiv \theta_{ijk} \tag{3}$$

where $\boldsymbol{pa}_i^{1,S}, \ldots, \boldsymbol{pa}_i^{q_i,S}$ denotes the values of $\boldsymbol{Pa}_i^S$, that is the set of parents of the variable X_i in the structure S; q_i is the number of different possible instantiations of the parent variables of X_i. Thus, $q_i = \prod_{X_g \in \boldsymbol{Pa}_i} r_g$. The local parameters are given by $\boldsymbol{\theta}_i = ((\theta_{ijk})_{k=1}^{r_i})_{j=1}^{q_i})$. In other words, the parameter θ_{ijk} represents the conditional probability that variable X_i takes its kth value, knowing that the set of its parent variables take its jth value. We assume that every θ_{ijk} is greater than zero.

All the EDAs are classified depending on the maximum number of dependencies between variables that they accept (maximum number of parents that a variable X_i can have in the probabilistic graphical model).

Without Interdependencies. The Univariate Marginal Distribution Algorithm (UMDA) [20] is a representative example of this category, which can be written as:

$$p_l(\boldsymbol{x}; \boldsymbol{\theta}^l) = \prod_{i=1}^{n} p_l(x_i; \boldsymbol{\theta}_i^j) \tag{4}$$

where $\boldsymbol{\theta}^l = \left\{ \theta_{ijk}^l \right\}$ is recalculated every generation by its maximum likelihood estimation, i.e. $\widehat{\theta}_{ijk}^l = \frac{N_{ijk}^{l-1}}{N_{ij}^{l-1}}$. N_{ijk}^l is the number of cases on which the variable X_i takes the value x_i^k when its parents are on their j^{th} combination of values for the lth generation, and $N_{ij}^{l-1} = \sum_k N_{ijk}^{l-1}$.

Pairwise Dependencies. An example of this second category is the greedy algorithm called MIMIC (Mutual Information Maximization for Input Clustering) [21]. The main idea in MIMIC is to describe the true mass joint probability as closely as possible by using only one univariate marginal probability and $n-1$ pairwise conditional probability functions.

Multiple Interdependencies. We will use EBNA (Estimation of Bayesian Network Algorithm) [22] as an example of this category. The EBNA approach was introduced for the first time in [23], where the authors use the Bayesian Information Criterion (BIC) [24] as the score to evaluate the goodness of each structure found during the search. Following this criterion, the corresponding BIC score $-BIC(S, D)-$ for a Bayesian network structure S constructed from a database D and containing N cases can be proved to be as follows:

$$BIC(S, D) = \sum_{i=1}^n \sum_{j=1}^{q_i} \sum_{k=1}^{r_i} N_{ijk} \log \frac{N_{ijk}}{N_{ij}} - \frac{\log N}{2} \sum_{i=1}^n (r_i - 1) q_i \qquad (5)$$

where N_{ijk} denotes the number of cases in D in which the variable X_i has the value x_i^k and $\boldsymbol{Pa}_i$ is instantiated as its jth value, and $N_{ij} = \sum_{k=1}^{r_i} N_{ijk}$.

Unfortunately, to obtain the best model all possible structures must be searched through, which has been proved to be NP-hard [25]. Even if promising results have been obtained through global search techniques [26–28], their computation cost makes them impractical for our problem. As the aim is to find a model as good as possible –even if not the optimal– in a reasonable period of time, a simpler algorithm is preferred. An example of the latter is the so called Algorithm B [29], which is a greedy search heuristic that begins with an arc-less structure and adds iteratively the arcs that produce maximum improvement according to the BIC approximation –but other measures can also be applied. The algorithm stops when adding another arc would not increase the score of the structure.

Local search strategies are another way of obtaining good models. These begin with a given structure, and every step the addition or deletion of an arc that improves most the scoring measure is performed. Local search strategies stop when no modification of the structure improves the scoring measure. The main drawback of local search strategies is their strong dependence on the initial structure. Nevertheless, since it has been shown in [30] that local search strategies perform quite well when the initial structure is reasonably good, the model of the previous generation could be used as the initial structure.

The initial model M_0 in EBNA, is formed by its structure S_0 which is an arc-less DAG and the local probability distributions given by the n unidimensional marginal probabilities $p(X_i = x_i) = \frac{1}{r_i}$, $i = 1, \ldots, n$ –that is, M_0 assigns the same probability to all individuals. The model of the first generation $-M_1-$ is learned using Algorithm B, while the rest of the models are learned following a local search strategy that received the model of the previous generation as the initial structure.

Simulation in Bayesian Networks. In EDAs, the simulation of Bayesian networks is used merely as a tool to generate new individuals for the next population based on the structure learned previously. The method used in this work is the *Probabilistic Logic Sampling* (PLS) proposed in [31]. Following this method, the instantiations are done one variable at a time in a forward way, that is, a variable is not sampled until all its parents have already been so.

2.3   EDAs in Continuous Domains

In this section we introduce an example of the probabilistic graphical model paradigm that assumes the joint density function to be a multivariate Gaussian density.

The local density function for the ith variable is computed as the linear-regression model

$$f(x_i \mid \boldsymbol{pa}_i^S, \boldsymbol{\theta}_i) \equiv \mathcal{N}(x_i; m_i + \sum_{x_j \in \boldsymbol{pa}_i} b_{ji}(x_j - m_j), v_i) \qquad (6)$$

where $\mathcal{N}(x; \mu, \sigma^2)$ is a univariate normal distribution with mean μ and variance σ^2.

Local parameters are given by $\boldsymbol{\theta}_i = (m_i, \boldsymbol{b}_i, v_i)$, where $\boldsymbol{b}_i = (b_{1i}, \ldots, b_{i-1i})^t$ is a column vector. Local parameters are as follows: m_i is the unconditional mean of X_i, v_i is the conditional variance of X_i given $\boldsymbol{Pa}_i$, and b_{ji} is a linear coefficient that measures the strength of the relationship between X_j and X_i. A probabilistic graphical model built from these local density functions is known as a *Gaussian network* [32]. Gaussian networks are of interest in continuous EDAs because the number of parameters needed to specify a multivariate Gaussian density is smaller.

Next, an analogous classification of continuous EDAs as for the discrete domain is done, in which these continuous EDAs are also classified depending on the number of dependencies they take into account.

Without Dependencies. In this case, the joint density function is assumed to follow a n–dimensional normal distribution, and thus it is factorized as a product of n unidimensional and independent normal densities. Using the mathematical notation $\boldsymbol{X} \equiv \mathcal{N}(\boldsymbol{x}; \boldsymbol{\mu}, \sum)$, this assumption can be expressed as:

$$f_{\mathcal{N}}(\boldsymbol{x}; \boldsymbol{\mu}, \textstyle\sum) = \prod_{i=1}^{n} f_{\mathcal{N}}(x_i; \mu_i, \sigma_i) = \prod_{i=1}^{n} \frac{1}{\sqrt{2\pi}\sigma_i} e^{-\frac{1}{2}(\frac{x_i - \mu_i}{\sigma_i})^2}. \qquad (7)$$

An example of continuous EDAs in this category is UMDA$_c$ [33].

Bivariate Dependencies. An example of this category is MIMIC$_c^G$ [33], which is basically an adaptation of the MIMIC algorithm [21] to the continuous domain.

Multiple Dependencies. Algorithms in this section are approaches of EDAs for continuous domains in which there is no restriction in the learning of the density function every generation. An example of this category is EGNA$_{BGe}$ (Estimation of Gaussian Network Algorithm) [33]. The method used to find the Gaussian network structure is a Bayesian score+search. In EGNA$_{BGe}$ a local search is used to search for good structures.

Simulation of Gaussian Networks. A general approach for sampling from multivariate normal distributions is known as the conditioning method, which generates instances of X by sampling X_1, then X_2 conditionally to X_1, and so on. The simulation of a univariate normal distribution can be done with a simple method based on the sum of 12 uniform variables.

3 Graph Matching as a Combinatorial Optimization Problem with Constraints

3.1 Traditional Representation of Individuals

The choice of an adequate individual representation is a very important step in any problem to be solved with heuristics that will determine the behavior of the search. An individual represents a point in the search space that has to be evaluated, and therefore is a solution. For a graph matching problem, each solution represents a match between the nodes of a data graph G_2 and those of model graph G_1.

A possible representation that has already been used either in GAs or discrete EDAs [34] consists of individuals with $|V_2|$ variables, where each variable can take any value between 1 and $|V_1|$. More formally, the individual as well as the solution it represents could be defined as follows: for $1 \leq k \leq |V_1|$ and $1 \leq i \leq |V_2|$, $X_i = k$ means that the ith node of G_2 is matched with the kth node of G_1.

3.2 Representing a Matching as a Permutation

Permutation-based representations have been typically applied to problems such as the Travelling Salesman Problem (TSP), but they can also be used for inexact graph matching. In this case the meaning of the individual is completely different, as an individual does not show directly which node of G_2 is matched with each node of G_1. In fact, what we obtain from each individual is the order in which nodes will be analyzed and treated so as to compute the matching solution that it is representing.

For the individuals to contain a permutation, the individuals will have the same size as the *traditional* ones described in Section 3.1 (i.e. $|V_2|$ variables long). However, the number of values that each variable can take will be $|V_2|$, and not $|V_1|$ as in that representation. In fact, it is important to note that a permutation is a list of numbers in which all the values from 1 to n have to appear in an individual of size n. In other words, our new representation of individuals needs to satisfy a strong constraint in order to be considered as correct, that is, they all have to contain every value from 1 to n, where $n = |V_2|$.

More formally, for $1 \leq k \leq |V_2|$ and $1 \leq i \leq |V_2|$, $X_i = k$ means that the kth node of G_2 will be the ith node that is analyzed for its most appropriate match.

Now it is important to define a procedure to obtain the solution that each permutation symbolizes. As this procedure will be done for each individual, it is important that this translation is performed by a fast and simple algorithm. A way of doing this is introduced next.

A solution for the inexact graph matching problem can be calculated by comparing the nodes to each other and deciding which is more similar to which using a similarity function $\varpi(i,j)$ defined to compute the similarity between nodes i and j. The similarity measures used so far in the literature have been applied to two nodes, one from each graph, and their aim was to help in the computation of the fitness of a solution, that is, the final value of a fitness function. However, the similarity measure $\varpi(i,j)$ proposed in this work is quite different, as these two nodes to be evaluated are both in the data graph $(i, j \in V_2)$ –see Section 4.3 for more details. With these new similarity values we will identify for each particular node of G_2 which other nodes in the data graph are most similar to it, and try to group it with the best set of already matched nodes.

Given an individual $\boldsymbol{x} = (x_1, \ldots, x_{|V_1|}, x_{|V_1|+1}, \ldots, x_{|V_2|})$, the procedure to do the translation is performed in two phases as follows:

1. The first $|V_1|$ values $(x_1, \ldots, x_{|V_1|})$ that directly represent nodes of V_2 will be matched to nodes $1, 2 \ldots, |V_1|$ (that is, the node $x_1 \in V_2$ is matched with the node $1 \in V_1$, the node $x_2 \in V_2$ is matched with the node $2 \in V_1$, and so on, until the node $x_{|V_1|} \in V_2$ is matched with the node $|V_1| \in V_1$).
2. For each of the following values of the individual, $(x_{|V_1|+1}, \ldots, x_{|V_2|})$, and following their order of appearance in the individual, the most similar node will be chosen from all the previous values in the individual by means of the similarity measure ϖ. For each of these nodes of G_2, we assign the matched node of G_1 that is matched to the most similar node of G_2.

The first phase is very important in the generation of the individual, as this is also the one that ensures the correctness of the solution represented by the permutation: all the values of V_1 are assigned from the beginning, and as we assumed $|V_2| > |V_1|$, we conclude that all the nodes of G_1 will have at least a occurrence in the solution represented by any permutation.

Looking for correct individuals

As explained in Section 2.2, the simulation process is PLS [31]. But a simple PLS algorithm will not take into account any restriction the individuals must have for a particular problem. The interested reader can find a more exhaustive review of this topic in [34], where the authors propose different methods to obtain only correct individuals that satisfy the particular constraints of the problem.

3.3   Obtaining a Permutation with Continuous EDAs

Continuous EDAs provide the search with other types of EDA algorithms that can be more suitable for some problems. But again, the main goal is to find a representation of individuals and a procedure to obtain an univocal solution to the matching from each of the possible permutations.

In this case we propose a strategy based on the previous section, trying to translate the individual in the continuous domain to a correct permutation in the discrete one, evaluating it as explained in Section 3.2. This procedure has to be performed for each individual in order to be evaluated. Again, this process has to be fast enough in order to reduce computation time.

With all these aspects in mind, individuals of the same size ($n = |V_2|$) will be defined, where each of the variables of the individual can take any value following a Gaussian distribution. This new representation of individuals is a continuous value in $\mathbb{R}^n$ that does not provide directly the solution it symbolizes: the values for each of the variables only show the way to translate from the continuous world to a permutation, and it does not contain similarity values between nodes of both graphs. This new type of representation can also be regarded as a way to focus the search from the continuous world, where the techniques that can be applied to the estimation of densities are completely different.

In order to obtain a translation to a discrete permutation individual, we propose to order the continuous values of the individual, and to set its corresponding discrete values by assigning to each $x_i \in \{1, \ldots, |V_2|\}$ the respective order in the continuous individual. The procedure described in this section is further described in [35].

4   Experimental Results. The Human Brain Example

4.1   Overview of the Human Brain Example

The example chosen to test the performance of the different EDAs for permutation-based representations in inexact graph matching is a problem of recognition of regions in 3D Magnetic Resonance Images (MRI) of the brain. The data graph $G_2 = (V_2, E_2)$ is generated after over-segmenting an image and contains a node for each segmented region (subset of a brain structure). The model graph $G_1 = (V_1, E_1)$ contains a node for each of the brain regions to be recognized. The experiments carried out in this chapter are focused on this type of graphs, but could similarly be adapted to any other inexact graph matching problem.

More specifically, the model graph was obtained from the main structures of the the inner part of the brain (the brainstem). This example is a reduced version of the brain images recognition problem in [1]. In our case the number of nodes of G_2 (number of structures of the image to be recognized) is 94, and contains 2868 arcs. The model graph contains 13 nodes and 84 arcs.

4.2   Description of the Experiment

This section compares EDA algorithms each other and to a broadly known GA, the GENITOR [36], which is a steady state type algorithm (ssGA).

Both EDAs and GENITOR were implemented in ANSI C++ language, and the experiment was executed on a two processor Ultra 80 Sun computer under Solaris version 7 with 1 GByte of RAM.

The initial population for all the algorithms was created using the same random generation procedure based on a uniform distribution. The fitness function used is described later in Section 4.4.

In the discrete case, all the algorithms were set to finish the search when a maximum of 100 generations or when uniformity in the population was reached. GENITOR, as it is a ssGA algorithm, only generates two individuals at each iteration, but it was also programmed in order to generate the same number of individuals as in discrete EDAs by allowing more iterations (201900 individuals). In the continuous case, the ending criterion was to reach 301850 evaluations (i.e. number of individuals generated).

In EDAs, the following parameters were used: a population of 2000 individuals ($N = 2000$), from which a subset of the best 1000 are selected ($S_e = 1000$) to estimate the probability, and the elitist approach was chosen (that is, always the best individual is included for the next population and 1999 individuals are simulated). In GENITOR a population of 2000 individuals was also set, with a mutation rate of $p_m = \frac{1}{|V_2|}$ and a crossover probability of $p_c = 1$. The operators used in GENITOR where CX [37] and EM [38].

4.3   Definition of the Similarity Function

Speaking about the similarity concept, we have used only a similarity measure based on the grey level distribution, so that the function ϖ returns a higher value for two nodes when the grey level distribution over two segments of the data image is more similar. In addition, no clustering process is performed, and therefore the similarity measure ϖ is kept constant during the generation of individuals. These decisions have been made knowing the nature and properties of an MRI image. More formally, the function ϖ can be defined as the set of functions that measure the correspondence between the two nodes of the data graph G_2: $\varpi = \{\rho_\sigma^{u_2} : V_2 \to [0,1], u_2 \in V_2\}$.

4.4   Definition of the Fitness Function

We have chosen a function proposed in [1] as an example. Following this function, an individual $\boldsymbol{x} = (x_1, \ldots, x_{|V_2|})$ will be evaluated as follows:

$$f(\boldsymbol{x}; \rho_\sigma, \rho_\mu, \alpha) = \alpha \left[\frac{1}{|V_2||V_1|} \sum_{i=1}^{|V_2|} \sum_{j=1}^{|V_1|} \left(1 - |c_{ij} - \rho_\sigma^{u_1^i}(u_2^j)| \right) \right] +$$

Table 1. Mean values of experimental results after 10 executions for each algorithm of the inexact graph matching problem of the Human Brain example.

	Best fitness value	Execution time	Number of evaluations
UMDA	0.718623	00:53:29	85958
UMDA$_c$	0.745036	03:01:05	301850
MIMIC	0.702707	00:57:30	83179
MIMIC$_c$	0.747970	03:01:07	301850
EBNA	0.716723	01:50:39	85958
EGNA	0.746893	04:13:39	301850
ssGA	0.693575	07:31:26	201900
	$p < 0.001$	$p < 0.001$	$p < 0.001$

$$(1-\alpha) \left[\frac{1}{|E_2||E_1|} \sum_{e_1^l=(u_1^i,v_1^{i'})\in E_1} \sum_{e_2^k=(u_2^j,v_2^{j'})\in E_2} \left(1 - |c_{ij}c_{i'j'} - \rho_\mu^{e_1^l}(e_2^k)|\right) \right] \quad (8)$$

where

$$c_{ij} = \begin{cases} 1 \text{ if } X_i = j \\ 0 \text{ otherwise,} \end{cases}$$

α is a parameter used to adapt the weight of node and arc correspondences in f. For each $u_1^i \in V_1$, $\rho_\sigma^{u_1^i}$ is a function from V_2 into $[0,1]$ that measures the correspondence between u_1^i and each node of V_2. Similarly, for each $e_1 \in E_1$, ρ_μ is the set of functions from E_2 into $[0,1]$ that measure the correspondence between the arcs of both graphs G_1 and G_2. The value of f associated for each variable returns the goodness of the matching. Typically ρ_σ and ρ_μ are related to the similarities between node and arc properties respectively.

Node properties are described as attributes on grey level and size, while edge properties correspond to spatial relationships between nodes.

4.5   Experimental Results

Results such as the best individual obtained, the computation time, and the number of evaluations to reach the final solution were recorded for each of the experiments. The computation time obtained is the CPU time of the process for each execution, and therefore it is not dependent on the load of the system. The latter is given as a measure to illustrate the different computation complexity of all the algorithms.

Each algorithm was executed 10 times. The non-parametric tests of Kruskal-Wallis and Mann-Whitney were used to test the null hypothesis of the same distribution densities for all –or some– of them. This task was done with the statistical package S.P.S.S. release 9.00. The results for the tests applied to all the algorithms are shown in Table 1. The study of particular algorithms gives the following results:

– Between algorithms of similar complexity only:

- UMDA vs. UMDA$_c$. Fitness value: $p < 0.001$; CPU time: $p < 0.001$; Evaluations: $p < 0.001$.
- MIMIC vs. MIMIC$_c$. Fitness value: $p < 0.001$; CPU time: $p < 0.001$; Evaluations: $p < 0.001$.
- EBNA vs. EGNA. Fitness value: $p < 0.001$; CPU time: $p < 0.001$; Evaluations: $p < 0.001$.

These results show that the differences between EDAs in the discrete and continuous domains are significant in all the cases analyzed, meaning that the behavior of selecting a discrete learning algorithm or its equivalent in the continuous domain is very different. It is important to note that the number of evaluations was expected to be different, as the ending criteria for the discrete and continuous domains were also different. In all the cases, continuous EDAs obtained a fitter individual, but the CPU time and number of individuals created was also bigger.

- Between discrete algorithms only:
  - Fitness value: $p < 0.001$. CPU time: $p < 0.001$. Evaluations: $p < 0.001$.

In this case significant results are also obtained in fitness value, CPU time, and number of evaluations. The discrete algorithm that obtained the best result was UMDA, closely followed by EBNA. The differences in the CPU time are also according to the complexity of the learning algorithm they apply. Finally, the results show that MIMIC required significantly less individuals to converge (to reach the uniformity in the population), whereas the other two EDA algorithms require nearly the same number of evaluations to converge. The genetic algorithm GENITOR is far behind the performance of EDAs. The computation time is also a factor to consider: the fact that GENITOR requires about 7 hours for each execution shows the complexity of the graph matching problem.

- Between continuous algorithms only:
  - Fitness value: $p = 0.342$. CPU time: $p < 0.001$. Evaluations: $p = 1.000$.

Differences between all the continuous EDAs appear to be not significant. As expected, the CPU time required for each of them is according to the complexity of the learning algorithm. On the other hand, the fact of having the same number of evaluations is due to the same ending criterion. Speaking about the differences in computation time between discrete and continuous EDA algorithms, it is important to note that the latter ones require all the 300000 individuals to be generated before they finish the search. The computation time for the continuous algorithms is also longer than the discrete equivalents as a result of several factors: firstly, due to the higher number of evaluations they perform each execution, secondly because of the longer individual-to-solution translation procedure that has to be done for each of the individuals generated, and lastly, as a result of the longer time required to learn the model in continuous spaces.

We can conclude from the results that generally speaking continuous algorithms perform better than discrete ones, either when comparing all of them in general or only with algorithms of equivalent complexity.

5   Conclusions and Further Work

This work describes the application of the EDA approach to graph matching. Different individual representations have been shown in order to allow the use of discrete and continuous representation and algorithms.

In an experiment with real data a comparison of the performance of this new approach between the discrete and continuous domains has been done, and continuous EDAs have shown a better performance looking at the fittest individual obtained, however a longer execution time and more evaluations were required. Additionally, other fitness functions should be tested with this new approach. Techniques such as [39, 40] could also help to introduce better similarity measures and therefore improve the results obtained considerably.

For the near future there are several tasks to be done. The most important is to perform more experiments with more data images (more data graphs) in order to evaluate the effectiveness of the proposed matching heuristic with more examples. In addition, a deeper study on the influence of node and arc correspondences requires also to be done. These new experiments are expected to highlight the importance of the structural aspects (the edges) as appreciated in our recent work.

Acknowledgments

This work has been partially supported by the University of the Basque Country, the Spanish Ministry for Science and Education, and the French Ministry for Education, Research and Technology with the projects 9/UPV/EHU 00140.226-12084/2000, HF1999-0107, and Picasso-00773TE respectively. The authors would also like to thank Ramon Etxeberria, Iñaki Inza and Jose A. Lozano for their useful advice and contributions to this work.

References

1. A. Perchant and I. Bloch. A New Definition for Fuzzy Attributed Graph Homomorphism with Application to Structural Shape Recognition in Brain Imaging. In *IMTC'99, 16th IEEE Instrumentation and Measurement Technology Conference*, pages 1801–1806, Venice, Italy, May 1999.
2. A. Perchant, C. Boeres, I. Bloch, M. Roux, and C. Ribeiro. Model-based Scene Recognition Using Graph Fuzzy Homomorphism Solved by Genetic Algorithm. In *GbR'99 2nd International Workshop on Graph-Based Representations in Pattern Recognition*, pages 61–70, Castle of Haindorf, Austria, 1999.
3. Aymeric Perchant. *Morphism of graphs with fuzzy attributes for the recognition of structural scenes (In French)*. PhD thesis, Ecole Nationale Supérieure des Télécommunications, Paris, France, September 2000.
4. A. D. J. Cross and E. R. Hancock. Convergence of a hill climbing genetic algorithm for graph matching. In *Lecture notes in Computer Science 1654*, pages 220–236, York, UK, 1999. E. R. Hancock, M. Pelillo (Eds.).

5. A. D. J. Cross, R. C. Wilson, and E. R. Hancock. Inexact graph matching using genetic search. *Pattern Recognition*, 30(6):953–70, 1997.

6. M. Singh and A. Chatterjeeand S. Chaudhury. Matching structural shape descriptions using genetic algorithms. *Pattern Recognition*, 30(9):1451–62, 1997.

7. A. W. Finch, R. C. Wilson, and E. R. Hancock. Matching Delaunay graphs. *Pattern Recognition*, 30(1):123–40, 1997.

8. S. Gold and A. Rangarajan. A graduated assignment algorithm for graph matching. *IEEE Transactions on Pattern Analysis and Machine Intelligence*, 18(4):377–88, 1996.

9. E. R. Hancock and J. Kittler. Edge-labeling using dictionary-based relaxation. *IEEE Transactions on Pattern Analysis and Machine Intelligence*, 12(2):165–181, 1990.

10. R. C. Wilson and E. R. Hancock. Bayesian compatibility model for graph matching. *Pattern Recognition Letters*, 17:263–276, 1996.

11. R. C. Wilson and E. R. Hancock. Structural matching by discrete relaxation. *IEEE Transactions on Pattern Analysis and Machine Intelligence*, 19(6):634–648, 1997.

12. A. D. J. Cross and E. R. Hancock. Graph matching with a dual-step EM algorithm. *IEEE Transactions on Pattern Analysis and Machine Intelligence*, 20(11):1236–53, 1998.

13. A. W. Finch, R. C. Wilson, and E. R. Hancock. Symbolic graph matching with the EM algorithm. *Pattern Recognition*, 31(11):1777–90, 1998.

14. C. Boeres, A. Perchant, I. Bloch, and M. Roux. A genetic algorithm for brain image recognition using graph non-bijective correspondence. Unpublished manuscript, 1999.

15. R. Myers and E.R. Hancock. Least committment graph matching with genetic algorithms. *Pattern Recognition*, 34:375–394, 2001.

16. P. Larrañaga and J. A. Lozano. *Estimation of Distribution Algorithms. A New Tool for Evolutionary Computation*. Kluwer Academic Publishers, 2001.

17. I. Inza, P. Larrañaga, R. Etxeberria, and B. Sierra. Feature subset selection by Bayesian networks based optimization. *Artificial Intelligence*, 123 (1–2):157–184, 2000.

18. I. Inza, M. Merino, P. Larrañaga, J. Quiroga, B. Sierra, and M. Girala. Feature subset selection by genetic algorithms and estimation of distribution algorithms. a case study in the survival of cirrhotic patients treated with TIPS. *Artificial Intelligence in Medicine*, Accepted for publication, 2001.

19. J. Pearl. *Probabilistic Reasoning in Intelligent Systems*. Morgan Kaufmann, Palo Alto, CA, 1988.

20. H. Mühlenbein. The equation for response to selection and its use for prediction. *Evolutionary Computation*, 5:303–346, 1998.

21. J. S. De Bonet, C. L. Isbell, and P. Viola. MIMIC: Finding optima by estimating probability densities. In *Advances in Neural Information Processing Systems*, volume 9. M. Mozer, M. Jordan and Th. Petsche eds., 1997.

22. P. Larrañaga, R. Etxeberria, J. A. Lozano, and J. M. Peña. Combinatorial optimization by learning and simulation of Bayesian networks. In *Proceedings of the Conference in Uncertainty in Artificial Intelligence, UAI 2000*, pages 343–352, Stanford, CA, USA, 2000.

23. R. Etxeberria and P. Larrañaga. Global optimization with Bayesian networks. In *Special Session on Distributions and Evolutionary Optimization*, pages 332–339. II Symposium on Artificial Intelligence, CIMAF99, 1999.

24. G. Schwarz. Estimating the dimension of a model. *Annals of Statistics*, 7(2):461–464, 1978.

25. D. M. Chickering, D. Geiger, and D. Heckerman. Learning Bayesian networks is NP–hard. Technical report, Technical Report MSR-TR-94-17, Microsoft Research, Redmond, WA, 1994.

26. R. Etxeberria, P. Larrañaga, and J. M. Picaza. Analysis of the behaviour of the genetic algorithms when searching Bayesian networks from data. *Pattern Recognition Letters*, 18(11–13):1269–1273, 1997.

27. P. Larrañaga, C. M. H. Kuijpers, R. H. Murga, and Y. Yurramendi. Searching for the best ordering in the structure learning of Bayesian networks. *IEEE Transactions on Systems, Man and Cybernetics*, 41(4):487–493, 1996.

28. P. Larrañaga, M. Poza, Y. Yurramendi, R. H. Murga, and C. M. H. Kuijpers. Structure learning of Bayesian networks by genetic algorithms. A performance analysis of control parameters. *IEEE Transactions on Pattern Analysis and Machine Intelligence*, 18(9):912–926, 1996.

29. W. Buntine. Theory refinement in Bayesian networks. In *Proceedings of the Seventh Conference on Uncertainty in Artificial Intelligence*, pages 52–60, 1991.

30. D. M. Chickering, D. Geiger, and D. Heckerman. Learning Bayesian networks: Search methods and experimental results. In *Preliminary Papers of the Fifth International Workshop on Artificial Intelligence and Statistics*, pages 112–128, 1995.

31. M. Henrion. Propagating uncertainty in Bayesian networks by probabilistic logic sampling. *Uncertainty in Artificial Intelligence*, 2:149–163, 1988. J.F. Lemmer and L.N. Kanal eds., North-Holland, Amsterdam.

32. R. Shachter and C. Kenley. Gaussian influence diagrams. *Management Science*, 35:527–550, 1989.

33. P. Larrañaga, R. Etxeberria, J.A. Lozano, and J.M. Peña. Optimization in continuous domains by learning and simulation of Gaussian networks. In *Proceedings of the Workshop in Optimization by Building and using Probabilistic Models. A Workshop within the 2000 Genetic and Evolutionary Computation Conference, GECCO 2000*, pages 201–204, Las Vegas, Nevada, USA, 2000.

34. E. Bengoetxea, P. Larrañaga, I. Bloch, A. Perchant, and C. Boeres. Inexact graph matching using learning and simulation of Bayesian networks. An empirical comparison between different approaches with synthetic data. In *Proceedings of CaNew workshop, ECAI 2000 Conference, ECCAI*, Berlin, aug 2000.

35. E. Bengoetxea, P. Larrañaga, I. Bloch, and A. Perchant. Solving graph matching with EDAs using a permutation-based representation. In P. Larrañaga and J. A. Lozano, editors, *Estimation of Distribution Algorithms. A new tool for Evolutionary Computation*. Kluwer Academic Publishers, 2001.

36. D. Whitley and J. Kauth. GENITOR: A different genetic algorithm. In *Proceedings of the Rocky Mountain Conference on Artificial Intelligence*, volume 2, pages 118–130, 1988.

37. J.M. Oliver, D.J. Smith, and J.R.C. Holland. A study of permutation crossover operators on the TSP. In Lawrence Erlbaum, editor, *Genetic Algorithms and their applications: Proceedings of the Second International Conference*, pages 224–230, Hillsdale, New Jersey, 1987. Grefenstette, J.J. (Ed.).

38. W. Banzhaf. The molecular traveling salesman. *Biological Cybernetics*, 64:7–14, 1990.

39. I. Bloch. On fuzzy distances and their use in image processing under imprecision. *Pattern Recognition*, 32:1873–1895, 1999.

40. I. Bloch. Fuzzy relative position between objects in image processing: a morphological approach. *IEEE Transactions on Pattern Analysis and Machine Intelligence*, 21(7):657–664, 1999.

A Complementary Pivoting Approach to Graph Matching

Alessio Massaro and Marcello Pelillo

Dipartimento di Informatica
Università Ca' Foscari di Venezia
Via Torino 155, 30172 Venezia Mestre, Italy

Abstract. Graph matching is a problem that pervades computer vision and pattern recognition research. During the past few decades, two radically distinct approaches have been pursued to tackle it. The first views the matching problem as one of explicit search in state-space. A classical method within this class consists of transforming it in the equivalent problem of finding a maximal clique in a derived "association graph." In the second approach, the matching problem is viewed as one of energy minimization. Recently, we have provided a unifying framework for graph matching which is centered around a remarkable result proved by Motzkin and Straus in the mid-sixties. This allows us to formulate the maximum clique problem in terms of a continuous quadratic optimization problem. In this paper we propose a new framework for graph matching based on the linear complementarity problem (LCP) arising from the Motzkin-Straus program. We develop a pivoting-based technique to find a solutions for our LCP which is a variant of Lemke's well-known method. Preliminary experiments are presented which demonstrate the effectiveness of the proposed approach.

1 Introduction

Graph matching is a fundamental problem in computer vision and pattern recognition, and a great deal of effort has been devoted over the past decades to devise efficient and robust algorithms for it (see [8] for an update on recent developments). Basically, two radically distinct approaches have emerged, a distinction which reflects the well-known dichotomy originated in the artificial intelligence field between "symbolic" and "numerical" methods. The first approach views the matching problem as one of explicit search in state-space (see, e.g., [15, 24, 25]). The pioneering work of Ambler et al. [1] falls into this class. Their approach is based on the idea that graph matching is equivalent to the problem of finding maximal cliques in the so-called association graph, an auxiliary graph derived from the structures being matched. This framework is attractive because it casts the matching problem in terms of a pure graph-theoretic problem, for which a solid theory and powerful algorithms have been developed [7]. Since its introduction, the association graph technique has been successfully applied to a variety of computer vision problems (e.g., [4, 12]).

M.A.T. Figueiredo, J. Zerubia, A.K. Jain (Eds.): EMMCVPR 2001, LNCS 2134, pp. 469–479, 2001.

In the second approach, the relational matching problem is viewed as one of energy minimization. In this case, an energy (or objective) function is sought whose minimizers correspond to the solutions of the original problem, and a dynamical system, usually embedded into a parallel relaxation network, is used to minimize it [11, 13, 23, 26]. Typically, these methods do not solve the problem exactly, but only in approximation terms. Energy minimization algorithms are attractive because they are amenable to parallel hardware implementation and also offer the advantage of biological plausibility.

In a recent paper [17], we have developed a new framework for graph matching which does unify the two approaches just described, thereby inheriting the attractive features of both. The approach is centered around a remarkable result proved by Motzkin and Straus in the mid-1960s, and more recently expanded by many authors [5, 10, 20, 6], which allows us to map the maximum clique problem onto the problem of extremizing a quadratic form over a linearly constrained domain (i.e., the standard simplex in Euclidean space). Local gradient-based search methods such as *replicator dynamics* [19] have proven to be remarkably effective when we restrict ourselves to simple version of the problem, such as tree matching [21] or graph isomorphism [18]. However, for more difficult problems the challenge remains to develop powerful heuristics.

It is a well-known fact that stationary points of quadratic programs can be characterized in terms of solutions of a linear complementarity problem (LCP), a class of inequality systems for which a rich theory and a large number of algorithms have been developed [9]. Hence, once that the graph matching is formulated in terms of a quadratic programming problem, the use of LCP algorithms naturally suggests itself, and this is precisely the idea proposed in the present paper. Among the many LCP methods presented in the literature, pivoting procedures are widely used and within this class Lemke's method is certainly the best known. Unfortunately, like other pivoting schemes, its finite convergence is guaranteed only for non-degenerate problems, and ours is indeed degenerate. The inherent degeneracy of the problem, however, is beneficial as it leaves freedom in choosing the driving variable, and we exploited this property to develop a variant of Lemke's algorithm which uses a new and effective "look-ahead" pivot rule. The procedure depends critically on the choice of a vertex in the graph which identifies the driving variable in the pivoting process. Since there is no obvious way to determine such a vertex in an optimal manner, we resorted to iterate this procedure over most, if not all, vertices in the graph. The resulting *pivoting-based heuristic* has been tested on various instances of random graphs and the preliminary results obtained confirm the effectiveness of the proposed approach.

2   Graph Matching and Linear Complementarity

Given two graphs $G_1 = (V_1, E_1)$ and $G_2 = (V_2, E_2)$, an *isomorphism* between them is any bijection $\phi : V_1 \to V_2$ such that $(i, j) \in E_1 \Leftrightarrow (\phi(i), \phi(j)) \in E_2$, for all $i, j \in V_1$. Two graphs are said to be isomorphic if there exists an isomorphism between them. The maximum common subgraph problem consists of finding the largest isomorphic subgraphs of G_1 and G_2. A simpler version of this problem is to find a maximal common subgraph, i.e., an isomorphism between subgraphs which is not included in any larger subgraph isomorphism.

The *association graph* derived from $G_1 = (V_1, E_1)$ and $G_2 = (V_2, E_2)$ is the undirected graph $G = (V, E)$ defined as follows:

$$V = V_1 \times V_2$$

and

$$E = \{((i, h), (j, k)) \in V \times V \; : \; i \neq j, \; h \neq k, \; \text{and } (i, j) \in E_1 \Leftrightarrow (h, k) \in E_2\} \; .$$

Given an arbitrary undirected graph $G = (V, E)$, a subset of vertices C is called a *clique* if all its vertices are mutually adjacent, i.e., for all $i, j \in C$, with $i \neq j$, we have $(i, j) \in E$. A clique is said to be *maximal* if it is not contained in any larger clique, and *maximum* if it is the largest clique in the graph. The *clique number*, denoted by $\omega(G)$, is defined as the cardinality of the maximum clique.

The following result establishes an equivalence between the graph matching problem and the maximum clique problem (see, e.g., [2]).

Theorem 1. *Let $G_1 = (V_1, E_1)$ and $G_2 = (V_2, E_2)$ be two graphs, and let G be the corresponding association graph. Then, all maximal (maximum) cliques in G are in one-to-one correspondence with maximal (maximum) common subgraph isomorphisms between G_1 and G_2.*

Now, let $G = (V, E)$ be an arbitrary graph of order n, and let S_n denote the standard simplex of $\mathbb{R}^n$:

$$S_n = \{ \, x \in \mathbb{R}^n \; : \; e^T x = 1 \text{ and } x_i \geq 0, \; i = 1 \ldots n \, \}$$

where e is the vector whose components equal 1, and a "T" denotes transposition. Given a subset of vertices C of G, we will denote by x^c its *characteristic vector* which is the point in S_n defined as

$$x_i^c = \begin{cases} 1/|C|, & \text{if } i \in C \\ 0, & \text{otherwise} \end{cases}$$

where $|C|$ denotes the cardinality of C.

Consider the following quadratic program

$$\begin{aligned} \min \; & f_G(x) = x^T A_G x \\ \text{s.t. } \; & x \in S_n \end{aligned} \tag{1}$$

where $A_G = (a_{ij})$ is the $n \times n$ symmetric matrix defined as

$$a_{ij} = \begin{cases} \frac{1}{2}, & \text{if } i = j \\ 0, & \text{if } i \neq j \text{ and } (i, j) \in E \\ 1, & \text{if } i \neq j \text{ and } (i, j) \notin E \end{cases} \tag{2}$$

The following theorem, recently proved by Bomze [5], expands on the Motzkin-Straus theorem [16], a remarkable result which establishes a connection between the maximum clique problem and certain standard quadratic programs. This has an intriguing computational significance in that it allows us to shift from the discrete to the continuous domain in an elegant manner.

Theorem 2. *Let C be a subset of vertices of a graph G, and let x^c be its characteristic vector. Then, C is a maximal (maximum) clique of G if and only if x^c is a local (global) solution of program (1). Moreover, all local (and hence global) solutions of (1) are strict.*

Unlike the original Motzkin-Straus formulation, which is plagued by the presence of "spurious" solutions [20], the previous result guarantees us that *all* solutions of (1) are strict, and are characteristic vectors of maximal/maximum cliques in the graph. In a formal sense, therefore, a one-to-one correspondence exists between maximal cliques and local minimizers of f_G in S_n on the one hand, and maximum cliques and global minimizers on the other hand.

The following result, which is a straightforward consequence of Theorems 1 and 2, establishes an elegant connection between graph matching and quadratic programming.

Theorem 3. *Let $G_1 = (V_1, E_1)$ and $G_2 = (V_2, E_2)$ be two graphs, and let G be the corresponding association graph. Then, all local (global) solutions to (1) are in one-to-one correspondence with maximal (maximum) common subgraph isomorphisms between G_1 and G_2.*

Computing the stationary points of (1) can be done by solving the LCP (q_G, M_G), which is the problem of finding a vector x satisfying the system

$$y = q_G + M_G x \geq 0, \quad x \geq 0, \quad x^T y = 0$$

where

$$q_G = \begin{bmatrix} 0 \\ \vdots \\ 0 \\ -1 \\ 1 \end{bmatrix} \qquad M_G = \begin{bmatrix} A_G & -e & e \\ e^T & 0 & 0 \\ -e^T & 0 & 0 \end{bmatrix}. \tag{3}$$

With the above definitions, it is well known that if z is a complementary solution of (q_G, M_G) with $z^T = (x^T, y^T)$ and $x \in \mathbb{R}^n$, then x is a stationary point of (1). Indeed, the matrix A_G is always strictly copositive, hence so is M_G and that is enough to assure that (q_G, M_G) always has a solution [9][1]. Of course, a stationary point of (1) is not necessarily a local minimum, but in practice this is not a problem since there are several techniques that, starting from a stationary point can reach a nearby local optimum. An example is given by the replicator dynamics [19], but see [14] for a complete discussion on this topic.

---

[1] Recall that, given a cone $\Gamma \subseteq \mathbb{R}^n$, a symmetric matrix Q is said to be Γ-*copositive* if $x^T Q x \geq 0$ for all $x \in \Gamma$. If the inequality holds strictly for all $x \in \Gamma \setminus \{o\}$, then Q is said to be *strictly Γ-copositive*.

3   A Pivoting-Based Heuristic for Graph Matching

Technical literature supplies a large number of algorithms to go about solving an LCP [9]. The most popular is probably Lemke's method, largely for its ability to provide a solution for a large number of matrix classes. Lemke's "Scheme I" belongs to the family of pivoting algorithms. Given the generic LCP (q, M), it deals with the augmented problem (q, d, M) defined by

$$y = q + [M, d] \begin{bmatrix} x \\ \theta \end{bmatrix} \geq 0, \quad \theta \geq 0, \quad x \geq 0, \quad x^T y = 0. \tag{4}$$

A solution of (q, d, M) with $\theta = 0$ promptly yields a solution to (q, M), and Lemke's method intends to compute precisely such a solution. We refer to [9] for a detailed description of Lemke's algorithm. In our implementation, we chose $d = e$, as our problem does not expose peculiarities that would justify a deviation from this common practice.

As usually done for outlining pivoting algorithms, we will use an exponent for the problem data. In practice q^ν and M^ν will identify the situation after ν pivots and A_G^ν will indicate the $n \times n$ leading principal submatrix of M^ν. Consistently, y^ν and x^ν will indicate the vectors of basic and non-basic variables, respectively, each made up of a combination of the original x_i and y_i variables. The notation $\langle x_i^\nu, y_j^\nu \rangle$ will be used to indicate pivoting transformations. The index set of the basic variables that satisfy the min-ratio test at iteration ν will be denoted with Ω^ν, i.e.

$$\Omega^\nu = \arg\min_i \left\{ \frac{-q_i^\nu}{m_{is}^\nu} : m_{is}^\nu < 0 \right\}$$

where s is the index of the driving column. Also, in the sequel the auxiliary column that contains the covering vector d in (4) will be referred to as the column $n + 3$ of matrix $M = M_G$.

In general, assuming an LCP non-degenerate is a strategy commonly taken to prove finiteness of pivoting schemes. This assumption amounts to having $|\Omega^\nu| = 1$ for all ν, thereby excluding any cycling behavior. In particular, Lemke's method is guaranteed to process any non-degenerate problem (q, M) where M is strictly $\mathbb{R}_+^n$-copositive, and to do so without terminating on a secondary ray [9]. Unfortunately our LCP (q_G, M_G) is degenerate and standard degeneracy resolution strategies have proven to yield unsatisfactory results [14].

The proposed degeneracy resolution technique makes use of the so-called *least-index rule* which amounts to blocking the driving variable with a basic one that has minimum index within a certain subset of Ω^ν, i.e. $r = \min \Phi^\nu$ for some $\Phi^\nu \subseteq \Omega^\nu$. The least-index rule per se does not guarantee convergence. In fact we can ensure termination by choosing the blocking variable only among those that make the number of degenerate variables decrease as slowly as possible, i.e. among the index-set

$$\Phi^\nu = \arg\min_i \left\{ |\Omega^\nu| - |\Omega_i^{\nu+1}| > 0 : i \in \Omega^\nu \right\} \subseteq \Omega^\nu$$

where $\Omega_i^{\nu+1}$ is the index-set of those variables that would satisfy the min-ratio test at iteration $\nu + 1$ if the driving variable at iteration ν was blocked with y_i^ν as $i \in \Omega^\nu$. The previous conditional implies that a pivot step is taken and then reset in a sort of "look-ahead" fashion, hence we will refer to this rule as the *look-ahead (pivot) rule*.

Before actually proceeding to illustrate a version of Lemke's algorithm applied to our matching problem, let us take a look at the tableaus that it generates. This will help us to identify regularities that are reflected in the behavior of the algorithm itself. The initial tableau follows:

	1	x_1	$\cdots$	x_n	x_{n+1}	x_{n+2}	θ
y_1	0				-1	1	1
$\vdots$	$\vdots$		A_G		$\vdots$	$\vdots$	$\vdots$
y_n	0				-1	1	1
y_{n+1}	-1	1	$\cdots$	1	0	0	1
y_{n+2}	1	-1	$\cdots$	-1	0	0	1

As q_{n+1} is the only negative entry for the column of q, the first pivot to occur during initialization is $\langle y_{n+1}, \theta \rangle$ thereby producing the following transformation:

	1	x_1	$\cdots$	x_n	x_{n+1}	x_{n+2}	y_{n+1}
y_1	1				-1	1	1
$\vdots$	$\vdots$		$A_G - ee^T$		$\vdots$	$\vdots$	$\vdots$
y_n	1				-1	1	1
θ	1	-1	$\cdots$	-1	0	0	1
y_{n+2}	2	-2	$\cdots$	-2	0	0	1

The driving variable for the second pivot is x_{n+1}. Since $m_{i,n+1}^1 = -1$ for all $i = 1, \ldots, n$ it is immediate to see that the relative blocking variable can be any one of $y_1, \ldots, y_n$. In this case we apply no degeneracy resolution criterion, but rather allow for user intervention by catering for the possibility of deciding the second driving variable a priori. Let thus y_p be the (arbitrary) variable that shall block x_{n+1}. After performing $\langle y_p, x_{n+1} \rangle$, we have the following tableau:

	1	x_1	$\cdots$	x_n	y_p	x_{n+2}	y_{n+1}
y_1	0				1	0	0
$\vdots$	$\vdots$				$\vdots$	$\vdots$	$\vdots$
y_{p-1}	0				1	0	0
x_{n+1}	1		$A_{G,p}$		-1	1	1
y_{p+1}	0				1	0	0
$\vdots$	$\vdots$				$\vdots$	$\vdots$	$\vdots$
y_n	0				1	0	0
θ	1	-1	$\cdots$	-1	0	0	1
y_{n+2}	2	-2	$\cdots$	-2	0	0	1

Algorithm 3.1 Lemke's "Scheme I" with the look-ahead rule.

Input: A graph $G = (V, E)$ and $p \in V$.
Let (q_G, e, M_G) be the augmented LCP, where q_G and M_G are defined in (3).
$\nu \leftarrow 0$, $\langle y_{n+1}, \theta \rangle$, $\nu \leftarrow \nu + 1$, $\langle x_p, x_{n+1} \rangle$
The driving variable is x_p.
Infinite loop
      $\nu \leftarrow \nu + 1$
      Let x_s^ν denote the driving variable.
      $\Omega^\nu = \arg \min_i \left\{ \frac{-q_i^\nu}{m_{is}^\nu} : m_{is}^\nu < 0 \right\}$
      If $|\Omega^\nu| = 1$ then $r = \min \Omega^\nu$
      else $\Phi^\nu = \arg \min_i \left\{ |\Omega^\nu| - |\Omega_i^{\nu+1}| > 0 : i \in \Omega^\nu \right\}$, $r = \min \Phi^\nu$.
      $\langle y_{r \in \Omega^\nu}^\nu, x_s^\nu \rangle$
      If $y_r^\nu \equiv \theta$ then
            Let $\bar{x}$ denote the complementary solution of (q_G, M_G).
            The result is $\text{supp}(\bar{x}) \cap V$
      The new driving variable is the complementary of y_r^ν.

Algorithm 3.2 The *pivoting-based heuristic* (PBH) for graph matching.

Input: Two graphs G_1 and G_2.
Construct the association graph $G = (V, E)$ of G_1 and G_2.
Let $G' = (V', E')$ be a permutation of G
with $\deg(u') \geq \deg(v')$ for all $u', v' \in V'$ with $u' < v'$.
$K^\star \leftarrow \emptyset$
For $v' = 1, \ldots, n : \deg(v') > |K^\star|$ do
      Run Algorithm 3.1 with G' and v' as input.
      Let K be the obtained result.
      If $|K| > |K^\star|$, then $K^\star \leftarrow K$.
The result is the mapping of $K^\star$ in G.

---

where $A_{G,p}$ denotes the matrix whose rows are defined as

$$(A_{G,p})_i = \begin{cases} (A_G)_p - e^T & \text{if } i = p \\ (A_G)_i - (A_G)_p & \text{otherwise.} \end{cases}$$

Algorithm 3.1 formalizes the previous statements.

Empirical evidence indicated p as a key parameter for the quality of the final result of Algorithm 3.1. Unfortunately we could not identify any effective means to restrict the choice of values in V that can guarantee a good sub-optimal solution. We thus had to consider iterating for most, if not all, vertices of V as outlined in Algorithm 3.2. There we employ a very simple criterion to avoid considering those nodes that cannot drive to larger cliques than the one we already have because they have a too small degree. Clearly such a criterion is effective only for very sparse graphs.

We also observed that the schema is sensitive to the ordering of nodes and found that the best figures were obtained by reordering G by decreasing node degrees. This feature too is formalized in Algorithm 3.2. We will refer to that scheme by the name Pivoting Based Heuristic (PBH).

4   Experimental Results

In this section we present some experimental results of applying PBH to the problem of matching pairs of random graphs. Random structures represent a useful benchmark not only because they are not constrained to any particular application, but also because it is simple to replicate experiments and hence to make comparisons with other algorithms.

We generated random 50-nodes graphs using edge-probablities (i.e. densities) ranging from 0.1 to 0.95. For each density value, 20 graphs were constructed so that, overall, 200 graphs were used in the experiments. Each graph had its vertices permuted and was then subject to a corruption process which consisted of randomly deleting a fraction of its nodes. In so doing we in fact obtain a graph isomorphic to a proper subgraph of the original one. Various levels of corruption (i.e., percentage of node deletion) were used, namely 0% (the pure isomorphism case), 10%, 20% and 30%. In other words, the order of the corrupted graphs ranged from 50 to 35.

PBH was applied on each pair of graphs thus constructed and, after convergence, the percentage of matched nodes was recorded. Replicator dynamics, a class of dynamical systems developed in evolutionary game theory and other branches of mathematical biology, have recently proven remarkably powerful on simple versions of the graph matching problem, despite their inherent inability to escape from local optima [17–19]. For the sake of comparison, we therefore tested their effectiveness on our (more difficult) subgraph isomorphim task.

Figure 1 plots the results obtained with both PBH and replicator dynamics. As can be seen, whenever no corruption was applied on the original graphs (i.e. in the case of isomorphic graphs), both methods found sistematically a maximum isomorphism, i.e. a maximum clique in the association graph (as far as replicator equations are concerned, this is indeed not surprising, as shown in [18]). The emerging picture did not change significantly for PBH when we did delete some nodes, whereas the replicator equations underwent a notable deterioration of performance. For the latter case, in fact, the curves (b)-(d) of Figure 1 have a peculiar "w" shape with a performance peak on 0.5-density graphs, where the corresponding association graphs have minimum density.

It is also possible to compare our approach with the well-known Graduated Assignment method (GA) of Gold and Rangarajan [11]. Their algorithm is based on the minimization of an objective function which is significantly different from ours. In [11] (Figure 8) they present results of applying GA on 100-node random graphs with density values ranging from 4% to 28%, and various corruption levels up to 30%. From their results a significant sensitivity of GA to node deletion emerges, similarly to what happens for the replicator dynamics, but

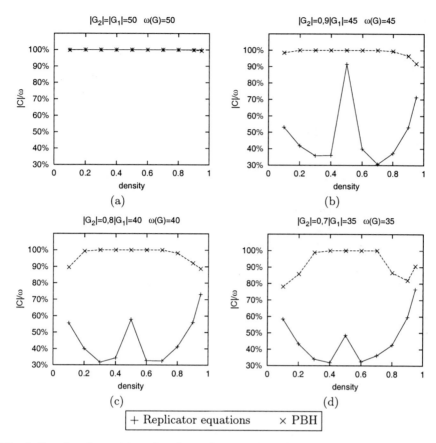

Fig. 1. Results of matching 50-node random graphs, with varying levels of corruption, using PBH and replicator dynamics. The x-axis represents the (approximate) density of the matched graphs, while the y-axis represents the percentage of correct matches. Here ω is the size of the maximum clique of the association graph, i.e. the size of the maximum isomorphism, and $|C|$ is the size of the isomorphism returned by the algorithms, i.e., the size of the maximal clique found. Figures (a) to (d) correspond to different levels of corruption, i.e. 0%, 10%, 20% and 30%, respectively. All curves represent averages over 20 trials.

in a less pronounced manner. In contrast, the performance of PBH (on smaller graphs) seems to be more insensitive to the corruption level, a feature which is clearly desirable. Notice, however, that the results tend to degrade slowly for the denser association graphs that arise for densities close to 0 and 1. This phenomenon tends to strengthen up slowly as more nodes are deleted, but the average efficiency never goes below 85%. This figure is superior to those obtained with replicator dynamics and GA.

A remarkable empirical finding was that Algorithm 3.1 never failed to return a maximal clique. We then never needed to perturb the final point in order to reach a nearby local minimizer. We tried to find exceptions by running PBH on random graphs with non-clique regular subgraphs. The latter subgraphs correspond in fact to stationary points of program (1) as shown in [5]. Hundreds of experiments were conducted on random instances with different degrees of noise, but PBH never failed to return a maximal clique. At the moment we cannot give a formal proof of this fact.

5   Conclusions

Motivated by a recent quadratic formulation, we have presented a pivoting-based heuristic for the graph matching problem based on the corresponding linear complementarity problem. The preliminary results obtained are very encouraging and indicate the proposed framework as a new promising way to tackle graph matching and related combinatorial problems. Note also that our algorithm is completely devoid of working parameters, a valuable feature which distinguishes it from other heuristics proposed in the literature

Clearly, more experimental work needs to be done in order to fully assess the potential of the method. Also, generalizations of the proposed approach to attributed graph and error-tolerant (many-to-many) matching problems are possible, along the lines suggested in [17, 3, 22]. All this will be the subject of future work.

References

1. A. P. Ambler and et al. A versatile computer-controlled assembly system. In *Proc. 3rd Int. J. Conf. Artif. Intell.*, pages 298–307. Stanford, CA, 1973.
2. H. G. Barrow and R. M. Burstall. Subgraph isomorphism, matching relational structures and maximal cliques. *Inform. Process. Lett.*, 4(4):83–84, 1976.
3. M. Bartoli, M. Pelillo, K. Siddiqi, and S. W. Zucker. Attributed tree homomorphism using association graphs. In *Proc. 15th Int. Conf. Pattern Recognition*, volume 2, pages 133–136. IEEE Computer Society Press, 2000.
4. R. C. Bolles and R. A. Cain. Recognizing and locating partially visible objects: The locus-feature-focus method. *Int. J. Robotics Res.*, 1:57–82, 1982.
5. I. M. Bomze. Evolution towards the maximum clique. *J. Global Optim.*, 10:143–164, 1997.
6. I. M. Bomze. On standard quadratic optimization problems. *J. Global Optim.*, 13:369–387, 1998.
7. I. M. Bomze, M. Budinich, P. M. Pardalos, and M. Pelillo. The maximum clique problem. In D.-Z. Du and P. M. Pardalos, editors, *Handbook of Combinatorial Optimization - suppl. vol. A*, pages 1–74. Kluwer Academic Publishers, 1999.
8. H. Bunke. Recent developments in graph matching. In *Proc. 15th Int. Conf. Pattern Recognition*, volume 2, pages 117–124. IEEE Computer Society Press, 2000.
9. R. W. Cottle, J. Pang, and R. E. Stone. *The Linear Complementarity Problem.* Academic Press, Boston, MA, 1992.
10. L. E. Gibbons, D. W. Hearn, P. M. Pardalos, and M. V. Ramana. Continuous characterizations of the maximum clique problem. *Math. Oper. Res.*, 22:754–768, 1997.

11. S. Gold and A. Rangarajan. A graduated assignment algorithm for graph matching. *IEEE Trans. Pattern Analysis and Machine Intelligence*, 18(4):377–388, 1996.

12. R. Horaud and T. Skordas. Stereo correspondence through feature grouping and maximal cliques. *IEEE Trans. Pattern Analysis and Machine Intelligence*, 11:1168–1180, 1989.

13. S. Z. Li. Matching: Invariant to translations, rotations, and scale changes. *Pattern Recognition*, 25:583–594, 1992.

14. A. Massaro, M. Pelillo, and I. M. Bomze. A complementary pivoting approach to the maximum weight clique problem. *SIAM J. Optim.*, in press.

15. B. Messmer and H. Bunke. A new algorithm for error tolerant subgraph isomorphism. *IEEE Trans. Pattern Anal. Machince Intell.*, 20:493–505, 1998.

16. T. S. Motzkin and E. G. Straus. Maxima for graphs and a new proof of a theorem of Turán. *Canad. J. Math.*, 17(4):533–540, 1965.

17. M. Pelillo. A unifying framework for relational structure matching. In *Proc. 14th Int. Conf. Pattern Recognition*, pages 1316–1319. IEEE Computer Society Press, 1998.

18. M. Pelillo. Replicator equations, maximal cliques, and graph isomorphism. *Neural Computation*, 11:1933–1955, 1999.

19. M. Pelillo. Replicator dynamics in combinatorial optimization. In P. M. Pardalos and C. A. Floudas, editors, *Encyclopedia of Optimization*. Kluwer Academic Publishers, Boston, MA, 2001. in press.

20. M. Pelillo and A. Jagota. Feasible and infeasible maxima in a quadratic program for the maximum clique problem. *J. Artif. Neural Networks*, 2(4):411–420, 1995.

21. M. Pelillo, K. Siddiqi, and S. W. Zucker. Matching hierarchical structures using association graphs. *IEEE Trans. Pattern Anal. Machince Intell.*, 21(11):1105–1120, 1999.

22. M. Pelillo, K. Siddiqi, and S. W. Zucker. Many-to-many matching of attributed trees using association graphs and game dynamics. In C. Arcelli, L. P. Cordella, and G. Sanniti di Baja, editors, *Visual Form 2001*, pages 583–593. Springer, Berlin, 2001.

23. A. Rangarajan and E. Mjolsness. A lagrangian relaxation network for graph matching. *IEEE Trans. Neural Networks*, 7:1365–1381, 1996.

24. L. G. Shapiro and R. M. Haralick. Structural descriptions and inexact matching. *IEEE Trans. Pattern Anal. Machine Intell.*, 3:504–519, 1981.

25. W.-H. Tsai and K.-S. Fu. Subgraph error-correcting isomorphisms for syntactic pattern recognition. *IEEE Trans. Syst. Man Cybern.*, 13:48–62, 1983.

26. R. C. Wilson and E. R. Hancock. Structural matching by discrete relaxation. *IEEE Trans. Pattern Anal. Machince Intell.*, 19(6):634–648, 1997.

Application of Genetic Algorithms to 3-D Shape Reconstruction in an Active Stereo Vision System

Sanghyuk Woo, Albert Dipanda*, and Franck Marzani

Université de Bourgogne, Laboratoire LE2I, Aile des Sciences de l'Ingénieur, 9, Avenue
Alain Savary BP 47870 – 21078 DIJON CEDEX, FRANCE
adipanda@u-bourgogne.fr

Abstract. In this paper, a new method for reconstructing 3-D shapes is
proposed. It is based on an active stereo vision system composed of a camera
and a light system which projects a set of structured laser rays on the scene to
be analyzed. The depth information is provided by matching the laser rays and
the corresponding spots appearing in the image. The matching task is performed
by using Genetic Algorithms (GAs). The process converges towards the
optimum solution which proves that GAs can effectively be used for this
problem. An efficient 3-D reconstruction method is introduced. The
experimental results demonstrate that the proposed approach is stable and
provides high accuracy 3-D object reconstruction.

1 Introduction

Reconstructing 3-D shapes is a very important issue for many applications in
computer vision and computer graphics, namely object recognition for robotic vision,
virtual environment construction, and so on. In order to obtain the three-dimensional
surface information of an object, a passive or active stereovision method is usually
used. The most commonly employed passive method consists in taking two images of
a scene at two different shooting angles by using either two cameras or only one
camera from two different positions. Then, two-dimensional coordinates in the two
images are determined. Supposing that both, the geometrical relationship between the
two cameras (or the displacement of the unique camera) and their intrinsic parameters
are known, 3-D coordinates of a point can be deduced from the two-dimensional
coordinates by triangulation. Although this method is accurate and often used, it
requires high-performance image processing tasks such as extracting the points to be
reconstructed from one of the two images and searching along the epipolar line for
their corresponding points in the second image [1]. This process is defined as stereo
image matching and remains one of the bottlenecks in computer vision [2][3][4][5].

Active stereovision systems offer an alternative approach to the use of two
cameras. They consist in replacing one of the two cameras by a light system (a laser
emitter) which projects either one light ray or a set of structured light rays onto the
scene. In the first case, a sequence of images is taken by the camera as the light ray

---

* Corresponding author : e-mail : adipanda@u-bourgogne.fr ; fax : +33 3 80 39 58 83

M.A.T. Figueiredo, J. Zerubia, A.K. Jain (Eds.): EMMCVPR 2001, LNCS 2134, pp. 480–493, 2001.
© Springer-Verlag Berlin Heidelberg 2001

scans the scene whereas in the second case, only one image is taken. In this study, we are concerned with the second case. An image thus obtained has many spots created by the laser rays. Supposing that both the geometrical relationship between the camera and the light projection system, and the intrinsic parameters of the system are known, 3-D coordinates of a spot in the image can be determined and provide the corresponding depth information. This requires identifying the laser ray from which the 2-D spot originates. In this case, the stereo matching problem boils down to matching the laser rays and their corresponding spots in the image reference. It is a hard combinatorial search problem which is difficult to solve with a conventional optimization method. We propose to tackle this problem by using Genetic Algorithms (GAs).

The remainder of this paper is organized as follows: In the next section, we briefly present our active stereovision system, then we describe the calibration of the system and the 3-D reconstruction process. In section 3, we present the principal elements of the proposed GAs for matching laser rays and points. In section 4, we describe the partitioning process. Data are distributed into regions and GAs are independently applied in each cluster. In section 5, we show experimental results and in section 6 the conclusion.

2   The Active Stereovision System

2.1   System Description and Calibration

Our active stereovision system is composed of the following elements: A CCD camera connected to a PC which allows image acquisitions, and a laser diode connected to a diffraction grid for the generation of a laser array composed of 361 (19×19) rays directed so that the angle between two consecutive rays is equal to 0.77°. Each ray is indexed by two indices m and n which vary from –9 to 9. In order to reconstruct the 3-D surface of an object, one only needs to take an image of the object illuminated by the laser array. The intersection of each ray with the object produces a spot on the object. Thus, the camera provides an image in which many points are lit (see Fig. 1).

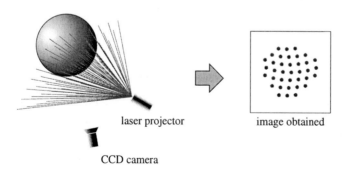

laser projector   image obtained

CCD camera

Fig. 1. An outlook of the active stereo vision system.

3-D coordinate points on the illuminated scene can be determined only if the system is calibrated. Instead of using a classical calibration method that requires the determination of the matrices which characterize the intrinsic and extrinsic parameters of the system [1], we use a simpler methodology. It consists in taking a sequence of images of an illuminated plane which moves between two fixed positions. During the translation the plane must stay perpendicular to the main ray ($m = n = 0$) (see Fig. 2). Knowing both the characteristics of the acquisition system, the position of the plane for each image of the sequence, and the spot coordinates in each image, a set of calibration parameters can be deduced [6]. Thus, for each ray $(m, n)_{(-9 \leq m \leq 9, -9 \leq n \leq 9)}$ of the beam we will have:

1) the parameters A_{mn} and B_{mn} of the straight line Δ_{mn} which is the projection of the ray (m, n) on the image reference;

2) the parameters C_{mn}, D_{mn} and E_{mn} which model the hyperbolic curve F_{mn}. It describes the depth of the successive spots created by the ray (m, n) along the image sequence. F_{mn} is a function of the spot projections on Δ_{mn}.

The calibration is performed only one time before acquiring images of objects to be analyzed. The parameters then provided will be used for 3-D reconstruction.

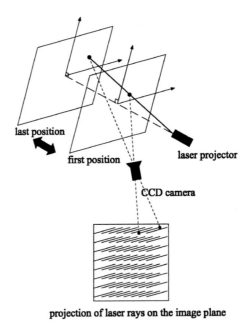

projection of laser rays on the image plane

Fig. 2. The calibration process.

2.2 3-D Reconstruction

For each spot visible on an image, the 2-D coordinates of its center are measured. The corresponding three-dimensional coordinates of the spot can be calculated as follows [7]: Let p_k be the center of a given spot. If p_k is connected to the straight line Δ_{mn}, we calculated p_k', the orthogonal projection of p_k on the straight line Δ_{mn}. Substituting the coordinates of p_k' in the function F_{mn} gives the depth Z_k of the 3-D point P_k whose projection in the image is p_k. The 3-D coordinates (X_k, Y_k, Z_k) of P_k are expressed in the absolute referential $(OXYZ)$ linked to the illuminated scene (the Z-axis corresponds to the main laser ray $(m = n = 0)$). If φ is the inter-ray angle, the indices of the straight lines Δ_{mn} can be chosen so that the corresponding ray be at an angle $m \cdot \varphi$ around Y and at an angle $n \cdot \varphi$ around X (see Fig. 3).

From these hypotheses, we have:

$$X_k = (L_0 - Z_k)\tan(m\varphi) \tag{1a}$$

$$Y_k = (L_0 - Z_k)\tan(n\varphi) \tag{1b}$$

where L_0 is the distance between the plane (XOY) and the laser emitter.

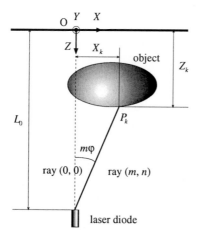

Fig. 3. Three dimensional reconstruction

By scanning the image, this operation is repeated for all the spots appearing in the image. The 3-D points calculated serve as a basis for 3-D object shape reconstruction.

The problem at hand is then to match each spot in the image with its corresponding laser ray. We propose to solve this matching task by using GAs.

3 Matching Laser Rays and Points Using GAs

GAs proposed by Holland [8] are adaptive procedures that find solutions to problems by using an evolutionary process based on natural selection. Their application in image processing and pattern recognition has become widespread in the last decade [4][5][9][10][11].

A GA is an iterative procedure which uses a *population* of potential solutions to a problem. Each individual solution is encoded as a *chromosome* made up of a string of *genes* which may take one of several values called *alleles*.

Each iteration consists of three main stages, namely evaluation, selection and mating. In the evaluation stage, each chromosome is assigned a *fitness* value which represents its ability to solve the problem.

In the selection stage, chromosomes are picked based on their fitness in such a way that the better chromosomes are more likely to be selected. In the mating stage two processes are performed: pairs of selected chromosomes, also called *parent* chromosomes, are recombined by the *crossover* operation to form two new *offspring*.

New offspring are also created by modifying one or more genes on the chromosomes randomly chosen in the mating pool. This operation is called *mutation*.

From generation to generation, this process leads to increasingly better chromosomes and to near-optimal solutions.

3.1 Coding

In our study, the original data is made up of a set of points $P_{i\,(1\,\leq\,i\,\leq\,M)}$ which are the centers of spots in the image reference and a set of lines $\Delta_{j\,(1\,\leq\,j\,\leq\,N)}$ which represent the 2-D projections, in the image, of the laser rays cast by the light system. In order to constrain the solutions even further, we use a set of segments $S_{j\,(1\,\leq\,j\,\leq\,N)}$ rather than lines. A segment is a part of a line limited by the two points on the two planes located on the first and the last position introduced during the calibration process (see Fig. 2). The object to be analyzed must be placed within the region delimited by these two planes. It can be noted that the set of segments does not vary regardless of the object to be analyzed (the number of segments is always equal to the number of laser rays and each segment is always located in the same position). By contrast, the set of points depends on the object to be analyzed. In fact, the position of a given point on the image depends on the depth of its corresponding real object point and furthermore some rays can be missed due to the shape of the object and the position of the camera. By scanning the image, each point and each segment are sequentially labeled.

Given N segments and M points ($N \geq M$), the chromosome of an individual is encoded as a permutation of N integers whose values are between one and N. The ith gene is the number of the point to be matched with the ith segment. Overlooked points are replaced by *virtual* points which are not taken into account for the fitness value.

3.2 Fitness

Our goal, therefore, is to match a point with its closest segment. In theory, the point must be located exactly along the segment, but in practice, there is an error due to the noise effects and the process used to determine the spot center coordinates. Before the fitness function is stated formally, the error between a segment and its matched point needs to be defined.

Given a segment S and its matched point P, we consider two cases for calculating the error:

1) if the point is *within* the segment (see Figure 4a), the error is obtained by:

$$e = \left| mx^* + b - y^* \right| \tag{2}$$

where m is the slope, b is the y-intercept of the segment, and x^* and y^* are the coordinates of the corresponding point.

2) if the point is *outside* the segment (see Figure 4b), a penalty is applied to the error which is given by:

$$e = \left| mx^* + b - y^* \right| \times \left(Min(l_1, l_2) + 1 \right) \tag{3}$$

where l_1 and l_2 are the distances between the point and the two edges of the segment.

Finally, the fitness function of a kth chromosome is the sum of the errors of all its genes and is expressed by the following equation:

$$f_k = \sum_{i=1}^{M} e_i \tag{4}$$

where k is the index of a chromosome, M is the number of points to be matched.

According to this fitness function, the better the chromosome the lower its fitness value.

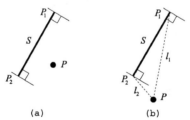

(a)   (b)

Fig. 4. Determination of the error between a segment and its matched point. (a) The point P is within its matched segment S. (b) The point P is outside its matched segment S.

3.3 Selection and Surviving Strategy

We have applied a modified version of the selection strategy proposed by Z. Michalewicz [12]. This process can be described as follows:

First, we select N_g survivors among the N_p individuals of the current generation for the next generation. This selection is based on a criterion called the "Surviving Test" and is defined by:

$$(f_i \times c) < \bar{f} \tag{5}$$

where f_i is the fitness of the ith chromosome, $\bar{f}$ is average fitness and $c \in [0.5, 1.5]$ is the survival testing coefficient randomly obtained.

Thus, the number of survivors of each generation varies. Moreover, the above surviving test provides more variations of chromosomes in a population since a chromosome with a high fitness value and a chromosome with an average fitness value have almost the same chance to survive.

Secondly, by a tournament selection [13], $(N_p - N_g)$ parents are picked from the whole population of the current generation to conduct the crossover operation described below. The number of offspring produced depends on the crossover rate p_c and is equal to $(N_p - N_g) \times p_c$.

3.4 Crossover

In this study, we have applied the PMX operation [13]. Two parents are selected in the mating pool. First two locations are randomly chosen. Then the chosen portion of each parent is swapped with each other. And finally, the rest of the chromosome is copied preventing gene repetitions (see Fig. 5).

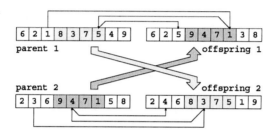

Fig. 5. PMX operator

3.5 Mutation

Mutation is used to prevent a convergence to a local optimum. In fact, crossover loses its role when the greater part of the population is centered around a local optimum of the fitness function. In this case, individuals at the same peak are often identical. So, the crossover operation does not significantly modify a chromosome. The mutation operation is a local mutation that shuffles the loci of genes in a randomly chosen block within the chromosome.

4   Partitioning Method

When using GAs, the size of chromosome is a drawback for computional time. The curve in Fig. 12 shows that the execution time of the crossover operation grows exponentially with the chromosome size. In [14] we have introduced a deterministic step to cope with this problem. However, since we can't backtrack after matching some segments and points, an error occurring in this step may not be corrected in the GAs step.

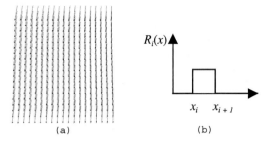

Fig. 6. (a) Superimposed view of segments and points. (b) the member function.

In a real acquisition process, according to a chosen configuration of the camera and the laser ray system, the segments and the points form a vertical (or horizontal) stripe pattern, and ambiguities in the matching process only occur in the vertical (or horizontal) direction (see Fig. 6a). So, the data can be partitioned into independent regions. There are always 19 clusters since the laser array projects 19×19 beams on the scene which gives 19 independent matching problems to solve.

This partitioning process provides two main advantages: First, the size of a chromosome is always the same (a chromosome is composed of 19 genes) whatever the complexity of the object to be analyzed. Second, the search space is limited since the matching process is performed locally in each cluster which increases the convergence.

4.1 Clustering the Data

The simplest way of getting regions is by using lines, referred to as the *dividers*, that pass through the center of each cluster of segments. Since these dividers are not parallel, we have defined a customized member function for each region for the purpose of clustering the points.

The customized member function $R_i(x)$ of the *ith* region is expressed as (see Fig. 6b):

$$R_i(x) = \begin{cases} 1, & x_{i-1} \leq x < x_i \quad with \ 1 \leq i \leq 19 \\ 0, & otherwise \end{cases} \tag{6}$$

where x_{i-1} and x_i are the x-values of respective corresponding points on the dividers. Note that $x_0 = 0$ and $x_{19} = \infty$.

For example, let's consider a point P and its coordinates (p, q). The equation of the *ith* divider is expressed as $y_i = m_i x + b_i$. By replacing y_i with q in the above formula, we obtain the corresponding x_i. Then, x_{i-1} is calculated in the same way by considering the equation of the $(i - 1)$th divider. According to the value of p which corresponds to x in the member function (eq. 6), P may be included or not in the *ith* region.

4.2 Chromosome Coding and Multi-Population

The points have been distributed into 19 independent regions which have, for each one, 19 points and 19 segments. Thus a chromosome consists of a permutation of 19 integers that represent the indices of points. Note that if there are some overlooked

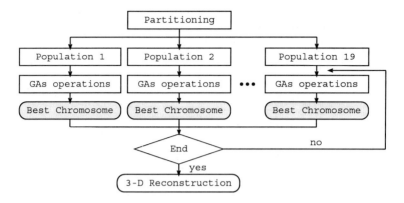

Fig. 7. Outlook of the partitioning method

points, we introduce *virtual* points to complete the chromosome. So we have 19 problems that can be solved in parallel. We work with a population PP partitioned into $PP_{i\,(i\,\in\,[1,\,19])}$ sub-populations whose size is the same (*pop_size*). Thus we have the following organization: $PP=\{PP_1,PP_2,PP_3,\ldots,PP_{18},PP_{19}\}$, $PP_i=\{C_{i1},C_{i2},\ldots,C_{ipop\_size}\}$, and $C_{ij}=\{S_1,S_2,\ldots,S_{18},S_{19}\}$, where $C_{i,j}$ is the jth chromosome of the ith sub-population, S_l are the segments of the ith region, $i\in[1,19]$ and $j\in[1,19]$.

The Genetic operations described above are then applied to each sub-population independently (see Fig. 7).

5   Experimental Results

In this section, we present experimental results of our method. A large number of experiments were conducted to show the validity of our approach for 3-D shape reconstruction.

Fig. 9, Fig. 10, and Fig. 11 illustrate 3-D reconstruction of three objects: a biplane, a computer mouse and a human face, which constitute a meaningful sample of the objects we used. We have placed a plane behind the biplane and the computer mouse during their image acquisition. The objective was to recover all the laser spots. Whereas face image acquisitions were done in a more realistic context, i.e. without any additional plane. Thus, only the laser rays which intersect the face may appear on the images. Moreover, we have acquired an image sequence of the face during a rotation movement.

There were 3 overlooked points on the biplane image and 11 overlooked points on the computer mouse image. But on the face images, about 200 spots, out of the 361 possible, were visible.

The experiments were always conducted until an optimal solution was reached. Since GAs are stochastic, the number of generations may vary at different runs. The mean generation number was 200 whatever the object to reconstruct since all the matching problems were similar.

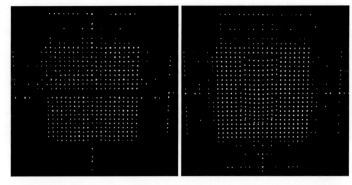

Fig. 8. Images obtained with the active stereo vision system – aperture of the camera is chosen in order to viewing only the spots. The biplane (left) and the computer mouse (right).

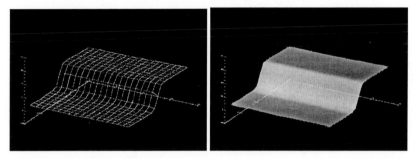

Fig. 9. 3-D Reconstruction of a biplane – A mesh view (left) and a shaded surface view (right) in a different angle

The major concern in our approach is the selection of GAs parameters to obtain the final results with high speed convergence. An experimental study shows that the population size is the most important parameter. On one hand, if the population size is too small, it may cause a premature convergence to a suboptimal solution. On the other hand, a large population size requires more evaluations per generation but allows better convergence to an optimal solution. Fig. 13 shows the curve of execution time versus the population size. It appears that the optimal population size is 30. According to our experimental study, the importance of the other parameters is not very significant. The crossover rate was set to 0.8 and the mutation rate was set to 0.1.

For each object, more than 100 different runs for 3-D reconstruction were carried out giving the same final result, which proves that our method is stable. Fig. 14 represents an example of the evolution of the fitness of the best chromosome in each of the 19 sub-populations. Fig. 15 illustrates the fitness value evolution, until convergence, of all individuals in a sub-population at each generation. It appears that the process converges rapidly.

The different results obtained show that our approach permits the recovery of 3-D coordinates of spots and consequently it enables 3-D object reconstruction with high accuracy.

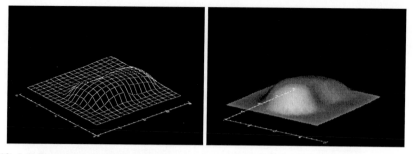

Fig. 10. 3-D Reconstruction of a computer mouse – A mesh view (left) and a shaded surface view (right) in a different angle.

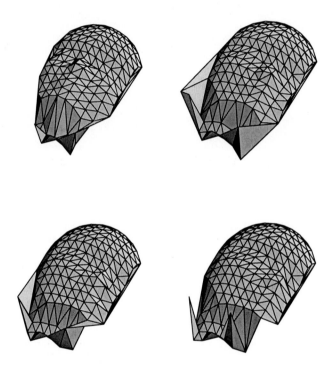

Fig. 11. 3-D Reconstruction of a face which is rotating

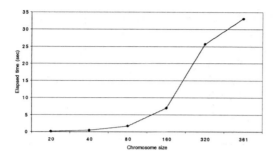

Fig. 12. Execution time for 500 crossover operations vs. chromosome size (PMX)

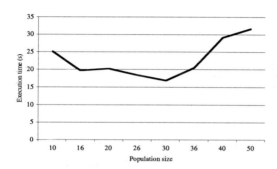

Fig. 13. Plot of average execution time versus population size for computer mouse.

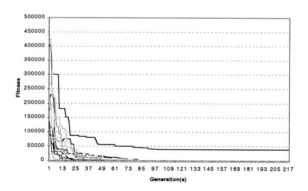

Fig. 14. Plot of fitness evolution of the best chromosome in each subpopulation

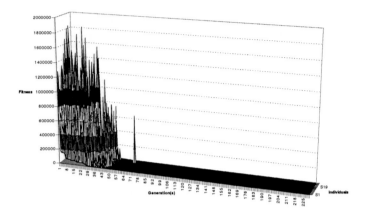

Fig. 15. Plot of the fitness evolution of all individuals in a subpopulation

6   Conclusion

In this paper, a new method for reconstructing 3-D shapes is proposed. It is based on an active stereo vision system composed of a camera and a light system which projects a set of structured laser rays on the scene to be analyzed. The image acquired by the system has many spots created by the laser rays. These spots are the basis of the 3-D shape reconstruction. The determination of the depth information on a point, represented by a spot in the image, requires to identify the laser ray from which the spot originates. The matching task is performed using GAs. Data is partitioned into independent clusters and GAs are performed independently in the different clusters. In all cases, the matching processes converge towards the optimum solution which proves that GAs can effectively be used to this matching problem. The 3-D reconstruction is performed by an efficient method. The experimental results confirm that the proposed approach is stable and provides high accuracy 3-D object reconstruction. Consequently, it can be used efficiently as the first stage in a global 3-D shape system analysis.

References

1.   Faugeras, O., Toscani, G.: The Calibration Problem for Stereo, Computer Vision & Pattern Recognition, Miami Beach, Florida, (1986) 15-20
2.   Weng, J., Huang, T., Ahuja, N.: Motion on Structure from Perspective Views: Algorithms, Error Analysis and Error Estimation, IEEE Trans. on Pattern Anal. and Mach. Intell. Vol. 11(5), (1989) 451-476

3. Deriche, R., Faugeras, O.: 2D-curves Matching Using High Curvatures Points: Applications to Stereovision, In Proc. of 10th ICPR, Atlantic City, Vol.1 (1990) 240-242

4. Kanade, T., Okutomi, T.: A Stereo Matching Algorithm with an Adaptive Window: Theory and Experiments, IEEE Trans. on Pattern Anal. and Mach. Intell. Vol. 16(9), (1994) 920-932

5. Saito. H., Mori, M.: Application of Genetic Algorithms to Stereo Matching of Images, Pattern Recognition Letters Vol. 16, (1995) 815-821

6. Voisin, Y., Marzani, F., Diou, A.: Calibration d'un Système de Vision par Lumière Structurée, *Graphics/Vision Interface*, Montréal, Canada, (2000) 128-135

7. Marzani, F., Voisin, Y., Lew Yan Voon, LFC., Diou, A.: Active Stereo Vision System: a Fast and easy calibration method, In Proc. of ICARCV, Singapour, (2000)

8. Holland, J.H.: Adaptation in Natural and Artificial System, MIT Press, Cambridge, MA, (1975)

9. Roth, G., Levine, M.: Geometric Primitive Extraction Using a Genetic Algorithm, IEEE Trans. on Pattern Anal. and Mach. Intell. Vol. 16(9), (1994) 901-905

10. Huang, Y., Palaniappan, K., Zhuang, X., Cavanaugh, J.E.: Optic Flow Field Segmentation and Motion Estimation Using a Robust Genetic Partitioning Algorithm, IEEE Trans. on Pattern Anal. and Mach. Intell. Vol. 17(12), (1995)

11. Fan., K.C., Wang, Y.K.: A Genetic Sparse Distributed Memory Approach to The Application of Handwritten Character Recognition, Pattern Recognition, Vol. 30(12), (1997) 2015-2022

12. Michalewicz, Z.: Genetic Algorithms + Data Structures = Evolution Programs. 3rd, Extended Edition, Springer-Verlag, (1995)

13. Goldberg, D. E.: Genetic Algorithms in Search, Optimization & Machine Learning, Addison-Wesley, (1989)

14. S. Woo, A. Dipanda,: Matching Lines and Points in an Active Stereovision System Using Genetic Algorithms , In Proc. of IEEE ICIP'2000, Vancouver, Canada, Septembre 2000, Vol.3, (2000) 332-335

Part V

Shapes, Curves, Surfaces, and Templates

A Markov Process Using Curvature
for Filtering Curve Images

Jonas August and Steven W. Zucker

Center for Computational Vision and Control
Departments of Electrical Engineering and Computer Science
Yale University
51 Prospect Street, New Haven, CT 06520
{jonas.august,steven.zucker}@yale.edu

Abstract. A Markov process model for contour curvature is introduced via a stochastic differential equation. We analyze the distribution of such curves, and show that its mode is the Euler spiral, a curve minimizing changes in curvature. To probabilistically enhance noisy and low contrast curve images (e.g., edge and line operator responses), we combine this curvature process with the curve indicator random field, which is a prior for ideal curve images. In particular, we provide an expression for a nonlinear, minimum mean square error filter that requires the solution of two elliptic partial differential equations. Initial computations are reported, highlighting how the filter is curvature-selective, even when curvature is absent in the input.

1   Introduction

Images are ambiguous. One unpleasant consequence of this singular fact is that we cannot compute contours without making assumptions about image structure. Inspired by Gestalt psychology [16], most previous work has defined this structure as good continuity in orientation, that is to say, curves with varying orientation—high curvature—are rejected, and, conversely, straighter curves are enhanced. This is naturally phrased in terms of an energy functional on curves that minimizes curvature. In this paper, we present a stochastic model that instead aims to enforce good continuation in curvature, and thus minimizes *changes* in curvature.

To understand why we believe that good continuation in curvature is important, imagine the situation of a bug trying to "track" the contour in Fig. 1. Suppose the bug is special in that it can only "search" for its next piece of contour in a cone in front of it centered around its current predicted position and direction (i.e., orientation with polarity) [24, 6]. This strategy is appropriate so long as the contour is relatively straight. However, when the bug is on a portion of the contour veering to the right, it will constantly waste time searching to the left, perhaps even mistracking completely if the curvature is too large. In estimation terms, the errors of our searching bug are correlated, a tell-tale clue that the assumption that the contour is straight is biased. A good model would

M.A.T. Figueiredo, J. Zerubia, A.K. Jain (Eds.): EMMCVPR 2001, LNCS 2134, pp. 497–512, 2001.

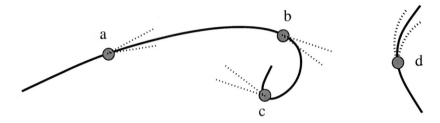

Fig. 1. Mistracking without curvature. A bug (grey dot) attempts to track the contour, "looking" in the cone of search directions centered around its current direction. At point (a), the curve is straight and the bug is successful, although at (b), curve is veering to the right and the bug can barely still track. At (c), the curvature is so high that tracking fails. A better model would explicitly include the curvature of the contour, giving rise to a "bent" search cone (d) for the bug. The same difficulty arises in contour enhancement, which is the application considered in this paper.

only lead to an unavoidable "uncorrelated" error. We present a Markov process that models not only the contour's direction, but also its local curvature.

It may appear that one may avoid these problems altogether by allowing a higher bound on curvature. However, this forces the bug to spend more time searching in a larger cone. In stochastic terms, this larger cone is amounts to asserting that the current (position, direction) state has a weaker influence on the next state; in other words, the prior on contour shape is weaker (less peaked or broader). But a weaker prior will be less able to counteract a weak likelihood (high noise): it will not be robust to noise. Thus we must accept that *good continuation models based only on contour direction are forced to choose between allowing high curvature or high noise*; they cannot have it both ways[1].

Although studying curvature is hardly new in vision, modeling it probabilistically is. In [3, 25, 15] and [8, 361 ff.], measuring curvature in images was the key problem. In [14], curvature is used for smooth interpolations, following on the work on elastica in [20, 10] and later [18]. The closest work in spirit to this is relaxation labeling [26], several applications of which include a deterministic form of curvature [19, 11]. Markov random fields for contour enhancement using orientation [17] and co-circularity [9, 21] have been suggested, but these have no complete stochastic model of individual curves. The explicit study of stochastic but direction-only models of visual contours was initiated by Mumford [18] and has been an extended effort of Williams and co-workers [22, 23].

This paper is organized as follows. We first introduce a curvature random process and its diffusion equation; we then present example impulse responses, which act like the "bent" search cones. Second, we relate the mode of the distribution for the curvature process to an energy functional on smooth curves. Next we review a model of an ideal curve image (e.g., "perfect" edge operator

---

[1] Observe in the road-tracking examples in [6] how all the roads have fairly low curvature. While this is realistic in flat regions such as the area of France considered, others, more mountainous perhaps, have roads that wind in the hillsides.

responses) called the curve indicator random field (CIRF), which was introduced in [2] and theoretically developed in [1], but in the context of Mumford's direction process [18]. Here we apply the CIRF to the curvature process, and then report a minimum mean square error filter for enhancing image contours. We conclude with some example computations.

2   A Brownian Motion in Curvature

Recall that a planar curve is a function taking a parameter $t \in \mathbb{R}$ to a point $(x(t), y(t))$ in the plane $\mathbb{R}^2$. Its direction is defined as $\theta = \arg(\dot{x} + \sqrt{-1}\,\dot{y})$, where the dot denotes differentiation with respect to the arc-length parameter t ($\dot{x}^2 + \dot{y}^2 = 1$ is assumed). Curvature κ is equal to $\dot{\theta}$, the rate of change of direction.

Now we introduce a Markov process that results from making curvature a Brownian motion. Let $R(t) = (X, Y, \Theta, K)(t)$ be random[2], with realization $r = (x, y, \theta, \kappa) \in \mathbb{R}^2 \times \mathbb{S} \times \mathbb{R}$. Consider the following stochastic differential equation:

$$\dot{X} = \cos\Theta, \qquad \dot{Y} = \sin\Theta, \qquad \dot{\Theta} = K, \qquad dK = \sigma dW,$$

where $\sigma = \sigma_{\dot{\kappa}}$ is the "standard deviation in curvature change" (see §3) and W denotes standard Brownian motion. The corresponding Fokker-Plank partial differential equation (PDE), describing the diffusion of a particle's probability density, is

$$\frac{\partial p}{\partial t} = \frac{\sigma^2}{2}\frac{\partial^2 p}{\partial \kappa^2} - \cos\theta\frac{\partial p}{\partial x} - \sin\theta\frac{\partial p}{\partial y} - \kappa\frac{\partial p}{\partial \theta} \tag{1}$$

$$= \frac{\sigma^2}{2}\frac{\partial^2 p}{\partial \kappa^2} - (\cos\theta, \sin\theta, \kappa, 0) \cdot \nabla p,$$

where $p = p(x, y, \theta, \kappa, t) = p(R(t) = r | R(0) = r_0)$, the conditional probability density that the particle is located at r at time t given that it started at r_0 at time 0. Observe that this PDE describes probability transport in the $(\cos\theta, \sin\theta, \kappa, 0)$-direction at point $r = (x, y, \theta, \kappa)$, and diffusion in κ. An extra decay term [18, 22] is also included to penalize length (see §3). We have solved this parabolic equation by first analytically integrating the time variable and then discretely computing the solution to the remaining elliptic PDE. Details will be reported in [1]. See Fig. 2 for example time-integrated transition densities.

3   What Is the Mode of the Distribution of the Curvature Random Process?

To get more insight into our random process in curvature, consider one of the simplest aspects of its probability distribution: its mode. First, let us consider the situation for Mumford's direction-based random process in[3] $\mathbb{R}^2 \times \mathbb{S}$, or

---

[2] Capitals will often be used to denote random variables, with the corresponding letter in lower case denoting a realization. However, capitals are also used to denote operators later in the paper.

[3] $\mathbb{R}^2 \times \mathbb{S}$ is also called (x, y, θ)-space, the unit tangent bundle, and orientation space [13].

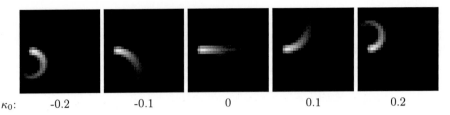

κ_0: -0.2 -0.1 0 0.1 0.2

Fig. 2. Curvature diffusions for various initial curvatures. For all cases the initial position of the particle is an impulse centered vertically on the left, directed horizontally to the right. Shown is the time integral of the transition density of the Markov process in curvature (1), integrated over direction θ and curvature κ; therefore, the brightness displayed at position (x, y) indicates the expected time that the particle spent in (x, y). (Only a linear scaling is performed for displays in this paper; no logarithmic or other nonlinear transformation in intensity is taken.) Observe that the solution "veers" according to curvature, as sought in the Introduction. Contrast this with the straight search cone in Fig. 3. The PDE was solved on a discrete grid of size $32 \times 32 \times 32 \times 5$, with $\sigma_{\dot{\kappa}} = 0.01$ and an exponential decay of characteristic length $\lambda = 10$ (see §3 for length distribution).

$$\dot{X} = \cos\Theta, \qquad \dot{Y} = \sin\Theta, \qquad d\Theta = \sigma_\kappa \, dW,$$

where σ_κ is the "standard deviation in curvature" and W is standard Brownian motion. This process has the following Fokker-Planck diffusion equation:

$$\frac{\partial p}{\partial t} = \frac{\sigma_\kappa{}^2}{2}\frac{\partial^2 p}{\partial \theta^2} - \cos\theta \frac{\partial p}{\partial x} - \sin\theta \frac{\partial p}{\partial y}, \tag{2}$$

where $p = p(x, y, \theta, t)$ is the transition density for time t. As Mumford has shown [18], the mode of the distribution of this direction process is described by *elastica*, or planar curves that minimize the following functional:

$$\int (\alpha\kappa^2 + \beta)dt, \tag{3}$$

where α and β are nonnegative constants. With such an elegant expression for the mode of the Mumford process, we ask: Is there a corresponding functional for the curvature process? If so, what is its form?

To answer these questions, we follow a line of analysis directly analogous to Mumford [18]. First, we discretize our random curve into N subsections. Then we write out the distribution and observe the discretization of a certain integral that will form our desired energy functional.

Suppose our random curve from the curvature process has length T, distributed with the exponential density $p(T) = \lambda^{-1}\exp(-\lambda^{-1}T)$, and independent of the shape of the contour. Each step of the N-link approximation to the curve has length $\Delta t := T/N$. Using the definition of the t-derivatives, for example,

$$\dot{X} = \frac{dX}{dt} = \lim_{N \to \infty} \frac{X_{i+1} - X_i}{T/N},$$

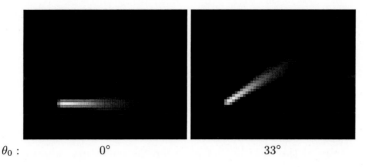

θ_0 : $0°$ $33°$

Fig. 3. Solutions to Mumford's diffusion. Equation (2) was integrated over time and then solved for a slightly blurred impulse on a $80 \times 80 \times 44$ grid, with parameters $\sigma_\kappa = 1/24, \lambda = 100$, and at discrete directions 0 (left) and 4 (right). Depicted is the integral over θ, cropped slightly. The method used [1] responds accurately at all directions. Note that these responses are straight, analogous the search cone described in the Introduction. Given their initial direction, particles governed by the direction process move roughly straight ahead, in contrast to those described by our curvature process (Fig. 2).

we can make the approximation $X_{i+1} \approx X_i + \Delta t \dot{X}$. Recalling the stochastic differential equation (1), we therefore let the curvature process be approximated in discrete time by

$$X_{i+1} = X_i + \Delta t \cos \Theta_i, \qquad Y_{i+1} = Y_i + \Delta t \sin \Theta_i, \qquad \Theta_{i+1} = \Theta_i + \Delta t K_i,$$

where $i = 1, \ldots, N$. Because Brownian motion has independent increments whose standard deviation grows with the square root $\sqrt{\Delta t}$ of the time increment Δt, the change in curvature for the discrete process becomes

$$K_{i+1} = K_i + \sqrt{\Delta t}\, \epsilon_i,$$

where $\{\epsilon_i\}$ is an independent and identically distributed set of 0-mean, Gaussian random variables of standard deviation $\sigma = \sigma_{\dot\kappa}$. Let the discrete contour be denoted by

$$\Gamma_N = \{(X_i, Y_i, \Theta_i, K_i) : i = 0, \ldots, N\}.$$

Given an initial point $p_0 = (x_0, y_0, \theta_0, \kappa_0)$, the probability density for the other points is

$$p(\Gamma_N | p_0) = \lambda^{-1} \exp(-\lambda^{-1} T) \cdot (\sqrt{2\pi}\sigma)^{-N} \exp\left(-\sum_i \frac{\epsilon_i^2}{2\sigma^2}\right),$$

which, by substitution, is proportional to

$$\exp\left[-\sum_i \frac{1}{2\sigma^2}\left(\frac{\kappa_{i+1} - \kappa_i}{\Delta t}\right)^2 \Delta t - \lambda^{-1} T\right].$$

We immediately recognize $\frac{\kappa_{i+1}-\kappa_i}{\Delta t}$ as an approximation to $\frac{d\kappa}{dt} = \dot{\kappa}$, and so we conclude that

$$p(\Gamma_N|p_0) \to p(\Gamma|p_0) \propto e^{-E(\Gamma)} \text{ as } N \to \infty,$$

where the energy $E(\Gamma)$ of (continuous) curve Γ is

$$E(\Gamma) = \int (\alpha\dot{\kappa}^2 + \beta)dt, \tag{4}$$

where $\alpha = (2\sigma^2)^{-1}$ and $\beta = \lambda^{-1}$.

Maximizers of the distribution $p(\Gamma)$ for the curvature random process are planar curves that minimize of the energy functional $E(\Gamma)$. Such curves are known as Euler spirals, and have been studied recently in [14]. A key aspect of the Euler spiral functional (4) is that it penalizes *changes* in curvature, preferring curves with slowly varying curvature. In contrast, the elastica functional (3) penalizes curvature itself, and therefore allows only relatively straight curves, to the dismay of the imaginary bug of the Introduction.

4   Filtering and the Curve Indicator Random Field

Given our stochastic shape model for contours, we now introduce the *curve indicator random field* (CIRF), which naturally captures the notion of an ideal curve image, and provides a precise definition for the kind of output we would like from an edge operator, for example. Roughly, this random field is non-zero-valued along the true contours, and zero-valued elsewhere. The actually measured edge/line map is then viewed as an *imperfect* CIRF, corrupted by noise, blur, etc. The goal of filtering, then, is to estimate the true CIRF given the imperfect one. For completeness, we review the theory of the CIRF now; proofs and more details can be found in [1].

4.1   Definitions

For generality, we shall define the curve indicator random field for any continuous-time Markov process $R_t, 0 \le t < T$ taking values in a finite (or at most countable) set $\mathcal{I}$ of cardinality $|\mathcal{I}|$. As in §3, the random variable T is exponentially-distributed with mean value $\lambda > 0$, and represents the length of a contour. To ensure the finiteness of the expressions that follow, we assume $\lambda < \infty$. Sites or states within $\mathcal{I}$ will be denoted i and j. (Think of $\mathcal{I}$ as a discrete approximation to the state space $\mathcal{R} = \mathbb{R}^2 \times \mathbb{S} \times \mathbb{R}$ where the curvature random process takes values.) Let $\mathbb{1}\{condition\}$ denote the (indicator) function that takes on value 1 if *condition* is true, and the value 0 otherwise. With these notations we define the *curve indicator random field V for a single curve* to be

$$V_i := \int_0^T \mathbb{1}\{R_t = i\}dt, \qquad \forall i \in \mathcal{I}.$$

Observe that V_i is the (random) amount of time that the Markov process spent in state i. In particular, V_i is zero unless the Markov process passed through site i. In the context of Brownian motion or other symmetric processes, V is variously known as the occupation measure or the local time of R_t [4, 5].

Generalizing to multiple curves, we pick a random number $\mathcal{N}$, Poisson distributed with average value $\bar{\mathcal{N}}$. We then choose $\mathcal{N}$ independent copies $R_{t_1}^{(1)}, \ldots,$ $R_{t_{\mathcal{N}}}^{(\mathcal{N})}$ of the Markov process R_t, with independent lengths $T_1, \ldots, T_{\mathcal{N}}$, each distributed as T. To define the (multiple curve) CIRF, we take the superposition of the single-curve CIRFs $V^{(1)}, \ldots, V^{(\mathcal{N})}$ for the $\mathcal{N}$ curves.

Definition 1. *The curve indicator random field U is defined to be*

$$U_i := \sum_{n=1}^{\mathcal{N}} V_i^{(n)} = \sum_{n=1}^{\mathcal{N}} \int_0^{T_n} \mathbb{1}\{R_{t_n}^{(n)} = i\} dt_n, \qquad \forall i \in \mathcal{I}.$$

Thus U_i is the total amount of time that all of the Markov processes spent in site i. Again, observe that this definition satisfies our desiderata for an ideal edge/line map: (1) non-zero value where the contours are, and (2) zero-value elsewhere. The probability distribution of U will become our prior for inference.

4.2   Statistics of the Curve Indicator Random Field

Probabilistic models in vision and pattern recognition have been specified in a number of ways. For example, Markov random field models [7] are specified via clique potentials and Gaussian models are specified via means and covariances. Here, instead of providing the distribution of the curve indicator random field itself, we report its moment generating functional, from which all moments can be computed straightforwardly.

Before doing so, we need to develop more Markov process theory. We first define the inner product $(a, b) = \sum_{i \in \mathcal{I}} a_i b_i$. The *generator* of the Markov process R_t is the $|\mathcal{I}| \times |\mathcal{I}|$ matrix $L = (l_{ij})$, and is the instantaneous rate of change of the probability transition matrix $P(t) = (p_{ij})(t)$ for R_t. For the curvature process, we let L be a discretization of the partial differential operator on the right hand side of (1), or

$$L \approx \frac{\sigma_\kappa^2}{2} \frac{\partial^2}{\partial \kappa^2} - \cos \theta \frac{\partial}{\partial x} - \sin \theta \frac{\partial}{\partial y} - \kappa \frac{\partial}{\partial \theta} \qquad \text{(curvature process)},$$

and for the direction process, L is the discretization of the corresponding operator in (2), or

$$L \approx \frac{\sigma_\kappa^2}{2} \frac{\partial^2}{\partial \theta^2} - \cos \theta \frac{\partial}{\partial x} - \sin \theta \frac{\partial}{\partial y} \qquad \text{(direction process)}.$$

To include the exponential distribution over T (the lifetime of each particle), we construct a *killed* Markov process with generator $Q = L - \lambda^{-1} I$. (Formally, we do this by adding a single "death" state $\dagger$ to the discrete state space $\mathcal{I}$. When $t \geq T$, the process enters $\dagger$ and it cannot leave.) Slightly changing our notation, we shall now use R_t to mean the killed Markov process with generator Q. The Green's function matrix $G = (g_{ij})$ of the Markov process is the matrix $\int_0^\infty e^{Qt}dt = \int_0^\infty P(t)e^{-t/\lambda}dt$, where $P(t) = e^{Lt}$ (e^A denotes the matrix exponential of matrix A). The (i, j)-entry g_{ij} in the Green's function matrix G represents the expected amount of time that the Markov process spent in j before death, given that the process started in i. One can show that $G = -Q^{-1}$. Given a vector $c \in \mathbb{R}^{|\mathcal{I}|}$ having sufficiently small entries c_i, we define the Green's function matrix $G(c)$ with spatially-varying "creation" c as the Green's function matrix for the killed Markov process with extra killing $-c$, i.e., having generator $Q(c) := Q + \text{diag}\, c$, where $\text{diag}\, c$ is a diagonal matrix with the entries of vector c along the diagonal; in particular, $G(c) = -Q(c)^{-1} = -(Q + \text{diag}\, c)^{-1}$.

Recalling that each Markov process $R_{t_1}^{(1)}, \ldots, R_{t_N}^{(N)}$ is distributed as R_t, let the joint distribution of the initial and final states of R_t be

$$\mathbb{P}\{R_0 = i, R_{T-} = j\} = \mu_i g_{ij} \nu_j, \qquad \forall i, j \in \mathcal{I},$$

where $\mu = (\mu_i)$ and $\nu = (\nu_i)$ are vectors in $\mathbb{R}^{|\mathcal{I}|}$ weighting initial and final states, respectively, and $f(T-)$ is the limit of $f(t)$ for t approaching T from below. Therefore, vectors μ and ν must satisfy the *normalization constraint* $(\mu, G\nu) = 1$. For general purpose contour enhancement, we typically have no a-priori preference for the start and end locations of each contour, and so we set these vectors proportional to the constant vector $\mathbf{1} = (1, \ldots, 1)$. For example, by setting $\mu = |\mathcal{I}|^{-1}\mathbf{1}, \nu = \lambda^{-1}\mathbf{1}$, the normalization constraint is satisfied.

The following key theoretical result is used in this paper but is developed in [1], and is most closely related to the work of Dynkin [4].

Proposition 1. *The moment generating functional of the curve indicator random field U is*

$$\mathbb{E}\exp(c, U) = \exp(\mu, \bar{\mathcal{N}}(G(c) - G)\nu).$$

While this result may seem abstract, it is actually very useful. Let G^* denote the transpose of G. From Prop. 1 we obtain the first two cumulants of the CIRF [2]:

Corollary 1. *Suppose the $\mu = |\mathcal{I}|^{-1}\mathbf{1}, \nu = \lambda^{-1}\mathbf{1}$. The mean of the curve indicator random field U is $\mathbb{E}\, U_i = \bar{\mathcal{N}}\lambda|\mathcal{I}|^{-1}, \forall i \in \mathcal{I}$. The covariance matrix of U is* $\text{cov}\, U = \bar{\mathcal{N}}\lambda|\mathcal{I}|^{-1}(G + G^*)$.

Several "columns" of the covariance matrix for the curvature process are illustrated in Fig. 4, by taking its impulse response for several positions, directions and curvatures. In addition, using Prop. 1 one can compute the higher-order cumulants of U, and they are generally *not* zero, which shows that *the curve indicator random field is non-Gaussian* [1]. Despite that, its moment generating functional has a tractable form that we shall directly exploit next.

5   Minimum Mean Square Error Filtering

Instead of the unknown random field U, what we actually observe is some realization m of a random field M of (edge or line) *measurements*. Given m, we seek that approximation $\tilde{u}$ of U that minimizes the mean square error (MMSE), or

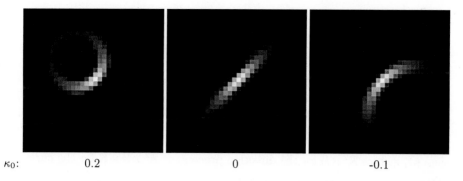

κ_0:   0.2   0   -0.1

Fig. 4. Impulse responses of the covariance matrix for the curve indicator random field for the curvature process. Impulses are located at the center of each image, directed at discrete direction 4 out of 32, with 5 curvatures. Parameters are $\sigma_{\dot{\kappa}} = 0.01, \lambda = 10$.

$$\tilde{u} \triangleq \arg\min_{u} \mathbb{E}_m ||u - U||^2,$$

where $\mathbb{E}_m$ the denotes taking an expectation conditioned on the measurement realization m. It is well-known that the posterior mean is the MMSE estimate

$$\tilde{u} = \mathbb{E}_m U,$$

but in many interesting, non-Gaussian, cases this is extremely difficult to compute. In our context, however, we are fortunate to be able to make use of the moment generating functional to simplify computations.

Before developing our MMSE estimator, we must define our likelihood function $p(M|U)$. First let H_i be the binary random variable taking the value 1 if one of the contours passed through (or "hit") site i, and 0 otherwise, and so H is a binary random field on $\mathcal{I}$. In this paper we consider conditionally independent, local likelihoods: $p(M|H) = p(M_1|H_1)\cdots p(M_{|\mathcal{I}|}|H_{|\mathcal{I}|})$. Following [6, 24], we consider two distributions over measurements at site i: $p_{\mathrm{on}}(M_i) := p(M_i|H_i = 1)$ and $p_{\mathrm{off}}(M_i) := p(M_i|H_i = 0)$. It follows [24] that $\ln p(M|H) = \sum_i \ln(p_{\mathrm{on}}(M_i)/p_{\mathrm{off}}(M_i))H_i$. Now let τ be the average amount of time spent by the Markov processes in a site, given that the site was hit; observe that U_i/τ and H_i are therefore equal on average. This suggests that we replace H with U/τ above to generate a likelihood in U, in particular,

$$\ln p(M|U) \approx \sum_i c_i U_i = (c, U), \text{ where } c_i = c_i(M_i) = \tau^{-1} \ln \frac{p_{\mathrm{on}}(M_i)}{p_{\mathrm{off}}(M_i)}.$$

As shown in [1], the posterior mean in this case becomes

$$\mathbb{E}_m U_i \approx \frac{\partial}{\partial c_i}(\mathbb{E}\exp(c, U))(c) = \bar{\mathcal{N}} f_i b_i, \qquad \forall i \in \mathcal{I}, \tag{5}$$

where $f = (f_1, \ldots, f_{|\mathcal{I}|})$ is the solution to the forward equation

$$(Q + \mathrm{diag}\, c)f + \nu = 0 \tag{6}$$

and $b = (b_1, \ldots, b_{|\mathcal{I}|})$ is the solution to the backward equation

$$(Q^* + \operatorname{diag} c)b + \mu = 0. \tag{7}$$

Note that equations (6) and (7) are linear systems in $\mathbb{R}^{|\mathcal{I}|}$; however, since $Q = L - \lambda^{-1}$, where the generator L is the discretization of an (elliptic) partial differential operator, we view the forward and backward equations as (linear) elliptic partial differential equations, by replacing L with its undiscretized counterpart, and c, f, b, μ, and ν with corresponding (possibly generalized) functions on a continuum, such as $\mathbb{R}^2 \times \mathbb{S}$ for the direction process, or $\mathbb{R}^2 \times \mathbb{S} \times \mathbb{R}$ for the curvature process.

Observe that two nonlinearities arise in this posterior mean in equation (5). First, there is a product of the forward and backward solutions[4]. Second, although both the forward and backward equations are linear, they represent nonlinear mappings from input (c) to output $(f$ or $b)$. For example, it follows that $f = (I - G \operatorname{diag} c)^{-1} G\nu = \sum_{k=0}^{\infty} (G \operatorname{diag} c)^k G\nu$, i.e., f is a polynomial—and thus nonlinear—function of the input c.

5.1   Example Computations

We have implemented a preliminary version of the CIRF posterior mean filter. For our initial experimentation, we adopted a standard additive white Gaussian noise model for the likelihood $p(M|U)$. As a consequence, we have $c(m) = \gamma_1 m - \gamma_2$, a simple transformation of the input m, where γ_1 and $\gamma_2 = 3$ are constants. The direction-dependent input m was set to the result of logical/linear edge and line operators [12]. The output of the logical/linear operator was linearly interpolated to a many directions as necessary. For direction-only filtering, this input interpolation was sufficient, but not for the curvature-based filtering, as *curvature was not directly measured in the image*; instead, the directed logical/linear response was simply copied over all curvature values, i.e., the input m was constant as a function of curvature. The limit of the invertibility of $Q + \operatorname{diag} c$ and its transpose was used to set γ_1 [1]. The technique used to solve the forward and backward CIRF equations for the curvature process in (x, y, θ, κ) will be reported in [1], and are a generalization of the method used for the forward and backward CIRF equations for the Mumford (direction) process in (x, y, θ) [1], which is also used here. Parameter settings were $\bar{N} = 1, \mu = |\mathcal{I}|^{-1}\mathbf{1}, \nu = \lambda^{-1}\mathbf{1}$. The direction-process based CIRF was solved on a grid the size of the given image but with 32 directions. For the curvature-based CIRF filtering, very few curvatures were used (3 or 5) in order to keep down computation times in our unoptimized implementation. Unless we state otherwise, all filtering responses (which are fields over either discrete (x, y, θ)-space or discrete (x, y, θ, κ)-space) are shown summed over all variables except (x, y).

For our first example, we considered a blood cell image (Fig. 5, top). To illustrate robustness, noise was added to a small portion of the image that contained

---

[4] This is analogous to the source/sink product in the stochastic completion field [22].

two cells (top left), and was processed with the logical/linear edge operator at the default settings[5]. The result was first filtered using the CIRF posterior mean based on Mumford's direction process (top center). Despite using two very different bounds on curvature, the direction-based filtering cannot close the blood cell boundaries appropriately. In contrast, the CIRF posterior mean with the curvature process (top right) was more effective at forming a complete boundary. To illustrate in more detail, we plotted the filter responses for the direction-based filter at $\sigma_\kappa = 0.025$ for 8 of the 32 discrete directions in the middle of Fig. 5. The brightness in each of the 8 sub-images is proportional to the response for that particular direction as a function of position (x, y). Observe the over-straightening effect shown by the elongated responses. The curvature filter responses were plotted as a function of direction and curvature (bottom). Despite the input having been constant as a function of curvature, the result shows *curvature selectivity*. Indeed, one can clearly see in the $\kappa > 0$ row (Fig. 5, bottom) that the boundary of the top left blood cell is traced out in a counter-clockwise manner. In the $\kappa < 0$ row, the same cell is traced out in the opposite manner. (Since the parameterization of the curve is lost when forming its image, we cannot know which way the contour was traversed; our result is consistent with both ways.) The response for the lower right blood cell was somewhat weaker but qualitatively similar. Unlike the direction-only process, the curvature process can effectively deal with highly curved contours.

For our next example, we took two sub-images of a low-contrast angiogram (top of Fig. 6; sub-images from left and top right of original). The first sub-image (top left) contained a straight structure, which was enhanced by our curvature-based CIRF filter (summed responses at top right). The distinct responses at separate directions and curvatures show curvature selectivity as well, since the straight curvature at 45° had the greatest response (center). The second sub-image (bottom left) of a loop structure also produced a reasonable filter response (bottom right); the individual responses (bottom) also show some curvature selectivity.

As argued in the Introduction, the bug with a direction-only search cone would mistrack on a contour as curvature builds up. To make this point computationally, we consider an image (top left of Fig. 7) of an Euler spiral extending from a straight line segment[6]. Observe that the contour curvature begins at zero (straight segment) and then builds up gradually. To produce a 3-dimensional input to our direction-based filter, this original (2-d) image was copied to all directions (i.e., $m(x, y, \theta) = \text{image}(x, y)$, for all θ). Similarly, the image was copied to all directions and curvatures to produce a 4-d input to the curvature-based filter. For this test only, our 2-dimensional outputs were produced by taking, at each position (x, y), the maximum response over all directions (for the

---

[5] Code and settings available at http://www.ai.sri.com/~leei/loglin.html.

[6] We used formula (16.7) of Kimia et al [14], and created the plot in Mathematica with all parameters 0, except $\gamma = 0.1$ (Kimia et al's notation). The resulting plot was grabbed, combined with a line segment, blurred with a Gaussian, and then subsampled.

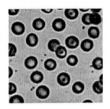

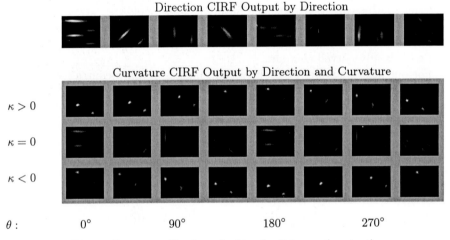

Original	Direction CIRF		Curvature CIRF
	$\sigma_\kappa = 0.025$	$\sigma_\kappa = 0.33$	$\sigma_{\dot{\kappa}} = 0.01$

Direction CIRF Output by Direction

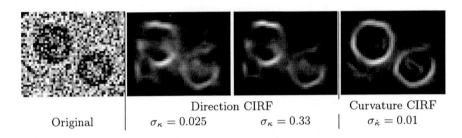

Curvature CIRF Output by Direction and Curvature

$\kappa > 0$

$\kappa = 0$

$\kappa < 0$

$\theta:$ $0°$ $90°$ $180°$ $270°$

Fig. 5. Curvature filtering of a blood cell image (see text).

direction-based filtering) or over all directions and curvatures (for the curvature-based filtering). The direction-based CIRF posterior mean (with parameters $\sigma_\kappa = 0.025, \lambda = 10$, with 64 directions) was computed (center), showing an undesirable reduction in response as curvature built up. The curvature-based CIRF posterior mean (right, with parameters $\sigma_{\dot{\kappa}} = 0.05, \lambda = 10$, 64 directions, and 7 curvatures $(0, \pm 0.05, \pm 0.1, \pm 0.15)$) shows strong response even at the higher curvature portions of the contour. To test robustness, 0-mean Gaussian noise of standard deviation 0.4 was added (bottom left) to the image (0 to 1 was the signal range before adding noise). The results (bottom center and right) show that the curvature-based filter performs better in high curvature regions despite noise.

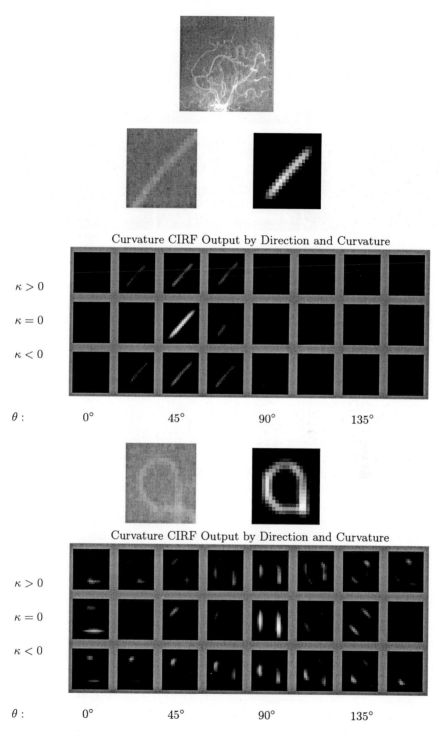

Fig. 6. Curvature filtering for an angiogram (see text).

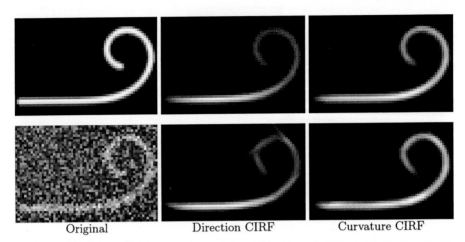

| Original | Direction CIRF | Curvature CIRF |

Fig. 7. Filtering an Euler spiral without noise (top) and with noise (bottom). The original images are on the left; the result after filtering using the curve indicator random field based on Mumford's direction-based Markov process (center) and our curvature-based Markov process (right). Notice that the direction CIRF result tends to repress the signal at high curvatures, while the curvature process has more consistent performance, even at higher curvatures. See text for details.

Computations were conveniently performed using the Python scripting language with numerical extensions in a GNU/Linux environment.

6   Conclusion

In this paper we introduced a new stochastic model for contour curvature to more faithfully capture the shape of image curves. Whereas most contour models penalize large curvatures, our curvature Markov process allows highly curving contours, and only penalizes changes in curvature. The curvature process can be used directly in the curve indicator random field [2, 1] to construct a prior for curve images. To enhance noisy images of contours, we present a nonlinear filter (details in [1]) that approximates the posterior mean of the curve indicator random field. Our initial computations show that the filter responds well along smooth contours, even those having large curvature.

Acknowledgements

We thank Patrick Huggins, Athinodoros Georghiades, Ohad Ben-Shahar, and the reviewers for their helpful comments. This work was supported by AFOSR.

References

1. J. August. *The Curve Indicator Random Field*. PhD thesis, Yale University, 2001.
2. J. August and S. W. Zucker. The curve indicator random field: curve organization via edge correlation. In K. Boyer and S. Sarkar, editors, *Perceptual Organization for Artificial Vision Systems*, pages 265–288. Kluwer Academic, Boston, 2000.

3. A. Dobbins, S. W. Zucker, and M. S. Cynader. Endstopped neurons in the visual cortex as a substrate for calculating curvature. *Nature*, 329(6138):438–441, 1987.

4. E. B. Dynkin. Markov processes as a tool in field theory. *Journal of Functional Analysis*, 50:167–187, 1983.

5. E. B. Dynkin. Gaussian and non-gaussian fields associated with markov processes. *Journal of Functional Analysis*, 55:344–376, 1984.

6. D. Geman and B. Jedynak. An active testing model for tracking roads in satellite images. *IEEE Transactions on Pattern Analysis and Machine Intelligence*, 18(1):1–14, 1996.

7. S. Geman and D. Geman. Stochastic relaxation, gibbs distributions, and the bayesian restoration of images. *IEEE Transactions on Pattern Analysis and Machine Intelligence*, 6(6):721–741, 1984.

8. G. H. Granlund and H. Knutsson. *Signal Processing for Computer Vision*. Kluwer Academic, Dordrecht, 1995.

9. L. Herault and R. Horaud. Figure-ground discrimination: A combinatorial optimization approach. *IEEE Transactions on Pattern Analysis and Machine Intelligence*, 15(9):899–914, 1993.

10. B. K. P. Horn. The Curve of Least Energy. *ACM Transactions on Mathematical Software*, 9:441–460, 1983.

11. L. A. Iverson. *Toward Discrete Geometric Models for Early Vision*. PhD thesis, McGill University, Montreal, 1994.

12. L. A. Iverson and S. W. Zucker. Logical/linear operators for image curves. *IEEE Transactions on Pattern Analysis and Machine Intelligence*, 17(10):982–996, 1995.

13. S. N. Kalitzin, B. M. ter Haar Romeny, and M. A. Viergever. Invertible orientation bundles on 2d scalar images. In *Proc. Scale-Space '97*, LICS, pages 77–88. Springer, 1997.

14. B. B. Kimia, I. Frankel, and A.-M. Popescu. Euler spiral for shape completion. In K. Boyer and S. Sarkar, editors, *Perceptual Organization for Artificial Vision Systems*, pages 289–309. Kluwer Academic, Boston, 2000.

15. J. J. Koenderink and W. Richards. Two-dimensional curvature operators. *J. Opt. Soc. Am. A*, 5(7):1136–1141, 1988.

16. K. Koffka. *Principles of Gestalt Psychology*. Harcourt, Brace & World, New York, 1963.

17. J. L. Marroquin. A markovian random field of piecewise straight lines. *Biological Cybernetics*, 61:457–465, 1989.

18. D. Mumford. *Algebraic Geometry and Its Applications*, chapter Elastica and Computer Vision, pages 491–506. Springer-Verlag, 1994.

19. P. Parent and S. W. Zucker. Trace inference, curvature consistency, and curve detection. *IEEE Transactions on Pattern Analysis and Machine Intelligence*, 11(8):823–839, August 1989.

20. S. Ullman. Filling-in gaps: The shape of subjective contours and a model for their generation. *Biological Cybernetics*, 25:1–6, 1976.

21. S. Urago, J. Zerubia, and M. Berthod. A markovian model for contour grouping. *Pattern Recognition*, 28(5):683–693, 1995.

22. L. Williams and D. Jacobs. Stochastic completion fields: A neural model of illusory contour shape and salience. *Neural Computation*, 9(4):837–858, 1997.

23. L. Williams, T. Wang, and K. Thornber. Computing stochastic completion fields in linear-time using a resolution pyramid. In *Proc. of 7th Intl. Conf. on Computer Analysis of Images and Patterns*, Kiel, Germany, 1997.

24. A. L. Yuille and J. M. Coughlan. Fundamental bounds of bayesian inference: Order parameters and phase transitions for road tracking. *IEEE Transactions on Pattern Analysis and Machine Intelligence*, 22(2):160–173, 2000.
25. S. W. Zucker, A. Dobbins, and L. Iverson. Two stages of curve detection suggest two styles of visual computation. *Neural Computation*, 1:68–89, 1989.
26. S. W. Zucker, R. Hummel, and A. Rosenfeld. An application of relaxation labelling to line and curve enhancement. *IEEE Trans. Computers*, C-26:393–403, 922–929, 1977.

Geodesic Interpolating Splines

Vincent Camion and Laurent Younes

CMLA, ENS de Cachan, CNRS UMR 0876
94235 Cachan CEDEX, France
email: younes@cmla.ens-cachan.fr
fax: 33 1 47 40 59 01
tel: 33 1 47 40 59 18

Abstract. We propose a simple and efficient method to interpolate landmark matching by a non-ambiguous mapping (a diffeomorphism). This method is based on spline interpolation, and on recent techniques developed for the estimation of flows of diffeomorphisms. Experimental results show interpolations of remarkable quality. Moreover, the method provides a Riemannian distance on sets of landmarks (with fixed cardinality), which can be defined intrinsically, without refering to diffeomorphisms. The numerical implementation is simple and efficient, based on an energy minimization by gradient descent. This opens important perspectives for shape analysis, applications in medical imaging, or computer graphics

1 Introduction

This paper proposes a new, efficient and consistent method for generating dense diffeomorphisms within an image from sparse information on the displacements of a finite number of points (landmarks). This is an important issue for image processing and computer graphics, and the problem has generated a large number of publications, starting with the seminal papers of Bookstein (see [3] and references therein). There are numerous applications: generating deformations from the position of control points is used, for example, to synthesize facial expressions, or to compute morphings; analyzing variations of shape has application in medical imaging or face recognition, matching is essential for the construction of anatomical atlases. Jointly with the purpose of interpolating from landmark-matching, comes the issue of measuring the discrepancy between two groups of matched landmarks. This is not an obvious problem, and it seems quite intuitive that the smoothness of the underlying, unobserved, global displacement comes as an essential part for the perceptive impression of discrepancy. A third, important, feature is the consistency of the interpolated displacement, in the sense that it should be one-to-one, ensuring that there cannot be two distinct parts of the original picture which are matched to the same zone in the target.

The method which is described here addresses the three problems simultaneously. It does provide a way to interpolate from landmark-matching, while providing a distance between configurations of landmarks which takes into account the smoothness of the underlying warping, generated as a diffeomorphism

M.A.T. Figueiredo, J. Zerubia, A.K. Jain (Eds.): EMMCVPR 2001, LNCS 2134, pp. 513–527, 2001.

defined on the image grid. As a fourth, non-negligible property, comes the fact that this method is easy to implement, and numerically efficient.

To fix notations, let Ω be a bounded set in the plane. When $(x_1, \ldots, x_N)$, $(y_1, \ldots, y_N)$, two sets of N labeled landmarks in Ω, are given, we shall deal with the problem of finding a diffeomorphism g of Ω, with minimal size (in a sense to be defined), such that, for all i, $g(x_i) \simeq y_i$ (*inexact matching*).

The method which is developed in the sequel takes its roots from three main ideas:

- Interpolating splines, as pioneered by Bookstein in computer vision ([3]), and widely used to generate dense warpings from sparse information.
- Generation of diffeomorphisms as flows (solutions of an ODE), in a framework which guarantees smoothness and consistency, as in [10, 4]
- Computation of geodesic distances (minimal path length) on deformable data, as used in [11, 8].

The analysis results in a simple algorithm to compute diffeomorphisms from landmark data.

The paper is organized as follows. We start by reviewing the elements of spline theory which will be needed, and relate them to the (non-diffeomorphic) interpolation introduced by Bookstein. This forms the first ingredient for our method. In a second step, we give a presentation of the theory of groups of diffeomorphisms, generated as flows (solutions of ODEs) on a set Ω, and show how this framework can be used to generate geodesic distances on structures acted on by diffeomorphisms (ie. deformable patterns). The last step will be to use this framework on the very simple deformable structure which are sets of landmarks, to derive an efficient algorithm for simultaneously computing distances between sets of landmarks and generating a diffeomorphism to interpolate the pointwise matching. The paper ends with a presentation of some experimental facts and data.

2   Landmark matching and splines

2.1   Splines

Like for all landmark-matching methods, the numerical efficiency of the algorithm that we propose relies on spline interpolation theory. For completeness of the presentation, we spend some time in describing the foundations of this theory, exhibiting in particular its remarkable algebraic simplicity.

Formally speaking, spline fitting can be considered a particular case of what follows. let $\mathcal{H}$ be a Hilbert space, let $f_1, \ldots, f_N \in \mathcal{H}$, and $c_1, \ldots, c_N \in \mathbb{R}$ be given. Denote by $\langle . , . \rangle$ the inner product on $\mathcal{H}$. Consider the following problems:

1. Find $h \in \mathcal{H}$ such that $\|h\|$ is minimum subject to the constraints $\langle f_i , h \rangle = c_i$ for $i = 1, \ldots, N$.

2. Fixing $\lambda > 0$, find h such that $\|h\|^2 + \lambda \sum_{i=1}^{N}(\langle f_i\,, h \rangle - c_i)^2$ is minimum.

The first problem corresponds to interpolation, or exact matching, the second one to smoothing, or approximate matching, and both are solved by elementary linear algebra. It is indeed clear that, in both cases, the constraints are not affected if h is replaced by $h + v$ where v is orthogonal to all the f_i, so that the solution must in fact be searched in the linear space spanned by $f_1, \ldots, f_N$: so, introduce the $N \times N$ matrix S with $S_{ij} = \langle f_i\,, f_j \rangle$, and express the unknown h as a linear combination $h = \sum_{i=1}^{N} \alpha_i f_i$.

Problem 1 now requires to minimize ${}^t\alpha S \alpha$ subject to the constraint $S\alpha = c$ (where α and c are vectors with components α_i and c_i respectively), and problem 2 to minimize ${}^t\alpha S \alpha + \lambda\, {}^t(S\alpha - c)(S\alpha - c)$

Assume that S is invertible, so that no linear constraint can be deduced one from another [1]. The solution of problem 1 is in fact uniquely specified by the constraint: it is $\alpha = S^{-1}.c$. For the second problem, routine computations shows that it is $\alpha = S_\lambda^{-1}.c$ with $S_\lambda = S + I/\lambda$ (the invertibility of S is here not required).

Let us see how this applies to splines. In this context, a set of points $(x_1, \ldots, x_N)$ in Ω is given, together with real numbers $c_1, \ldots, c_N$, and spline interpolation corresponds to finding a real-valued function h (defined on Ω), as smooth as possible, such that $h(x_i) = c_i$ or $h(x_i) \simeq c_i$. The smoothness of h is evaluated through a norm of the kind

$$\|h\|_L = \int_\Omega |Lh|^2 dx$$

where L is, say, a differential operator. This norm defines a Hilbert space of functions $\mathcal{H}_L$, with inner-product

$$\langle h\,, g \rangle_L = \int_\Omega LhLg\, dx\,.$$

The constraints $h(x_i) = c_i$ are linear in h, and the issue, to fit in the previous abstract setting, is whether there exists an element f_{x_i} in $\mathcal{H}_L$ such that, for all $h \in \mathcal{H}_L$ $h(x_i) = \langle f_{x_i}\,, h \rangle_L$. If this can be done[2], the solution of the interpolation problem is given by a linear combination of the f_{x_i}, the coefficients of which are simply obtained by applying the inverse of the matrix of inner-products of the f_{x_i} to the values of the constraints c_i. A similar conclusion can be drawn if we replace this exact interpolation problem by an inexact form, which consists in minimizing

$$\|h\|_L + \lambda \sum_{i=1}^{N}(h(x_i) - c_i)^2$$

---

[1] Problem 1 may have no solution when S is not invertible

[2] This is equivalent, by the Riesz representation theorem, to the continuity of the evaluation mapping $h \mapsto h(x)$ for the norm $\|.\|_L$

It must be noted that the inner-products $\langle f_{x_i}, f_{x_j} \rangle$ are, by construction, given by $f_{x_i}(x_j)$ (f is self-reproducing), so that their computation is immediate.

So everything depends on the existence of f_x. Theoretical arguments for proving this existence can be given (linked, for example, to Sobolev's inclusion theorems when L is a differential operator) but, for practical purposes, it is also necessary to have an analytical and computable expression for them. The functions f are obtained from the Green kernel of the operator $L^*.L$. [3] So, practical applicability of spline interpolation depends on whether the Green kernel of K is known or not, provided of course it exists at all.

Well-know cases in which explicit expressions for Green functions are available are when L is a variant of the Laplacian (with simple enough boundary conditions). However, this can be too specific in some applications, and noting that the method never requires explicit knowledge of L, it is possible to start directly with a function $(x, y) \mapsto f_x(y)$ provided that one knows that f is the Green kernel of some positive operator K (not necessarily a differential operator), which needs not be specified. Non constructive existence assumptions exist, for example one may require that f is symmetric ($f_x(y) = f_y(x)$), continuous, squared-integrable and induces a positive operator on $\mathcal{L}^2$, the last requirement being satisfied when $f_x(y) = F(x - y)$, F being the Fourier transform of a positive, even function.

In [2], [1], these requirements are further specialized to ensure that f a radial basis function: $f_x(y) = G(|x - y|)$, the simplest example being the Gaussian $G(t) = \exp(-t^2/\sigma^2)$. This additional assumption has the advantage to provide rotation invariant interpolation (which is also true when L is a linear combination of powers of the Laplacian).

2.2   Landmark matching and Bookstein's splines

For diffeomorphic matching, it must be taken into account, to apply the previous, that the unknown function is vector valued. In fact, if $x_1, \ldots, x_N$ and $y_1, \ldots, y_N$ are two matched sets of landmarks, one should find a diffeomorphism $h : \Omega \to \Omega$ such that $h(x_i) = y_i$ (equivalently, one searches a displacement $u = h - \mathrm{id}$ such that $u(x_i) = y_i - x_i$).

Bookstein (see [3]) proposes to apply spline interpolation to each component of u. This is the simplest approach, and we will keep to this setting in this

---

[3] Let L^* be the dual operator of L, which is such that, for all g and h with compact support in Ω,

$$\int_\Omega (Lh)g = \int_\Omega (L^*g)h$$

and let $K = L^*.L$. For all x, one has

$$h(x) = \langle f_x, h \rangle_L = \int_\Omega Lf_x Lh \, dy = \int_\Omega f_x K h \, dy$$

which is precisely the definition of the fact that the function $(x, y) \mapsto f_x(y)$ is the Green kernel K. (K is also affected by boundary conditions, but we omit the complications here).

paper. But it must be remarked that this is not a general point of view, the Green function being, in this context, naturally expressed as a *matrix* of kernels.

Returning to Bookstein splines, consider the inner-product

$$\langle h\,,\,g\rangle = \int_{\mathbb{R}^2} \Delta h \Delta g \, dx\,. \tag{1}$$

$\mathcal{H}$ being the space of functions with square integrable second derivatives (a Beppo-Levi space). This space is not, strictly speaking, a Hilbert space, because the inner product is degenerate (it vanishes for affine functions), but can considered as one provided one consideres that functions which only differ by an affine function are equal.

With this in mind, let $U(r) = r^2 \log r$: this function is such that, for any smooth function $h \in \mathcal{H}$,

$$h(x) = \int_{\mathbb{R}^2} U(|x-y|)\Delta^2 h(y) dy$$

where Δ^2 is the iterated Laplacian, and equality being up to the addition of an affine function (cf [7]). Letting $f_x(y) = U(|x-y|)$, this is $\langle f_x\,,\,h\rangle = h(x)$ (up to an affine function). So let c_i be one of the components of $y_i - x_i$, so that the constraints $h(x_i) = c_i$ for $i = 1$ to N write: there exist $a = (a^1, a^2) \in \mathbb{R}^2$, $b \in \mathbb{R}$ such that, for all i : $\langle h\,,\,f_{x_i}\rangle = c_i - {}^t a x_i - b$.

Let $S_{ij} = \langle f_{x_i}\,,\,f_{x_j}\rangle = U(|x_i - x_j|)$. The interpolation problem becomes: minimize ${}^t\alpha S\alpha$ with the constraint $S\alpha + Q\gamma = c$ where $\gamma = {}^t(a^1 a^2 b)$ is a 3×1 matrix and Q is a $N \times 3$ matrix, given by, letting $x_i = (x_i^1, x_i^2)$:

$$Q = \begin{pmatrix} x_1^1 & x_1^2 & 1 \\ \vdots & \vdots & \vdots \\ x_N^1 & x_N^2 & 1 \end{pmatrix}$$

solving this problem in (α, γ) yields $\hat{\gamma} = \left({}^t Q S^{-1} Q\right)^{-1} {}^t Q c$ and $\hat{\alpha} = S^{-1}(c - Q\hat{\gamma})$.

The smoothing problem requires minimizing

$${}^t\alpha S\alpha + \lambda {}^t(S\alpha + {}^t a x_i + b - c)(S\alpha + {}^t a x_i + b - c)$$

and its solution is formally similar to the previous one, simply replacing S by $S_\lambda = S + (1/\lambda)I$ in the formulas.

When this is applied to both components of $y_i - x_i$, one obtains a function u such that $u(x_i) = y_i - x_i$ for exact matching, which thus provides a smooth interpolation of the landmark correspondence. However, *there is no constraint in this approach, which ensures that* $h(x) = x + u(x)$ *is one-to-one*: folding is indeed possible, and examples will be given in the last section of this paper. We shall obtain a rigorous one-to-one matching using flows of diffeomorphisms, as introduced in the next section.

3   Diffeomorphic landmark matching

One way to introduce the groups of diffeomorphisms we shall be dealing with starts from standard methods for generating metrics and distances on sets acted on by groups. We address this in the next section.

3.1   Distances and group actions

General facts We start with a short algebraic section in which basic facts on how inducing a distance from a group action are obtained, introducing in particular a "least-action principle". First recall that a distance on a set $\mathcal{I}$ is a mapping $d : \mathcal{I}^2 \mapsto \mathbb{R}_+$ such that, for all $I, I', I'' \in \mathcal{I}$: D1) $d(I, I') = 0 \Leftrightarrow I = I'$, D2) $d(I, I') = d(I', I)$, D3) $d(I, I'') \leq d(I, I') + d(I', I'')$.

If D1) is not true and $d(I, I) = 0$ for all I, we use the term *pseudo-distance*.

A group G is acting on $\mathcal{I}$ if an operation $(g, I) \to g.I$ is defined on $G \times \mathcal{I}$ with values in $\mathcal{I}$ such that $\mathrm{id}_G.I = I$ and $g.(h.I) = (gh).I$ for all $I \in \mathcal{I}$ and all $g, h \in G$. If G is a group acting on $\mathcal{I}$, one says that a distance d on $\mathcal{I}$ is G-equivariant if and only if, for all $g \in G$, for all $I, I' \in \mathcal{I}$, $d(g.I, g.I') = d(I, I')$.

We shall be dealing with the following construction. Let G act on $\mathcal{I}$, and consider the product $\mathcal{O} = G \times \mathcal{I}$, so that G also acts on $\mathcal{O}$ (simply letting, for $k \in G$, $o = (h, I) \in \mathcal{O}$: $k.o = (kh, k.I)$).

For $o = (h, I) \in \mathcal{O}$, let $\pi(o) = h^{-1}.I$. Assume that $d_{\mathcal{O}}$ is a distance on $\mathcal{O}$, and let, for $I, I' \in \mathcal{I}$

$$d(I, I') = \inf\{d_{\mathcal{O}}(o, o'), o, o' \in \mathcal{O}, \pi(o) = I, \pi(o') = I'\} \qquad (2)$$

Proposition 1. *If $d_{\mathcal{O}}$ is G-equivariant, then d in (2) is a pseudo-distance on $\mathcal{I}$*

We shall use these results for landmarks, letting diffeomorphisms act on them. This however asks the problem of building an invariant distance on $\mathcal{O}$: one simple approach for this is to use geodesics in this space, as presented in the next section.

Infinitesimal approach A standard way for building distances on sets like $\mathcal{O}$ is to compute shortests paths. Assume that we are able to give a meaning of the speed $V_{\mathbf{o}}(t) = \frac{d\mathbf{o}}{dt}$ of a path $\mathbf{o} : t \mapsto \mathbf{o}(t)$ on $\mathcal{O}$. Assume also that, for each $o \in \mathcal{O}$, we have a way to quantify the speeds of paths passing through o with the help of a norm $V \mapsto \|V\|_o$ (the norm depends on o). Then, let the associated path energy be given by

$$E(\mathbf{o}) = \int_0^1 \|V_{\mathbf{o}}(t)\|^2_{\mathbf{o}(t)} \, dt \qquad (3)$$

and the *geodesic distance* on $\mathcal{O}$ be then defined by

$$d_{\mathcal{O}}(o, o') = \inf\{\sqrt{E(\mathbf{o})}, \mathbf{o}(0) = o, \mathbf{o}(1) = o'\} . \qquad (4)$$

To build a G-equivariant distance (as required by proposition 1), it suffices to start with a family of norms $(\|.\|_o, o \in \mathcal{O})$ which shares this property, in the sense that, if $\mathbf{o}$ is a path on $\mathcal{O}$ and $h \in G$, then the translated path $h.\mathbf{o}$ and $\mathbf{o}$ both have the same speeds at the same times: this writes

$$\|V_{h.\mathbf{o}}(t)\|_{h.\mathbf{o}(t)} = \|V_{\mathbf{o}}(t)\|_{\mathbf{o}(t)} \tag{5}$$

One can interpret this formula with the help of the differential of the action of G on $\mathcal{O}$, but the meaning and the consequences of (5) will be easily derived, and we will not need to introduce the usual machinery of differential geometry.

It is important to notice that this condition provides norms of velocities at translated objects $h.o$ as soon as these norms are known at o. Since $\mathcal{O} = G \times \mathcal{I}$, it thus suffices to define $\|.\|_o$ for $o \in \mathcal{O}$ of the kind $o = (\mathrm{id}_G, I)$.

3.2   Mixing deformations and object variations: landmark matching

We specialize the point of view of section 3.1, by letting G be a group of diffeomorphisms of Ω and $\mathcal{I}$ be the set of all collections of N landmarks on Ω. An element of $\mathcal{I}$ is thus a N-tuple $I = (p_1, \dots, p_N) \in \Omega^N$. We use on G the product $gh = h \circ g$ and define the action of G on $\mathcal{I}$ to be

$$g.I = (g^{-1}(p_1), \dots, g^{-1}(p_N))$$

which does provide a left-action: $(gh).I = g.(h.I)$.

Following the lines of section 3.1, we consider paths on $\mathcal{O}$. Such a path takes the form $\mathbf{o}(t) = (\mathbf{g}(t,.), \mathbf{p}_1(t), \dots, \mathbf{p}_N(t))$ where $\mathbf{g}(t,.)$ is a time dependent diffeomorphism and $\mathbf{p}_i(t)$ is a curve in Ω for $i = 1, \dots, N$ (landmark trajectory). The velocity at $\mathbf{o}(t)$ is

$$V_{\mathbf{o}}(t) = \left(V_{\mathbf{g}}(t), \frac{d\mathbf{p}_1}{dt}(t), \dots, \frac{d\mathbf{p}_N}{dt}(t) \right)$$

with $V_{\mathbf{g}}(t) = \frac{\partial \mathbf{g}}{\partial t}$.

Let h be a diffeomorphism; the path $h.\mathbf{o}$ is given by

$$h.\mathbf{o}(t) = (\mathbf{g}(t, h(.)), h^{-1}(\mathbf{p}_1(t)), \dots, h^{-1}(\mathbf{p}_N(t)))$$

and its speed is

$$V_{h.\mathbf{o}}(t) = \left(V_{\mathbf{g}} \circ h(t), D_{\mathbf{p}_1(t)} h^{-1} \frac{d\mathbf{p}_1}{dt}(t), \dots, D_{\mathbf{p}_N(t)} h^{-1} \frac{d\mathbf{p}_N}{dt}(t) \right)$$

where $D_p h^{-1}(t)$ is the differential of $h^{-1}(.)$ with respect to spatial coordinates, evaluated at a point $p \in \Omega$. Equation (5), requires that

$$\|V_{h.\mathbf{o}}(t)\|_{h.\mathbf{o}(t)} = \|V_{\mathbf{o}}(t)\|_{\mathbf{o}(t)}$$

This is true in particular when h is the inverse of $\mathbf{g}(t,.)$, yielding

$$\|V_{\mathbf{o}}(t)\|_{\mathbf{o}(t)} = \|V_{\mathbf{g}^{-1}\mathbf{o}}(t)\|_{\mathbf{g}^{-1}.\mathbf{o}(t)}$$

so that it is only necessary to define norms at elements $o = (id, p_1, \ldots, p_N)$. We have,

$$V_{g^{-1}o}(t) = \left(\mathbf{v_g}(t), D_{\mathbf{p}_1(t)}\mathbf{g}(t)\frac{d\mathbf{p}_1}{dt}(t), \ldots, D_{\mathbf{p}_N(t)}\mathbf{g}(t)\frac{d\mathbf{p}_N}{dt}(t)\right)$$

in which we have let $\mathbf{v_g}(t, y) = \mathbf{V_g}(t, \mathbf{g}^{-1}(t, y))$. Making the change of variables $\mathbf{q}_i(t) = \mathbf{g}(t, \mathbf{p}_i(t))$, this writes

$$\mathbf{V}_{g^{-1}o}(t) = \left(\mathbf{v_g}(t), \frac{d\mathbf{q}_1}{dt}(t) + \mathbf{v_g}(t, \mathbf{q}_1(t)), \ldots, \frac{d\mathbf{q}_N}{dt}(t) - \mathbf{v_g}(t, \mathbf{q}_N(t))\right)$$

and the energy of the path $o(t)$ takes the form

$$E(\mathbf{o}) = \int_0^1 \left\|\mathbf{v_g}(t), \frac{d\mathbf{q}_1}{dt}(t) + \mathbf{v_g}(t, \mathbf{q}_1(t)), \ldots, \frac{d\mathbf{q}_N}{dt}(t) - \mathbf{v_g}(t, \mathbf{q}_N(t))\right\|^2 dt$$

with a certain norm, which may depend on the current position $(\mathbf{q}_1(t), \ldots, \mathbf{q}_N(t))$.

The essential trick, for building diffeomorphisms (in theory and in practice), is to replace the unknown time-dependent diffeomorphism $\mathbf{g}$ by its so-called Eulerian velocity $\mathbf{v_g}$ on which everything now depends. Noting that, by definition:

$$\frac{\partial \mathbf{g}}{\partial t} = \mathbf{v_g}(t, \mathbf{g}(t))$$

knowing $\mathbf{v}$ allows to compute $\mathbf{g}$ by integration of an ODE, providing in that way a flow of diffeomorphisms (under smoothness conditions on $\mathbf{v}$ which have been studied in detail in [10] and [4]).

So, we know think in terms of $\mathbf{v}$ rather of $\mathbf{g}$. To compute the distance between two elements of $\mathcal{O}$, it suffices to minimize the energy of the paths which link them. We now restrict to the particular case when

$$E(\mathbf{o}) = \int_0^1 \int_\Omega |L\mathbf{v_g}(t)|^2 dt dx + \sum_{i=1}^N \int_0^1 \left|\frac{d\mathbf{q}_i}{dt}(t) - \mathbf{v_g}(t, \mathbf{q}_i(t))\right|^2 dt$$

and L being some operator acting on $v(t)$ for all t. We are interested by the distance between two sets of landmarks I and I', which is given, according to (2)

$$d(I, I') = \inf\{d_\mathcal{O}(o, o'), o, o' \in \mathcal{O}, \pi(o) = I, \pi(o') = I'\}$$

where $\pi(g, p_1, \ldots, p_N) = g^{-1}(p_1, \ldots, p_N) = (g(p_1), \ldots, g(p_N))$. It is not difficult to check that in fact, $d(I, I')$ is the infimum of

$$\int_0^1 \int_\Omega |L\mathbf{v}(t)|^2 dt dx + \sum_{i=1}^N \int_0^1 |\frac{d\mathbf{q}_i}{dt}(t) - \mathbf{v}(t, \mathbf{q}_i(t))|^2 dt \qquad (6)$$

over all time dependent velocities $\mathbf{v}$ on Ω, and over all curves $\mathbf{q}_1(.), \ldots, \mathbf{q}_N(.)$ such that $I = (\mathbf{q}_1(0), \ldots, \mathbf{q}_N(0))$ and $I' = (\mathbf{q}_1(1), \ldots, \mathbf{q}_N(1))$. We thus obtain a new landmark-based matching formula, which only involves the velocity, and which, in the same time, provides a distance between sets of landmarks. For fixed trajectories $\mathbf{q}_i(.), i = 1, \ldots, N$, the optimal $\mathbf{v}$ can be explicitly computed at each time t, in function of the Green kernel of L^*L, as developed in section 2.1: this is the basis of the numerical algorithm which is detailed in section 4.

The final form of the energy is somehow reminiscent from S. Joshi's landmark matching method, which is also based on flows of diffeomorphisms ([6]). The main difference comes from the fact that Joshi's method does not optimize landmark trajectories, but rather uses an end-point matching penalty which leads to an optimal control formulation. There are two consequences of this: the first one is that this does not provide a metric between landmark configurations, whereas the methods derived here provides this feature as an initial motivation. The second one is that the numerical problem in our case is much simpler, as will be seen in section 4.

3.3   A Riemannian metric on deformable landmark configurations

An interesting feature of the previous construction can be pointed out here: it is that minimizing (6) with boundary conditions only in $\mathbf{q}$ is equivalent to compute a *geodesic path* for a specific metric on the set of configurations of N landmarks. Indeed, for $I = (q_1, \ldots, q_N) \in \Omega^N$, and for $h = (h_1, \ldots, h_N) \in \left(\mathbb{R}^2\right)^N$, define

$$\|h\|_I^2 = \min_v \int_\Omega |Lv|\, dx + \lambda \sum_{i=1}^N |h_i - v(q_i)|^2$$

It is easy to prove that $\|h\|_I$ is a norm as a function of h, which therefore provides a Riemannian metric on Ω^N, and to check that the optimal trajectories $\mathbf{I}(.) = (\mathbf{q}_1(.), \ldots, \mathbf{q}_N(.))$ minimize the energy

$$E(\mathbf{I}) = \int_0^1 \left\| \frac{d\mathbf{I}}{dt} \right\|_{\mathbf{I}(t)}^2 dt$$

with fixed boundary conditions at time 0 and at time 1, yielding the fact that they are geodesics. Noting, moreover, that, for a given h, the minimizing v in the definition of $\|h\|_I$ can be explicitly computed, provided that the Green function of L^*L is known (cf section 2.1), we finally obtain an explicit view of Ω^N as a Riemanian manifold, in which diffeomorphisms are now only implicit.

4   Experiments

4.1   Implementation details

The simplest numerical scheme is not to directly work with the geodesic energy of the previous section. We give ourselves a Green function, denoted f, as in section 2.1, associated to some operator L we do not need to compute. For each t, the optimal $\mathbf{v}$ must have the form

$$\mathbf{v}(t, x) = \sum_{k=1}^{N} \alpha_k(t) f(q_k(t), x)$$

where for each k and t, $\alpha_k(t)$ is a 2D vector. The energy in (6) writes, as a function of α and q:

$$E(\alpha, q) = \sum_{k,l=1}^{N} \int_0^1 \langle \alpha_k(t), \alpha_l(t) \rangle f(q_k(t), q_l(t)) dt$$

$$+ \lambda \sum_{k=1}^{n} \int_0^1 \left\| \frac{dq_k}{dt} - \sum_{l=1}^{N} \alpha_l(t) f(q_l(t), q_k(t)) \right\|^2 dt \quad (7)$$

in which we use norms and inner products in $\mathbb{R}^2$. Now, for fixed q, the optimal α is explicit. Let $S(t)$ be the $N \times N$ matrix with coefficients $f(q_l(t), q_k(t))$, and let $S_\lambda(t) = S(t) + I/\lambda$. Letting $\alpha^i = (\alpha_1^i, \dots, \alpha_N^i)$ and $q^i = (q_1^i, \dots, q_N^i)$, $i = 1, 2$, we have, for all t

$$\alpha^i(t) = [S_\lambda(t)]^{-1} . q^i(t)$$

Minimizing in q with fixed α is not explicit, but the gradient of E in q can be computed. We assume a time discretization of order T, and set, for $t = 0, \dots, T-1$: $D_t u = T(u(t+1) - u(t))$ for a time dependent function u. The discretized energy takes the form

$$E(\alpha, q) = \sum_{k,l=1}^{N} \sum_{t=0}^{T} \langle \alpha_k(t), \alpha_l(t) \rangle f(q_k(t), q_l(t))$$

$$+ \lambda \sum_{k=1}^{N} \sum_{t=0}^{T-1} \left\| D_t q_k - \sum_{l=1}^{N} \alpha_l(t) f(q_l(t), q_k(t)) \right\|^2 \quad (8)$$

Introduce the notation $Z_k(t) = D_t q_k - \sum_{l=1}^{N} \alpha_l(t) f(q_l(t), q_k(t))$.

The partial derivative of E with respect to $q_k(t)$ is a 2D vector, given by, for $t = 1, \dots T-1$:

$$\frac{\partial E}{\partial q_k(t)} = 2 \sum_{l=1}^{N} \langle \alpha_k(t), \alpha_l(t) \rangle \nabla_1 f(q_k(t), q_l(t)) - 2\lambda T D_{t-1} Z_k$$

$$- 2\lambda \sum_{l=1}^{N} (\langle \alpha_k(t), Z_l(t) \rangle + \langle \alpha_l(t), Z_k(t) \rangle) \nabla_1 f(q_k(t), q_l(t)) \quad (9)$$

where $\nabla_1 f \in \mathbb{R}^2$ denotes the gradient of f with respect to one of its variables (it does not matter which one, f is symmetric). Note that $q(0)$ and $q(T)$ are clamped to the boundary conditions.

The optimal landmark trajectories are computed by iterating the following steps until convergence (initializing with $\alpha = 0$ and linear trajectories)

1. Gradient step for q: for all $t = 2, \ldots T - 1$, substract to $q_k(t)$ a quantity proportional to $\dfrac{\partial E}{\partial q_k(t)}$

2. Velocity updating: set $\alpha^i(t) = [S_\lambda(t)]^{-1} . q^i(t)$, $t = 1, \ldots, T - 1$, $i = 1, 2$

Thin-plate generalization We now show how this can be modified to incorporate affine invariance as in the thin-plate case. If L is the Laplacian, we have seen in section 2.2 that, for each t, $v(t, x)$ is defined up to an affine component which may in turn be optimized. This yields an expression

$$\mathbf{v}(t, x) = a(t)x + b(t) + \sum_{k=1}^{N} \alpha_k(t) f(q_k(t), x)$$

for the unknown velocity field, $a(t)$ being a 2×2 matrix and $b(t) \in \mathbb{R}^2$. Let $\gamma^i(t)$ be a column of the 3×2 matrix ${}^t[a(t)b(t)]$, $i = 1, 2$. When trajectories are fixed, the optimal coefficients are given like in section 2.2 by

$$\gamma^i(t) = \left({}^t Q(t) S_\lambda^{-1}(t) Q(t) \right)^{-1} {}^t Q(t) \frac{dq^i}{dt}$$

and $\alpha^i(t) = S_\lambda^{-1} \left(\dfrac{dq^i}{dt} - Q(t) \gamma^i(t) \right)$ where S_λ is as above and

$$Q(t) = \begin{pmatrix} q_1^1(t) & q_1^2(t) & 1 \\ \vdots & \vdots & \vdots \\ q_N^1(t) & q_N^2(t) & 1 \end{pmatrix}$$

The modification of the gradient equation in $q(t)$ is almost straightforward and we only give the result in discretized form, letting

$$Z_k(t) = D_t q_k - a(t) q_k(t) - b(t) - \sum_{l=1}^{N} \alpha_l(t) f(q_l(t), q_k(t))$$

so that the minimized energy is

$$E(\alpha, q) = \sum_{k,l=1}^{N} \sum_{t=0}^{T} \langle \alpha_k(t), \alpha_l(t) \rangle f(q_k(t), q_l(t)) + \lambda \sum_{k=1}^{N} \sum_{t=0}^{T-1} \|Z_k(t)\|^2 . \quad (10)$$

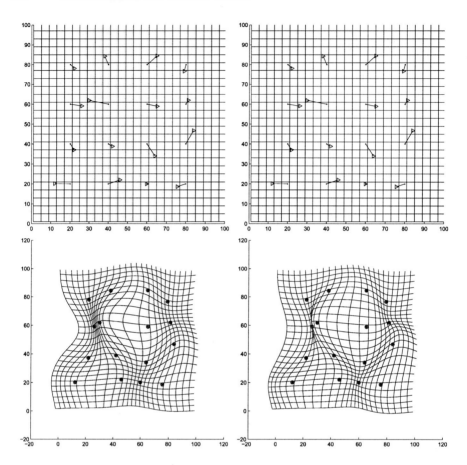

Fig. 1. Random point displacements: small deformations; upper-left: evenly spaced points and random displacements ; upper-right: optimal trajectories ; down-left: estimated diffeomorphism ; down-right: interpolated displacement field by classical splines.

We have

$$\frac{\partial E}{\partial q_k(t)} = 2 \sum_{l=1}^{N} \langle \alpha_k(t) , \alpha_l(t) \rangle \nabla_1 f(q_k(t), q_l(t)) - 2\lambda T D_{t-1} Z_k$$

$$- 2\lambda \sum_{l=1}^{N} (\langle \alpha_k(t) , Z_l(t) \rangle + \langle \alpha_l(t) , Z_k(t) \rangle) \nabla_1 f(q_k(t), q_l(t)) - 2\lambda \, {}^t a(t) Z_k(t) .$$

$$(11)$$

Note that we wrote everything for 2D matching, but that the formulas can obviously generalize to any number of dimensions.

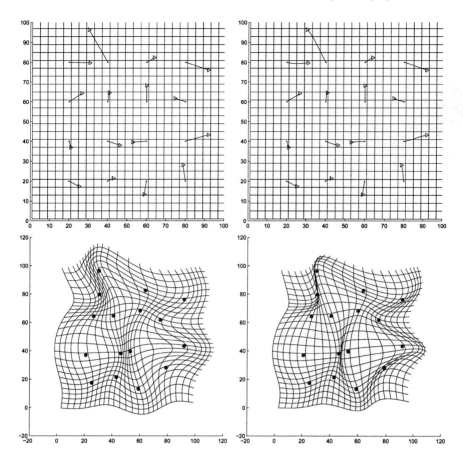

Fig. 2. Random point displacements: average deformations; upper-left: evenly spaced points and random displacements ; upper-right: optimal trajectories ; down-left: estimated diffeomorphism ; down-right: interpolated displacement field by classical splines

4.2   Experiments

In the proposed experiments, random displacements are attributed to points evenly distributed on a grid. Interpolated deformation and landmark trajectories are computed. This is compared to classical spline interpolation (which just corresponds to $T = 2$ in the previous algorithm). The Green kernel, f is Gaussian: $f(x, y) = \exp\left(-|x - y|^2/2\sigma^2\right)$.

Three experiments are presented. The first one generates small displacements, the last one very large ones. Progressively, one sees the singularities generated by classical interpolating splines increase, foldings being created, while geodesic splines remain one-to-one, and of rather impressive smoothness. The estimated landmarks trajectories start to bend in the second experiments, and are clearly curved in the last one.

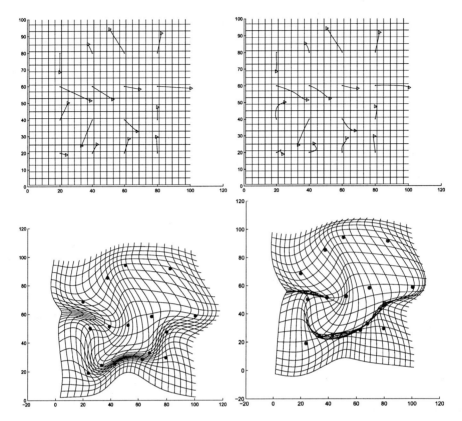

Fig. 3. Random point displacements: large deformations; upper-left: evenly spaced points and random displacements ; upper-right: optimal trajectories ; down-left: estimated diffeomorphism ; down-right: interpolated displacement field by classical splines

References

1. N. ARAD, N. DYN, D. REISFELD, AND Y. YESHURUN, *Image warping by radial basis functions: application to facial expressions*, CVGIP: Graphical Models and Image Processing, 56 (1994), pp. 161–172.
2. N. ARAD AND D. REISFELD, *Image warping using few anchor points and radial functions*, Computer Graphics forum, 14 (1995), pp. 35–46.
3. L. BOOKSTEIN, F, *Morphometric tools for landmark data; geometry and biology*, Cambridge University press, 1991.
4. P. DUPUIS, U. GRENANDER, AND M. MILLER, *Variational problems on flows of diffeomorphisms for image matching*, Quaterly of Applied Math., (1998).
5. S. HELGASON, *Differential Geometry, Liie groups and Symmetric spaces*, Academic Press, 1978.
6. S. JOSHI AND M. MILLER, *Landmark matching via large deformation diffeomorphisms*, IEEE transactions in image processing, 9 (2000), pp. 1357–1370.

7. J. MEINGUET, *Multivariate interpolation at arbitrary points made simple*, J. Appliet Math. and Physics, 30 (1979), pp. 292–304.

8. I. MILLER, M AND L. YOUNES, *Group action, diffeomorphism and matching: a general framework*, in Proceeding of SCTV 99, 1999.   http://www.cis.ohio-state.edu/ szhu/SCTV99.html.

9. P. OLVER, *Equivalence, Invarians and Symmetry*, Cambridge University Press, 1995.

10. A. TROUVÉ, *Infinite dimensional group action and pattern recognition*, Quaterly of Applied Math. (to appear), (2000).

11. L. YOUNES, *Computable elastic distances between shapes*, SIAM J. Appl. Math, 58 (1998), pp. 565–586.

Averaged Template Matching Equations

Anil N. Hirani, Jerrold E. Marsden, and James Arvo

California Institute of Technology, Pasadena, CA, USA

Abstract. By exploiting an analogy with averaging procedures in fluid dynamics, we present a set of averaged template matching equations. These equations are analogs of the exact template matching equations that retain all the geometric properties associated with the diffeomorphism group, and which are expected to average out small scale features and so should, as in hydrodynamics, be more computationally efficient for resolving the larger scale features. From a geometric point of view, the new equations may be viewed as coming from a change in norm that is used to measure the distance between images. The results in this paper represent first steps in a longer term program: what is here is only for binary images and an algorithm for numerical computation is not yet operational. Some suggestions for further steps to develop the results given in this paper are suggested.

1 Introduction

1.1 Previous Work

Deformable template matching is a technique for comparing images with applications in computer vision, medical imaging and other fields. It has been reported on extensively in the literature. See for example, Younes (2000), Trouvé (1995, 1998), Grenander and Miller (1998) and the references therein.

Template matching is based on the notion of computing a deformation induced distance between two images. The "energy" required to do a deformation that takes one image to the other defines the distance between them. The deformations are often taken to be diffeomorphisms of the image rectangle, i.e smooth maps with smooth inverse. The energy can be defined using various metrics on the space of diffeomorphisms. In addition to diffeomorphisms, which are merely a change of coordinates of the underlying image rectangle, one can also allow changes to the pixel values. Trouvé (1995, 1998) develops such a theory and gives several numerical examples. He gives conditions on the metric that are sufficient to make the space of deformations a complete metric space. He works with a subgroup of homeomorphisms as the space of deformations and allows pixel value changes by using a semidirect product with a group that acts on the pixel values. The paper by Dupuis, Grenander and Miller (1998) also derives conditions for existence of template matching solutions.

Recently a partial differential equation for template matching was derived by Ratnanather, Baigent, Mumford and Miller (2000), for both exact and inexact matching. In exact matching the two images being compared have to be

M.A.T. Figueiredo, J. Zerubia, A.K. Jain (Eds.): EMMCVPR 2001, LNCS 2134, pp. 528–543, 2001.

diffeomorphic and in inexact matching they need not be. Their derivation was done using Euler-Poincaré reduction theory and also using classical calculus of variations. For an early version, which does not use the Euler-Poincaré theory, see Mumford (1998b). For Euler-Poincaré reduction theory, see Marsden and Ratiu (1999, Chapters 1 and 13). This technique is useful for computing Euler-Lagrange equations when the Lagrangian is invariant under the action of some Lie group. For example, it is possible to do a variational derivation of the Euler equations of rigid bodies and fluid mechanics using Euler-Poincaré reduction theory.

In their most general form as given in Mumford (1998b), the exact template matching equations (TME) depend on the choice of a self-adjoint operator that appears in the definition of the metric on the group of diffeomorphisms. When this metric is L^2 we will refer to the equations as L^2-TME.

1.2   Contributions

In this paper we derive the isotropic averaged template matching equations, (H_α^1-ATME), which we hope will be a version of the exact template matching equations that average out small scale features, yet retain the larger scale features. The H_α^1 refers to a weighted Sobolev metric that we use instead of the L^2 metric on the group of diffeomorphisms.

Thus the H_α^1-ATME are derived by making a special choice for the self-adjoint operator that appears in the derivation of Ratnanather, Baigent, Mumford and Miller (2000). We expect that the averaged equations and even their anisotropic counterparts may also be of interest in computer vision. These might allow template matching while ignoring features smaller than a chosen size (α in equation (13)). The H_α^1-ATME derivation was inspired by recent work on Lagrangian averaged equations in fluid mechanics as described in Marsden and Shkoller (2001) and references there in.

By analogy with fluid mechanics the H_α^1-ATME may be much more amenable to numerical solution than the L^2-TME. Finally, by allowing the ignorable feature size to vary it may be possible to perform template matching more robustly using a multiscale approach.

1.3   Overview

We first set up the framework of template matching. For this paper, the main task of template matching reduces to defining distance between binary images. After describing the framework we give the definitions and facts that are needed for our derivation. These preliminaries include a brief summary of Euler-Poincaré reduction in Section 3.3. Before giving a derivation of H_α^1-ATME we repeat the derivation of the TME of Mumford (1998b) for the special case of the L^2 metric. The main result in this paper is the derivation of the isotropic averaged template matching equations for the exact matching case and this derivation is in Section 6.

2   Our Framework

The basic element of template matching is the computation of a distance between two images and the computation of a deformation that takes one image to the other. For concreteness and simplicity we will limit our attention to binary images, i.e. an image will be a characteristic function on some bounded open subset M of $\mathbb{R}^n$, $n \geq 1$. Thus our space of images is $\mathcal{P} = \{f \mid f : M \to \{0,1\}\}$. We do the derivations for a general n since those are just as easy as derivations for the case $n = 2$. For $n = 2$, M will typically be a rectangle in the plane.

In order to define a metric on $\mathcal{P}$, given two images f and g one finds the "smallest" map $\varphi : M \to M$ such that $f = g \circ \varphi$. In Section 3.2 we show that this smallest map φ induces a pseudometric on $\mathcal{P}$. This approach does not allow one to modify the range of the images, φ is just a change of coordinates for M. A more general framework that allows one to modify the range of the images (i.e. modify the pixel values) by using semidirect products is described in Trouvé (1995).

In order to define the "smallest" map φ mentioned above, one must define a metric on the space to which φ belongs. In addition one has a choice of what space to use as the source of the maps φ. These choices and an analysis of their implications require extensive and subtle analysis that uses many mathematical tools. A nice discussion and use of these subtleties is in Trouvé (1995). In this paper, to keep things simple, we will ignore these subtleties. We will take the space to which the maps φ belong to be the space of all diffeomorphisms of M fixing its boundary pointwise and denote this space by $\text{Diff}(M)$.

3   Preliminaries

3.1   Facts about Diff(M)

We will require some basic facts about $\text{Diff}(M)$ and its tangent spaces which we state here, some without proof. We will ignore the difficulties associated with defining a differentiable structure on $\text{Diff}(M)$. For details on this, see Ebin and Marsden (1970). See also Marsden and Ratiu (1999) for an elementary discussion. The most important fact is that a vector in the tangent space of $\text{Diff}(M)$ is a vector field on M. This is stated more formally in Facts 1 and 2 below.

Fact 1. *The tangent space of* $\text{Diff}(M)$ *at the point* $\varphi \in \text{Diff}(M)$, *is the space of all material (i.e Lagrangian) velocity vector fields* $\boldsymbol{V}_\varphi$ *over* φ *on* M *that vanish on the boundary* ∂M *of* M. *This tangent space is denoted by* $T_\varphi(\text{Diff}(M))$.

Fact 2. *The tangent space of* $\text{Diff}(M)$ *at identity* $e \in \text{Diff}(M)$, *i.e.* $T_e(\text{Diff}(M))$ *is the space* $\mathfrak{X}(M)$ *of all spatial (i.e Eulerian) velocity vector fields on* M *that vanish on the boundary* ∂M *of* M.

We also need some facts about the tangent map (derivative) of the action of $\text{Diff}(M)$ acting on itself. Let $\text{Diff}(M)$ act on itself on the right by function composition. Thus for $\varphi, \eta \in \text{Diff}(M)$ the right action of η on φ is $\varphi \cdot \eta = R_\eta(\varphi) = \varphi \circ \eta$, where R_η denotes right multiplication of the argument by η. Now we compute the tangent lifted action, i.e TR_η which is the derivative of the right action described above. We show that

Fact 3. *If R_η is the right action defined above, then its derivative is*

$$T_\varphi R_\eta(\boldsymbol{V}_\varphi) = \boldsymbol{V}_\varphi \circ \eta$$

for all $\boldsymbol{V}_\varphi \in T_\varphi(\text{Diff}(M))$. This is called the right action by η on $\boldsymbol{V}_\varphi$.

We recall the proof of this standard fact for the reader's convenience.

Proof. The proof essentially consists of checking definitions. Let $\varphi_t \subset \text{Diff}(M)$ be a smooth curve such that $\varphi_0 = \varphi$ and $d/dt|_{t=0}\varphi_t = \boldsymbol{V}_\varphi$. Thus for every $X \in M$, $\partial/\partial t|_{t=0}\varphi(X,t) = \boldsymbol{V}_\varphi(X)$. Then by definition of derivative $T_\varphi R_\eta(\boldsymbol{V}_\varphi) = d/dt|_{t=0}(\varphi_t \circ \eta)$. Thus, $T_\varphi R_\eta(\boldsymbol{V}_\varphi)(X) = d/dt|_{t=0}\varphi_t(\eta(X)) = \boldsymbol{V}_\varphi(\eta(X))$. $\quad\square$

Definition 1. *An inner product on $\text{Diff}(M)$ is said to be right invariant under action by $\text{Diff}(M)$ if $(\boldsymbol{V}_\varphi, \boldsymbol{U}_\varphi) = (T_\varphi R_\eta(\boldsymbol{V}_\varphi), T_\varphi R_\eta(\boldsymbol{U}_\varphi)) = (\boldsymbol{V}_\varphi \circ \eta, \boldsymbol{U}_\varphi \circ \eta)$ for all $\varphi, \eta \in \text{Diff}(M)$ and $\boldsymbol{V}_\varphi, \boldsymbol{U}_\varphi \in T_\varphi(\text{Diff}(M))$. Here $(\cdot,\cdot)$ denotes an inner product on $\text{Diff}(M)$.*

3.2 Pseudometric Using Diffeomorphisms

We induce a pseudometric (Abraham, Marsden and Ratiu (1988)) on the space of images $\mathcal{P}$ from a metric defined on $\text{Diff}(M)$ as follows.

Definition 2. *The positive valued function $\text{d}_\mathcal{P} : \mathcal{P} \times \mathcal{P} \to \mathbb{R}$, is called a **pseudometric induced on $\mathcal{P}$ from** $\text{Diff}(M)$, if for any $f, g \in \mathcal{P}$*

$$\text{d}_\mathcal{P}(f, g) = \inf\{d(e, \varphi) \,|\, \varphi \in \text{Diff}(M) \text{ and } f = g \circ \varphi\} \;,$$

where e is the identity diffeomorphism, $d(e, \varphi)$ is the geodesic distance between e and φ and inf stands for infimum, or greatest lower bound.

As usual, the geodesic distance on $\text{Diff}(M)$, is defined in terms of the inner product on the tangent spaces of $\text{Diff}(M)$, i.e. the Riemannian metric on $\text{Diff}(M)$. One must prove that $\text{d}_\mathcal{P}$ as defined above is actually a pseudometric, i.e. that it satisfies the symmetry and triangle inequality properties as well as the property that $\text{d}_\mathcal{P}(f, f) = 0$ for all $f \in \mathcal{P}$. This is stated in the following Fact 4. See Miller and Younes (1999) for a sketch of a proof or Hirani, Marsden and Arvo (2001), which is the technical report version of the present paper, for a more detailed proof.

Fact 4. *If the Riemannian metric on $\text{Diff}(M)$ is right invariant under action by $\text{Diff}(M)$, then the function $\text{d}_\mathcal{P}$ of Definition 2 satisfies the pseudometric axioms, namely that*

1. $\text{d}_\mathcal{P}(f, f) = 0$ for all $f \in \mathcal{P}$;

2. $d_\mathcal{P}(f,g) = d_\mathcal{P}(g,f)$ *for all* $f, g \in \mathcal{P}$ *(symmetry) ; and*
3. $d_\mathcal{P}(f,h) \le d_\mathcal{P}(f,g) + d_\mathcal{P}(g,h)$ *for all* $f, g, h \in \mathcal{P}$ *(triangle inequality)* .

Furthermore, if the infimum in Definition 2 is achieved, then $d_\mathcal{P}$ *is a metric on* $\mathcal{P}$, *in which case property 1 becomes*

1. $d_\mathcal{P}(f,g) = 0 \iff f = g$ *(definiteness)* .

One can also show the same result when right invariance is replaced by left invariance or bi-invariance.

Thus to compute $d_\mathcal{P}(f,g)$ we need to find the smallest diffeomorphism φ in $\mathrm{Diff}(M)$ such that $f = g \circ \varphi$. The definition of *smallest* depends on the chosen metric on $\mathrm{Diff}(M)$. The typical strategy for this is to find a geodesic on $\mathrm{Diff}(M)$, from the identity map to the unknown diffeomorphism φ. The unknown diffeomorphism satisfies the constraint $f = g \circ \varphi$. Any such φ will be the smallest, since it will be the diffeomorphism closest to identity, which also satisfies $f = g \circ \varphi$.

There may or may not be many such smallest diffeomorphisms, but it is sufficient to find one, in order to solve the template matching problem. The lack of uniqueness, if present, may have practical implications for numerical solvers, which is an issue we have not yet addressed. Moreover, there may not exist any such φ ; for example this is the case when the image corresponding to f is not homemorphic to that corresponding to g. The existence issue also requires further investigation. Trouvé (1995, 1998) gives conditions that a metric must satisfy for existence and uniqueness of minimizers in inexact matching.

3.3   Euler-Poincaré Reduction

We now recall some facts about Euler-Poincaré reduction theorem that we will need. For details, see Chapter 13 of Marsden and Ratiu (1999). Euler-Poincaré reduction is useful in mechanics. For example, it is possible to do a variational derivation of the Euler equations of rigid bodies and fluid mechanics using Euler-Poincaré reduction theory. Consider a Lagrangian L i.e. a map $L : T(\mathrm{Diff}(M)) \to \mathbb{R}$, so L is a function of $\varphi \in \mathrm{Diff}(M)$ and $\dot{\varphi} \in T_\varphi(\mathrm{Diff}(M))$. If this Lagrangian is invariant under right action by $\mathrm{Diff}(M)$ then we can use the Euler-Poincaré reduction theorem (Marsden and Ratiu (1999) Theorem 13.5.3). According to this theorem, the following two statements are equivalent :

1. The variational principle $\delta \int_a^b L(\varphi(X,t), \dot{\varphi}(X,t))\,dt = 0$ holds for variations of curves $\varphi(X,t)$ with fixed end points, i.e. for $\delta\varphi(X,a) = \delta\varphi(X,b) = 0 \; \forall X \in M$;
2. The variational principle $\delta \int_a^b l(\boldsymbol{u}(x,t))\,dt = 0$ holds on $\mathfrak{X}(M)$, i.e. on the tangent space at the identity of $\mathrm{Diff}(M)$, using variations of the form $\delta\boldsymbol{u} = \dot{\boldsymbol{w}} + [\boldsymbol{w}, \boldsymbol{u}]_L$. This is called the reduced variational principle.

Here $\dot{\varphi}(X,t) = \partial/\partial t \varphi(X,t)$ (keeping X fixed). The vector $\boldsymbol{u}$ is the tangent vector $\dot{\varphi}$ moved to identity $e \in \mathrm{Diff}(M)$ by right action by φ_t^{-1}, i.e. $\boldsymbol{u} = \dot{\varphi} \circ$

φ_t^{-1}. Subscript t here denotes fixed time t not derivative w.r.t t. More precisely, if $x = \varphi(X, t) = \varphi_t(X)$ then $\boldsymbol{u}(x, t) = \dot{\varphi}(\varphi_t^{-1}(x), t)$. By this we mean that first the time derivative of $\varphi(X, t)$ is computed keeping X fixed and *then* one substitutes $X = X(x, t) = \varphi_t^{-1}(x)$ into the resulting expression. The function $l : T_e(\text{Diff}(M)) \to \mathbb{R}$ is simply the restriction of L to the tangent space at identity e.

The vector $\boldsymbol{w}$ is the vector $\delta\varphi$ moved to identity in $\text{Diff}(M)$. Thus $\boldsymbol{w} = \delta\varphi_t \circ \varphi_t^{-1}$. The notation $[\boldsymbol{w}, \boldsymbol{u}]_L \equiv (\boldsymbol{u} \cdot \nabla)\boldsymbol{w} - (\boldsymbol{w} \cdot \nabla)\boldsymbol{u}$ is the Jacobi Lie bracket. Note that $\boldsymbol{w}(x, a) = \boldsymbol{w}(x, b) = 0 \ \forall x \in M$ since $\delta\varphi(X, a) = \delta\varphi(X, b) = 0 \ \forall X \in M$.

3.4   Gauss-Green Theorem and Its Corollary

We will need some basic facts from vector calculus, for the derivation of the L^2-TME and H_α^1-ATME. We state these facts here.

Fact 5. (Gauss-Green Theorem) *Let M be an open bounded subset of $\mathbb{R}^n$ and suppose that the boundary ∂M is C^1. Suppose $u \in C^1(\overline{M})$. Then*

$$\int_M \frac{\partial u}{\partial x_i} \, dx = \int_{\partial M} u\nu^i \, dS$$

for all $i = 1, \ldots, n$ and where $\hat{\nu} = (\nu^1, \ldots, \nu^n)$ is the outward pointing unit normal field on ∂M.

A simple corollary of the Gauss-Green theorem is the following fact which we will use several times.

Fact 6. *Let M be an open bounded subset of $\mathbb{R}^n$ and suppose that ∂M is C^1. Let $\mathbf{u}, \mathbf{v}, \mathbf{w}$ be vector fields on $\overline{M}$. Then*

$$\int_M \text{div}\,\boldsymbol{v}\langle\boldsymbol{u}, \boldsymbol{w}\rangle + \langle\boldsymbol{u}, (\boldsymbol{v} \cdot \nabla)\boldsymbol{w}\rangle + \langle(\boldsymbol{v} \cdot \nabla)\boldsymbol{u}, \boldsymbol{w}\rangle \, dx = \int_{\partial M} \langle\boldsymbol{u}, \boldsymbol{w}\rangle\langle\boldsymbol{v}, \hat{\nu}\rangle \, dS \quad (1)$$

where $\hat{\nu} = (\nu^1, \ldots, \nu^n)$ is the outward pointing unit normal field of ∂M.

Proof. We will use the Gauss-Green theorem (Fact 5) stated above. By this theorem we have that for all i, j in $\{1, \ldots, n\}$, $\int_M \partial/\partial x_j(u^i w^i v^j) dx = \int_{\partial M} u^i w^i v^j \nu^j \, dS$. Thus

$$\sum_{i,j=1}^n \int_M u^i w^i \frac{\partial v^j}{\partial x_j} + u^i v^j \frac{\partial w^i}{\partial x_j} + w^i v^j \frac{\partial u^i}{\partial x_j} dx = \sum_{i,j=1}^n \int_{\partial M} u^i w^i v^j \nu^j \, dS \ ,$$

which proves equation (1). □

4   Metrics on $\text{Diff}(M)$

We need to define two different Riemannian metrics on $\text{Diff}(M)$, i.e. inner products on its tangent spaces. One is for the L^2-TME derivation and the other one is for the H_α^1-ATME derivation.

Definition 3. *Let* $V_\varphi, U_\varphi \in T_\varphi(\text{Diff}(M))$, *i.e.* V_φ, U_φ *are tangent vectors, tangent to* $\text{Diff}(M)$ *at the point* $\varphi \in \text{Diff}(M)$. *Let* $J(\varphi)(X)$ *be the determinant of the derivative of (i.e. the Jacobian determinant of)* φ *evaluated at point* $X \in M$. *The* L^2 *Riemannian metric on* $\text{Diff}(M)$ *we will use for the* L^2-*TME derivation is defined as*

$$(V_\varphi, U_\varphi)_{\text{L}^2} \equiv \int_M \langle V_\varphi(X), U_\varphi(X) \rangle J(\varphi)(X) \, dX \ . \tag{2}$$

Here $\langle \cdot, \cdot \rangle$ *is the standard inner product on* $\mathbb{R}^n$.

The H^1_α metric on $\text{Diff}(M)$ is defined by first defining it on the tangent space at identity and then extending it to all of $\text{Diff}(M)$ right invariantly.

Definition 4. *Let* v, u *be vectors in the tangent space at identity* $e \in \text{Diff}(M)$ *i.e.* $v, u \in T_e(\text{Diff}(M))$. *For any* $\alpha > 0$, $\alpha \in \mathbb{R}$, *define*

$$(v, u)_{\text{H}^1_\alpha} \equiv \int_M \langle v(x), u(x) \rangle + \alpha^2 \sum_{i=1}^n \langle D_i \, v(x), D_i \, u(x) \rangle \, dx \ . \tag{3}$$

where $D_i \, v = \partial/\partial x_i(v(x))$. *The inner products inside the integral are the standard inner products (dot products) on* $\mathbb{R}^n$.

To compute the inner product at a point $\varphi \in \text{Diff}(M)$ different from identity, define $(V_\varphi, U_\varphi)_{\text{H}^1_\alpha} = (V_\varphi \circ \varphi^{-1}, U_\varphi \circ \varphi^{-1})_{\text{H}^1_\alpha}$. Note that $V_\varphi \circ \varphi^{-1}, U_\varphi \circ \varphi^{-1} \in T_e(\text{Diff}(M))$ because right action by φ^{-1} moves the vectors at φ to identity on $\text{Diff}(M)$. Thus we can use (3) to compute the inner product. Note that we defined the L^2 inner product at a general point of $\text{Diff}(M)$ but defined the H^1_α inner product at identity and showed how it can be computed at a general point. This is done for simplicity. The expression for the L^2 inner product at a general point is simple but not so for the H^1_α inner product. We will write the corresponding norms as follows. The L^2 norm of $U_\varphi \in T_\varphi(\text{Diff}(M))$ is written as $\|U_\varphi\|_{\text{L}^2} \equiv (U_\varphi, U_\varphi)_{\text{L}^2}^{1/2}$ and similarly for the H^1_α norm.

The geodesic distance between φ_a and φ_b on $\text{Diff}(M)$ is defined as

$$d(\varphi_a, \varphi_b) \equiv \inf \left\{ \int_a^b (\dot\varphi(t), \dot\varphi(t))^{1/2} \, dt \ \middle| \ \varphi(a) = \varphi_a, \varphi(b) = \varphi_b \right\}$$

and the infimum is taken over all smooth parametric curves $\varphi : [a, b] \to \text{Diff}(M)$ from φ_a to φ_b. Here $(\cdot, \cdot)$ is any Riemannian metric on $\text{Diff}(M)$. Thus $d(\varphi_a, \varphi_b) = \int_a^b (\dot\varphi(t), \dot\varphi(t))^{1/2} \, dt$, where φ is the curve between the endpoints that makes $\int_a^b (\dot\varphi(t), \dot\varphi(t))^{1/2} \, dt$ stationary.

The same curve makes the functional $\int_a^b (\dot\varphi(t), \dot\varphi(t)) \, dt$ stationary. This fact is sometimes stated as "minimizing length is the same as minimizing kinetic energy". One way to prove this fact is by computing the Euler-Lagrange equations for both the integrals and noting that the equations are the same.

4.1   Right Invariance of $\mathbf{L}^2$ Metric

We now prove the right invariance property of the L^2 metric in Definition 3. This property is crucial for application of the Euler-Poincaré reduction theorem.

Claim 1. *The metric defined by (2) is right invariant under action of the group* $\mathrm{Diff}(M)$ *acting on* $\mathrm{Diff}(M)$, *i.e. for any* $\eta \in \mathrm{Diff}(M)$

$$(T_\varphi R_\eta(\boldsymbol{V}_\varphi), T_\varphi R_\eta(\boldsymbol{U}_\varphi))_{\mathrm{L}^2} = (\boldsymbol{V}_\varphi, \boldsymbol{U}_\varphi)_{\mathrm{L}^2} \ .$$

Proof. By the computation of the tangent lifted group action in Fact 3, this is equivalent to showing that $(\boldsymbol{V}_\varphi \circ \eta, \boldsymbol{U}_\varphi \circ \eta)_{\mathrm{L}^2} = (\boldsymbol{V}_\varphi, \boldsymbol{U}_\varphi)_{\mathrm{L}^2}$. The left hand side above is equal to $\int_M \langle \boldsymbol{V}_\varphi(\eta(X)), \boldsymbol{U}_\varphi(\eta(X)) \rangle J(\varphi \circ \eta)(X) \, dX$. Note that the argument $\varphi \circ \eta$ of J is the base point of $T_\varphi R_\eta(\boldsymbol{V}_\varphi)$ and $T_\varphi R_\eta(\boldsymbol{U}_\varphi)$ as required by the definition of the metric. Using chain rule for $J(\varphi \circ \eta)(X)$ the above integral becomes $\int_M \langle \boldsymbol{V}_\varphi(\eta(X)), \boldsymbol{U}_\varphi(\eta(X)) \rangle J(\varphi)(\eta(X)) J(\eta)(X) \, dX$. Now use the change of variable $Y = \eta(X)$. By the change of variables theorem then $dY = J(\eta)(X)dX$ and the above integral becomes $\int_{\eta(M)} \langle \boldsymbol{V}_\varphi(Y), \boldsymbol{U}_\varphi(Y) \rangle J(\varphi)(Y) \, dY$. Since $\eta(M) = M$ the above is equal to $(\boldsymbol{V}_\varphi, \boldsymbol{U}_\varphi)_{\mathrm{L}^2}$ as desired. □

We now give the intuition behind the form of the L^2 inner product. Specifically we address the question of why the Jacobian determinant term appears in the L^2 inner product definition (Definition 2). It appears so that the inner product can be made right invariant. Right invariance of the metric on $\mathrm{Diff}(M)$ implies that the induced function $d_\mathcal{P}$ is a pseudometric (Fact 4). Thus right invariance (or left- or bi-invariance for that matter) is a convenient assumption. Moreover, the distance between two images should not change if they are both distorted by the same change of variables. This also makes the requirement of invariance attractive.

4.2   Right Invariance of $\mathbf{H}^1_\alpha$ Metric

Since the H^1_α metric was defined at identity and extended in a right invariant fashion, the check for right invariance is easy. For completeness we give it below.

Claim 2. *The* H^1_α *metric defined by (3) is right invariant under action of the group* $\mathrm{Diff}(M)$ *acting on* $\mathrm{Diff}(M)$, *i.e. for any* $\eta \in \mathrm{Diff}(M)$

$$(T_\varphi R_\eta(\boldsymbol{V}_\varphi), T_\varphi R_\eta(\boldsymbol{U}_\varphi))_{\mathrm{H}^1_\alpha} = (\boldsymbol{V}_\varphi, \boldsymbol{U}_\varphi)_{\mathrm{H}^1_\alpha} \ .$$

Proof. By Fact 3, it is enough to show that $(\boldsymbol{V}_\varphi \circ \eta, \boldsymbol{U}_\varphi \circ \eta)_{\mathrm{H}^1_\alpha} = (\boldsymbol{V}_\varphi, \boldsymbol{U}_\varphi)_{\mathrm{H}^1_\alpha}$ for all $\eta \in \mathrm{Diff}(M)$. But by definition of H^1_α,

$$(\boldsymbol{V}_\varphi \circ \eta, \boldsymbol{U}_\varphi \circ \eta)_{\mathrm{H}^1_\alpha} = (\boldsymbol{V}_\varphi \circ \eta \circ (\varphi \circ \eta)^{-1}, \boldsymbol{U}_\varphi \circ \eta \circ (\varphi \circ \eta)^{-1})_{\mathrm{H}^1_\alpha}$$
$$= (\boldsymbol{V}_\varphi, \boldsymbol{U}_\varphi)_{\mathrm{H}^1_\alpha} \ .$$

□

5   Template Matching Equations

Both the exact and inexact TME, using Euler-Poincaré reduction theory, and also using classical calculus of variations, were derived recently, and communicated to us by Ratnanather, Baigent, Mumford and Miller (2000). An early version without the use of Euler-Poincaré theory appears in Mumford (1998b). We should note that although Trouvé (1995) does not mention Euler-Poincaré reduction, and does not give a PDE for template matching explicitly, he was certainly aware of, and used the idea of moving back and forth between the tangent space at identity and a general point of $\mathrm{Diff}(M)$. For completeness, we now give the Euler-Poincaré derivation of the L^2-TME in our notation. We do the derivation of the exact equations, i.e. it is assumed that the two images being compared are diffeomorphic.

5.1   Derivation of Exact L^2-TME

We have seen in Claim 1 that the L^2 metric of Definition 3 is right invariant. Thus if we define a Lagrangian $L : T(\mathrm{Diff}(M)) \to \mathbb{R}$ as

$$L(\varphi(t), \dot{\varphi}(t)) = \frac{1}{2}(\dot{\varphi}(t), \dot{\varphi}(t))_{L^2} \tag{4}$$

then it will also be right invariant under that action of $\mathrm{Diff}(M)$.

Let $\varphi : [0, 1] \to \mathrm{Diff}(M)$ be a smooth parameterized curve in $\mathrm{Diff}(M)$ between the points $e = \varphi(0)$ (identity map) and $\varphi(1) \in \mathrm{Diff}(M)$. The point $\varphi(1)$ is such that $f = g \circ (\varphi(1))$ for the given images f and g. Take a smooth family of curves φ_ϵ with the same end points $\varphi(0)$ and $\varphi(1)$ and such that $\varphi_0 = \varphi$. Define the variations of the curve φ to be the vector field $\delta\varphi = d/d\epsilon|_{\epsilon=0}\varphi_\epsilon$ along φ.

Consider the variational principle $\delta \int_0^1 L(\varphi(t), \dot{\varphi}(t)) \, dt = 0$, with the above variations. By the discussion in Section 3.2 the solution of the variational principle above is a geodesic on $\mathrm{Diff}(M)$ under the L^2 metric from the identity map $e \in \mathrm{Diff}(M)$ to the diffeomorphism $\varphi(1)$ which satisfies the condition of matching, i.e. $f = g \circ (\varphi(1))$. Due to the right invariance of the Lagrangian we can use the Euler-Poincaré reduction theorem (see Theorem 13.5.3, Page 437 of Marsden and Ratiu (1999) and Section 3.3 of this paper). By applying this theorem, we will get a variational principle on $\mathfrak{X}(M)$ (called the reduced variational principle) and hence a differential equation in terms of Eulerian veclocity vector fields on M. These are the exact L^2-TME derived by Ratnanather, Baigent, Mumford and Miller (2000).

The reduced variational principle uses the reduced Lagrangian l which is a function on the tangent space at identity of $\mathrm{Diff}(M)$, namely on $\mathfrak{X}(M)$, the space of all spatial or Eulerian velocity vector fields on M. As noted in Section 3.3 the function l is just the restriction of L to $T_e(\mathrm{Diff}(M))$. Furthermore, L as defined in equation (4) is right invariant under right action of $\mathrm{Diff}(M)$. As a result $L(\varphi, \dot{\varphi}) = L(e, \dot{\varphi} \circ \varphi^{-1}) = l(\boldsymbol{u})$ where $\boldsymbol{u} = \dot{\varphi} \circ \varphi^{-1}$. Thus by Definition 3

$$l(\boldsymbol{u}) = \frac{1}{2} \int_M \|\dot{\varphi}(X, t)\|^2 J(\varphi_t)(X) \, dX \ ,$$

where the overdot is time derivative keeping X fixed and the norm $\|\cdot\|$ is the standard norm in $\mathbb{R}^n$. Let $X = \varphi_t^{-1}(x)$. Then $dX = J(\varphi_t^{-1})(x)\,dx$. Thus,

$$l(u) = \frac{1}{2}\int_M \|\dot{\varphi}(\varphi_t^{-1}(x),t)\|^2 J(\varphi_t)(\varphi_t^{-1}(x))J(\varphi_t^{-1})(x)\,dx$$

$$= \frac{1}{2}\int_M \|u(x,t)\|^2\,dx = \frac{1}{2}\|u\|_{L^2}^2 \ .$$

Let us call the functional for the reduced variational principle $\mathcal{E}$, where

$$\mathcal{E}(u) = \int_0^1 l(u(t))\,dt = \frac{1}{2}\int_0^1 \|u(x,t)\|_{L^2}^2\,dt \ .$$

Then $\delta\mathcal{E} = \int_0^1 \int_M \langle u(x,t), \delta u(x,t)\rangle\,dx\,dt$, where the inner product inside the integral is the usual dot product in $\mathbb{R}^n$. Inserting the definition of δu from Section (3.3) in this integral and setting the resulting expression to 0 we get

$$\int_0^1 \int_M \langle u(x,t), \dot{w}(x,t) + [w,u]_L(x,t)\rangle\,dx\,dt = 0.$$

Now substitute the definition of $[w,u]_L$ from Section 3.3, or page 20 of Marsden and Ratiu 1999. With this the above equation becomes

$$\int_0^1 \int_M \langle u, \dot{w}\rangle - \langle u, (w\cdot\nabla)u\rangle + \langle u, (u\cdot\nabla)w\rangle\,dx\,dt = 0 \ . \tag{5}$$

Using integration by parts on the time variable for the first term, and the fact that $w(x,0) = w(x,1) = 0 \ \forall x \in M$ (see Section 3.3) implies that

$$\int_0^1 \int_M \langle u(x,t), \dot{w}(x,t)\rangle\,dx\,dt = -\int_0^1 \int_M \langle \dot{u}(x,t), w(x,t)\rangle\,dx\,dt \ . \tag{6}$$

For the second and third term of equation (5) also, the goal is to rewrite those in the form $\langle \cdot, w\rangle$. To bring the second term into the required form, note that $(w\cdot\nabla)u = \mathbf{D}\,u\cdot w$ where $\mathbf{D}$ denotes the spatial derivative. Thus

$$\langle u, (w\cdot\nabla)u\rangle = \langle u, \mathbf{D}\,u\cdot w\rangle = \langle (\mathbf{D}\,u)^T\cdot u, w\rangle \ . \tag{7}$$

For the third term, we use Fact 6. From Fact 2 $u|_{\partial M} = 0$ and so the RHS of equation (1) is 0. Thus

$$\int_M \langle u, (u\cdot\nabla)w\rangle\,dx = -\int_M \operatorname{div} u\langle w, u\rangle + \langle (u\cdot\nabla)u, w\rangle\,dx \ . \tag{8}$$

Using equations (6), (7) and (8) in equation (5) one gets that

$$\int_0^1 \int_M -\langle \dot{u}, w\rangle - \langle (\mathbf{D}\,u)^T\cdot u, w\rangle - \langle (\operatorname{div} u)u, w\rangle - \langle (u\cdot\nabla)u, w\rangle\,dx\,dt = 0 \ .$$

Then since w is arbitrary it follows that

$$\frac{\partial u}{\partial t} + (\mathbf{D}\,u)^T \cdot u + (\text{div}\,u)u + (u \cdot \nabla)u = 0 \ . \tag{9}$$

The above equation (9) is the template matching equation, for exact matching, i.e. the L^2-TME, as communicated to us by Ratnanather, Baigent, Mumford, Miller (2000). We have just repeated the derivation in our notation for completeness. Note that for all $(x, t) \in M \times [0, 1]$, $(\mathbf{D}\,u(x, t))^T \cdot u(x, t) = \frac{1}{2}\nabla(\|u(x, t)\|^2)$ where now, the norm on the RHS is the standard norm in $\mathbb{R}^n$. With this, the L^2-TME, equation (9) can be written in an alternative form as

$$\frac{\partial u}{\partial t} + (\text{div}\,u)u + (u \cdot \nabla)u = -\frac{1}{2}\nabla(\|u\|^2) \tag{10}$$

where $u = u(x, t)$ is the unknown time dependent spatial (Eulerian) velocity vector field on M that vanishes on the boundary ∂M of M.

These equations can be written more concisely, in the Lie derivative form as $\partial\beta/\partial t + \pounds_u\beta = 0$ where β is the *one form density* associated with u and where $\pounds$ is the Lie derivative. In $\mathbb{R}^n$, $\beta = \sum_{i=1}^{n} u^i dx^i \otimes d^n x$. These are the Euler-Poincaré equations associated with the right invariant L^2 metric of Definition 3 on the diffeomorphism group. The advantage of this form is that it can accomodate other metrics, simply by changing β. This will become clear when we derive the H^1_α-ATME in Section 6.1.

6   Averaged Template Matching Equations

We now derive H^1_α-ATME, which are a set of averaged template matching equations. These equations are analogs of the exact template matching equations that retain all the geometric properties associated with the diffeomorphism group and which are expected to average out small scale features and so should, as in hydrodynamics, be more computationally efficient for resolving the larger scale features. From a geometric point of view, the new equations may be viewed as coming from a change in norm that is used to measure the distance between images.

6.1   Derivation of H^1_α-ATME

The steps in deriving the H^1_α-ATME are almost identical to those used for L^2-TME, except that we use the H^1_α metric (Definition 4) on $\text{Diff}(M)$, instead of the L^2 metric. Thus we start with a Lagrangian $L : T(\text{Diff}(M)) \to \mathbb{R}$ defined as

$$L(\varphi(t), \dot\varphi(t)) = \frac{1}{2}(\dot\varphi(t), \dot\varphi(t))_{H^1_\alpha} \ . \tag{11}$$

The initial and final value conditions are the same as in the L^2-TME case, i.e. $f = g \circ (\varphi(1))$. By Claim 2 this Lagrangian is invariant under the right action of

Diff(M). Thus, as in Section 5.1, Euler-Poincaré reduction can be applied but with a different norm. The reduced Lagrangian is $l(\boldsymbol{u}) = \frac{1}{2}\|\boldsymbol{u}\|_{H^1_\alpha}^2$. By Definition 4 of the H^1_α norm, this implies that $l(\boldsymbol{u}) = \frac{1}{2}\int_M \langle \boldsymbol{u}, \boldsymbol{u} \rangle + \alpha^2 \sum_{i=1}^n \langle \mathbf{D}_i\,\boldsymbol{u}, \mathbf{D}_i\,\boldsymbol{u} \rangle\, dx$. The functional that appears in the reduced variational principle is

$$\mathcal{E}(\boldsymbol{u}) = \int_0^1 l(\boldsymbol{u})\, dt = \frac{1}{2}\int_0^1 \int_M \langle \boldsymbol{u}, \boldsymbol{u} \rangle + \alpha^2 \sum_{i=1}^n \langle \mathbf{D}_i\,\boldsymbol{u}, \mathbf{D}_i\,\boldsymbol{u} \rangle\, dx\, dt\ .$$

Let $\boldsymbol{u}_\epsilon$ be a one parameter family of spatial vector fields on M, depending smoothly on ϵ such that $\boldsymbol{u}_0 = \boldsymbol{u}$ and as usual $\delta\boldsymbol{u} \equiv \partial\boldsymbol{u}_\epsilon/\partial\epsilon|_{\epsilon=0}$. The variations $\delta\mathcal{E}(\boldsymbol{u})$ are given by

$$\delta\mathcal{E}(\boldsymbol{u}) = \int_0^1 \langle \frac{\delta l}{\delta \boldsymbol{u}}, \delta\boldsymbol{u} \rangle\, dt\ . \tag{12}$$

We now compute the above expression. The integrand is

$$\langle \frac{\delta l}{\delta \boldsymbol{u}}, \delta\boldsymbol{u} \rangle \equiv \frac{d}{d\epsilon}\Big|_{\epsilon=0} l(\boldsymbol{u}_\epsilon) = \int_M \langle \boldsymbol{u}_\epsilon, \frac{\partial\boldsymbol{u}_\epsilon}{\partial\epsilon} \rangle + \alpha^2 \sum_{i=1}^n \langle \frac{\partial\boldsymbol{u}_\epsilon}{\partial x_i}, \frac{\partial^2\boldsymbol{u}_\epsilon}{\partial\epsilon\partial x_i} \rangle\Big|_{\epsilon=0}\, dx\ .$$

But

$$\sum_{i=1}^n \langle \frac{\partial\boldsymbol{u}_\epsilon}{\partial x_i}, \frac{\partial^2\boldsymbol{u}_\epsilon}{\partial\epsilon\partial x_i} \rangle = \sum_{i=1}^n \sum_{j=1}^n \frac{\partial u_\epsilon^j}{\partial x_i}\frac{\partial^2 u_\epsilon^j}{\partial\epsilon\partial x_i}$$

$$= \sum_{j=1}^n \sum_{i=1}^n \frac{\partial u_\epsilon^j}{\partial x_i}\frac{\partial^2 u_\epsilon^j}{\partial\epsilon\partial x_i} = \sum_{j=1}^n \langle \frac{\partial u_\epsilon^j}{\partial x}, \frac{\partial^2 u_\epsilon^j}{\partial x\partial\epsilon} \rangle\ .$$

Now

$$\int_M \sum_{i=1}^n \langle \frac{\partial u_\epsilon^i}{\partial x}, \frac{\partial^2 u_\epsilon^i}{\partial x\partial\epsilon} \rangle\Big|_{\epsilon=0}\, dx = \int_M \sum_{i=1}^n \langle \frac{\partial u^i}{\partial x}, \frac{\partial(\delta u^i)}{\partial x} \rangle\, dx\ .$$

Then using integration by parts,

$$\int_M \langle \frac{\partial u^i}{\partial x}, \frac{\partial(\delta u^i)}{\partial x} \rangle\, dx \equiv \int_M \sum_{j=1}^n \frac{\partial u^i}{\partial x_j}\frac{\partial(\delta u^i)}{\partial x_j}\, dx$$

$$= -\int_M \sum_{j=1}^n \frac{\partial^2 u^i}{\partial x_j^2}\delta u^i\, dx + \int_{\partial M} \sum_{j=1}^n \frac{\partial u^i}{\partial x_j}\delta u^i \nu^j\, dS$$

where $\nu = (\nu^1, \ldots, \nu^n)$ is the outward pointing normal field on the boundary ∂M of M. But by Fact 2, $\boldsymbol{u}|_{\partial M} = 0$ so we get that

$$\int_M \langle \frac{\partial u^i}{\partial x}, \frac{\partial(\delta u^i)}{\partial x} \rangle\, dx = -\int_M \sum_{j=1}^n \frac{\partial^2 u^i}{\partial x_j^2}\delta u^i\, dx = -\int_M (\Delta u^i)\delta u^i\, dx\ .$$

Thus

$$\langle \frac{\delta l}{\delta \boldsymbol{u}}, \delta \boldsymbol{u} \rangle = \int_M \langle \boldsymbol{u}, \delta \boldsymbol{u} \rangle - \alpha^2 \sum_{i=1}^{n} (\Delta u^i) \delta u^i \, dx \ .$$

Substituting this into equation (12) we get that

$$\delta \mathcal{E}(\boldsymbol{u}) = \int_0^1 \int_M \langle \boldsymbol{u}, \delta \boldsymbol{u} \rangle - \alpha^2 \sum_{i=1}^{n} (\Delta u^i) \delta u^i \, dx \, dt$$

$$= \int_0^1 \int_M \langle \boldsymbol{u} - \alpha^2 \Delta \boldsymbol{u}, \delta \boldsymbol{u} \rangle \, dx \, dt \ .$$

Now substituting the expression for $\delta \boldsymbol{u}$ from Section 3.3 we get

$$\delta \mathcal{E}(\boldsymbol{u}) = \int_0^1 \int_M \langle \boldsymbol{u} - \alpha^2 \Delta \boldsymbol{u}, \dot{\boldsymbol{w}} - (\boldsymbol{w} \cdot \nabla)\boldsymbol{u} + (\boldsymbol{u} \cdot \nabla)\boldsymbol{w} \rangle \, dx \, dt \ .$$

We move the derivative operators away from $\boldsymbol{w}$, as in the L^2-TME derivation in Section 5.1, to get an integrand of the form $\langle \cdot, \boldsymbol{w} \rangle$. Because of the arbitrariness of $\boldsymbol{w}$, we get the isotropic averaged H^1_α template matching equations, i.e. the H^1_α-ATME as

$$\frac{\partial}{\partial t}\boldsymbol{u} - \alpha^2 \frac{\partial}{\partial t}\Delta \boldsymbol{u} + \boldsymbol{u}(\operatorname{div} \boldsymbol{u}) - \alpha^2 (\operatorname{div} \boldsymbol{u})\Delta \boldsymbol{u} + (\boldsymbol{u} \cdot \nabla)\boldsymbol{u} -$$
$$\alpha^2 (\boldsymbol{u} \cdot \nabla)\Delta \boldsymbol{u} + (\mathbf{D}\,\boldsymbol{u})^T \cdot \boldsymbol{u} - \alpha^2 (\mathbf{D}\,\boldsymbol{u})^T \cdot \Delta \boldsymbol{u} = 0 \ , \quad (13)$$

where Δ is the componentwise Laplacian and $\mathbf{D}\,\boldsymbol{u}$ is the spatial derivative of $\boldsymbol{u}$. Here $\boldsymbol{u} = \boldsymbol{u}(x, t)$ is the unknown time dependent spatial (Eulerian) velocity vector field on M which vanishes on the boundary ∂M of M. To make it easier to see the relationship between the structure of the H^1_α-ATME and L^2-TME we define $\boldsymbol{v} \equiv (1 - \alpha^2 \Delta)\boldsymbol{u}$. Then the H^1_α-ATME equation (13) becomes

$$\frac{\partial \boldsymbol{v}}{\partial t} + (\mathbf{D}\,\boldsymbol{u})^T \cdot \boldsymbol{v} + (\operatorname{div} \boldsymbol{u})\boldsymbol{v} + (\boldsymbol{u} \cdot \nabla)\boldsymbol{v} = 0 \ . \quad (14)$$

The Lie derivative form of these equations is $\partial \beta / \partial t + \mathcal{L}_{\boldsymbol{u}}\beta = 0$ where now β is the one form density associated with $\boldsymbol{v} = (1 - \alpha^2 \Delta)\boldsymbol{u}$.

7   Connections with Fluid Mechanics

We now give the analogy and connections with fluid mechanics which have inspired our present work. We start with the connection between TME and fluid mechanics. The L^2-TME in n spatial dimensions, namely equation (9) or equivalently (10), is a higher dimensional analogue of the inviscid Burger's equation. By this we mean that in one spatial dimension the L^2-TME reduce to the equation $u_t + 3uu_x = 0$ where the subscripts indicate derivatives and $u = u(x, t)$ is the velocity of the fluid at location x at time t. This fact is mentioned in Mumford

(1998). Burger's equation, at least in the initial value formulation, can develop shocks. The framework for L^2-TME sets this equation in higher dimensions, and as an initial-final value problem. It is possible that shocks may develop in this formulation also. The well-posedness and possibility of shocks in L^2-TME remain to be checked. However, as in the case of Burger's equation and incompressible fluid mechanics, they are well-posed for short time evolution; see Marsden, Ratiu and Shkoller (2000) and Marsden and Shkoller (2001) and references therein.

Our H^1_α-ATME, on the other hand, contain diffusive terms which may ameliorate some of the analytical problems of L^2-TME, and may be a reason to expect more stable numerics. In one spatial dimension our H^1_α-ATME, equations (13) reduce to the shallow water equations $u_t - u_{xxt} = -3uu_x + 2u_x u_{xx} + uu_{xxx}$ or equivalently $v_t + uv_x + 2vu_x = 0$ where $v = u - u_{xx}$ (here α of H^1_α-ATME has been set to unity). These equations are completely integrable and have peaked solitons, as was shown by Camassa and Holm (1993). The shallow water equations, like Burger's equation, also have a smooth spray, as was shown by Shkoller (1998) and hence one has local existence and uniqueness of geodesics. The L^2-TME are equations of geodesics on Diff(M) under the right invariant L^2 metric whereas the H^1_α-ATME are equations of geodesics under a right invariant H^1_α metric.

Recently, averaged Euler and Navier-Stokes equations for fluid mechanics have been developed. See for example Holm, Marsden and Ratiu (1998) and Marsden, Ratiu and Shkoller (2000). Besides having nice analytical properties, preliminary numerical experiments (see Mohseni et al (2000) and references therein) of these averaged Euler and Navier-Stokes equations show the possible advantages of an averaging approach in the context of numerical solution of nonlinear equations of fluid mechanics.

There is however a very important difference between the template matching framework and the usual fluid mechanics framework. In template matching the equations have to be solved as an initial-final value problem. Thus one is given image f and it has to be deformed to image g moving the pixels in such a way that the motion of the image during the deformation satisfies the template matching equations. In fluid mechanics one is typically interested in giving some initial velocity and studying how the particles move.

8   Discussion and Future Work

We have named the H^1_α equations *averaged* equations. This is with the expectation that they will have averaging properties like the averaged equations of hydrodynamics described in Marsden and Shkoller (2001). But we have not yet done an averaging derivation in the template matching context to see if the solution does indeed allow one to compare images while ignoring features smaller than α. This is the most important task that remains to be done. Furthermore, a condition like $f = g \circ (\varphi(1))$ will have to be modified in the averaging case possibly by preprocessing f and g.

It is our expectation that there will be considerable improvement in the numerical performance of the H_α^1-ATME. This expectation is based on the analogous situation in fluid dynamics in which averaging improves numerical simulation as demonstrated in Mohseni et. al (2000) and references therein. We also plan to investigate generalizations of the procedures here using inexact matching and semidirect product theory (used for *inhomogeneous* fluid problems, for example), to generalize beyond binary images. We also want to explore the role of the rotation group and reduction constructions. This is based on the fact that the notion of *shape space* is a technique common to both mechanics and computer vision.

Due to an initial-final value formulation, it appears that an optimization approach is one way to solve template matching type equations, as is done in Trouvé (1995, 1998). Thus when it comes to computations, the PDEs of template matching (9) or (13) may, or may not be used directly for some applications. In the optimization approach, one goes back to the Lagrangian (material) formulation on the group and finds geodesics directly, by a gradient descent type algorithm for example.

One benefit of the PDE formulation is theoretical, now one knows what equation is being solved. But more importantly, we emphasize that the very reason that we were able to arrive at an averaged version of L²-TME was because we knew how averaging worked in hydrodynamics by changing the metric on the group Diff(M), and we knew how to go back and forth between an arbitrary point on the group and identity using Euler-Poincaré theory. Finally, there may be other problems within computer vision or outside it, in which the PDEs are used directly in the computations.

As for the existence of minimizer of the energy functional, Trouvé (1995, 1998) uses a different definition of distance on Diff(M). He gives a sufficient condition on the metric on Diff(M) for the variational problem of template matching to have a minimizer. Roughly speaking, this condition (which is part of what he calls the admissibility criteria) is that the metric must be as strong as the C^1 metric. By Sobolev embedding theorem this implies that an H^s metric will satisfy this condition iff $s > n/2 + 1$. Thus for $n = 2$ or 3, an H^1 or H^2 metric, including the H_α^1 metric will not satisfy this condition. However, note that Trouvé's admissibility criteria is a sufficient condition. In practice in template matching sometimes the metric $\int_M \langle u, u \rangle + (\Delta u)^2 dx$ is used as mentioned in Grenander and Miller (1998). This metric also does not satisfy the admissibility criteria. This suggests that more work on the theory of existence of minimizer for template matching functionals is needed.

Finally we note that we have only shown that $d_\mathcal{P}$ is a pseudometric. If the infimum in Definition 2 in not achieved $d_\mathcal{P}$ is only a pseudometric and there can exist f and g, $f \neq g$, but $d_\mathcal{P}(f, g) = 0$. What do specific examples (if any) of such f, g pairs look like ? Even more interestingly one can ask if for some metrics on Diff(M), for example for the H_α^1 metric of Definition 4, $d_\mathcal{P}$ is a metric. We plan to investigate these questions.

Acknowledgements

We would like to thank J. Tilak Ratnanather for bringing the TME to our attention in 1999 and keeping us informed of their work since then. We would also like to thank Steve Shkoller, Antonio Hernandez, Sergey Pekarsky and Banavara Shashikanth for helpful discussions. Comments from the mutual review group in Caltech Computer Science, especially the detailed suggestions from Min Chen were very useful in improving the organization of the paper.

References

Abraham, R., Marsden, J. E. and Ratiu, T. S.: Manifolds, Tensor Analysis and Applications. Springer Verlag (1988)

Camassa, R. and Holm D. D.: An integrable shallow water equation with peaked solitons. Phys. Rev. Lett. **71** (1993) 1661–1664

Dupuis, P., Grenander, U. and Miller, M. I.: Variational problems on flows of diffeomorphisms for image matching. Quarterly of Applied Mathematics **LVI** (1998) 587–600

Ebin, D. E., Marsden, J. E.: Groups of diffeomorphisms and the motion of an incompressible fluid. Ann. of Math. **92** (1970) 102–163

Grenander, U. and Miller, M. I.: Computational anatomy: an emerging discipline. Quarterly of Applied Mathematics **LVI** (1998) 617–694

Hirani, A. N., Marsden, J. E. and Arvo, J.: Averaged template matching equations. California Institute of Tecnology, Computer Science Technical Report (2001)

Holm, D. D., Marsden, J. E. and Ratiu, T. S.: Euler-Poincaré models of ideal fluids with nonlinear dispersion. Phys. Res. Lett. **349** (1998) 4173–4177

Marsden, J. E. and Ratiu, T. S.: Introduction to Mechanics and Symmetry, Second Edition. Springer Verlag (1999)

Marsden, J. E., Ratiu, T. S. and Shkoller, S.: The geometry and analysis of the averaged Euler equations and a new diffeomorphism group. Geometric and Functional Analysis **10** (2000) 582–599

Marsden, J. E. and Shkoller, S.: Global well-posedness of the isotropic LANS equations. Proc. Royal Soc. London (to appear)

Miller, M. I. and Younes, L.: Group actions, homeomorphisms and matching : a general framework. Preprint (1999)

Mohseni, K., Shkoller, S., Kosović, B., Marsden, J. E., Carati, D., Wray, A. and Rogallo, R.: Numerical Simulations of Homogeneous Turbulence using the Lagrangian-Averaged Navier-Stokes Equations. Proc. CTR summer school (2000)

Mumford, D.: Unpublished note (1998)

Mumford, D.: Pattern theory and vision. Questions Mathématiques en Traitement du Signal et de L'Image, Institut Henri Poincaré (1998) 7–13

Ratnanather, J. T., Baigent, S. A., Mumford, D. and Miller, M. I.: Personal communication (2000)

Shkoller, S.: Geometry and curvature of diffeomorphism groups with H^1 metric and mean hydrodynamics. J. Funct. Anal. **160** (1998) 337–365

Trouvé, A.: An infinite dimensional group approach for physics based models in pattern recognition. Preprint (1995)

Trouvé, A.: Diffeomorphism groups and pattern matching in image analysis. Intl. J. Comp. Vis. **28** (1998) 213–221

Younes, L.: Deformations, warping and object comparison. Preprint (2000)

A Continuous Shape Descriptor by Orientation Diffusion

Hsing-Kuo Pao and Davi Geiger

Courant Institute, New York University, New York, NY 10012, USA
212-9983485, 212-9983235
{hsingkuo,geiger}@cs.nyu.edu

Abstract. We propose a continuous description for 2-D shapes that calculates convexity, symmetry and is able to account for size. Convexity and size are known to be critical in deciding figure/ground (F/G) separation, with the study initiated by the Gestalt school [9] [11]. However, few quantitative discussions were made before. Thus, we emphasize the convexity/size measurement for the purpose of F/G prediction. A Kullback-Leibler measure is introduced. In addition, the symmetry information is studied through the same platform. All these shape properties are collected for shape representations. Overall, our representations are given in a continuous manner. For convexity measurement, unlike the $1/0$ mathematical definition where shapes are categorized as convex or concave, we give a measure describing shapes as "more" or "less" convex than others. In symmetry information (skeleton) retrieval, a 2-D intensity map is provided with the intensity value specifying "strength" of the skeleton. The proposed representations are robust in the sense that small fine-scale perturbations on shape boundaries will cause minor effects on the final representations. All these shape properties are intergrated into one description. To apply to the F/G separation, the shape measure can be flexibly chosen between a size-invariant convexity measure or a convexity measure with the small size preference. The model is established on an orientation diffusion framework, where the local features, served as inputs, are intensity edge locations and their orientations . The approach is a variational one, rooted in a Markov random field (MRF) formulation. A quadratic form is used to assure simplicity and the existence of solution.

Key Words: Early Vision, Shape Analysis, Convexity, Symmetry, Orientation Diffusion.

1 Introduction

The convexity criteria has been argued to be important in F/G separation (Kanizsa [9] or Fig. 1), where a 2-D region can be recognized as figure due to the convexity property of its borders. However, the measurement for convexity was left as intuitive and no formalism was then offered. The mathematical definition of convexity[1] only allows for two class of shapes: convex or concave ones (not convex). There is an intuition that some shapes are "more convex" than others (Fig. 1 (a1) (a2), Fig. 6 (a1)-(a3)). To capture this intuition, we study a continuous measure of convexity.

---

[1] A shape is convex if given any pair of interior points, the segment connecting these points is completely inside the shape

M.A.T. Figueiredo, J. Zerubia, A.K. Jain (Eds.): EMMCVPR 2001, LNCS 2134, pp. 544–559, 2001.
© Springer-Verlag Berlin Heidelberg 2001

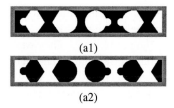

(a1)

(a2)

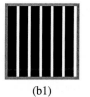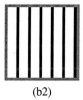

(b1)   (b2)

Fig. 1. The preference of convexity and size. In (a1)/(a2), white/black regions are reported as figures respectively which argues convexity playing an important role in such a decision. In (b1), white strips are likely to be perceived in front of black background which gives an example of (small) size preference.

First, the human visual system tends to ignore minor perturbation (protrusion) of shapes. Such robustness is therefore a desired feature for a model measuring convexity. By a measure with this consideration, figural regions can be selected. We will argue that this F/G selection can not be provided by a well-known continuous criteria, called *shape compactness*, defined by the ratio of the square of perimeter to the shape area [1]. A related topic is to study a size-invariant measure. Under this measure, shapes can be compared to each other, for shapes with or without similar size. However, because the human visual system prefers small size objects to be perceived as figures (Koffka [11], Fig. 1(b1) (b2)), our complete model of shapes should also be able to measure convexity integrated with a preference of small size shapes. Our model will provide a parameter that can be tuned to a size-invariant convexity measure or one that biases towards small size shapes.

We propose an orientation diffusion process defined in the space $\mathbf{R}^2 \times \mathbf{S}^1$. In our view, the elements/features detected at images at the first stage are intensity edge locations and their orientations. It is known that human visual perception is based on orientation filters (found in area V1 and V2 of the brain), providing the orientation of the edges detected. Afterwards, a scheme is designed by a computation of propagating the oriented boundary information through *local interactions*. The problem of propagation is formulated as a Markov random field. By our model, the problem of F/G can be studied in a wide range of imagery.

Besides the convexity measurement, the symmetry information (skeleton) can be derived through the computation of divergence of a vector field which is generated from the result of orientation diffusion. Overall, our model is able to (i) deliver simultaneously a convexity measure and symmetry information of shapes; (ii) adjust (via one parameter) the balance between convexity and size, i.e., it is able to bias to a size invariant model or to include size in its measure.

1.1   Previous Work

Mumford [13] used *Elastica* in the smooth curve finding. The line propagation was done via a diffusion process in orientation and a translation in the $(\cos\theta \frac{\partial}{\partial x} + \sin\theta \frac{\partial}{\partial y})$-direction (with an exponential decay). Therefore, our model is similar to his. The most important difference is that our consideration is made in $\mathbf{R}^2 \times \mathbf{S}^1$ rather than in $\mathbf{R}^2$, causing all orientations to be considered simultaneously in a minimization formulation. Also, we are proposing various shape measures, a topic beyond his work.

Another interesting technical work was given by Tang et al. [20]. They were only concerned with smoothing dense vector field. A technical difference is that their work was done in the space of maps with a unit vector for each 2-D point, while we work on the space of $\mathbf{R}^2 \times \mathbf{S}^1$. Their *direction diffusion* was used for image processing and noise removal. We use a different diffusion process to generate a field based on a local sparse input. Also, we are interested in obtaining various measures to describe 2-D shapes, by investigating this field.

Pao et al. [16] have proposed a continuous measure of convexity (let us call it the PGR model). However, various problems exist with their model, perhaps the most serious one is that the size of shapes dominates the convexity measure and so small concave shapes could be preferred over larger circles. Thus, not only the model did not separate convexity from size, but also the dominance of size might not be desired.

The work on diffusion and shapes by Kimia, Tannenbaum & Zucker [10] and Siddiqi & Kimia [19] are sources of inspiration. The main difference here is that we are examining a linear diffusion equation on a more complex space of positions and orientations. For searching the skeleton of a shape, we compute the "sinkage" of energy in the shape. It is similar to Dimitrov et al. [4], with the computation of divergence of a vector field. Although, our vector field is generated by a different method.

2   Orientation Diffusion

Given a 2-D region/shape Ω (boundary and its inside), or its boundary $\partial\Omega$, we discuss its convexity and other shape properties. The region/shape or its boundary can be complete, or partial where only part of it is visible through the image frame. We use Γ instead for the boundary when the shape/boundary is partially visible. On the boundary, the orientation information can be locally represented by unit normal vectors in the inward directions (Fig. 2(b1)). Given a set of detectors of the boundary and their orientations, we want to derive a field inside the boundary to describe various shape properties.

We adopt an *orientation diffusion / random walk* process to solve this problem. The approach is in part inspired by Kumaran et al. [12], Pao et al. [16] (PGR model or decay diffusion [15]) where their diffusion process was worked on the image space $\mathbf{I}$, and also inspired by Mumford [13], Tang [20] where they included the orientation space. We extend the PGR model to augment the space to $\mathbf{I} \times \Theta$ by adding an orientation dimension $\Theta \equiv \{\theta \cdot 2\pi/T : \theta = 0, 1, \ldots, T-1\}$.

We will show that our model can provide a more appropriate measure for convexity than previous works. Moreover, other properties of shapes such as their skeleton information will also be obtained.

2.1   Notations

For a given region Ω (represented by Γ) in an input image[2] $\mathbf{I} \equiv \{\mathbf{x} = (x, y) \in \{0, \ldots, L_1 - 1\} \times \{0, \ldots, L_2 - 1\}$, a set of useful information is collected. For an intensity function $I(\mathbf{x})$, the edge function

---

[2] We will use **bold** face, lower-case letters to denote vectors.

$$e(\mathbf{x};\theta) = \frac{1}{M_e} \left| \frac{\partial I(\mathbf{x})}{\partial \mathbf{u}_\theta} \right| \in [0,1], \quad \mathbf{x} \in \Gamma$$

records the normalized magnitude of the intensity change at pixel $\mathbf{x}$ in the direction of $\mathbf{u}_\theta = (\cos\theta, \sin\theta)$; namely, the (unsigned) directional derivative in $\mathbf{u}_\theta$, normalized by $M_e = \max\{|\frac{\partial I(\mathbf{x})}{\partial \mathbf{u}_\theta}| : \mathbf{x} \in \mathbf{I}, \theta \in \Theta\}$, the largest orientational intensity edge in the image $\mathbf{I}$. Also, on Γ, a hypothesis set (or inducers) is defined by

$$\sigma_0(\mathbf{x};\theta) = \begin{cases} e(\mathbf{x};\theta) & \text{if } \mathbf{u}_\theta \cdot \mathbf{n}(\mathbf{x}) \geq 0 \wedge \mathbf{x} \in \Gamma \\ 0 & \text{if } \mathbf{u}_\theta \cdot \mathbf{n}(\mathbf{x}) < 0 \wedge \mathbf{x} \in \Gamma. \end{cases} \tag{1}$$

On the boundary, the vector $\mathbf{n}(\mathbf{x})$ is the unit normal vector chosen the inward direction. We say that the directions closer to the inward side are in the source mode and the directions closer to the outward side are in the sink mode. Finally, a field

$$\sigma(\mathbf{x};\theta) : \Omega \times \Theta \to \mathbf{R}$$

will be evaluated by our orientation diffusion process.

2.2 Variational Model

We will create an orientation diffusion process worked in the field $\{\sigma(\mathbf{x};\theta) : \mathbf{x} \in \Omega, \theta \in \Theta\}$ by formulating it as a variational problem.

Local Hypotheses and Data Fitting. The field $\sigma(\mathbf{x};\theta)$ should take the local hypothesis values $\sigma_0(\mathbf{x};\theta)$, where they are available. In our model they are available at all intensity edge pixels (pixels on Γ) according to their strength $e(\mathbf{x};\theta)$. I.e., we seek the $\sigma(\mathbf{x};\theta)$ which minimizes

$$E_{\text{data}}(\sigma|\sigma_0) = \sum_{(\mathbf{x};\theta) \in \Gamma \times \Theta} e(\mathbf{x};\theta) \left(\sigma(\mathbf{x};\theta) - \sigma_0(\mathbf{x};\theta)\right)^2. \tag{2}$$

In most cases, the gradient direction is the one with the maximum value of $e(\mathbf{x};\theta)$, associated with either an inward ($\sigma_0 \geq 0$) or outward hypothesis ($\sigma_0 = 0$).

For the homogeneous regions (where no intensity edge is present), we extend the definition of the functions σ_0 and e by respectively assigning a local hypothesis of value 0 and a small constant strength,

$$\sigma_0(\mathbf{x};\theta) = 0 \quad \text{if } \mathbf{x} \in \Omega \wedge \mathbf{x} \notin \Gamma \tag{3}$$
$$e(\mathbf{x};\theta) = \lambda \quad \text{if } \mathbf{x} \in \Omega \wedge \mathbf{x} \notin \Gamma. \tag{4}$$

The index of the summation in Eq. 2 becomes $(\mathbf{x};\theta) \in \Omega \times \Theta$ now, taking the whole region. The small constant parameter $0 < \lambda \ll 1$, known as the decay coefficient[3], controlling the decay effect of the energy when σ is away from the inducers (hypothesis set). A larger λ has stronger effect to bring pixels away from the intensity edges to take the value 0 (See Fig. 3(d) & (e)).

---

[3] When this functional is analyzed as a Markov chain, the parameter λ plays the role of decay parameter, or the probability of "vanishing", of the random walk associated to this functional.

Smoothness. Propagation of the local hypothesis is done by adding a smoothness term that prefers neighboring pixels with similar orientations sharing the similar values. For instance, in Fig. 2(a), the vector in position P_0 with the orientation θ and its neighbor P_1 with the orientation $\theta + \psi$ are encouraged to share similar value of σ. A simple quadratic form is applied here by minimizing

$$\frac{1}{\kappa} \sum_{\psi=-\kappa}^{\kappa} M(\mathbf{x}; \theta, \psi)(\sigma(x + \cos\theta, y + \sin\theta, \theta + \psi) - \sigma(\mathbf{x}, \theta))^2, \tag{5}$$

for each $\mathbf{x}$ and θ. The function $M(\mathbf{x}; \theta, \psi)$ is simply provided by $\cos(\psi \frac{\pi}{2k})$, giving the cosine weighting for the smoothness that concentrates particularly on small deviations. A more complicated version of the function M may also depend on $\mathbf{x}$ (non-homogeneous) or θ (anisotropic). The parameter[4] $\kappa \in (0, \pi)$, called the underline{deviation factor} controlling the deviation of orientations for the moving particles. A continuous version of Eq. 5 is used here for computational purposes.

$$E_{\text{smooth}}(\sigma) = \int_{\Omega \times \Theta} \left[\frac{1}{\kappa} \int_{-\kappa}^{\kappa} M(\mathbf{x}; \theta, \psi)(\cos\theta \sigma_x + \sin\theta \sigma_y + \psi \sigma_\theta)^2 d\psi \right] d\mathbf{x} d\theta. \tag{6}$$

Energy Functional. The total energy functional is the summation of the data fitting term (a continuous form is applied by substituting a 2-D Dirac-delta function in Eq. 2 [15]) and the smoothness term

$$E(\sigma|\sigma_0) = E_{\text{data}}(\sigma|\sigma_0) + E_{\text{smooth}}(\sigma), \tag{7}$$

where the functional $\mathcal{H}(\sigma|\mathbf{x}; \theta)$ within the bracket in Eq. 6 can be abbreviated as

$$\mathcal{H}(\sigma|\mathbf{x}; \theta)$$

$$= (\cos\theta \sigma_x + \sin\theta \sigma_y)^2 \cdot \frac{1}{\kappa} \int_{-\kappa}^{\kappa} M(\mathbf{x}; \theta, \psi) \, d\psi$$

$$+ 2\sigma_\theta(\cos\theta \sigma_x + \sin\theta \sigma_y) \cdot \frac{1}{\kappa} \int_{-\kappa}^{\kappa} \psi M(\mathbf{x}; \theta, \psi) \, d\psi + \sigma_\theta^2 \cdot \frac{1}{\kappa} \int_{-\kappa}^{\kappa} \psi^2 M(\mathbf{x}; \theta, \psi) \, d\psi$$

$$= A (\cos\theta \sigma_x + \sin\theta \sigma_y)^2 + 2B \, \sigma_\theta(\cos\theta \sigma_x + \sin\theta \sigma_y) + C \sigma_\theta^2. \tag{8}$$

where $A = 4/\pi$, $B = 0$ and $C = 4\kappa^2/\pi$. Its Euler-Lagrange equation can be given by

$$\cos^2\theta \, \sigma_{xx} + 2\sin\theta\cos\theta \, \sigma_{xy} + \sin^2\theta \, \sigma_{yy} + \kappa^2(1 - \frac{8}{\pi^2})\sigma_{\theta\theta} = \frac{\lambda\pi}{4}\sigma, \tag{9}$$

with the boundary condition $\sigma(\mathbf{x}; \theta) = \sigma_0(\mathbf{x}; \theta)$, if $(\mathbf{x}, \theta) \in \Gamma \times \Theta$.

Numerically, the energy function is quadratic and the minimizer is straightforwardly obtained by rewriting Eq. 7 as a matrix form by the finite difference method, and solving it by a gradient-descent method. We call this minimizer $\sigma^*(\mathbf{x}; \theta)$. Some examples of $\sigma^*(\mathbf{x}; \theta)$ are shown in Fig. 3(a) & (b).

---

[4] We avoid the degenerate case, $\kappa = 0$, when the smoothness functional becomes $\sum_{\mathbf{x},\theta} M(\mathbf{x}, \theta, 0)(\sigma(\mathbf{x}, \theta) - \sigma(x + \cos\theta, y + \sin\theta, \theta))^2$, no longer depending on ψ, and the minimization process can be worked separately through different θ's.

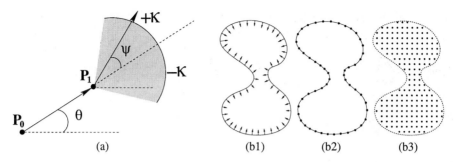

Fig. 2. (a) a particle moves from P_0 to P_1 with slightly changed in orientation. We say that the particle has the configuration changed from $(\mathbf{x}; \theta)$ to $(x + \cos\theta, y + \sin\theta; \theta + \psi)$ as it goes from the point P_0 to P_1 (assume $|P_0 - P_1| = 1$). The shadow area indicates the possible trails that the particle may choose, with different weighting according to the deviation angle ψ. (b1) one part of the hypothesis set σ_0 (Eq. 1: part 1) with inward vectors of length $e(\mathbf{x}; \theta)$ represented by vector notations. Only the normal directions are shown. Other parts includes (b2) set of vectors of length 0 with outward direction (Eq. 1: part 2) and (b3) decay vectors generally put all over the space $(\mathbf{I} - \varGamma) \times \Theta$ (Eq. 3).

2.3   Kullback-Leibler Measure

Once the field $\sigma^*(\mathbf{x}; \theta)$ is obtained, we can evaluate those shape properties, such as convexity or symmetry. First of all, from the solution space $\varOmega \times \Theta$ to the image space $\varOmega$, we perform a vector summation considering $\sigma^*(\mathbf{x}; \theta)$ as a vector in the direction of $\mathbf{u}_\theta = (\cos\theta, \sin\theta)$ with length $\sigma^*(\mathbf{x}; \theta)$ (always non-negative),

$$\hat{\sigma}^*(\mathbf{x}) = \hat{\sigma}^*_{cv}(\mathbf{x}) = \int_0^{2\pi} \sigma^*(\mathbf{x}; \theta)\,\mathbf{u}_\theta\,d\theta, \tag{10}$$

where direction of the resultant vector $\hat{\sigma}^*_{cv}$ will be recorded by θ^*, if it has non-zero length. We shall use $\hat{\sigma}^*$ to denote the resultant vectors if no confusion can be made. One example of the vector field $\hat{\sigma}^*(\mathbf{x})$ is in Fig. 3(f2). The idea is that this vector summation will remove the symmetry information of the solution field, and thus what is left is "convexity". For example, the center of a circle is perfectly symmetric and will result in $\hat{\sigma}^* = \mathbf{0}$ while other internal points will have the symmetry removed and still produce evidence of convexity. In our approach, convexity works on the complementary information as symmetry does. Detecting symmetry will be done by investigating which coordinates have a vector summation yield zero value (cancellations), while convexity examines the non-zero valued information of the vector summation. Indeed, the convexity measure we propose measures how well the "vector bundle" is accumulated around this summation vector. Let us be more precise.

At a fixed location $\mathbf{x}$, for each pair of opposite orientations θ and $\theta + \pi$, we compute the net effect, called the map $\tau^*(\mathbf{x}; \theta)$ by

$$\tau^*(\mathbf{x}; \theta) = \frac{1}{2}\left\{\sigma^*(\mathbf{x}, \theta) - \sigma^*(\mathbf{x}, \theta + \pi) + |\sigma^*(\mathbf{x}, \theta) - \sigma^*(\mathbf{x}, \theta + \pi)|\right\}$$

$$\tau^*(\mathbf{x}; \theta + \pi) = \frac{1}{2}\left\{\sigma^*(\mathbf{x}, \theta + \pi) - \sigma^*(\mathbf{x}, \theta) + |\sigma^*(\mathbf{x}, \theta + \pi) - \sigma^*(\mathbf{x}, \theta)|\right\}$$

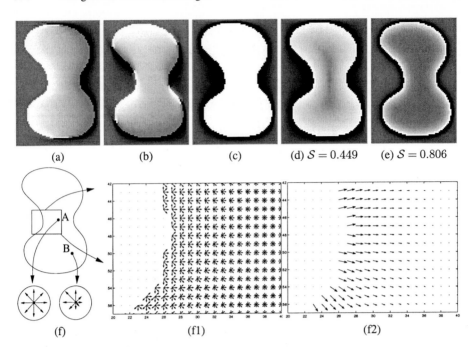

Fig. 3. Results of orientation diffusion process by two presentations. (a) $\sigma(x,y;0)$, (b) $\sigma(x,y;\frac{27}{16}\pi)$, (c) maximum magnitude among all orientations, and (d) (e) relative entropy $D(P_\mathbf{x}\|Q)$ (Eq. 12) with $\lambda = 0.1/|\Omega| = 2.876 \times 10^{-5}$, $500/|\Omega| = 0.144$ respectively. The difference shows effect of the energy decay. Larger λ gives stronger decay, less diffusion and larger convexity measure (Eq. 13). (f1) (f2) Vector presentations for part of the bell shape figure in (f). (f1) the vector bundles with choice of 8 orientations. We say that the point A has a more balanced (symmetry) result along different orientations than the bundle in B. (f2) the convexity vector $\hat{\sigma}^*$ (Eq. 10).

$$= \tau^*(\mathbf{x};\theta) - \sigma(\mathbf{x};\theta) + \sigma(\mathbf{x};\theta+\pi), \tag{11}$$

where a cyclic boundary condition $\theta = \theta + 2\pi$ is used. Note that Eq. 10 can be rewritten as $\hat{\sigma}^*(\mathbf{x}) = \int_0^{2\pi} \tau^*(\mathbf{x};\theta) \mathbf{u}_\theta \, d\theta$. The second step is to transform $\tau(\mathbf{x};\theta)$ to $P^*(\mathbf{x};\theta)$ or simply $P_\mathbf{x}(\theta)$, by a linear transformation. It is

$$P^*(\mathbf{x};\theta) = \frac{1}{2}(1 + \tau^*(\mathbf{x};\theta)).$$

Unlike any previous work, we propose a Kullback-Leibler distance (or relative entropy) to measure convexity. The map $P_\mathbf{x}(\theta)$ is compared to a Gaussian map in $\mathbf{S}^1$ (not normalized)

$$Q(\theta) = \frac{1}{1+\epsilon_N} \exp(-\frac{(\theta-\theta^*)^2}{2 \cdot (2.0)^2}), \qquad -\pi \leq \theta \leq \pi$$

where the center of Q is located in the direction θ^*, the direction of vector $\hat{\sigma}^*$. A small positive constant ϵ_N is added to avoid the case of $Q(\theta) = 1$. The Kullback-Leibler distance, computed at every point $\mathbf{x}$, between $Q(\theta)$ and $P_\mathbf{x}(\theta)$ is given by

$$D(P_{\mathbf{x}}\|Q) = \int_0^{2\pi} P_{\mathbf{x}}(\theta) \log \frac{P_{\mathbf{x}}(\theta)}{Q(\theta)} + (1 - P_{\mathbf{x}}(\theta)) \log \frac{1 - P_{\mathbf{x}}(\theta)}{1 - Q(\theta)}\, d\theta. \qquad (12)$$

Intuitively, it measures the inefficiency of assuming that the distribution is $Q(\theta)$ when the real distribution is $P_{\mathbf{x}}(\theta)$. That is, we assume the map in $\mathbf{S}^1$ has a sharp peak at θ^*. $D(P_{\mathbf{x}}\|Q)$ is always equal to or greater than 0, and it can be greater than 1. A smaller measure means a better fit.

This measure is given for each point $\mathbf{x}$. To obtain a global measure of a shape, we simply average this measure over the points on the figure. I.e., the final measure of a shape Ω is

$$\mathcal{S}(P_{\mathbf{x}}) = \frac{1}{|\Omega|} \int_\Omega D(P_{\mathbf{x}}\|Q)\, d\mathbf{x}, \qquad (13)$$

A shape with a smaller measure is considered more convex than others. A simple example can be seen in Fig. 4 as a F/G experiment. We use $\mathcal{S}/\overline{\mathcal{S}}$ to denote the measure for (conventional) figure/background area respectively.

3   Convexity Measurement

To examine the orientation model and the Kullback-Liebler measure, we conduct different set of experiments. One set of images refers to the F/G separation task and we test ability of the model to account for human visual perception. The second set displays shape figures and the task is to order and compare them. For each set of examples we illustrate the results with several prototypes. The prototype illustrations for the F/G set are Fig. 4, Fig. 5 and Kanizsa's figure of comparing convexity versus symmetry (Fig. 6). The prototypes for the second set are a (non-) perfect ellipse and a "bell" shape (shown on the right-hand side of Fig. 7).

In Sec. 4, we consider another set studying behavior of the model as we vary the parameter κ. This is particularly important to understand how the shape size plays a role in the model.

We are also interested in the convexity comparison of perfectly convex shapes. Shapes like circles, squares, and triangles are lined up by the Kullback-Liebler measure. Also, the comparison of squares to rectangles will favor squares than rectangles. They will be shown in Sec. 5.

In all cases we used synthesized binary images. The parameters we used are, the decay coefficient $\lambda = 0.1/|\Omega|$, divided by area of the region Ω and the deviation factor

(a)   (b)

Fig. 4. A simple experiment used for F/G separation and its relative entropy $D(P_{\mathbf{x}}\|Q)$. While right side is convex and left side is concave, we have $\mathcal{S}/\overline{\mathcal{S}} = \mathbf{0.605}/0.671$ respectively. Both regions are equally sized.

$\kappa = 0.4$ except in the cases that are said otherwise. The peak of the delta function is simulated by $1/\epsilon$ with $\epsilon = 10^{-5} \cdot |\partial \Omega|$, a constant normalized by the perimeter of Ω. The normalization of the parameters λ or ϵ according to area or perimeter of Ω respectively is not essential for the convexity measurement and can be removed.

3.1 Convexity as Salience

We test our measure for various prototypes. For a simple test in Fig. 4, the measure is given by $\mathcal{S}/\overline{\mathcal{S}} = \mathbf{0.605}/0.671$, favoring the white region. For another F/G image in Fig. 5, we have the consistent predictions through images with different ratios of bk/wt area. Also, we do observe the size effect from (a) to (c): the differences between figures and background become less as black/white regions get smaller/larger respectively. For a Kanizsa figure in Fig. 6(a3) where the white regions own the biggest area among (a1)-(a3), the result predicts that the white regions (convexity) prevail as the figure over the black regions (symmetry) with $\mathcal{S}/\overline{\mathcal{S}} = \mathbf{0.490}/0.497$. It can not be given by the model provided by [16] which gives $\mathcal{S}/\overline{\mathcal{S}} = 0.715/\mathbf{0.645}$, saying that the black regions will be figures and it is a "wrong" prediction.

The reason is that the decay model provided by Pao et al. [16] is too sensitive to the size and can not provide consistent predictions when we move the edge boundaries leftward or rightward, even the change is small and beyond the detection from our eyes. A better model, the oriented one will give correct predictions consistently, with shift of the edge boundaries.

4 Convexity versus Size

In the Euler-Lagrange equation in Eq. 9, the deviation factor κ serves as the diffusivity in the orientation space Θ. In the random walk formulation, a larger κ provides more noise and less deterministic behavior in orientation when it moves from one location to another neighboring location. A measure with small size preference is yielded in such a situation. On the other hand, a smaller κ has more control in orientation. The measure will have less size preference and be closer to ideal convexity measure than the one given in the less-deterministic case. The most extreme case gives the size invariance measure, provided by letting $\kappa \to 0$. It will be discussed later. Results related to different choices of κ will be studied in Sec. 4.1 for F/G separation and Sec. 4.2 for shape convexity comparison respectively. The choice of κ provides the flexibility of choosing convexity

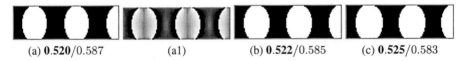

(a) $\mathbf{0.520}/0.587$ (a1)   (b) $\mathbf{0.522}/0.585$ (c) $\mathbf{0.525}/0.583$

Fig. 5. Colonnade with boundaries translated through the horizontal direction from (a), a size balanced one to (c), with white regions owning the largest area. The relative entropy of (a) is shown in (a1). Their differences between the measures in figure/ground get smaller from (a) to (c), as black/white regions get smaller/larger. It shows the size/proximity preference of the model.

measure between a size-invariant one and the one with small size preference. It cannot be achieved by the decay measure in [16]. We use the Kanizsa images in Fig. 6 (Sec. 4.1) and the ellipse/bell pair in Fig. 7 (Sec. 4.2) to illustrate our idea.

Size Invariance by Letting $\kappa \to 0$ Let us analyze the case when $\kappa \to 0$, where the walk is totally deterministic in orientation. By taking the limit $\kappa \to 0$, the functional in Eq. 8 becomes

$$\lim_{\kappa \to 0} \mathcal{H}(\sigma | \mathbf{x}; \theta) = \frac{4}{\pi}(\cos\theta\,\sigma_x + \sin\theta\,\sigma_y)^2.$$

We want to examine the effect of shape scaling in this limit for the whole functional in Eq. 7. After that, we study the scaling effect on the convexity measure $\mathcal{S}$.

Given two *similar* shapes Ω and Ω' in an image $\mathbf{I}$, indicated by two characteristic functions χ and χ' s.t. $\chi(\mathbf{x}) = 1$ or $\chi'(\mathbf{x}) = 1$ if $\mathbf{x} \in \Omega$ or Ω' respectively, and $\chi(\mathbf{x}) = 0$ or $\chi'(\mathbf{x}) = 0$ otherwise. Under an appropriately chosen coordinate system, we have $\chi(\mathbf{x}) = \chi'(r\mathbf{x}) = \chi'(\mathbf{x}')$, $\forall \mathbf{x}, \mathbf{x}' \in \mathbf{I}$. Given similar edge maps $e(\mathbf{x}; \theta) = e'(\mathbf{x}'; \theta) = |\mathbf{u}_\theta \cdot \mathbf{n}(\mathbf{x})|$, when $\kappa \to 0$ and $\lambda \to 0$, the decay term will vanish and we have

$$E(\sigma') = E(\sigma) = \int_{\Omega \times \Theta} \delta_2 \cdot e \cdot (\sigma - \sigma_0)^2 + \frac{4}{\pi}(\cos\theta\,\sigma_x + \sin\theta\,\sigma_y)^2 \, d\mathbf{x}\,d\theta,$$

if we assign $\sigma'(\mathbf{x}'; \theta) = \sigma(\mathbf{x}; \theta)$. So the minimizer for either functional can be obtained easily when the other one has been computed. Two minimizers are related by $\sigma^*(\mathbf{x}; \theta) = \sigma'^*(\mathbf{x}'; \theta)$. Different orientations are worked independently here.

Let us discuss the scaling effect on the convexity measure. For two similar maps σ^*, σ'^*, we can obtain the similarity between $P_\mathbf{x}$ and $P_{\mathbf{x}'}$ or $D(P_\mathbf{x} \| Q)$ and $D(P_{\mathbf{x}'} \| Q)$. Therefore, for the convexity measure, we have

$$\mathcal{S}(P_{\mathbf{x}'}) = -\frac{1}{|\Omega'|}\int_{\Omega'} D(P_{\mathbf{x}'} \| Q)\, d\mathbf{x}' = -\frac{1}{r^2|\Omega|} \cdot r^2 \int_\Omega D(P_\mathbf{x} \| Q)\, d\mathbf{x} = \mathcal{S}(P_\mathbf{x}).$$

It is an ideal case where we can achieve a measure with no sensitivity to the size. Examples in the discrete case can be found in Fig. 7 and Sec. 4.2. When λ is not zero, we need to set a new $\lambda' = \lambda/r^2$ to achieve the similarity $\sigma^*(\mathbf{x}; \theta) = \sigma'^*(\mathbf{x}'; \theta)$.

4.1   Figure/Ground Separation in Convexity-Symmetry Image and Tuning of κ

We will use the Kanizsa figures in Fig. 6 to illustrate our points. As we have discussed, the decay model cannot provide a consistent prediction when the area ratio of different regions is changed, even though the change is small and beyond the detection from our eyes. The orientation model will give a consistent prediction, with a small shift of the edge boundaries. The trick lies in the free parameter κ which on one hand (small κ or the extreme case with $\kappa \to 0$) gives a convexity measure without considering small size preference and on the other hand (big κ) gives a measure with the size preference. In Tab. 1, we have series (a1), balanced area for black and white regions, series (a2), larger white regions and (a3) white regions with the largest area. Several pairs of comparisons can be studied. When $\kappa = 0.1$, the purest convexity measure among them, gives the

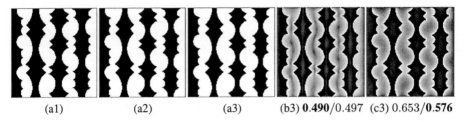

(a1)   (a2)   (a3)   (b3) **0.490**/0.497   (c3) 0.653/**0.576**

Fig. 6. Convexity measure for the Kanizsa figures (adapted from Kanizsa [9]). (b3) gives the relative entropy of (a3) and (c3) gives the decay diffusion field of (a3) (Pao et al. [16]). When the boundaries are translated from (a1) to (a3) with white regions getting bigger, the convexity measure from the orientation diffusion gives $S/\overline{S} = \mathbf{0.490}/0.497$ in (b3), by a test of $\kappa = 0.1$ while in (c3), the measure from the PGR model shows $S/\overline{S} = 0.653/\mathbf{0.576}$, a "wrong" prediction. Note that the (non-oriented) decay diffusion process will have more diffusion near the neck area while in (b3), a bad relative entropy will be given with help of the oriented process. More discussion related to size and the choice of κ can be seen in Tab. 1.

expected answer with white in the front, for all three cases. When $\kappa = \pi/2$, a case blended with the most size preference among them, white regions in (a1) & (a2) are preferred, but not for (a3) where the smaller black regions are preferred. The case of $\kappa = 0.4$ gives an intermediate transition. For the perceptual simulation, suppose a case where F/G is decided by both of the convexity and size preferences, we can tune the parameter κ to obtain the appropriate normalization of them, according to the preferences in human visual systems.

4.2   Convexity Comparison of Shapes and Tuning of κ

We study our convexity measure for different shapes with the same or different sizes. As shown in Fig. 7, the imperfect ellipses $A1$(large) & $A2$(small) represent convex shapes, and the bell shapes $B1$(large) & $B2$(small) represent non-convex shapes with "strong proximity" in the neck area. For the choice of κ, a similar scenario is used as in the F/G separation experiments. When κ is small, we pick shape by convexity and when κ is larger, we either pick the smaller size shapes or pick the bell shape with stronger proximity. The details are shown in Fig. 7.

Convexity Comparison of Shapes with the Same Size. When two shapes share the same size, we can easily pick up the ellipse as the more convex shape by choosing $\kappa \leq 0.6$. A large κ will favor proximity and therefore pick the bell as the more favorable shape. We have $S_{A1} < S_{B1}$ and $S_{A2} < S_{B2}$ when $\kappa \leq 0.6$.

Convexity Comparison of Shapes with Any Sizes. To make the measure capable to be applied in a wider range, we compare shapes with different sizes, achieved by using an even smaller $\kappa \leq 0.4$. In this case, no size/proximity issues need to be considered and the measure becomes a "convexity measure". We have $S_{A1}, S_{A2} < S_{B1}, S_{B2}$ if $\kappa \leq 0.4$ is provided. The smallest κ or $\kappa = 0.1$ provides a measure with the least sensitivity to the size. As we can see, the values of similar shapes with different sizes are coincided to each other in this situation.

Table 1. Kanizsa figures with various size ratios (Fig. 6), measured by the orientation diffusion and the PGR model [16]. The series from (a1) to (a3) gives the white region area from small to large. Series (a1) has balanced size. For the orientation diffusion, a smaller κ gives a purer convexity measure and a larger κ, meaning more uncertainty in orientation in walks, will cause a stronger size preference. The prediction for F/G is likely to be decided by convexity when κ is small and be decided by size/proximity when κ is large. We can get convex predictions for F/G when $\kappa \leq 0.1$. The measure collected by the PGR model (result of (a3) is shown in Fig. 6(c3)) is pretty much a size measure if we do not provide a size-balanced experiment.

Series (Area)	$\kappa = 0.1$	$\kappa = 0.4$	$\kappa = \pi/2$	Remark
Convexity Measure by Orientation Diffusion ($S/\bar{S}$)				
(a1) $(+0/-0\%)$	**0.487**/0.502	**0.490**/0.499	**0.560**/0.570	size balanced
(a2) $(+6/-0\%)$	**0.488**/0.500	**0.492**/0.497	**0.564**/0.565	
(a3) $(+28/-0\%)$	**0.490**/0.497	0.495/**0.491**	0.573/**0.555**	
Convexity Measure by PGR model ($S/\bar{S}$)				
(a1) $(+0/-0\%)$		**0.621**/0.653		size balanced
(a2) $(+6/-0\%)$		0.638/**0.635**		
(a3) $(+28/-0\%)$		0.671/**0.597**		

Large κ and Size/Proximity Preference. When κ is large, it is the case of diffusion with low certainty in orientation. We will have the result favoring smaller size shapes, as we have $S_{A2}, S_{B2} < S_{A1}, S_{B1}$. When similar size shapes are compared, a shape with stronger proximity will prevail. Therefore, the bell $B1$ is favored over the ellipse $A1$ and $B2$ is favored over $A2$, by having smaller measures.

5   Comparison of Convex Shapes

5.1   From Rectangle to Square

In Fig. 8, we run the model on a series of rectangles with ratio of side length from 0 to 1. As shown in the experiments, the closer to square the rectangle is, the better the convexity measure. The strong symmetry in the thin rectangles will be cancelled by the computation of Eq. 11.

5.2   From Triangle to Circle

In Fig. 9, we examine various regular shapes. Unlike the model provided by [16] giving a measure with the preference from triangle to circle, this orientation model gives a reverse order, prefers circle most, then, hexagon and triangle. By using the Kullback-Leibler measure, diffusion from neighboring inducers with *similar orientations* will accumulate around direction of the resulting vector θ^*, hence, giving a good score. For a cross check, the square in Fig. 8(d) has $S_{\text{hexagon}} < S_{\text{square}} < S_{\text{triangle}}$, falling between the triangle and hexagon. A preference similar to the one given by the PGR model [16] can be achieved by a simulation with a large κ.

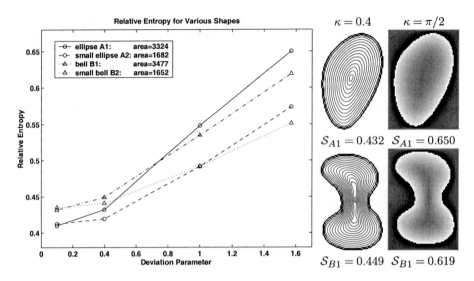

Fig. 7. A comparison between shapes with different sizes and convexity. Four curves listed in $\kappa = \pi/2$, from top to bottom are for the (imperfect) ellipse $A1$, bell $B1$, small ellipse $A2$ and small bell $B2$ (shapes $A1$, $B1$ are shown on the right). A measure with small κ will pick shapes by convexity. A measure with large κ will pick shapes by size/proximity; therefore, either small sized shapes or the bells which own strong proximity near the neck will be favored. When $\kappa = 0.1$, the case with the least size preference, the measures for all similar shapes with different sizes will coincide with each other. The level sets or the relative entropy for $A1$ and $B1$ with the simulations of $\kappa = 0.4$ and $\kappa = \pi/2$ are shown on the right-hand side. The preference between the ellipse and bell switches as we goes from a small κ to a large κ.

5.3   Convexity Is different from Shape Compactness

It is interesting to compare our measure with the compactness CP generally given by $\mathrm{CP}(\partial\Omega) = |\partial\Omega|^2/(4\pi \cdot |\Omega|)$. As we can easily find out, the same preference for regular shapes and the preference of squares over rectangles are also established by the compactness CP. However, the difference between them is shown in various viewpoints:

1. Unlike the shape convexity, the compactness will favor a region with large area instead of small area provided regions with the same perimeter. However, the small size preference does exsit in F/G selection, which can be simulated by our convexity measure (Fig. 5, Fig. 6 and Tab. 1).
2. A circle-like shape with fine scale perturbation may have larger compactness than a smooth-boundary, non-circular shape (Young et al. [21], Bribiesca [2], Fig. 10 (a) & (b)).
3. Our measure has the flexibility to switch between a size-invariant convexity measure or one with small size preference. Also, the freedom to choose the preference of circles over triangles (small κ) or triangles over circles (large κ), etc.
4. It is hard to generalize the shape compactness in the applications where the shape is partial or occluded.

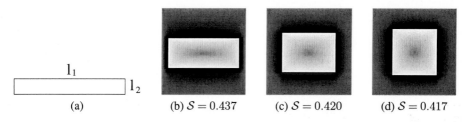

Fig. 8. (a) rectangle with ratio $l1$ to $l2$. (b) (c) (d) samples of different ratios $l2/l1$ and the relative entropy $D(P_{\mathbf{x}}\|Q)$. Their measures are shown, given the parameter $\kappa = 0.1$.

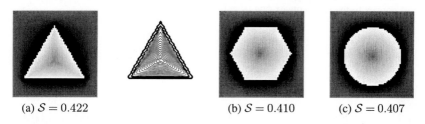

Fig. 9. The relative entropy or corresponding iso-contours derived by our orientation process. Their measures are shown, with the parameter set to be $\kappa = 0.1$. Note that the square in Fig. 8(d) falls between triangle and hexagon. The area information is provided as (a) triangle: 897, (b) hexagon: 1361, and (c) circle: 1469 pixels.

Some examples to illustrate the difference between the compactness and the convexity can be shown in Fig. 10. For the shape (a), perturbations in the fine scale cause a smaller change in the convexity measure, than in the compactness.

6 Symmetry Information

The idea that symmetry can be captured by our model is not particularly new or surprising. For example, based on the work of Siddiqi and Kimia [19], we know that the diffusion process over shapes will "meet" (yield shocks) at the symmetry axis. What is particular to our work, is that the diffusion is on the space $\mathbf{R}^2 \times \mathbf{S}^1$ and presented by a vector form, so the symmetry information can be extracted by a local computation method.

Let us collect the maximum vectors $\sigma_M^*(\mathbf{x})$ by

$$\hat{\sigma}_M^*(\mathbf{x}) = \sigma^*(\mathbf{x}; \theta_M) \cdot \mathbf{u}_M \qquad \text{where} \qquad \sigma^*(\mathbf{x}; \theta_M) = \max_{\theta \in [0, 2\pi]} \{\sigma^*(\mathbf{x}; \theta)\},$$

with $\mathbf{u}_M = (\cos\theta_M, \sin\theta_M)$. We would like to examine the field

$$\sigma_{\text{sym}}^* = \div\left(\frac{\hat{\sigma}_M^*}{\|\hat{\sigma}_M^*\|}\right). \tag{14}$$

The *shape axis* (different from the conventional symmetry axis [15]) is viewed as the place with most sinkage, in the normalized map of the maximum vectors. The map shows "how likely" a point can be on any axis or "how strong" the axis is. Examples of shape axis can be found in Fig. 11.

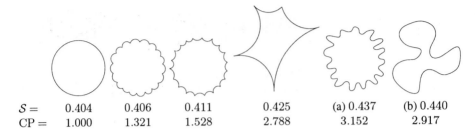

$S =$	0.404	0.406	0.411	0.425	(a) 0.437	(b) 0.440
$CP =$	1.000	1.321	1.528	2.788	3.152	2.917

Fig. 10. Convexity measure for various shapes with different convexity in different scales, from the most convex to the least convex one ($\kappa = 0.1$).

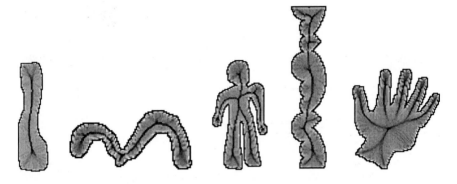

Fig. 11. Shape axis σ^*_{sym} (Eq. 14), computed by using the maximum vector σ^*_M, with $\kappa = \pi/2$.

6.1   Protrusion

To see what protrusion or noise on boundaries can affect the shape axis, we study the axes of shapes in Fig. 12. In (b1), the main axis stays the same as we perturbing the boundaries from (a) by a small protrusion. But a larger effect can (b2) eventually produce a new axis or (b3) even change location of the main axis. By this representation, any further pruning of the "sub-axis" will not be necessary. Because sub-axes are given in "lighter" representations and can be easily removed.

7   Conclusion

We have proposed a framework to capture critical shape information: namely convexity, symmetry and size. It is an orientation diffusion approach, rooted in Markov random fields. The focus of the paper was on demonstrating how the model evaluates convexity, and how size is integrated into the model depending upon a parameter κ. Although it is not surprising, we have indicated how symmetry can also be captured. The protrusion effect on boundaries was naturally solved by this approach. We have demonstrated the validity of the model on various examples and how it improves on previous works. We believe that this approach provides a wealth of information on shapes, and thus, will be used by other practitioners.

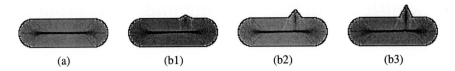

| (a) | (b1) | (b2) | (b3) |

Fig. 12. Shape axis with a protrusion on boundaries. We have the transition from (b1) ignored, (b2) having "sub-axis" to (b3) disturbing the main axis by a faction. We choose the maximum vector $\hat{\sigma}_M^*$, and select the deviation factor $\kappa = \pi/2$.

References

1. D. H. Ballard and C. M. Brown. *Computer Vision*, Prentice-Hall, New Jersey, 1982
2. E. Bribiesca. "Measuring 2D Shape Compactness using the Contact Perimeter", *Computers and Mathematics with Applications*, **33**(11): pp. 1–9, 1997.
3. V. Bruce, P. R. Green and M. A. Georgeson. *Visual Perception, Physiology, Psychology, and Ecology* (3rd ed.), Psychology Press, 1996.
4. P. Dimitrov, C. Philips and K. Sidiqi. "Robust and efficient Skeletal graphs", *CVPR*, South Carolina, June, 2000
5. D. Geiger, H. Pao and N. Rubin. Salient and multiple illusory surfaces. *Computer Vision and Pattern recognition*, June. 1998.
6. F. Heitger and R. von der Heydt. A computational model of neural contour processing: Figure-ground segregation and illusory contours. *Proceedings of the IEEE*, pp. 32–40, 1993.
7. D. Huttenlocher and P. Wayner, "Finding Convex Edge Groupings in an Image," *International Journal of Computer Vision*, **8**(1): pp. 7–29, 1992.
8. D. Jacobs. Robust and efficient detection of convex groups", *IEEE Trans. PAMI*, 1995.
9. G. Kanizsa. *Organization in Vision*. Praeger, New York, 1979.
10. B. Kimia, A. Tannenbaum, S. Zucker. "Shapes, Shocks, and Deformations I: The components of two-dimensional shape and the reaction-diffusion space", *Int. J. Comp. Vis.* **1**: pp. 189–224, 1995.
11. K. Koffka. *Principles of Gestalt Psychology*. New York: Harcourst. 1935.
12. K. Kumaran, D. Geiger, and L. Gurvits. Illusory surfaces and visual organization. *Network: Comput. in Neural Syst.*, **7**(1), Feb. 1996.
13. D. Mumford. Elastica and computer vision. In C. L. Bajaj, editor, *Algebraic Geometry and Its Applications*. Springer-Verlag, New York, 1993.
14. M. Nitzberg and D. Mumford. The 2.1-d sketch. In *ICCV*, pp. 138–144, 1990.
15. H. Pao. "A continuous model for shape selection and represenation", PhD thesis, 2001.
16. H. Pao, D. Geiger and N. Rubin. "Measuring convexity for figure/ground separation", *Int. Conf. on Comp. Vis.*, pp. 948–955, Sep. 1999.
17. S. Parent and S. W. Zucker, "Trace inference, curvature consistency and curve detection", *IEEE PAMI*, Vol. 11, No. 8, pp. 823–839, 1989.
18. E. Rubin, *Visuell wahrgenommene Figuren*, (Copenhagen: Gyldendals), 1921.
19. K. Siddiqi and B. B. Kimia. "A shock frammar for recognition", *Computer Vision and Pattern recognition*, 1996.
20. B. Tang, G. Sapiro and V. Caselles. "Direction diffusion", *International Conference on Computer Vision*, Sep. 1999.
21. I. Young, J. Walker and J. Bowie. "An Analysis technique for biological shape", *Information and Control*, **25**: pp. 357–370, 1974.

Multiple Contour Finding and Perceptual Grouping as a Set of Energy Minimizing Paths

Laurent D. Cohen[1] and Thomas Deschamps[2]

[1] CEREMADE, UMR 7534, Université Paris-Dauphine 75775 Paris cedex 16, France
cohen@ceremade.dauphine.fr
[2] Laboratoire d'Electronique Philips France
thomas.deschamps@philips.com

Abstract. We address the problem of finding a set of contour curves in an image. We consider the problem of perceptual grouping and contour completion, where the data is a set of points in the image. A new method to find complete curves from a set of contours or edge points is presented. Our approach is an extension of previous work on finding a set of contours as minimal paths between end points using the fast marching algorithm. Given a set of key points, we find the pairs of points that have to be linked and the paths that join them. We use the saddle points of the minimal action map. The paths are obtained by backpropagation from the saddle points to both points of each pair.

We also propose an extension of this method for contour completion where the data is a set of connected components. We find the minimal paths between each of these components, until the complete set of these "regions" is connected. The paths are obtained using the same backpropagation from the saddle points to both components.

Keywords: Perceptual grouping, salient curve detection, active contours, minimal paths, fast marching, level sets, weighted distance, reconstruction, energy minimization, medical imaging.

1 Introduction

We are interested in perceptual grouping and finding a set of curves in an image with the use of energy minimizing curves.

Since their introduction, active contours [12] have been extensively used to find the contour of an object in an image through the minimization of an energy. In order to get a set of contours of different objects, we need many active contours to be initialized on the image. The level sets paradigm [15, 1] allowed changes in topology. It enables to get multiple contours by starting with a single one. However, these do not give satisfying results when there are gaps in the data since the contour may propagate into a hole and then split to many curves where only one contour is desired. This is the problem encountered with perceptual grouping where a set of incomplete contours is given. For example, in a binary image like the ones in figure 1 with a drawing of a shape with holes and spurious edge points, human vision can easily fill in the missing boundaries, remove the

M.A.T. Figueiredo, J. Zerubia, A.K. Jain (Eds.): EMMCVPR 2001, LNCS 2134, pp. 560–575, 2001.

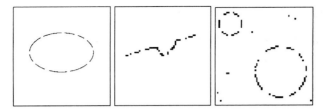

Fig. 1. Examples of incomplete contours

spurious ones and form complete curves. Perceptual grouping is an old problem in computer vision. It has been approached more recently with energy methods [17, 11, 18]. These methods find a criteria for saliency of a curve component or for each point of the image. In these methods, the definition of saliency measure is based indirectly on a second order regularization snake-like energy ([12]) of a path containing the point. However, the final curves are obtained generally in a second step as ridge lines of the saliency criteria after thresholding. In [19] a similarity between snakes and stochastic completion field is reported. Motivated by this relation between energy minimizing curves like snakes and completion contours, we are interested in finding a set of completion contours on an image as a set of energy minimizing curves.

In order to solve global minimization for snakes, the authors of [6] used the minimal paths, as introduced in [14, 13]. The goal was to avoid local minima without demanding too much on user initialization, which is a main drawback of classic snakes [4]. Only two end points were needed. The numerical method has the advantage of being consistent (see [6]) and efficient using the Fast Marching algorithm introduced in [16]. In this paper we propose a way to use this minimal path approach to find a set of curves drawn between points in the image. In order to find a set of most salient contour curves in the image, we draw the minimal paths between pairs of points.

We are also interested in finding a set of curves in an image between a set of connected components. This extension of our perceptual grouping technique finds its application in the completion of tube-like structures in images. The problem is here to complete a partially detected object, based on a number of connected components that belong to this object.

In our examples, the potential P to be minimized along the curves is usually an image of edge points that represent simple incomplete shapes. These edge points are represented as a binary image with small potential values along the edges and high values at the background. Such a potential can be obtained from real images by edge detection (see [5]). The potential could also be defined as edges weighted by the value of the gradient or as a function of an estimate of the gradient of the image itself, $P = g(\|\nabla I\|)$, like in classic snakes. In these cases the chosen function has to be such that the potential is positive everywhere, and it has to be decreasing in order to have edge points as minima of the potential. The potential could also be a grey level image as in [6]. It can also be a more complicated function of the grey level, as in [7] or in Section 4.4.

The problems we solve in this paper are presented as follows:

- Minimal path between two points: The solution proposed in [6] is reviewed in Section 2.
- Minimal paths between a given set of pairs of points is a simple application of the previous one.
- Minimal paths between a given set of unstructured points: a way to find the pairs of linked neighbors and paths between them is proposed in Section 3.
- Minimal paths between a given set of connected components: we propose to find the set of minimal paths that link altogether this set of regions, and we show an example for a medical image in section 4.
- Minimal paths between an unknown set of point: In [2] we propose the automatic finding of key points among a larger set of admissible points and the drawing of minimal paths that leads to completed curves.

2   Minimal Paths and Weighted Distance

2.1   Global Minimum for Active Contours

We present in this section the basic ideas of the method introduced in [6] to find the global minimum of the active contour energy using minimal paths. The energy to minimize is similar to classical deformable models (see [12]) where it combines smoothing terms and image features attraction term (Potential P):

$$E(C) = \int_{\Omega} \left\{ w_1 \|C'(s)\|^2 + w_2 \|C''(s)\|^2 + P(C(s)) \right\} ds \tag{1}$$

where $C(s)$ represents a curve drawn on a 2D image and Ω is its domain of definition. The authors of [6] have related this problem with the recently introduced paradigm of the level-set formulation. In particular, its Euler equation is equivalent to the geodesic active contours [1]. The method introduced in [6] improves energy minimization because the problem is transformed in a way to find the global minimum.

2.2   Problem Formulation

In [6], contrary to the classical snake model (but similarly to geodesic active contours), s represents the arc-length parameter, which means that $\|C'(s)\| = 1$, leading to a geometric energy form. Considering a simplified energy model without the second derivative term leads to the expression $E(C) = \int \{w\|C'\|^2 + P(C)\}ds$. Assuming that $\|C'(s)\| = 1$ leads to the formulation

$$E(C) = \int_{\Omega=[0,L]} \{w + P(C(s))\}ds \tag{2}$$

The regularization of this model is now achieved by the constant $w > 0$ (see [6] for details).

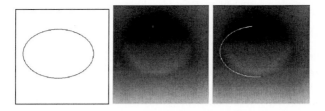

Fig. 2. Finding a minimal path between two points. On the left, the potential is minimal on the ellipse. In the middle, the minimal action or weighted distance to the marked point. On the right, minimal path using backpropagation from the second point

We now have an expression in which the internal energy can be included in the external potential. Given a potential $P \geq 0$ that takes lower values near desired features, we are looking for paths along which the integral of $\tilde{P} = P + w$ is minimal. The surface of minimal action $\mathcal{U}$ is defined as the minimal energy integrated along a path between a starting point p_0 and any point p:

$$\mathcal{U}(p) = \inf_{\mathcal{A}_{p_0,p}} E(C) = \inf_{\mathcal{A}_{p_0,p}} \left\{ \int_{\Omega} \tilde{P}(C(s)) ds \right\} \tag{3}$$

where $\mathcal{A}_{p_0,p}$ is the set of all paths between p_0 and p. The minimal path between p_0 and any point p_1 in the image can be easily deduced from this action map. Assuming that potential $P \neq 0$ (this is always the case for $\tilde{P}$), the action map has only one local minimum which is the starting point p_0. The minimal path is found by a simple back-propagation, that is a gradient descent on the minimal action map $\mathcal{U}$ starting from p_1 until p_0 is reached. Thus, contour initialization is reduced to the selection of the two extremities of the path. We explain in the next section how to compute efficiently the action map $\mathcal{U}$.

2.3 Fast Marching Resolution

In order to compute this map $\mathcal{U}$, a front-propagation equation related to Equation (3) is solved:

$$\frac{\partial C}{\partial t} = \frac{1}{\tilde{P}} \vec{n}. \tag{4}$$

It evolves a front starting from an infinitesimal circle shape around p_0 until each point inside the image domain is assigned a value for $\mathcal{U}$. The value of $\mathcal{U}(p)$ is the time t at which the front passes over the point p.

The *Fast Marching* technique, introduced in [16], was used in [6] noticing that the map $\mathcal{U}$ satisfies the Eikonal equation:

$$\|\nabla \mathcal{U}\| = \tilde{P} \quad \text{and} \quad \mathcal{U}(p_0) = 0. \tag{5}$$

Classic finite differences schemes for this equation tend to overshoot and are unstable. An up-wind scheme was proposed by [16]. It relies on a one-sided

Table 1. *Fast Marching* algorithm

Algorithm for 2D Fast Marching

- Definitions:
  - *Alive* set: all grid points at which the action value $\mathcal{U}$ has been reached and will not be changed;
  - *Trial* set: next grid points (4-connexity neighbors) to be examined. An estimate U of $\mathcal{U}$ has been computed using Equation (6) from alive points only (i.e. from $\mathcal{U}$);
  - *Far* set: all other grid points, there is not yet an estimate for U;
- Initialization:
  - *Alive* set: reduced to the starting point p_0, with $U(p_0) = \mathcal{U}(p_0) = 0$;
  - *Trial* set: reduced to the four neighbors p of p_0 with initial value $U(p) = \tilde{P}(p)$ $(\mathcal{U}(p) = \infty)$;
  - *Far* set: all other grid points, with $\mathcal{U} = U = \infty$;
- Loop:
  - Let $p = (i_{min}, j_{min})$ be the *Trial* point with the smallest action U;
  - Move it from the *Trial* to the *Alive* set (i.e. $\mathcal{U}(p) = U_{i_{min}, j_{min}}$ is frozen);
  - For each neighbor (i, j) (4-connexity in 2D) of (i_{min}, j_{min}):
    * If (i, j) is *Far*, add it to the *Trial* set and compute $U_{i,j}$ using Eqn. 6;
    * If (i, j) is *Trial*, update the action $U_{i,j}$ using Eqn. 6.

---

derivative that looks in the up-wind direction of the moving front, and thereby avoids the over-shooting associated with finite differences:

$$(\max\{u - \mathcal{U}_{i-1,j}, u - \mathcal{U}_{i+1,j}, 0\})^2 +$$
$$(\max\{u - \mathcal{U}_{i,j-1}, u - \mathcal{U}_{i,j+1}, 0\})^2 = \tilde{P}_{i,j}^2, \tag{6}$$

giving the correct viscosity-solution u for $\mathcal{U}_{i,j}$. The improvement made by the *Fast Marching* is to introduce order in the selection of the grid points. This order is based on the fact that information is propagating *outward*, because the action can only grow due to the quadratic Equation (6).

This technique of considering at each step only the necessary set of grid points was originally introduced for the construction of minimum length paths in a graph between two given nodes in [8].

The algorithm is detailed in Table 1. An example is shown in Figure 2. The *Fast Marching* technique selects at each iteration the *Trial* point with minimum action value. In order to compute this value, we have to solve Equation (7) for each trial point, as detailed in Table 2.

2.4   Algorithm for 2D Up-wind Scheme

Notice that for solving Equation (6), only alive points are considered. This means that calculation is made using current values of $\mathcal{U}$ for neighbors and not estimate U of other trial points. Considering the neighbors of grid point

(i, j) in 4-connexity, we note $\{A_1, A_2\}$ and $\{B_1, B_2\}$ the two couples of opposite neighbors such that we get the ordering $\mathcal{U}(A_1) \leq \mathcal{U}(A_2)$, $\mathcal{U}(B_1) \leq \mathcal{U}(B_2)$, and $\mathcal{U}(A_1) \leq \mathcal{U}(B_1)$. Considering that we have $u \geq \mathcal{U}(B_1) \geq \mathcal{U}(A_1)$, the equation derived is

$$(u - \mathcal{U}(A_1))^2 + (u - \mathcal{U}(B_1))^2 = \tilde{P}_{i,j}^2 \tag{7}$$

Computing the discriminant Δ of Equation (7) we have the steps described in Table 2.

Table 2. Solving locally the upwind scheme

1. – If $\Delta \geq 0$, u should be the largest solution of Equation (7);
        • If the hypothesis $u \geq \mathcal{U}(B_1)$ is wrong, go to 2;
        • If this value is larger than $\mathcal{U}(B_1)$, this is the solution;
    – If $\Delta < 0$, B_1 has an action too large to influence the solution. It means
      that $u \geq \mathcal{U}(B_1)$ is false. Go to 2;
  Simple calculus can replace case 1 by the test:
 	
 1bis. If $\tilde{P}_{i,j} > \mathcal{U}(B_1) - \mathcal{U}(A_1)$,
    $u = \dfrac{\mathcal{U}(B_1)+\mathcal{U}(A_1)+\sqrt{2\tilde{P}_{i,j}^2 - (\mathcal{U}(B_1)-\mathcal{U}(A_1))^2}}{2}$ is the largest solution of Equation (7)
    else go to 2;
 2. Considering that we have $u < \mathcal{U}(B_1)$ and $u \geq \mathcal{U}(A_1)$, we finally have
    $u = \mathcal{U}(A_1) + \tilde{P}_{i,j}$.

Thus it needs only one pass over the image. To perform efficiently these operations in minimum time, the *Trial* points are stored in a min-heap data structure (see details in [16]). Since the complexity of the operation of changing the value of one element of the heap is bounded by a worst-case bottom-to-top proceeding of the tree in $O(\log_2 P)$, the total work is bounded $O(P \log_2 P)$ for the *Fast Marching* on a grid with P nodes.

3   Finding Multiple Contours from a Set of Key Points p_k

The method of [6], detailed in the previous section allows to find a minimal path between two endpoints. We are now interested in finding many or all contours in an image. A first step for multiple contours finding in an image is to assume we have a set of points p_k given on the image and then find contours passing through these points. We assume the points are either given by a preprocessing or by the user. We propose to find the contours as a set of minimal paths that link pairs of points among the p_k's. If we also know which pairs of points have to be linked together, finding the whole set of contours is a trivial application of the previous section. This would be similar to the method in [10] which used a dynamic programming (non consistent, see [6]) approach to find the paths between successive points given by the user. The problem we are interested in here is also to find out which pairs of points have to be connected by a contour. Since the set of points p_k's is assumed to be given unstructured, we do not know in advance how the points connect. This is the key problem that is solved here using a minimal action map.

3.1   Main Ideas of the Approach

Our approach is similar to computing the distance map to a set of points and their Voronoi diagram. However, we use here a weighted distance defined through the potential P. This distance is obtained as the minimal action with respect to P with zero value at all points p_k. Instead of computing a minimal action map for each pair of points, as in Section 2, we only need to compute one minimal action map in order to find all paths. At the same time the action map is computed we determine the pairs of points that have to be linked together. This is based on finding meeting points of the propagation fronts. These are *saddle points* of the minimal action $\mathcal{U}$. In Section 2, we said that calculation of the minimal action can be seen as the propagation of a front through equation (4). Although the minimal action is computed using fast marching, the level sets of $\mathcal{U}$ give the evolution of the front. During the fast marching algorithm, the boundary of the set of alive points also gives the position of the front. In the previous section, we had only one front evolving from the starting point p_0. Since all points p_k are set with $\mathcal{U}(p_k) = 0$, we now have one front evolving from each of the starting points p_k. In what follows when we talk about front meeting, we mean either the geometric point where the two fronts coming from different p_k's meet, or in the discrete algorithm the first alive point which connects two components from different p_k's (see Figures 3 and 4).

Our problem is related to the approach presented at the end of [6] in order to find a closed contour. Given only one end point, the second end point was found as a saddle point. This point is where the two fronts propagating both ways meet. Here we use the fact that given two end points p_1 and p_2, the saddle point S where the two fronts starting from each point meet can be used to find the minimal path between p_1 and p_2. Indeed, the minimal path between the two points has to pass by the meeting point S. This point is the point half way (in energy) on the minimal path between p_1 and p_2. Backpropagating from S to p_1 and then from S to p_2 gives the two halves of the path. This is in fact an approximation, due to some discretization error in finding the meeting point S. If high precision is needed, a subpixel location of *saddle points* can be made based on the final energy map. In order to get the precise minimal path between the two points, we could also backpropagate from the second point to the first as in Section 2, but computation time would be then much increased.

3.2   Some Definitions

Here are some definitions that will be used in what follows.

- For a point p in the image, we note $\mathcal{U}_p$ the minimal action obtained by Fast Marching with potential $\tilde{P}$ and starting point p.

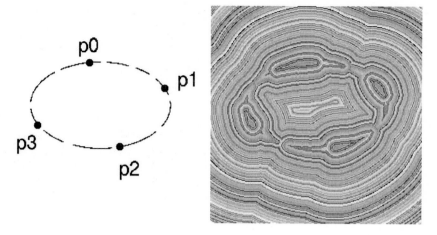

Fig. 3. Ellipse example with four points. On the left the incomplete ellipse as potential and four given points; on the right the minimal action map (random LUT to show the level sets) from these points

- X being a set of points in the image, $\mathcal{U}_X$ is the minimal action obtained by Fast Marching with potential $\tilde{P}$ and starting points $\{p, p \in X\}$. This means that all points of X are initialized as alive points with value 0 and all their 4-connexity neighbors are *trial* points. This is easy to see that $\mathcal{U}_X = \min_{p \in X} \mathcal{U}_p$.
- The *region* R_k associated with a point p_k is the set of points p of the image closer in energy to p_k than to other points p_j. This means that minimal action $\mathcal{U}_{p_k} \leq \mathcal{U}_{p_j}, \forall j \neq k$. Thus, if $X = \{p_j, 0 \leq j \leq N\}$, we have $\mathcal{U}_X = \mathcal{U}_{p_k}$ on R_k and the computation of $\mathcal{U}_X$ is the same as the simultaneous computation of each $\mathcal{U}_{p_k}$ on each region R_k. These are the simultaneous fronts starting from each p_k.
- The *region index* r is $r(p) = k, \forall p \in R_k$. (Voronoi Diagram for weighted distance).
- A *saddle point* $S(p_i, p_j)$ between p_i and p_j is the first point where the front starting from p_i to compute $\mathcal{U}_{p_i}$ meets the front starting from p_j to compute $\mathcal{U}_{p_j}$; At this point, $\mathcal{U}_{p_i}$ and $\mathcal{U}_{p_j}$ are equal and this is the smallest value for which they are equal.
- Two points among the p_k's will be called *linked neighbors* if they are selected to be linked together. The way we choose to link two points is to select some *saddle points*. Thus points p_i and p_j are *linked neighbors* if their *saddle point* is among the selected ones.

3.3   Saddle Points and Reconstruction of the Set of Curves

The main goal of our method is to obtain all significant paths joining the given points. However, each point should not be connected to all other points, but

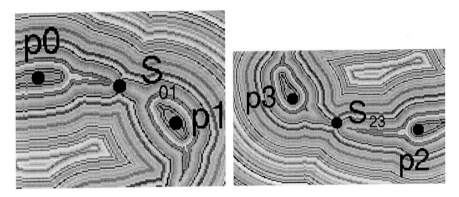

Fig. 4. Zoom on a *saddle point* between two key points

only to those that are closer to them in the energy sense. In order to form closed curves, each point p_k should not have more than two *linked neighbors*. The criteria for two points p_i and p_j to be connected is that their fronts meet before other fronts. It means that their *saddle point* $S(p_i, p_j)$ has lower action $\mathcal{U}$ than the *saddle points* between these points and other points p_k. The fact that we limit each p_k to have no more than two connections makes it possible that some points will have only one or no connection. This helps removing some isolated spurious points or getting different closed curves not being connected together. We illustrate this in the example of Figure 6 where one of the p_k is not linked to any other point since all the other points already have two linked neighbors. In case we also need to have T-junctions, the algorithm can be used with a higher number of linked neighbors allowed for each endpoint or we may connect together all possible points as in Section 4.3. A non symmetric relation may also be used to link each point to the closest or the two closest ones, regardless of whether these have already two or more neighbors. In the example of Figure 6, such an approach would link the spurious points with the circles. Postprocessing would be needed to remove undesired links, based on high energy for example.

Once a *saddle point* $S(p_i, p_j)$ is found and selected, backpropagation relatively to final energy $\mathcal{U}$ should be done both ways to p_i and to p_j to find the two halves of the path between them. We see in Figure 5 this backpropagation at each of the four *saddle points*. At a saddle point, the gradient is zero, but the direction of descent towards each point are opposite. For each backpropagation, the direction of descent is the one relative to each region. This means that in order to estimate the gradient direction toward p_i, all points in a region different from R_i have their energy put artificially to ∞. This allows finding the good direction for the gradient descent towards p_i. However, as mentioned earlier, these backpropagations have to be done only for selected *saddle points*. In the fast marching algorithm we have a simple way to find *saddle points* and update the *linked neighbors*.

As defined above, the *region* R_k associated with a point p_k is the set of points p of the image such that minimal energy $\mathcal{U}_{p_k}(p)$ to p_k is smaller than all

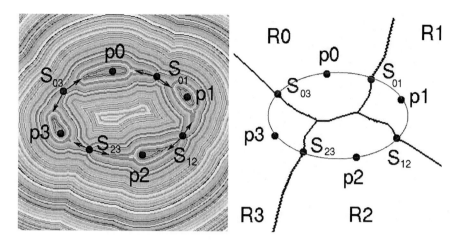

Fig. 5. Ellipse example with four points. On the left the *saddle points* are found, and backpropagation is made from them to each of the two points from where the front comes; on the right, the minimal paths and the Voronoi diagram obtained

the $\mathcal{U}_{p_j}(p)$ to other points p_j. The set of such *regions* R_k covers the whole image, and forms the Voronoi diagram of the image (see figure 5). All *saddle points* are at a boundary between two *regions*. For a point p on the boundary between R_j and R_k, we have $\mathcal{U}_{p_k}(p) = \mathcal{U}_{p_j}(p)$. The *saddle point* $S(p_k, p_j)$ is a point on this boundary with minimal value of $\mathcal{U}_{p_k}(p) = \mathcal{U}_{p_j}(p)$. This gives us a rule to find the *saddle points* during the fast marching algorithm.

Each time two fronts coming from p_k and p_j meet for the first time, we define the meeting point as $S(p_k, p_j)$. This means that we need to know for each point of the image from where it comes. This is easy to keep track of its origin by generating an index map updated at each time a point is set as alive in the algorithm. Each point p_k starts with index k. Each time a point is set as alive, it gets the same index as the points it was computed from in formula (6). In that formula, the computation of $U_{i,j}$ depends only on at most two of the four pixels involved. These two pixels, said A_1 and B_1, have to be from the same *region*, except if (i, j) is on the boundary between two regions. If A_1 and B_1 are both alive and with different indexes k and l, this means that regions R_k and R_l meet there. If this happens for the first time, the current point is set as the saddle point $S(p_k, p_l)$ between these regions. A point on the boundary between R_k and R_l is given the index of the neighbor point with smaller action A_1. At the boundary between two regions there can be a slight error on indexing. This error of at most one pixel is not important in our context and could be refined if necessary.

3.4   Algorithm and Results

The algorithm for this section is described in Table 3 and illustrated in figures 3 and 5. When there is a large number of p_k's, this does not change much the

Table 3. Algorithm of Section 3

Algorithm with previously defined p_k

- Initialization:
  - p_k's are given
  - $\forall k, V(p_k) = 0; r(p_k) = k;$ p_k alive.
  - $\forall p \notin \{p_k\}, V(p_k) = \infty; r(p) = -1;$ p is far except 4-connexity neighbors of p_k's that are *trial* with estimate U using Eqn. (6).
- Loop for computing $V = \mathcal{U}_{\{p_k, 0 \leq k \leq N\}}$:
  - Let $p = (i_{min}, j_{min})$ be the *Trial* point with the smallest action U;
  - Move it from the *Trial* to the *Alive* set with V(p) = U(p);
  - Update $r(p)$ with the same index as point A_1 in formula (6). If $r(A_1) \neq r(B_1)$ and we are in case 1 of Table 2 where both points are used and if this is the first time regions $r(A_1)$ and $r(B_1)$ meet, $S(p_{r(A_1)}, p_{r(B_1)}) = p$ is set as a *saddle point* between $p_{r(A_1)}$ and $p_{r(B_1)}$. If these points have not yet two *linked neighbors*, they are put as *linked neighbors* and $S(p_{r(A_1)}, p_{r(B_1)}) = p$ is selected,
    For each neighbor (i, j) (4-connexity) of (i_{min}, j_{min}):
    * If (i, j) is Far, add it to the *Trial* set and compute U using Eqn. (6);
    * If (i, j) is *Trial*, recompute the action $U_{i,j}$, and update it.
- Obtain all paths between selected *linked neighbors* by backpropagation each way from their *saddle point* (see Section 3.3).

---

computation time of the minimal action map, but this makes more complex dealing with the list of linked neighbors and *saddle points*. This may generate more conflicting neighbor points, and due to the constraint of having at most two linked neighbors, some gaps may remain between contours. The method can be applied to a whole set of edge points or points obtained through a preprocessing. However, choosing few key points simplifies the computation of *saddle points* and *linked neighbors* and the geometry of the paths. When there are few key points, they are not too close to each other. Finding all paths from a given set of points is interesting in the case of a binary potential defined, like in Figure 3, for perceptual grouping. It can be used as well when a special preprocessing is possible, either on the image itself to extract characteristic points or on the geometry of the initial set of points to choose more relevant points. In [2] we give a way to find automatically a set of key points from a larger set of "admissible points".

We show in figure 6 the results of the approach for the data given in figure 1. We show in figure 7 an application of our approach combined with the saliency map of [11]. In such an example, the given dots are too few to enable finding the ellipse as a minimal path. Indeed, taking two opposite points on the ellipse, the minimal path between them will not be along the ellipse but rather along a straight line. By passing through low potential points (in black) along the ellipse, the path will also pass through more points with high potential (background in white). Thus applying the method of [11] gives a saliency map that is much more dense than the original image. Taking the saliency map as potential, our

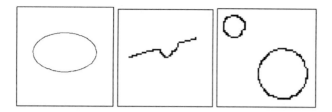

Fig. 6. Final paths obtained for images of Figure 1

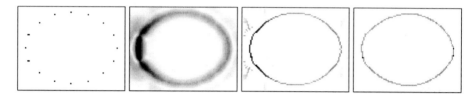

Fig. 7. Finding a set of minimal path using a saliency map as potential. From left to right, original data, saliency map, ridge lines and minimal paths

approach allows finding the whole ellipse as a set of minimal paths between points determined automatically. The set of points to be linked here can be either the initial set of points of the original image or the set of points obtained by thresholding the saliency map. We can also find the ellipse by looking for ridge curves on the saliency map but there are many spurious ridge curves obtained.

4   Extension to Finding Multiple Contours from a Set of Connected Components

4.1   Minimal Path between Two Regions

The method of [6], detailed in the previous section allows to find a minimal path between two endpoints. This is a straightforward extension to define a minimal path between two regions of the image. Given two connected regions of the image R_0 and R_1, we consider R_0 as the starting region and R_1 as a set of end points. The problem is then finding a path minimizing energy among all paths with start point in R_0 and end point in R_1. The minimal action is now defined by

$$\mathcal{U}(p) = \inf_{\mathcal{A}_{R_0,p}} E(C) = \inf_{p_0 \in R_0} \inf_{\mathcal{A}_{p_0,p}} E(C) \tag{8}$$

where $\mathcal{A}_{R_0,p}$ is the set of all paths starting at a point of R_0 and ending at p. This minimal action can be computed the same way as before in Table 1, with the alive set initialized as the whole set of points of R_0, with $\mathcal{U} = 0$ and trial points being the set of 4-connexity neighbors of points of R_0 that are not in R_0. Backpropagation by gradient descent on $\mathcal{U}$ from any point p in the image will give the minimal path that join this point with region R_0.

In order to find a minimal path between region R_1 and region R_0, we determine a point $p_1 \in R_1$ such that $\mathcal{U}(p_1) = \min_{p \in R_1} \mathcal{U}(p)$. We then backpropagate from p_1 to R_0 to find the minimal path between p_1 and R_0, which is also a minimal path between R_1 and R_0.

4.2   Minimal Paths from a Set of Connected Components

Here, our approach is to compute the distance map to a set of unstructured set of points where connected points are considered as regions, using a weighted distance defined through the potential P. The set of paths is obtained with the minimal action with respect to P with zero value at all regions R_k. This method has the same possibilities as the one presented in section 3, as we only need to compute one minimal action map in order to find all paths. In the same way, we find the *saddle points* between each pair of propagating fronts from two regions R_1 and R_2. And we compute the minimal paths between two regions R_1 and R_2 by back-propagating from each selected saddle-point until we meet a pixel belonging respectively to regions R_1 and R_2. The notion of linked neighbors is extended to linked regions. More details can be found in [3].

4.3   Connecting All Regions with Minimal Paths

The goal here is to connect all regions, but only to those that are closer to them in the energy sense. In Section 3, we were looking for closed contours from a set of points, and had constraints on the maximal number of linked neighbors. In the application we show below, we are interested in connecting all initial given points through a path. In this case we also need to have T-junctions, for reconstructing tree-like structures, therefore the algorithm can be used with a higher number of linked regions allowed for each region, as said for the end points in Subsection 3.3. The constraint we use now is to avoid creating a closed contour when connecting two regions. This is obtained through the definition of cycles and cycle tests.

A *cycle* is a sequence of different regions $R_k, 1 \le k \le K$, such that for $1 \le k \le K - 1$, R_k and R_{k+1} are *linked regions* and R_K and R_1 are also *linked regions*. A cycle test can be easily implemented using a recursive algorithm. When two regions R_i and R_j are willing to be connected - ie that their fronts meet - a table storing the connectivity between each region enables to detect if a connection already exists between those regions. Having N different regions, we fill a matrix $M(N, N)$ with zeros, and each time two regions R_i and R_j meet for the first time, we set $M(i, j) = M(j, i) = 1$. Thus, when two regions meet, we apply the algorithm detailed in Table 4.

If two regions are already connected, the pixel where their fronts meet is not considered as a valuable candidate for back-propagation.

The algorithm stops automatically when all regions are connected.

Once a *saddle point* between any region R_i and R_j is found and selected, back-propagation relatively to final energy $\mathcal{U}$ should be done both ways to p_i

Table 4. Cycle detection

Algorithm for Cycle detection when a region R_i meets a region R_j:
$Test(i, j, M, i);$ *with*
$Test(i, j, M, l);$

- if $M(l, j) = 1$, return 1;
- else
  - count=0;
  - for $k \in [1, N]$ with $k \neq i, k \neq j, k \neq l$:
    if $M(k, j) = 1$, count $+ = Test(j, k, M, l);$
  - return count;

---

and to p_j, the first points belonging to respectively R_i and R_j, during the back-propagation algorithm.

4.4   Medical Application

The method can be applied to connected components from a whole set of edge points or points obtained through a preprocessing. Finding all paths from a given set of points is interesting in the case of a binary potential defined, like in Figure 3, for perceptual grouping. It can be used as well when a special preprocessing is possible, either on the image itself to extract characteristic points or on the geometry of the initial set of points to choose more relevant points. We show in Figure 8 an example of application for a hip medical image where we are looking for vessels. Potential P is defined using ideas from [9] on vesselness filter.

For this, we propose to extract valuable information from this dataset, computing a multiscale vessel enhancement measure, based on the work of [9] on ridge filters. Having extracted the two eigenvalues of the Hessian matrix computed at scale σ, ordered $|\lambda_1| \leq |\lambda_2|$, we define at each pixel a vesselness function

$$\nu(\sigma) = \begin{cases} 0, & \text{if } \lambda_2 \geq 0 \\ \exp{\frac{-R_B^2}{2\beta^2}}(1 - \exp{\frac{-S^2}{2c^2}}) \end{cases}$$

where $R_B = \frac{|\lambda_1|}{|\lambda_2|}$, and $S = \sqrt{\lambda_1^2 + \lambda_2^2}$. See [9] for a detailed explanation of the settings of each parameter in this measure. Using this information computed at several scales, we can take as new image the maximum of the response of the filter across all scales. In figure 8-top right you can observe the response of the filter, based on the Hessian information.

And we can easily give a very constrained threshold of this image, that will lead to sets of unstructured pixels that surely belong to the anatomical object of interest, as shown in figure 8-bottom left. Figure 8-bottom right shows the set of completion paths obtained that link all given connected components together.

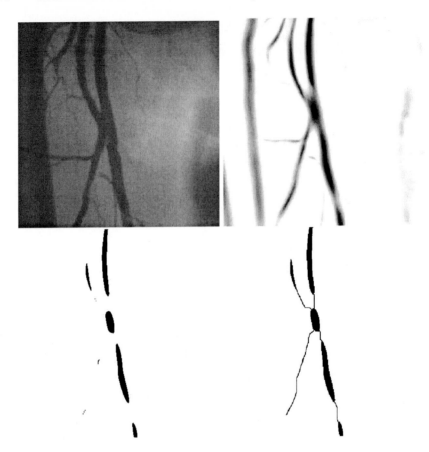

Fig. 8. Medical Image. First line: original image and vesselness potential; Second line: from the set of regions obtained from thresholding of potential image, our method finds links between these regions as minimal paths with respect to the potential

5 Conclusion

We presented a new method that finds a set of contour curves in an image. It was applied to perceptual grouping to get complete curves from a set of noisy contours or edge points with gaps. The technique is based on previous work of finding minimal paths between two end points [6]. However, in our approach, we do not need to give the start and end points as initialization. In a first method, given a set of key points, we found the pairs of key points that had to be linked by minimal paths. Once *saddle points* between pairs of points are found, paths are drawn on the image from the selected *saddle points* to both points of each pair. This gives the minimal paths between selected pairs of points. The whole set of paths completes the initial set of contours and allows to close these contours. In a second method, we compute the whole set of paths between unstructured regions in the image. We illustrate this approach with a medical image application.

References

1. V. Caselles, R. Kimmel, and G. Sapiro. Geodesic active contours. *International Journal of Computer Vision*, 22(1):61–79, 1997.
2. L. D. Cohen. Multiple contour finding and perceptual grouping using minimal paths. *Journal of Mathematical Imaging and Vision*, 14(3), May 2001. CERE-MADE TR 0101, Jan 2001. To appear.
3. L. D. Cohen and T. Deschamps. Grouping connected components using minimal path techniques. Technical report, CEREMADE, 2001. To appear.
4. Laurent D. Cohen. On active contour models and balloons. *CVGIP: Image Understanding*, 53(2):211–218, March 1991.
5. Laurent D. Cohen and Isaac Cohen. Finite element methods for active contour models and balloons for 2-D and 3-D images. *IEEE Transactions on Pattern Analysis and Machine Intelligence*, PAMI-15(11):1131–1147, November 1993.
6. Laurent D. Cohen and R. Kimmel. Global minimum for active contour models: A minimal path approach. *International Journal of Computer Vision*, 24(1):57–78, August 1997.
7. T. Deschamps and L.D. Cohen. Minimal paths in 3D images and application to virtual endoscopy. In *Proc. sixth European Conference on Computer Vision (ECCV'00)*, Dublin, Ireland, 26th June - 1st July 2000.
8. E. W. Dijkstra. A note on two problems in connection with graphs. *Numerische Mathematic*, 1:269–271, 1959.
9. A. Frangi, W. Niessen, K. L. Vincken, and M. A. Viergever. Multiscale vessel enhancement filtering. In *Proc. Medical Image Computing and Computer-Assisted Intervention, MICCAI'98, Cambridge*, pages 130–137, 1998.
10. D. Geiger, A. Gupta, L. Costa, and J. Vlontzos. Dynamic programming for detecting, tracking, and matching deformable contours. *IEEE Transactions on Pattern Analysis and Machine Intelligence*, 17(3):294–302, March 1995.
11. G. Guy and G. Medioni. Inferring global perceptual contours from local features. *International Journal of Computer Vision*, 20(1/2):113–133, October 1996.
12. Michael Kass, Andrew Witkin, and Demetri Terzopoulos. Snakes: Active contour models. *International Journal of Computer Vision*, 1(4):321–331, January 1988.
13. R. Kimmel, A. Amir, and A. Bruckstein. Finding shortest paths on surfaces using level sets propagation. *IEEE Transactions on Pattern Analysis and Machine Intelligence*, PAMI-17(6):635–640, June 1995.
14. R. Kimmel, N. Kiryati, and A. M. Bruckstein. Distance maps and weighted distance transforms. *Journal of Mathematical Imaging and Vision*, 6:223–233, May 1996. Special Issue on Topology and Geometry in Computer Vision.
15. R. Malladi, J. A. Sethian, and B. C. Vemuri. Shape modeling with front propagation: A level set approach. *IEEE Trans. on PAMI*, 17(2):158–175, February 1995.
16. J. A. Sethian. *Level Set Methods: Evolving Interfaces in Geometry, Fluid Mechanics, Computer Vision and Materials Sciences*. Cambridge Univ. Press, 1996.
17. A. Shaashua and S. Ullman. Structural saliency: The detection of globally salient structures using a locally connected network. In *Proc. Second IEEE International Conference on Computer Vision (ICCV'88)*, pages 321–327, December 1988.
18. L. R. Williams and D. W. Jacobs. stochastic completion fields: a neural model of illusory contour shape and salience. In *Proc. Fifth IEEE International Conference on Computer Vision (ICCV'95)*, pages 408–415, Cambridge, USA, June 1995.
19. L. R. Williams and D. W. Jacobs. Local parallel computation of stochastic completion field. In *Proc. IEEE CVPR'96*, San Francisco, USA, June 1996.

Shape Tracking Using Centroid-Based Methods

Arnaldo J. Abrantes[1] and Jorge S. Marques[2]

[1] Department of Electrical and Computer Engineering
Instituto Superior de Engenharia de Lisboa
Lisbon, Portugal
aja@isel.pt
[2] Institute for Systems and Robotics
Instituto Superior Técnico
Lisbon, Portugal
jsm@isr.ist.utl.pt

Abstract. Algorithms for tracking generic 2D object boundaries in a video sequence should not make strong assumptions about the shapes to be tracked. When only a weak *prior* is at hand, the tracker performance becomes heavily dependent on its ability to detect image features; to classify them as informative (i.e., belonging to the object boundary) or as outliers; and to match the informative features with corresponding model points. Unlike simpler approaches often adopted in tracking problems, this work looks at feature classification and matching as two unsupervised learning problems. Consequently, object tracking is converted into a problem of dynamic clustering of data, which is solved using competitive learning algorithms. It is shown that competitive learning is a key technique for obtaining accurate local motion estimates (avoiding aperture problems) and for discarding the outliers. In fact, the competitive learning approach shows several benefits: (i) a gradual propagation of shape information across the model; (ii) the use of shape and noise models competing for explaining the data; and (iii) the possibility of adopting high dimensional feature spaces containing relevant information extracted from the image. This work extends the unified framework proposed by the authors in [1].

1 Introduction

Object tracking has attracted the attention of researchers over the last three decades. Several approaches have been proposed to address this problem. One popular approach consists of using a continuous description of the object boundary (e.g., using a parametric curve) attracted by discrete features detected in the image (e.g., edge points) [2, 7]. Two problems make this approach difficult. First, it is not easy to associate image points to model points. This matching problem is usually addressed by recursive suboptimal techniques [4]. Second, only a subset of the detected features is associated to the boundary of the object to be tracked. Many of the detected features are associated to inner edges or to the background edges, and should therefore be considered as outliers. The outlier

M.A.T. Figueiredo, J. Zerubia, A.K. Jain (Eds.): EMMCVPR 2001, LNCS 2134, pp. 576–591, 2001.

classification is not easy. This problem is similar to the false alarm problem in radar processing [3], although there are some differences: in tracking, the percentage of outliers is usually higher and they are not uniformly distributed in space. In fact, they tend to cluster along strokes.

One way to circumvent the matching problem is by using model driven feature detection methods. In this case, the model boundary is sampled and an image feature is searched in the vicinity of each model sample (e.g., using a unidirectional search along a direction orthogonal to the object boundary) [16, 6]. This approach avoids the matching problem but it makes feature detection dependent on the initial estimate of the model boundary, obtained by prediction. The tracker will perform well while the object motion and shape is highly predictable but it fails in the presence of rapid motion or shape changes [13].

The presence of invalid features (outliers) is also a major source of difficulties. Most trackers use *ad hoc* techniques to separate good features from the outliers e.g., by discarding those features which are far from the object boundary [8]. Again, since we do not know the exact location of the object boundary and rely on estimates only, the performance of such techniques becomes dependent on the initial model obtained by prediction and fails in the case of inaccurate prediction results.

This paper addresses data matching and outlier segmentation using unsupervised learning techniques. A class of methods is presented which extends several well known algorithms (Kohonen maps, elastic nets, snakes, fuzzy c-means) and allows the design of new methods. All these methods represent the image features by a small number of centroids which are easily associated to model points. Matching is therefore achieved in this way while the outlier segmentation is performed during the unsupervised learning process.

This paper extends the work presented in [1] and is organized as follows: section 2 formulates the problem; section 3 describes a unified framework for shape estimation, which adopts centroid-based approaches for data matching; outlier rejection is discussed in section 4; experimental results are presented in sections 3 and 4; section 5 concludes the paper with a discussion of the proposed techniques.

2   Problem Formulation

Let $x(s) = (x_1(s), x_2(s))$ denote a 2D curve belonging to the admissible shape space

$$\mathcal{A} = \{x(s) : x(s) = H(s)\,\theta\} \tag{1}$$

where $H(s)$ is a known $2 \times N$ matrix with shape basis functions and θ is a $N \times 1$ vector of coefficients. Since the curve x depends on θ, it will be denoted as $x(s, \theta)$. Several sets of basis functions can be used to define the admissible shape space, such as splines, sinc or sinusoidal functions [5]. Furthermore, this model also allows to represent the object boundary as a geometric transformation (e.g., affine transformation) of a reference shape [6].

In dynamic problems, it will be assumed that the object shape describes a trajectory in the admissible shape space, $x(s, \theta^t)$. The evolution of θ^t is described by a dynamic model, e.g., a stochastic difference equation. The estimation of the model parameters from an image sequence is achieved by solving an optimization problem

$$\hat{\theta}^t = \arg\min_\theta E(\theta, Y^t) \tag{2}$$

where

$$E(\theta, Y^t) = E_r(\theta) + E_d(\theta, Y^t) \tag{3}$$

is an energy function with a data dependent term and a regularization term, and $Y^t = \{y_1, \cdots, y_P\}$ denotes the visual features detected at time t, e.g., the 2D coordinates of boundary points detected in the image.

The energy function is the sum of two competing terms: a regularization term and a data dependent term. The regularization term is low as long as the shape trajectory is well described by the dynamic model (i.e., while the object shape is close to the predicted shape) and increases as the shape evolution deviates from the predicted shape. The role of the data dependent term, E_d, is to evaluate the ability of the model to represent the observed data Y^t.

The optimization problem defined above can also be interpreted as a MAP estimation of the object shape, assuming a Gibbs model for the joint density $p(\theta, Y)$ [15].

2.1 Regularization Energy

It is often assumed that the object shape in a new frame t is close to a predicted shape, $\bar{x}$, with an isotropic and Gaussian uncertainty. In this case, the L_2 norm is used to define the regularization energy,

$$E_r = \alpha_r \int \|x(s) - \bar{x}(s)\|^2 ds \tag{4}$$

where α_r is a constant which controls the uncertainty level of the dynamic model. Using (1) and (4) it can be shown that

$$E_r = \alpha_r (\theta - \bar{\theta})^T \mathcal{H} (\theta - \bar{\theta}) \tag{5}$$

where

$$\mathcal{H} = \int H(s)^T H(s) ds \tag{6}$$

is usually denoted as the metric matrix of the admissible shape space $\mathcal{A}$.

2.2 Data Energy

Denote Y^t as the set of edge points detected in the t-th image. Ideally, we would like to detect image points belonging to the object boundary only. However, every practical edge detector also yields edge points produced by other objects

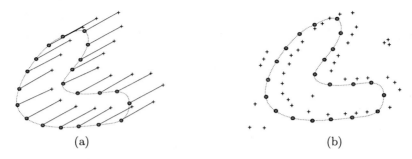

Fig. 1. Shape estimation problem. (a) Known data matching; and (b) unknown data matching (predicted model shape is represented by the dashed line; model samples are represented by the circles and data features by cross marks).

present in the scene as well as inner edges produced by the object to be tracked. These points will be considered as outliers.

The data energy should measure the match between the image features and the object model (see fig. 1b)

$$E_d = d(Y^t, x(\theta)) \qquad (7)$$

where d is a distortion measure between both sets of points.

This raises two difficulties: first we should be able to discard the influence of outliers; second we should be able to define a 1-1 match between image features and model points. Both operations are difficult. We will address each of these problems in the next two sections.

3   Shape Estimation

This section addresses shape estimation from a set of edge points detected in the image. For the sake of simplicity, it will be assumed first that all the points belong to the boundary of the object to be tracked. Furthermore, the object boundary is assumed to be represented by a set of samples $x(s_i), i = 1, \cdots, M$.

Two cases will be considered below (see fig. 1). First we will assume that there is a known 1-1 matching between the model points and the image features, i.e., each edge point detected in the image is matched to a known contour sample. This situation occurs when feature extraction is model driven, e.g., when the image features are detected by unidimensional search procedures along directions normal to the object contour. Second, we will discuss the case of unknown matching. This situation occurs in image driven feature detection methods in which the number of image features is much higher than the number of model samples.

3.1   Known Matching

Let $x(s_i), i = 1, \cdots, M$ be the samples of the predicted contour and let $y_i \in \mathcal{R}^2, i = 1, \cdots, M$ be the corresponding image features (see fig. 1a). Several metrics have been used to measure the difference between both sets of points, a popular solution being a weighted sum of the squared errors

$$E_d = \sum_{i=1}^{M} \frac{1}{2\sigma_i^2} \|y_i - x(s_i, \theta)\|^2 \tag{8}$$

Parameters σ_i assign a confidence degree to each observed feature. The estimation of the unknown vector parameters, θ, is obtained by minimizing (8). Since the gradient of (8) is

$$\frac{\partial E_d}{\partial \theta} = \sum_i \frac{1}{\sigma_i^2} H(s_i)^T \left(H(s_i)\theta - y_i\right) \tag{9}$$

the optimal solution is

$$\hat{\theta}_d = S^{-1}Z \tag{10}$$

with

$$S = \sum_i \frac{1}{\sigma_i^2} H(s_i)^T H(s_i) \tag{11}$$

and

$$Z = \sum_i \frac{1}{\sigma_i^2} H(s_i)^T y_i \tag{12}$$

A minimum of $N/2$ features are needed to obtain a solution for the shape estimation problem (non singular matrix S). The minimization of the weighted least squares criterion (8) is equivalent to a maximum likelihood estimation of the unknown parameters, assuming that the image features are independent random variables with Gaussian distribution and omnidirectional uncertainty.

This model has two drawbacks: (i) it is not robust with respect to the presence of outliers (this problem will be addressed later); (ii) it can not be used in the case of unmatched data. The use of the regularization energy allows to alleviate these drawbacks when the number of outliers is small and most of the observations are correctly matched with model points.

The solution of the optimization problem (3) with regularization is given by

$$\hat{\theta} = (\alpha_r \mathcal{H} + S)^{-1} \left(\alpha_r \mathcal{H}\bar{\theta} + Z\right) \tag{13}$$

where matrices S and Z are defined in (11) and (12), respectively.

3.2   Unknown Matching

Let us now address the problem of shape estimation from a set of unmatched data points (see fig. 1b). This problem has been addressed by several authors [11, 7, 4]. We will focus on an unsupervised learning strategy, developed by the authors, denoted as Unified Framework [1]. This framework extends several well known algorithms such as snakes [11], Kohonen maps [12], elastic nets [10], fuzzy c-means [9], and allows the development of new ones.

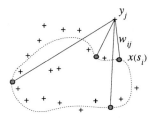

Fig. 2. Tentative matching between data points and model samples (only a few samples are shown).

Let $x(s_i), i = 1, \cdots, M$ and $y_i, i = 1, \cdots, P$ be the unmatched contour samples and image features, respectively. Since matching is unknown we will assume that each data feature is associated with all model samples with different confidence degrees (see fig. 2). The data energy adopted in this framework is given by (compare with (8))

$$E_d = \frac{1}{2} \sum_{i=1}^{M} \sum_{j=1}^{P} w_{ij} \|y_j - x(s_i, \theta)\|^2 \tag{14}$$

where w_{ij} is the confidence degree associated to the tentative match between $x(s_i)$ and y_j. This expression includes, as special cases, the objective functions minimized by snakes, Kohonen maps, elastic nets and fuzzy c-means, i.e., all these methods belong to the unified framework (see details in [1]). The weights w_{ij} associated with these methods are defined in table 1. Other choices for w_{ij} are also possible allowing the development of other shape estimation algorithms. The optimization of energy (14) can be achieved by evaluating its gradient,

$$\frac{\partial E_d}{\partial \theta} = \sum_i \mu_i \, H(s_i)^T \left(H(s_i)\, \theta - \xi_i \right) \tag{15}$$

where ξ_i and μ_i are the centroid and the mass of the data associated with the i-th model sample, defined by

$$\xi_i = \frac{\sum_j \vartheta_{ij} y_j}{\sum_j \vartheta_{ij}} \qquad\qquad \mu_i = \sum_j \vartheta_{ij} \tag{16}$$

The weight ϑ_{ij} represents the influence of the j-th feature on the i-th model sample. The influence functions for each of the previous methods are defined in table 1. They are related with the confidence degrees by

$$\vartheta_{ij} = w_{ij} + \sum_k d_{kj} \frac{\partial w_{kj}}{\partial d_{ij}} \tag{17}$$

where $d_{ij} = \|y_j - x(s_i)\|^2$.

Table 1. Weighting functions of snakes, Kohonen maps, elastic nets, fuzzy c-means and crisp c-means. Note that $d_{ij} = \|x(s_i) - y_j\|^2$, $\phi_\sigma(d_{ij}) = \exp(-d_{ij}/2\sigma^2)$, $i^*(j)$ denotes the index of the model sample nearest to y_j, q controls the degree of fuzzyness, δ is the Kronecker function and Λ_r is the neighborhood function used in Kohonen maps.

	w_{ij}	ϑ_{ij}
Snakes	$2\sigma^2 \frac{1-\phi_\sigma(d_{ij})}{d_{ij}}$	$\phi_\sigma(d_{ij})$
Kohonen maps	$\Lambda_r(i, i^*(j))$	$\Lambda_r(i, i^*(j))$
Elastic nets	$\frac{-2\sigma^2}{M} \frac{\log \sum_k \phi_\sigma(d_{kj})}{d_{ij}}$	$\frac{\phi_\sigma(d_{ij})}{\sum_k \phi_\sigma(d_{kj})}$
Fuzzy C-means	$\left(\sum_k \left(\frac{d_{ij}}{d_{kj}}\right)^{\frac{1}{q-1}}\right)^{-q}$	$\left(\sum_k \left(\frac{d_{ij}}{d_{kj}}\right)^{\frac{1}{q-1}}\right)^{-q}$
C-means	$\delta(i - i^*(j))$	$\delta(i - i^*(j))$

Table 2. Pseudo-code for the centroid-based tracking algorithm.

```
Predict model shape
Repeat
    Compute M samples of the model shape.
    Evaluate centroids and masses using (16)
    Estimate model parameters using (18, 19) in (13) (or in (10)).
Until a pre-defined number of iterations is performed
```

Figure 3 shows the influence functions and corresponding attraction regions (level set regions) in the case of a contour with a few samples. While the snake algorithm has omnidirectional attraction regions, the attraction regions of the other algorithms are no longer omnidirectional since they are influenced by the location of the neighboring contour samples. This is due to presence of competitive learning mechanisms — the model samples compete to represent the data.

Comparing (15) with (9) it can be concluded that the centroids play the role of the observations, y_i, and the masses play the role of $(\sigma_i^2)^{-1}$, in the known matching case. Therefore, the solution for the minimization problem (14) is still given by (10), with

$$S = \sum_i \mu_i H(s_i)^T H(s_i) \tag{18}$$

and

$$Z = \sum_i \mu_i H(s_i)^T \xi_i \tag{19}$$

Since the μ_i, ξ_i depend on the initial contour estimate, an iterative process is usually adopted to estimate the object boundary. The algorithm is summarized in table 2.

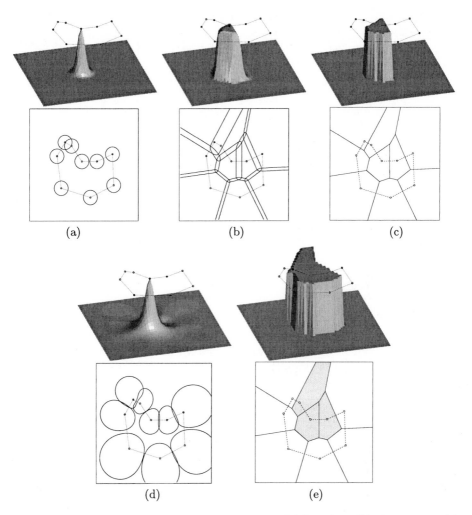

Fig. 3. Influence functions and attraction regions of (a) snakes, (b) elastic nets, (c) c-means, (d) fuzzy c-means and (e) Kohonen maps.

The next two examples illustrate the role played by the competitive learning mechanisms in shape estimation. It is emphasized that the use of competitive learning improves the solution of the matching problem.

Example 1

Figure 4a shows the example of an object undergoing a uniform motion. The samples of the predicted shape are represented by small circles and the observed data by a solid line representing a large number of edge points. The motion vector is represented by an arrow. Figure 4b shows a tentative matching between the model points and observed data using the nearest neighbor criterion, used

motion vector:

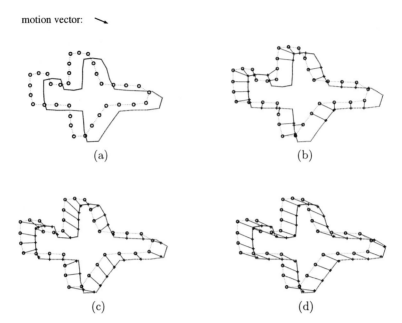

(a)   (b)

(c)   (d)

Fig. 4. Tracking example: (a) initial contour (dashed line) and data points (solid line); (b) nearest neighbor matching; and (c, d) centroid based matching (fuzzy c-means) after (c) 6 and (d) 200 iterations (the updated shapes are not shown).

for example in the ICP algorithm [4]. The displacement vectors associated with each match are not consistent, therefore leading to erroneous alignment results. Figures 4c,d show the centroid locations obtained with the fuzzy c-means after 6 and 200 iterations. Although the shape estimate was updated during the optimization process, only the initial position of the model is shown for the sake of simplicity. It is stressed that consistent displacement vectors are now obtained (see fig. 4d) due to the presence of the competitive learning mechanisms which avoid having the same data represented by different model samples.

Example 2

Figure 5 compares the ability of 6 different data association methods to recover (or not) from a large prediction error. In this figure the initial model configuration (predicted shape) is represented by a dashed line, the edge data is represented by a solid line and the association process is visualized by the segments joining model samples with data centroids (small circles). It is observed that the methods without competitive learning (snakes and nearest neighbor; see figs. 5a,f) fail to match the data points with the correct model samples. In fact, different model points are attracted toward the same data features and the shape of the model configuration (not shown in the figure) will collapse after a few iterations. Data association methods with competitive learning show clear improvements. All these methods manage to attract the upper and lower boundary

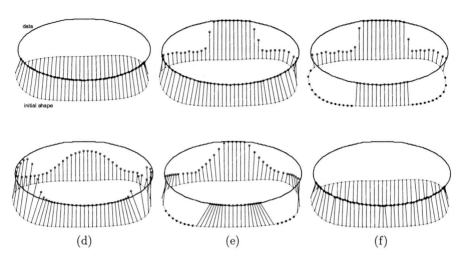

Fig. 5. Data matching after the first iteration for (a) snakes, (b) elastic nets, (c) c-means, (d) fuzzy c-means, (e) Kohonen maps and (f) nearest neighbor.

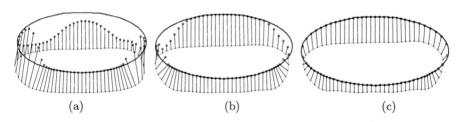

Fig. 6. Data matching after (a) first; (b) second; and (c) third iteration (fuzzy c-means).

of the model towards centroids located in the correct directions (see figs. 5b-e). As the number of iterations increases the matching accuracy gradually improves (see fig. 6 for the case of fuzzy c-means).

4   Robust Data Association

Previous methods work well when the boundary edges are segmented from background and inner edges (outliers). However, these methods fail when such edges are not removed (see fig. 7). The problem is even more severe in the case of competitive learning methods with unbounded attraction regions.

Two methods will be used in the sequel to overcome these difficulties. The first consists of segmenting the data as valid or invalid. This will be performed by a soft decision process involving the concept of noise plane. The second approach consists of using extended features i.e., feature vectors with dimension higher

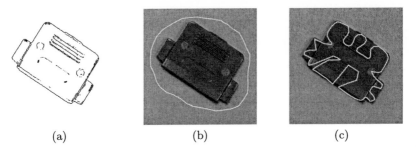

(a)	(b)	(c)

Fig. 7. Shape estimation failure in the presence of large number of outliers. (a) detected edge points; (b) initial contour; (c) final contour obtained with Kohonen maps.

than two which contain the edge coordinates as before and additional properties of the image in the vicinity of the edge point (e.g., color, gradient direction). A feature will attract a model point if they are close in the high dimension space i.e., if they are close in the image plane and furthermore if the other properties match. This provides an additional criterion which allows to discard the influence of the outliers. The use of extended features was advocated by a number of authors [17, 14]. Both methods can be implemented in the scope of the unified framework as shown below by introducing minor changes in the energy function (14).

4.1   Noise Plane

The detected edges which are far from the predicted contour should have a low confidence degree since the probability of belonging to the object boundary is low. Methods with unbounded attraction regions cannot cope with this situation: far away edges will have a strong influence on the final shape estimate. To overcome this difficulty a virtual model sample, $x(s_{M+1})$, will be defined in such a way that $d_{M+1,j} = \eta$, i.e., the distance of this additional sample to all image features is constant. The virtual sample $x(s_{M+1})$ is not a 2D point. Instead, it can be interpreted as a plane parallel to the image plane, which competes with the model samples to represent the data (see fig. 8). Points which are close to the object model will be represented by ordinary model samples while points far from the predicted shape will be best approximated by the noise plane. Therefore, the data energy becomes

$$E_d = \frac{1}{2} \sum_{i=1}^{M+1} \sum_{j=1}^{P} w_{ij} \|y_j - x(s_i)\|^2 \tag{20}$$

where the confidence degrees w_{ij} are still given by the expressions in table 1.

Figure 9 shows the effect of the noise plane on the attraction regions of fuzzy c-means for three values of η. It is observed that the practical influence of the noise plane is to bound the attraction regions while it preserves their shape in the vicinity of the predicted contour.

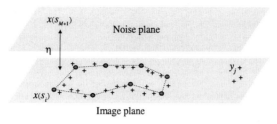

Fig. 8. Noise model represented by a plane parallel to the image plane.

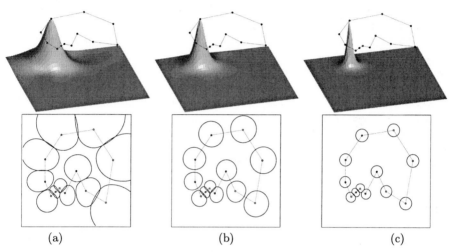

Fig. 9. Effect of the noise plane on the attraction regions of fuzzy c-means for different values of η: (a) large, (b) medium and (c) small.

Figure 10 shows the oval shape estimation problem, previously discussed in this section (see figs. 5 and 6), but now with an additional difficulty: the presence of outliers. This problem is not easy since the predicted shape is far from the true object boundary and it is closer to outliers detected in the image. Furthermore, we can not benefit from imposing a rigid model shape since we allow the predicted shape to deform. Despite these difficulties the fuzzy c-means algorithm with noise plane manages to estimate the object boundary well and to discard the incorrect data. These results were obtained in two stages, each one with a different value for η: a large value during the first 20 iterations and a much smaller one during the last 20. The first stage (with large η) allows a global convergence of the model towards the data, while the second stage (with small η) refines the solution.

4.2   Extended Features

The noise plane efficiently discards edges which are far from the predicted shape but it is useless for discarding close edge points. An additional technique must be devised for dealing with such cases.

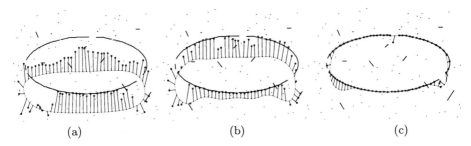

Fig. 10. Data matching in the presence of outliers. Fuzzy c-means after (a) one, (b) 10 and (c) 30 iterations.

Until this point only edge information was used to estimate the object boundary. The unified framework is easily extended to feature spaces of arbitrary dimension which may include color, texture and gradient information as well. The energy function in such case is given by

$$E_d = \frac{1}{2} \sum_i \sum_j w_{ij} \|\tilde{y}_j - \tilde{x}(s_i, \theta)\|^2 \tag{21}$$

where $\tilde{x}(s_i, \theta) \in \mathcal{R}^{2+K}$ and $\tilde{y}_j \in \mathcal{R}^{2+K}$, K being the number of additional features associated with each model or image point, respectively. To be more specific, $\tilde{x}(s_i) = [x(s_i)^T \, t_i^1 \ldots t_i^K]^T$ and $\tilde{y}_j = [y_j^T \, f_j^1 \ldots f_j^K]^T$, where $t_i^1, \ldots, t_i^K$ denote the K feature values associated with the i-th model point, $x(s_i, \theta)$, and $f_j^1, \ldots, f_j^K$, the corresponding feature values, obtained at y_j, using a set of adequate image feature extractors.

Since the gradient of the new energy (21) is similar to (15), the centroids and masses being computed by (16) as before, parameter estimation is still performed by the algorithm described in section 3.2 (see table 2). The weights ϑ_{ij} are defined in table 1 with d_{ij} replaced by $\tilde{d}_{ij} = \|\tilde{y}_j - \tilde{x}(s_i, \theta)\|^2$. We note that the centroids are still 2D vectors. The additional features only influence the weighting functions ϑ_{ij}, e.g., if the properties associated with an image feature and a model sample are different, then the weighting function ϑ_{ij} will be negligible, even if they are close in the image plane. For example, the RGB components or the gradient direction in the vicinity of an edge point can be used as extended features. In that case, the model samples $\tilde{x}(s_i, \theta)$ will only be attracted by image features with similar color and gradient direction. This allows to discriminate among features belonging to different objects present in the scene, therefore increasing the ability of the model to discard outliers.

Figure 11 shows an example of grain boundary estimation in a ceramic material using extended features. These images were obtained with a scanning electron microscope (SEM images). This is an example in which the use of noise plane is not enough to succeed in estimating the grain boundaries. In this case, the feature vector was extended with two additional components: $\cos(\theta), \sin(\theta)$, θ being the gradient direction i.e., a unit vector orthogonal to the iso-intensity

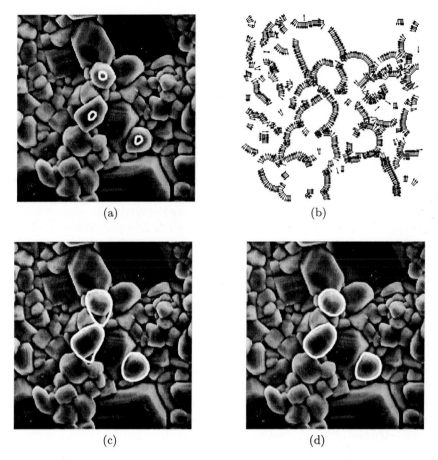

(a)   (b)

(c)   (d)

Fig. 11. Segmentation of microscope image of ceramic material. (a) contour seeds; (b) extended features (edge points and gradient direction); (c, d) results obtained with (c) edge points only and with (d) extended features.

curve at each edge point. It can be observed from this example that the use of extended features allows to discriminate the edge points belonging to each grain from the edges of neighboring grains.

5   Conclusion

This paper addresses the tracking of moving objects from a set of visual features detected in the image. Most tracking systems rely on three basic steps: shape prediction, feature detection and contour update. Several methods have been proposed for each of these operations. Two key difficulties concern the association of image features to model points and the presence of outliers i.e., detected features which do not belong to the object to be tracked and should be eliminated.

To circumvent these difficulties many trackers adopt a model driven feature detection in which the predicted shape is used to guide the image analysis operations. This approach solves the matching problem since a single image feature is obtained for each model sample. However, it is strongly dependent on the prediction results. Therefore, good tracking results can only be obtained when the object motion and shape evolve according to slowly varying trajectories. This approach is suitable in some practical applications but it can not cope with the shape variability which occurs in many other problems.

In this work, a set of centroids is used to represent the data features detected in the image (e.g., edge points) using competitive learning techniques. The centroids are initialized by sampling the boundary of the predicted contour model. The initialization procedure creates a natural association among the centroids and model points, therefore circumventing the need of an explicit matching technique. It has been shown that competitive learning procedures used for the update of centroids play a key role in the improvement of the consistency of local matching between data features and model points.

A second problem which has been addressed in this paper concerns the robustness of the shape estimate in the presence of outliers. To alleviate this difficulty two techniques were proposed. The first method consists of using a noise model, denoted as noise plane, which reduces the scope of the attraction regions associated with each centroid: far away features will be discarded since they will not be able to attract the centroids. The second method consists of using extended features. A set of features, such as color, texture or gradient information, is associated with each model point. Only the image features with similar properties will be able to attract the corresponding model points. Therefore, the attraction mechanisms become much more selective allowing the elimination of outliers. This provides an efficient ground for performing data fusion in the scope of shape estimation and tracking.

Acknowledgment

This work was partially supported by program PRAXIS XXI, in the scope of project P/EEI/12050/1998.

References

1. A. Abrantes and J. Marques. A class of constrained clustering algorithms for object boundary extraction. *IEEE Transactions on Image Processing*, 5(11):1507–1521, 1996.
2. A. Amini, T. Weymouth, and R. Jain. Using dynamic programming for solving variational problems in vision. *IEEE Trans. Pattern Analysis and Machine Intell.*, 12(9):855–867, 1990.
3. Y. Bar-Shalom and T. Fortmann. *Tracking and Data Association*. Academic Press, 1988.
4. P. Besl and N. McKay. A method for registration 3-D shapes. *IEEE Trans. Pattern Analysis and Machine Intell.*, 14(2):239–256, 1992.

5. J. Bioucas. Adaptive Bayesian contour estimation: A vector space representation approach. In *Workshop on Energy Minimization Methods in Computer Vision and Pattern Recognition*, pages 157–172, York, UK, 1999.

6. A. Blake and M. Isard. *Active Contours*. Springer-Verlag, 1998.

7. L. Cohen. NOTE on active contour models and balloons. *CVGIP: Image Understanding*, 53(2):211–218, 1991.

8. T. Cootes, C. Taylor, D. Cooper, and J. Graham. Active shape models — their training and application. *Computer Vision and Image Understanding*, 61(1):38–59, 1995.

9. J. Dunn. A fuzzy relative of the ISODATA process and its use in detecting compact well-separated clusters. *Journal of Cybernetics*, 3(3):32–57, 1973.

10. R. Durbin and D. Willshaw. An analogue approach to the travelling salesman problem using an elastic net method. *Nature*, 326(16):689–691, 1987.

11. M. Kass, A. Witkin, and D. Terzopoulos. Snakes: Active contour models. *International Journal of Computer Vision*, 1(4):321–331, 1987.

12. T. Kohonen. The self-organizing map. *Proc. IEEE*, 78(9):1464–1480, 1990.

13. J. Marques and J. Lemos. Optimal and suboptimal shape tracking based on multiple switched dynamic models. *Image and Vision Computing*, 2001.

14. X. Pardo and P. Radeva. Discriminant snakes for 3D reconstruction in medical images. In *Proc. Int. Conf. on Pattern Recognition*, volume 4, pages 336–339, Barcelona, 2000.

15. G. Storvik. A Bayesian approach to dynamic contours through stochastic sampling and simulated annealing. *IEEE Trans. Pattern Analysis and Machine Intell.*, 16(10):976–986, 1994.

16. H. Tagare. Deformable 2-D template matching using orthogonal curves. *Trans. Medical Imaging*, pages 108–117, 1997.

17. C. Wren, A. Azarbayejani, T. Darrell, and A. Pentland. Pfinder: Real-time tracking of the human body. *IEEE Trans. Pattern Analysis and Machine Intell.*, 19(7):780–785, 1997.

Optical Flow and Image Registration: A New Local Rigidity Approach for Global Minimization

Martin Lefébure[1] and Laurent D. Cohen[2]

[1] Current address: 69 rue Perronet, 92200 Neuilly Sur Seine, France
was with Poseidon Technologies
`mlefebure@compaqnet.fr`
[2] CEREMADE, Université Paris-Dauphine, 75775 Paris cedex 16, France
`cohen@ceremade.dauphine.fr`

Abstract. We address the theoretical problems of optical flow estimation and image registration in a multi-scale framework in any dimension. Much work has been done based on the minimization of a distance between a first image and a second image after applying deformation or motion field. We discuss the classical multiscale approach and point out the problem of validity of the motion constraint equation (MCE) at lower resolutions. We introduce a new local rigidity hypothesis allowing to write proof of such a validity. This allows us to derive sufficient conditions for convergence of a new multi-scale and iterative motion estimation/registration scheme towards a global minimum of the usual nonlinear energy instead of a local minimum as did all previous methods. Although some of the sufficient conditions cannot always be fulfilled because of the absence of the necessary a priori knowledge on the motion, we use an implicit approach. We illustrate our method by showing results on synthetic and real examples (Motion, Registration, Morphing), including large deformation experiments.

Keywords: motion estimation, registration, optical flow, multi-scale, motion constraint equation, global minimization, stereo matching

1 Introduction

Registration and motion estimation are one of the most challenging problems in computer vision, having uncountable applications in various domains [17, 18, 6, 4, 13, 30]. These problems occur in many applications like medical image analysis, recognition, visual servoing, stereoscopic vision, satellite imagery or indexation. Hence they have constantly been addressed in the literature throughout the development of image processing techniques. For example (Figure 1) consider the problem of finding the motion in a two-dimensional images sequence. We then look for a displacement $(h_1(x_1, x_2), h_2(x_1, x_2))$ that minimizes an energy functional:

$$\int \int |I_1(x, y) - I_2(x + h_1(x, y), y + h_2(x, y))|^2 dx dy.$$

M.A.T. Figueiredo, J. Zerubia, A.K. Jain (Eds.): EMMCVPR 2001, LNCS 2134, pp. 592–607, 2001.
© Springer-Verlag Berlin Heidelberg 2001

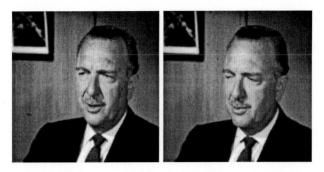

Fig. 1. Finding the motion in a two-dimensional images sequence

Next consider the problem of finding $(f_1(x_1, x_2), f_2(x_1, x_2))$ a rigid or non rigid deformation between two images (Figure 2), minimizing an energy functional:

$$\int \int |I_1(x, y) - I_2(f_1(x, y), f_2(x, y))|^2 dx dy.$$

Although most papers deal only with motion estimation or matching depending on the application in view, both problems can be formulated the same way and be solved with the same algorithm. Thus the work we present can be applied both to registration for a pair of images to match (stereo, medical or morphing) or motion field / optical flow for a sequence of images. In this paper we will focus our attention on these problems assuming grey level conservation between both images to be matched. Let us denote by $I_1(x)$ and $I_2(x)$ respectively the study and target images to be matched, where $x \in D = [-M, M]^d \subset \mathbb{R}^d$, and $d \geq 1$. In the following I_1 and I_2 are supposed to belong to the space $C_0^1(D)$ of continuously differentiable functions vanishing on the domain boundary ∂D. We will then assume there exists a homeomorphism f^* of D which represents the deformation such that:

$$I_1(x) = I_2 \circ f^*(x), \forall x \in D.$$

In the context of optical flow estimation, let us denote by h^* its associated motion field defined by $h^* = f^* - Id$ on D. We thus have:

$$I_1(x) = I_2(x + h^*(x)). \tag{1}$$

h^* is obviously a global minimum of the nonlinear functional

$$E_{NL}(h) = \frac{1}{2} \int_D |I_1(x) - I_2(x + h(x))|^2 dx. \tag{2}$$

We can deduce from (1) the well known Motion Constraint Equation (also called Optical Flow Constraint):

$$I_1(x) - I_2(x) \simeq < \nabla I_2(x), h^*(x) > , \forall x \in D. \tag{3}$$

E_{NL} is classically replaced in the literature by its quadratic version substituting the integrand with the squared difference between both left and right terms of the MCE, yielding the classical energy for the optical flow problem:

$$E_L(h) = \frac{1}{2} \int_D |I_1(x) - I_2(x) - \langle \nabla I_2(x), h(x) \rangle|^2 dx.$$

Here ∇ denotes the gradient operator. Since the work of Horn and Schunk [17], MCE (3) has been widely used as a first order differential model in motion estimation and registration algorithms. In order to overcome the too low spatio-temporal sampling problem which causes numerical algorithms to converge to the closest local minimum of the energy E_{NL} instead of a global one, Terzopoulos et al. [24, 30] and Adelson and Bergen [8, 29] proposed to consider it at different scales. This led to the popular coarse-to-fine minimizing technique [18, 11, 13, 25, 14]. It is based on the remark that MCE (3) is a first order expansion which is generally no longer valid with h^* searched for. The idea is then to consider images at a coarse resolution and to refine iteratively the estimation process.

Using a regularizing kernel G_σ at scale σ, Terzopoulos et al. [24, 30] and Adelson and Bergen [8] were led to consider the following modified MCE:

$$G_\sigma * (I_1 - I_2)(x) \simeq \langle G_\sigma * \nabla I_2(x), h^*(x) \rangle \qquad (4)$$

Remark.
One could also consider regularizing both left and right terms of the original MCE, yielding the following alternative:

$$G_\sigma * (I_1 - I_2)(x) \simeq G_\sigma * (\langle \nabla I_2, h^* \rangle)(x)$$

At finest scales it can be shown that these two propositions are equivalent.
To our knowledge and despite the huge literature on these approaches, no theoretical error analysis can be found when such approximations are done. Though it has been reported from numerical experiments that the modified MCE was not performing well at very coarse scales, thus betraying its progressive lack of sharpness, many authors pointed out convergence properties of such algorithms towards a dominant motion in the case of motion estimation [7, 11, 10, 21, 9, 16], or an acceptable deformation in the case of registration [13, 25, 26], even if the initial motion were large. It is widely assumed that deformation fields have some continuity or regularity properties, leading to the addition of some particular regularizing terms to the quadratic functional [17, 5, 30, 3, 2]. Let us emphasize on the modified MCE (4). We note $\hat{h}$ the value of h that reaches minimum for energy

$$\int |G_\sigma * (I_1 - I_2) - \langle G_\sigma * \nabla I_2, h \rangle|^2 dx. \qquad (5)$$

This multiscale approach assumes that Eqn. (4) is "valid" at lower resolutions, which ensures that $\hat{h}$ will be close to h^*.

Although it may come from the fact that flattened images are always "more similar", to our knowledge and despite the huge literature, no theoretical analysis can confirm this. Replacing G_σ by a particular low pass filter Π_σ (here

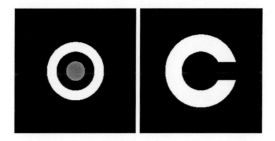

Fig. 2. Finding a non rigid deformation between two images

$\sigma \geq 0$ is proportional to the number of considered harmonics in the Fourier decomposition), we will address the problem of finding a linear operator $P_\sigma^{I_1}$ such that $P_\sigma^{I_1}(h^*)$ is close to $\Pi_\sigma\left(I_1 - I_2\right)$. The sharpness of this approximation will decrease with respect to both h^* norm and resolution parameter σ. This will lead us to introduce a new local rigidity hypothesis of deformations $f = Id + h$ with respect to image I_1. Hence such deformations allow to find the operator $P_\sigma^{I_1}$ satisfying our validity constraint on the modified MCE.

Considering general linear parametric motion models for h^*, we give sufficient conditions for asymptotic convergence of the sequence of combined motion estimations towards h^* together with the numerical convergence of the sequence of deformed templates towards the target I_2. Roughly speaking, the shape of the theorem will be the following:

Theorem: If

1. at each step the residual deformation is "locally rigid", and the associated motion can be linearly decomposed onto an "acceptable" set of functions the cardinal of which is not too large with respect to the scale,
2. the initial motion norm is not too large, and the systems conditionings do not decrease "too rapidly" when iterating,
3. the estimated deformations $Id + \hat{h}_i$ are invertible and "locally rigid",

Then the iterative scheme "converges" towards a global minimum of the energy E_{NL}.

The outline of the paper is as follows. In Section 2 we introduce a new local rigidity hypothesis and a low pass filter in order to derive a new MCE of the type of equation (6). In Section 3 we design an iterative motion estimation/registration scheme based on the MCE introduced in Section 2 and prove a convergence theorem. In order to avoid the a priori motion representation problem, we adopt an implicit approach in Section 4 and constrain each estimated deformation $Id + \hat{h}_i$ to be at least invertible. We show numerical results for large deformations problems in dimension 2. Section 5 gives a general conclusion to the paper.

2 Valid Modified MCE Upon a New Local Rigidity Hypothesis

Assuming a local rigidity hypothesis and adopting the Dirichlet low-pass operator Π_σ, we will find a different right hand side featuring a "natural" and unique linear operator $P_\sigma^{I_1}$ in the sense that:

$$\Pi_\sigma(I_1 - I_2)(x) \simeq P_\sigma^{I_1}(h^*)(x), \tag{6}$$

with remainder of the order of $\|h^*\|^2$ for some particular norm and vanishing as the scale is coarser (σ close to 0).

2.1 Local Rigidity Property

In this paragraph we introduce our local rigidity property of deformations. Notations in this context are to be understood as follows:

- $D = [-M, M]^d$ in $\mathbb{R}^d$.
- $I_{1,p}$, $I_{2,p}$, I_2, are functions from $\mathbb{R}^d$ to $\mathbb{R}$.
- $h(x)$, $\tilde{h}^*(x)$ are functions from $\mathbb{R}^d$ to $\mathbb{R}^d$.
- $<.,.>$ denotes the scalar product in $\mathbb{R}^d$.
- $[.,.]$ denotes the scalar product in L^2.

For technical reasons we assume that I_1 and I_2 belong to $C_0^1(D)$, and $I_1(x) = I_2(x + h^*(x))$, $x \in D$, $h^*(x) \in \mathbb{R}^d$.

Definition 1. $f \in Hom(D)$ is ξ-rigid for $I_1 \in C^1(D)$ iff:

$$Jac(f)^t.\nabla I_1 = det(Jac(f))\nabla I_1, \tag{7}$$

where $Jac(f)$ denotes the Jacobian matrix of f and $det(A)$ the determinant of matrix A, and $Hom(D)$ the space of continuously differentiable and invertible functions from D to D (homeomorphisms).

All ξ-rigid deformations have the following properties (see [19] for the proofs). Assume f^* is ξ-rigid for $I_1 \in C_0^1(D)$ and $I_1 = I_2 \circ f^*$. Then,

1. equation (7) is always true if dimension d is 1;
2. for all $d \geq 1$,
   (a) $\|\nabla I_1\|_{L^1} = \|\nabla I_2\|_{L^1}$, where L^1 denotes the space of integrable functions over D;
   (b) $\nabla I_1 \mathbin{/\!/} \nabla I_2 \circ f^*$.
   (c) relation $\sim$ defined by

$$[I_1 \sim I_2] \iff [\exists f\ \xi\text{-rigid for } I_1 \text{ s.t. } I_1 = I_2 \circ f]$$

   is an equivalence relation on $C_0^1(D)$;
3. suppose $d = 2$: then,
   (a) if $Jac(f^*)$ is symmetric, then (7) means that if $|\nabla I_1| \neq 0$,

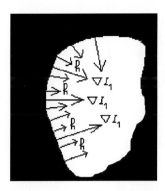

Fig. 3. An example of motion $h = f - Id$ of a ξ-rigid deformation f for image I_1. We show a level set of image I_1, and the fields ∇I_1 and h along its boundary. h varies only along the direction of ∇I_1.

- direction $\eta = \frac{\nabla I_1}{|\nabla I_1|}$ is eigenvector ($\lambda = det(Jac(f))$ is an eigenvalue);
- direction $\xi = \frac{\nabla I_1^{\perp}}{|\nabla I_1|}$ is "rigid" ($\lambda = 1$ is an eigenvalue);

This property can be seen as a non-sliding motion property. We illustrated this interesting property in Figure 3, where we show a level set of I_1, and a motion $h = f - Id$ of a ξ-rigid deformation f for image I_1. h can vary only along the direction of ∇I_1.

(b) $\kappa(I_1) = [Tr(Jac(f^*)) - det(Jac(f^*))].\kappa(I_2) \circ f^*$, where $\kappa(I)(x)$ stands for the curvature of the level line of I passing through x and $Tr(A)$ denotes the trace of matrix A;

4. if $d = 1$ or 2, and
   - h^* is known at
     - 1 point ($d = 1$).
     - each isolated critical point of I_1 and at one interior point of each connected constant set of I_1 ($d = 2$).
   - $h = h^*$ at this(ese) point(s), and

$$I_1 = I_2 \circ (Id + h) \text{ on } D,$$

then for all $x \in D$ where I_1 is not locally constant we have $h(x) = h^*(x)$.

Remark.

It is an important issue to know whether such h^* is unique. In case $d \in \{1, 2\}$, property 4 leads to uniqueness if h^* is known at some isolated points. Though it is not proved in the general case, we will assume uniqueness hereafter for simplicity.

As a consequence we can show that ξ-rigid deformations of images can be transfered to test functions. Indeed, we have the following

Lemma 1. *Suppose that*

1. I_1 and $I_2 \in C_0^1(D)$ are such that: $I_1 = I_2 \circ f$

2. f is ξ-rigid for I_1
3. $\phi \in C^\infty(D; I\!R)$, and $\Phi \in C^\infty(D; I\!R^d)$ s.t. $div\Phi = \phi$, where $C^\infty(D; I\!R)$ denotes the space of indefinitely differentiable function from D to $I\!R$.

Then, $\int_D (I_1 - I_2)\phi dx = \int_D < \nabla I_1, \Phi \circ f - \Phi > dx$.

Proof. See [20]   ∎

2.2   The Dirichlet Operator

One choice for the set of test functions in Lemma 1 is the Fourier basis, the simplest projection onto which is the Dirichlet projection operator. Let $D = [-M, M]^d$; $S_\sigma = \{k \in Z^d, \forall i \in [1, d], |k_i| \le M\sigma^2\}$; $c_k(I)$ denotes the Fourier coefficient of I defined by:

$$c_k(I) = \frac{1}{(2M)^{\frac{d}{2}}} \int_D I(x) e^{-\frac{i\pi <k,x>}{M}} dx.$$

Then the Dirichlet operator Π_σ is the linear mapping associating to each function $I \in C_0^1(D)$ the function $\Pi_\sigma(I) = G_\sigma * I$, where the convolution kernel G_σ is defined by its Fourier coefficients as follows:

$$c_k(G_\sigma) = \begin{cases} 1 \text{ if } k \in S_\sigma \\ 0 \text{ elsewhere} \end{cases}$$

2.3   New MCE by Linearization for the Dirichlet Projection

Now that we have introduced our rigidity property of deformations and the Dirichlet projection, let us choose the test functions of Lemma 1 in the Fourier basis. Defining $P_\sigma^{I_1}(h^*)(x)$ through its Fourier coefficients:

$$c_k(P_\sigma^{I_1}(h^*)) = \begin{cases} \frac{1}{d}c_0(< \nabla I_1, h^* >) \text{ if } k = 0 \\ c_k(\frac{<\nabla I_1, k><k, h^*>}{|k|^2}) \text{ if } k \in S_\sigma/\{0\} \\ 0 \text{ if } k \notin S_\sigma \end{cases}$$

we obtain the

Theorem 1. *If $f^* = Id + h^*$ is ξ-rigid for $I_1 = I_2 \circ f^* \in C_0^1(D)$, then we have:*

$$\|\Pi_\sigma(I_1 - I_2) - P_\sigma^{I_1}(h^*)\|_{L^2} \le \frac{\pi}{2}\sigma^{d+2}\|h^*|\nabla I_1|^{\frac{1}{2}}\|_{L^2}^2.$$

This inequality is nothing but the sharpness of MCE (6):

$$\Pi_\sigma(I_1 - I_2)(x) \simeq P_\sigma^{I_1}(h^*)(x), \tag{8}$$

at scale σ. It clearly expresses the fact that measuring the motion (e.g perceiving the optical flow) h^* is not relevant outside of the support of $|\nabla I_1|$.

Proof. See [20]   ∎

3 Theoretical Iterative Scheme and Convergence Theorem

In section 2 we found a new MCE and showed that we can control the sharpness of it. In this section we will make a rather general assumption on the motion in the sense that it should belong to some linear parametric motion model without being more specific on the model basis functions. Though it is somewhat restrictive to have motion fields in a finite dimensional functional space, this structural hypothesis will be a key to bounding the residual motion norm after registration in order to iterate the process. This makes it possible to consider a constraint on motion when there is a priori knowledge (like for rigid motion) or consider multi-scale decomposition of motion for an iterative scheme.

3.1 Linear Parametric Motion Models and Least Square Estimation

Let us assume the motion h^* has to be in a finite dimensional space of deformation generated by basis functions $\Psi(x) = (\psi_i(x))_{i=1..n}$. Thus h^* can be decomposed in the basis: $\exists \; \Theta^* = (\theta_i^*)_{i=1..n}$ unique, such that:

$$h^*(x) = < \Psi(x), \Theta^* > = \sum_{i=1..n} \theta_i^* \psi_i(x), \; \forall x \in Supp(|\nabla I_1|).$$

MCE (6) viewed as a linear model writes:

$$\Pi_\sigma(I_1 - I_2) = < P_\sigma^{I_1}(\Psi), \Theta^* > .$$

Now set, for σ s.t. the $P_\sigma^{I_1}(\psi_i)$ be mutually linearly independent in L^2:

$$M_\sigma = P_\sigma^{I_1}(\Psi) \otimes P_\sigma^{I_1}(\Psi), \;\; Y_\sigma = \Pi_\sigma(I_1 - I_2),$$

where $\otimes$ stands for the tensorial product in L^2. Then applying basic results from the classical theory of linear models yields: $\hat{h} = < \Psi, \hat{\Theta} > = < \Psi, M_\sigma^{-1} B_\sigma >$, where column B_σ's components are defined by $(B_\sigma)_i = < P_\sigma^{I_1}(\psi_i), Y_\sigma >$.

3.2 Estimation Error and Residual Motion

Given the least square estimation of the motion of last paragraph, we have

Lemma 2. *In this framework the motion estimation error is bounded by inequality*

$$\|(\hat{h} - h^*)|\nabla I_1|^{\frac{1}{2}}\|_{L^2} \leq \frac{\pi}{2}\sigma^{d+2}\left(Tr(M_\sigma^{-1})\right)^{\frac{1}{2}}\|h^*|\nabla I_1|^{\frac{1}{2}}\|_{L^2}^2.$$

Proof. See [20]   ∎

If $Id + \hat{h}$ is invertible, we can define:

$$I_{1,1} = I_1 \circ \left(Id + \hat{h}\right)^{-1}. \tag{9}$$

Letting r_1 denote the residual motion such that $I_{1,1} = I_2 \circ (Id + r_1)$, if $Id + \hat{h}$ is ξ-rigid for I_1 then a variable change yields equality

$$\||(\hat{h} - h^*)|\nabla I_1|^{\frac{1}{2}}\|_{L^2} = \|r_1|\nabla I_{1,1}|^{\frac{1}{2}}\|_{L^2},$$

thus giving by Lemma 2 the following bound on the residual motion norm:

$$\|r_1|\nabla I_{1,1}|^{\frac{1}{2}}\|_{L^2} \le \frac{\pi}{2}\sigma^{d+2}\left(Tr(M_\sigma^{-1})\right)^{\frac{1}{2}}\|h^*|\nabla I_1|^{\frac{1}{2}}\|_{L^2}^2. \tag{10}$$

In view of equality (9) and inequality (10), iterating the motion estimation/registration process looks completely natural and allows for pointing out sufficient conditions for convergence of such a process. Indeed, provided the same assumptions are made at each step, relations (9) and (10) can be seen as recurrence ones, yielding both r_p and $I_{1,p}$ sequences.

3.3   Theoretical Iterative Scheme

Having control on the residual motion after one registration step, we deduce the following theoretical iterative motion estimation / registration scheme:

1. Initialization: Enter accuracy $\epsilon > 0$ and the maximal number of iterations N. Set $p = 0$, and $I_{1,0} = I_1$.
2. Iterate while $(\|I_{1,p} - I_2\| \ge \epsilon \ \& \ p \le N)$
   (a) Enter the set of basis functions $\Psi_p = (\psi_{p,i})_{i=1..n_p}$ that linearly and uniquely decompose r_p on the support of $|\nabla I_{1,p}|$.
   (b) Enter scale σ_p and compute: $\hat{h}_p = < \Psi_p, M_{p,\sigma_p}^{-1} B_{\sigma_p} >$.
   (c) Set $I_{1,p+1} = I_{1,p} \circ (Id + \hat{h}_p)^{-1}$.

3.4   Convergence Theorem

Now that we have designed an iterative motion estimation / registration scheme, let us infer sufficient conditions for the residual motion to vanish. This leads us to state our following main result:

Theorem 2. *If:*

1. *For all $p \ge 0$, $I_{1,p} \sim I_2$ (as defined in Section 2.1), and the residual motion r_p can be linearly and uniquely decomposed on a set of basis functions $\{\psi_{p,i}, i = 1..n_p\}$;*
2. *For all $p \ge 0$, there exists a scale $\sigma_p > 0$ such that the set of functions $\{P_{\sigma_p}^{I_{1,p}}(\psi_{p,i}), i = 1..n_p\}$ be free in L^2 and, for $p = 0$, we assume that:*

$$\|h^*|\nabla I_1|^{\frac{1}{2}}\|_{L^2} < \left(\frac{\pi}{2}\sigma_0^{d+2}Tr(M_{0,\sigma_0})^{\frac{1}{2}}\right)^{-1};$$

Set $C_0 = \left(\frac{\pi}{2}\sigma_0^{d+2}Tr(M_{0,\sigma_0})^{\frac{1}{2}}\|h^*|\nabla I_1|^{\frac{1}{2}}\|_{L^2}\right)^{-1};$

3. *The sequence of conditioning ratios satisfy criteria:*

$$\forall p \geq 0, \; \frac{\sigma_{p+1}^{d+2} Tr(M_{p+1,\sigma_{p+1}})^{\frac{1}{2}}}{\sigma_p^{d+2} Tr(M_{p,\sigma_p})^{\frac{1}{2}}} \leq C_0;$$

4. *For all $p \geq 0$, the estimated deformations $Id + \hat{h}_p \in Hom(D)$ and are ξ-rigid for $I_{1,p}$;*

Then, $\lim_{p \to \infty} \||r_p|\nabla I_{1,p}|^{1/2}\|_{L^2} = 0.$

Proof. See [20] ∎

3.5   Numerical Algorithm Requirements

Firstly, due to the fact that h^* is unknown we have to make an arbitrary choice for the scale at each step. Secondly we at least have to ensure that $Id + \hat{h}$ be invertible at each step. Finally we are faced with the motion basis functions choice.

Multi-scale Strategy The scale choice expresses both a priori knowledge on the motion range and its structure complexity. Here we assume that $(\sigma_p)_p$ is an increasing sequence, starting from $\sigma_0 > 0$ such that:

$$\#S_{\sigma_0} \geq \#\{\text{expected independent motions}\}. \tag{11}$$

Then let $\alpha \in]0,1[$. In order to justify the minimization problem at new scale $\sigma_{p+1} > \sigma_p$, we will choose it such that:

$$\|(\Pi_{\sigma_{p+1}} - \Pi_{\sigma_p})(I_{1,p+1} - I_2)\|_{L^2} > \alpha \|I_{1,p+1} - I_2\|_{L^2}, \tag{12}$$

Invertibility of $Id + \hat{h}_p$ Let $\beta > 0$. We will apply to $I_{1,p}$ the inverse of the maximal invertible linear part of the computed deformation e.g. $\left(Id + t^*.\hat{h}_p\right)^{-1}$, where

$$t^* = \sup_{t \in [0,1]} \{t \; / \; det(Jac(Id + t.\hat{h}_p)) \geq \beta\}. \tag{13}$$

Remark.
Recursive version of the algorithm

Set $f^*(I_1, I_2)$ the solution to the correspondence problem between I_1 and I_2. Then, $f^*(I_{1,p}, I_2) = f^*(I_{1,p+1}, I_2) \circ (Id + \hat{h}_p)$. We thus deduce the following alternate recursive motion estimation / registration function $f^*(I_1, I_2)$ defined by:

$$\begin{cases} \text{If } \|I_1 - I_2\| > \epsilon, \\ \text{Then} \begin{cases} \text{Calculate } \hat{h}(I_1, I_2) \\ \text{Deform: } I_{1,1} = I_1 \circ (Id + \hat{h}(I_1, I_2))^{-1} \\ \text{Call } f = f^*(I_{1,1}, I_2) \\ \text{Return } f \circ (Id + \hat{h}(I_1, I_2)) \end{cases} \\ \text{Else return } Id \end{cases}$$

Choosing the Set of Basis Functions A major difficulty arising in the theoretical scheme comes from the lack of a priori knowledge on the finite set of basis
functions to be entered at each step. To alleviate this problem we proposed two
different approaches. In [20] we consider splitting both images into a collection
of pairs of level sets to be matched. In Section 4 we will use an implicit approach
via the optimal step gradient algorithm when minimizing the quadratic energy
associated to MCE (6).

4   Implicit Approach of Basis Functions

We now use the optimal step gradient algorithm for the minimization of the
quadratic functional associated to MCE (6). There are at least two good reasons
for doing this:

- the choice of base functions is implicit: it depends on the images I_1 and I_2,
  and the scale space.
- we can control and stop the quadratic minimization if the associated operator
  is no longer positive definite.

The general algorithm does not guaranty that the resulting matrix M_{p,σ_p} be
invertible. Hence we suggest to systematically use a stopping criteria to control
the quadratic minimization, based on the descent speed or simply a maximum
number of iterations N_G.

   In that case our final algorithm writes:

1. Initialization: Enter accuracy $\epsilon > 0$ and the maximal number of iterations
   N. Set $p = 0$, $I_{1,0} = I_1$, and choose first scale σ_0 according to (11).
2. Iterate while ($\|I_{1,p} - I_2\| \geq \epsilon$ & $p \leq N$ & $\sigma_p \leq 1$)
   (a) Choose σ_p satisfying (12).
   (b) Apply N_G iterations of the optimal step gradient algorithm for the min-
       imization of

$$E_p(h) = \|\Pi_{\sigma_p}(I_{1,p} - I_2) - P_{\sigma_p}^{I_{1,p}}(h)\|_{L^2}^2.$$

   (c) Compute $I_{1,p+1} = I_{1,p} \circ (Id + t^*.\hat{h}_p)^{-1}$ with t^* defined by (13) and
       increment p.

   In the following experiments we have fixed parameters to $\alpha = 2.5\%$, $N_G = 5$,
$\beta = 0.1$.

Running the Algorithm

We illustrate the algorithm on pairs of images with large deformation for registration applications and movies for motion estimation applications.

- **Registration problems involving large deformation:** In figures 4 and
  5 we show the different steps of the algorithm performing the registration

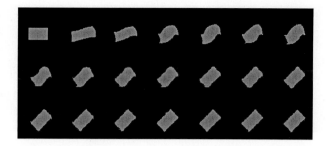

Fig. 4. Registration movie of a rotated rectangle: from left to right and from top to bottom we show the different steps of the algorithm performing the registration.

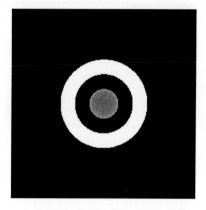

Fig. 5. Registration movie of a target to a 'C' letter. Again, each image corresponds to a step in the iterative scheme.

between the first and last images. In Figures 6 to 8, we show the study and target images, and the deformed study image after applying the estimated motion. This was applied for two examples of faces and a turbulence image featuring a vortex at two different states.

- **Optical Flow estimation examples**: in Figure 9 we show the sequence of the registered images of the original Cronkite sequence onto first image using the sequence of computed backward motions. The result is expected to be motionless. On top of Figure 10, we show the complete movie obtained by deforming iteratively only the first image of Cronkite movie. For that we use the sequence of computed motions between each pair of consecutive images of the original movie. In Figure 10 on the bottom, we see the error images.

5   Conclusion

We have addressed the theoretical problems of motion estimation and registration of images. We have introduced a new local ridigity hypothesis that we used to infer a unique Motion Constraint Equation with small remainder at coarse

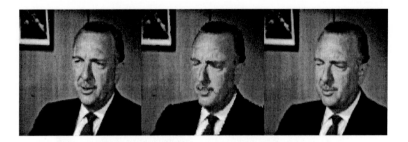

Fig. 6. Scene registration example: Study image (left), deformed Study image onto Target image (center), and Target image (right).

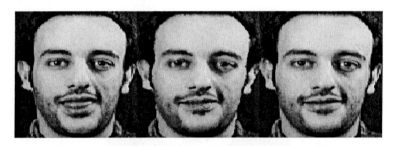

Fig. 7. Registration of a face with two different expressions: Study image (left), deformed Study image onto Target image (center), and Target image (right).

scales. We then showed that upon hypotheses on the motion norm and structure/scale tradeoff, an iterative motion estimation/registration scheme could converge towards the expected solution of the problem e.g. the global minimum of the nonlinear least square problem energy. Since each step of the theoretical scheme needs a set of motion basis functions which are not known, we have designed an implicit algorithm and illustrated the method with synthetic and real images, including large deformation examples.

References

1. L. Alvarez, J. Esclarin, M. Lefébure, J. Sanchez. A PDE model for computing the optical flow. *Proc. XVI Congresso de Ecuaciones Diferenciales y Aplicaciones*, Las Palmas, pp. 1349–1356, 1999.
2. L. Alvarez, J. Weickert, J. Sanchez, Reliable estimation of dense optical flow fields with large displacements. TR 2, Universidad de Las Palmas de Gran Canaria, November 1999.
3. G. Aubert, R. Deriche and P. Kornprobst. Computing optical flow via variational techniques. *SIAM J. Appl. Math.*, Vol. 60 (1), pp. 156–182, 1999.
4. N. Ayache. Medical computer vision, virtual reality and robotics. IVC (13), No 4, May 1995, pp 295-313.
5. Ruzena Bajcsy and Stane Kovacic. Multiresolution elastic matching. CVGIP, (46), No 1, pp. 1–21, 1989.
6. J.L. Barron, D.J. Fleet, and S.S. Beauchemin. Performance of optical flow. IJCV, 12(1):43–77, 1994.

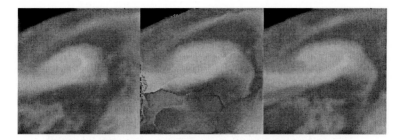

Fig. 8. Registration of a vortex at two different states: Study image (left), deformed Study image onto Target image (center), and Target image (right).

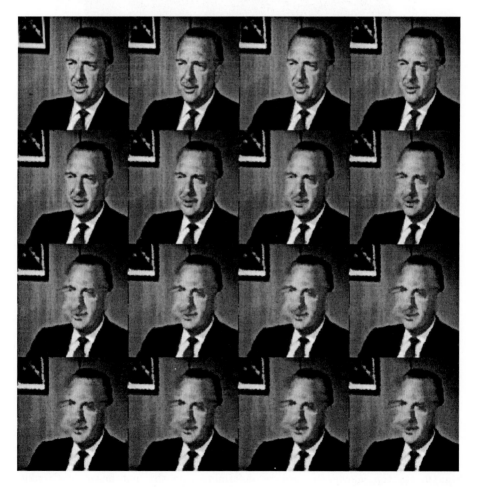

Fig. 9. Registered sequence of the original sequence onto first image using the computed backward motions.

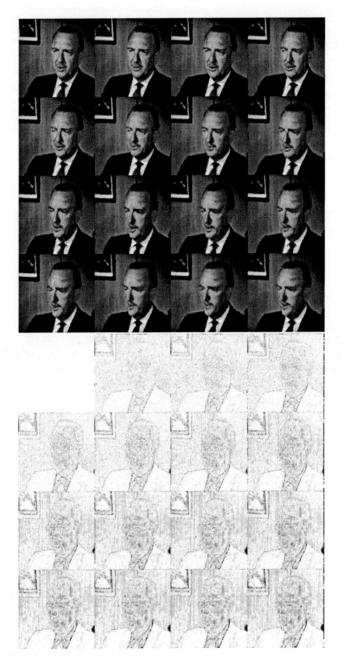

Fig. 10. On top, movie obtained by deforming only the first image of Cronkite movie using the sequence of computed motions. On the bottom, enhanced (applying $I' = 255.(1 - \sqrt{I/255})$) absolute difference between original and artificially deformed Cronkite sequences.

7. M. Ben-Ezra, B. Rousso, and S. Peleg. Motion segmentation using convergence properties. In *ARPA Im. Unders. Workshop*, pp II 1233-1235, 1994.

8. J.R. Bergen and E.H. Adelson. Hierarchical, computationally efficient motion estimation algorithm. *J. of the Optical Society Am.*, 4(35), 1987.

9. C. Bernard. Discrete wavelet analysis: a new framework for fast optic flow computation. *ECCV*, 1998.

10. M. Black and A. Rangajaran. On the unification of line processes, outlier rejection and robust statistics with applications in early vision. IJCV, Vol. 19, 1996.

11. P. Bouthemy and J.M. Odobez. Robust multiresolution estimation of parametric motion models. *J. of Vis. Comm. and Image Repres.*, 6(4):348–365, 1995.

12. M. Bro-Nielsen and C. Gramkow. Fast fluid registration of medical images. *VBC'96* Springer LNCS 1131, Hamburg, Germany, pp 267–276, Sept. 1996.

13. G. Christensen, R.D. Rabbitt, and M.I. Miller. 3D brain mapping using a deformable neuroanatomy. *Physics in Med and Biol*, (39), March:609–618, 1994.

14. D. Fleet, M. Black, Y. Yacoob and A. Jepson. Design and use of linear models for image motion analysis. *IJCV*, 36(3), 2000.

15. B. Galvin, B. McCane, K. Novins, D. Mason and S. Mills. Recovering Motion fields: An analysis of eight optical flow algorithms, *BMVC'98*, Sept. 1998.

16. P.R. Giaccone, D. Greenhill, G.A. Jones. Recovering very large visual motion fields. *SCIA97*, pp 917-922.

17. B.K.P. Horn and Brian Schunck. Determining optical flow. *Artificial Intelligence*, (17) (1-3):185–204, 1981.

18. M. Irani, B. Rousso, and S. Peleg. Detecting and tracking multiple moving objects using temporal integration. In *ECCV92*, pp 282–287, 1992.

19. M. Lefébure Estimation de Mouvement et Recalage de Signaux et d'Images: Formalisation et Analyse. PhD Thesis, Université Paris-Dauphine, 1998.

20. M. Lefébure and L. D. Cohen. Image Registration, Optical Flow and Local Rigidity. CEREMADE Technical Report, 0102, January 2001. To appear in Journal of Mathematical Imaging and Vision, 14 (2):131–147, March 2001.

21. E. Mémin and P. Pérez. Dense estimation and object-based segmentation of the optical flow with robust techniques. IEEE Trans. IP, 1998.

22. S. Srinivasan, R. Chellappa. Optical flow using overlapped basis functions for solving global motions problems. In *ECCV98*, pp 288–304, 1998.

23. C. Stiller and J. Konrad. Estimating motion in image sequences. In *IEEE Signal Processing Magazine*, Vol. 16, July, pp 70–91, 1999.

24. D. Terzopoulos. Multiresolution algorithms in computational vision. *Image Understanding*. S. Ullman, W. Richards, 1986.

25. J.P. Thirion. Fast non-rigid matching of 3D medical images. Technical Report 2547, INRIA, 1995.

26. A. Trouvé. Diffeomorphisms groups and pattern matching in image analysis. IJCV, 28(3), 1998.

27. B. C. Vemuri, J. Ye, Y. Chen and C. M. Leonard. A level-set based approach to image registration. *Proc. IEEE Workshop on Mathematical Methods in Biomedical Image Analysis, MMBIA'00*, Hilton Head Island, South Carolina, pp. 86–93, June 11-12 2000.

28. J. Weickert. On discontinuity-preserving optic flow. *Proc. Computer Vision and Mobile Robotics Workshop*, Santorini, pp. 115–122, Sept. 1998.

29. G. Whitten. A framework for adaptive scale space tracking solutions to problems in computational vision. In *ICCV'90, Osaka*, pp 210–220, Dec 1990.

30. A. Witkin, D. Terzopoulos, M. Kass. Signal matching through scale space. IJCV, 1(2):133–144, 1987.

Spherical Object Reconstruction Using Star-Shaped Simplex Meshes

Pavel Matula and David Svoboda

Faculty of Informatics, Masaryk University,
Botanická 68a, CZ-602 00 Brno, Czech Republic
{pam,xsvobod2}@fi.muni.cz

Abstract. Spherical object reconstruction is of great importance, especially in the field of cell biology, since cells as well as cell nuclei mostly have the shape of a deformed sphere. Fast, reliable and precise procedure is needed for automatic measuring of topographical parameters of the large number of cells or cell nuclei. This paper presents a new method for spherical object reconstruction. The method springs from Delingette general object reconstruction algorithm which is based on the deformation of simplex meshes. However, the unknown surface is searched only within the subclass of simplex meshes, which have the shape of a star. Star-shaped simplex meshes are suitable for modelling of spherical or ellipsoidal objects. In our approach, the law of motion was altered so that it preserves the star-shape during deformation. The proposed method is easier than the general method and therefore faster. In addition, it uses more computationally stable expressions than a method strictly implemented according to Delingette's paper. It is also shown how to partly avoid the occasional instability of the Delingette method. The accuracy of both methods is comparable. The star-shaped method achieves a stable state more often.

1 Introduction

Image analysis has recently become an essential part of many scientific disciplines. One of them is cytometry which performs measurements on cells and their components (cell nuclei, chromosomes, etc.). The shape of cell nuclei is mostly similar to a sphere or more generally to an ellipsoid. There is a need of having a general method for reconstruction of objects of this type.

Many techniques for reconstruction of cell nuclei are based on thresholding [12, 3, 9]. The resultant boundary of an object is often represented as a set of pixels (or a set of voxels in three-dimensional studies). Isosurfacing methods based on marching cubes algorithm [11] are also used [10, 7]. However, these methods do not handle missing and noisy data and can be hardly used for images with clusters of nuclei (e.g. tissue), because they make no assumption about the shape to recover.

Deformable modelling is capable of working with a priori knowledge about the shape of object and therefore it can deal with missing and noisy data. The

M.A.T. Figueiredo, J. Zerubia, A.K. Jain (Eds.): EMMCVPR 2001, LNCS 2134, pp. 608–620, 2001.

3D extension of Kass active contour model [8] has been applied to segmentation of CLSM tissue images [1]. However, the definition of minimised energy does not consider the spherical nature of nuclei. A priori knowledge about roundness is involved only in the shape of the initial model. Therefore the model can easily stick to artifacts or other objects in the neighbourhood.

The active contour method used in [2] is based on global minimisation. The search space is bounded by two concentric circles centralised upon a point found by an initial rough segmentation. The knowledge about the roundness is exploited during the construction of the search space and therefore it influences the energy minimisation. Unfortunately, this highly successful method for the automatic segmentation of cervical cell nuclei is designed only for two-dimensional space.

In this paper an original method for 2D and 3D reconstruction of cell nuclei boundaries (i.e circular or spherical objects) is described. However, this algorithm can be also used for reconstruction of some other "star-shaped" objects. The method is built on the Delingette general object reconstruction algorithm [5]. Delingette has used simplex meshes [4] for representation of surface. We discovered a new subclass of simplex meshes, which we call star-shaped simplex meshes. This subclass has some nice features and it is very convenient for spherical object reconstruction.

Simplex meshes and star-shaped simplex meshes are defined in Section 2.1. Section 2.2 introduces important notations and some geometric properties of simplex meshes. In Section 2.3 law of motion for star-shaped simplex meshes is presented, since it differs from the law of motion used for general simplex meshes. In Section 3 the biomedical application for which our method could be used is outlined.

2   Method

2.1   Definition of Simplex Meshes and Star-Shaped Simplex Meshes

Delingette's definition of k-simplex mesh embedded in an Euclidean space $\mathbb{R}^d$ is cited [4, 5] in the beginning of this section and then definition of star-shaped subclass follows.

A 0-*cell* of $\mathbb{R}^d$ also called *vertex* is a point of $\mathbb{R}^d$. A 1-*cell* of $\mathbb{R}^d$ also called *edge* is an unordered pair of distinct vertices of $\mathbb{R}^d$. A *p-cell* $(p \geq 2)$ $\mathcal{C}$ is recursively defined as a set of $(p-1)$-cells such that:

1. Every vertex belonging to $\mathcal{C}$ belongs to p distinct $(p-1)$-cells.
2. The intersection of two $(p-1)$-cells is either empty or is a $(p-2)$-cell.

A 2-cell is therefore a closed polygonal line of $\mathbb{R}^d$ and is called *face*. Examples of p-cells are shown in Fig. 1.

A k-*simplex mesh of* $\mathbb{R}^d$ is simply defined as a $(k+1)$-cell of $\mathbb{R}^d$.

We denote the convex hull of p-cell $\mathcal{C}$ by $CH(\mathcal{C})$. Let O be an arbitrary point of $\mathbb{R}^d$. The *cone of apex O with respect to p-cell $\mathcal{C}$ of* $\mathbb{R}^d$ is a union of all rays which begin at O and intersect $CH(\mathcal{C})$. This cone is denoted by $\mathcal{K}(O, \mathcal{C})$.

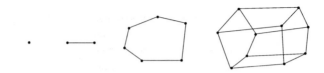

Fig. 1. Examples of some p-cells, from left to right are 0-cell (vertex), 1-cell (edge), 2-cell (face) and 3-cell.

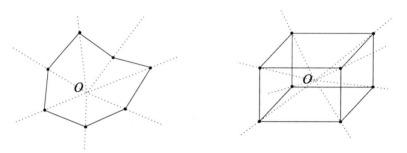

Fig. 2. Example of star-shaped 1-simplex mesh of $\mathbb{R}^2$ (left) and star-shaped 2-simplex mesh of $\mathbb{R}^3$ (right). There exists a point O inside the mesh such that any ray from O through any vertex P intersect the mesh only in point P. See text for exact definition.

Let the k-simplex mesh $\mathcal{M}$ consists of n k-cells $\mathcal{C}_i$, $i \in \{1, \ldots, n\}$.

The k-simplex mesh $\mathcal{M}$ is *star-shaped* if and only if there exists a point O in $\mathbb{R}^d$ such that

1. if two k-cells $\mathcal{C}_i$ and $\mathcal{C}_j$ intersect at $(k-1)$-cell $\mathcal{C}$ then the intersection of cones $\mathcal{K}(O, \mathcal{C}_i)$ and $\mathcal{K}(O, \mathcal{C}_j)$ is exactly the cone $\mathcal{K}(O, \mathcal{C})$.
2. if two k-cells $\mathcal{C}_i$ and $\mathcal{C}_j$ do not intersect then the intersection of cones $\mathcal{K}(O, \mathcal{C}_i)$ and $\mathcal{K}(O, \mathcal{C}_j)$ is exactly the point O.

The point O is called *centre*.

Examples of star-shaped simplex meshes are in Fig. 2.

Since the class of star-shaped k-simplex meshes is a subclass of k-simplex meshes, they have the same properties as the general k-simplex meshes [4]. Important property of k-simplex mesh is that each vertex has exactly $k+1$ neighbouring vertices. Another properties are recalled in section 2.2.

The short term *simplex mesh* will be used instead of 2-simplex mesh of $\mathbb{R}^3$ in the rest of this article.

2.2   Geometry of Simplex Meshes

Basic notation and important geometric quantities of simplex meshes (2-simplex meshes of $\mathbb{R}^3$) are introduced in this section. Similar results hold for 1-simplex meshes of $\mathbb{R}^3$ [5]. In our method the simplex angle is the most important quantity. It is used to control the desired shape of the simplex mesh.

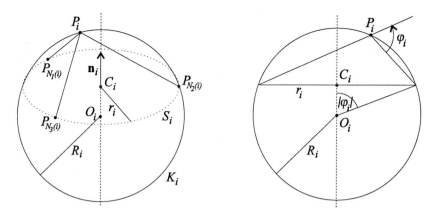

Fig. 3. (left) The circumscribed sphere K_i of radius R_i and of centre O_i. The circumscribed circle S_i of radius r_i and of centre C_i. Vector $\mathbf{n}_i$ is the unit normal vector of the plane defined by three neighbours of vertex P_i. (right) Projection of left figure. The geometrical meaning of the simplex angle φ_i is illustrated.

A vertex P_i of a simplex mesh has three neighbouring vertices $P_{N_1(i)}$, $P_{N_2(i)}$ and $P_{N_3(i)}$. These three points define a plane and the normal vector of this plane is denoted $\mathbf{n}_i$. Orientation of the normal vector is to the outer side of surface. We introduce the circumscribed circle S_i to the triangle $P_{N_1(i)}P_{N_2(i)}P_{N_3(i)}$. This circle is of centre C_i and of radius r_i. We introduce also the sphere K_i of centre O_i and radius R_i, which is circumscribed to the four vertices P_i, $P_{N_1(i)}$, $P_{N_2(i)}$, $P_{N_3(i)}$ (see Fig. 3).

The *simplex angle* $\varphi_i = \angle(P_i, P_{N_1(i)}, P_{N_2(i)}, P_{N_3(i)})$ at P_i is defined by following equations:

$$\varphi_i \in [-\pi, \pi]$$

$$sin(\varphi_i) = \frac{r_i}{R_i} sign((P_{N_1(i)} - P_i) \cdot \mathbf{n}_i) \tag{1}$$

$$cos(\varphi_i) = \frac{\|C_i - O_i\|}{R_i} sign((C_i - O_i) \cdot (P_i - C_i))$$

The simplex angle φ_i is independent of position of vertices $P_{N_1(i)}$, $P_{N_2(i)}$, $P_{N_3(i)}$ on the circle S_i and of P_i on a hemisphere of K_i. It is zero when P_i is on the plane defined by its three neighbours. The value of the simplex angle is invariant to rotation, translation and scale transformation. The geometric meaning of simplex angle is pictured in Fig. 3b.

There is a simple relationship between the simplex angle φ_i and the curvature $|H_i| = \frac{1}{R_i}$, also called the *mean curvature* at vertex P_i [4]:

$$H_i = \frac{sin\varphi_i}{r_i} \tag{2}$$

2.3   Deformation of Star-Shaped Simplex Meshes

Law of Motion. We have used the same law of motion that was used for general simplex meshes by Delingette [5]. Vertices of a simplex mesh are considered as a physical mass submitted to a Newtonian law of motion including internal and external forces:

$$m\frac{d^2 P_i}{dt^2} = -\gamma\frac{dP_i}{dt} + \mathbf{F}_{int} + \mathbf{F}_{ext} \tag{3}$$

where m is the vertex mass and γ is the damping factor. $\mathbf{F}_{int}$ is the internal force constraining the shape of the mesh. $\mathbf{F}_{ext}$ is the external force constraining the distance between the mesh and tridimensional dataset. The term $-\gamma\frac{dP_i}{dt}$ represents the counteraction of environment in which the mass is embedded.

The evolution of the simplex meshes under the law of motion (3) can be computed in the following manner [5]. Time t is discretized and using central finite differences with an explicit scheme, the law of motion has form:

$$P_i^{t+1} = P_i^t + (1 - \gamma)(P_i^t - P_i^{t-1}) + \alpha_i\mathbf{F}_{int} + \beta_i\mathbf{F}_{ext} \tag{4}$$

Both forces $\mathbf{F}_{int}$ and $\mathbf{F}_{ext}$ are computed at time t. This explicit scheme is conditionally stable and therefore parameters α_i and β_i must belong to a given interval to guarantee a stable scheme. In Eq. 4 the forces have the dimension of a displacement.

The motion of the star-shaped simplex mesh is confined in the following manner. We choose any proper centre O of the star-shaped simplex mesh and mark it as the *centre of deformation*. It means that the only allowed motion of vertices is along the rays from this centre. These rays are called *deformational rays*.

Deformation along the deformational rays preserves the star-shaped quality. The forces defined in [5] could be used with the only one change to achieve this type of deformation. Instead of the forces one can take their projections to the deformational rays. However, we will redefine this forces in order to make computations on the star-shaped simplex meshes faster and more stable.

Internal Force Computation. Internal force expressions for simplex meshes are not derived from minimisation of a global functional. The geometric parameters at a vertex are related to the vertex position with a complex non-linear relationship. Therefore, minimisation of a global functional expressed in terms of the geometric parameters would lead to unnecessarily complex force expressions [5]. Delingette proposed simplified regularising force formulae at the expense of not having a global functional for guiding the minimisation.

The internal force of deformable simplex meshes is defined as the composition of a tangential force and a normal force. The goal of the tangential force is to control the vertex position with respect to its three neighbours in the tangent plane[1]. The tangential force is not needed for deformation of star-shaped simplex meshes. The deformational rays play the role of this force.

---

[1] the plane which pass P_i and is parallel to the plane defined by three neighbours of P_i

The normal force is acting in order to change the mean curvature of surface according to the required geometrical continuity or the required local shape. These requirements are expressed by means of *reference simplex angle* $\tilde{\varphi}_i$. Remember that there is a simple relation between the simplex angle and the mean curvature (Eq. 2). The reference simplex angle is determined for each vertex before each iteration or at the beginning of minimisation process. Possibilities of computing $\tilde{\varphi}_i$ are discussed later.

Delingette used the following formula for computation of the normal force.

$$\mathbf{F}_{norm} = (L(r_i, d_i, \tilde{\varphi}_i) - L(r_i, d_i, \varphi_i)) \cdot \mathbf{n}_i \tag{5}$$

where

$$L(r_i, d_i, \varphi_i) = \frac{(r_i^2 - d_i^2)tan(\varphi_i)}{r_i + \delta\sqrt{r_i^2 + (r_i^2 - d_i^2)tan^2(\varphi_i)}} \tag{6}$$

Not yet defined symbol d_i is equal to distance between center C_i and the orthogonal projection of P_i onto the neighbouring triangle $(P_{N_1(i)}, P_{N_2(i)}, P_{N_3(i)})$. Factor $\delta = 1$ if $|\varphi_i| < \pi/2$ and $\delta = -1$ if $|\varphi_i| > \pi/2$. If the equation 6 is used for minimisation computation is unstable for φ_i near 0 or $\pi/2$ Since $L(r_i, d_i, \varphi_i)$ computes distance between P_i and the neighbouring triangle $(P_{N_1(i)}, P_{N_2(i)}, P_{N_3(i)})$, equation 5 can be evaluated to be more suitable for stable computation

$$\mathbf{F}_{norm} = (L(r_i, d_i, \tilde{\varphi}_i) - (P_{N_1(i)} - P_i) \cdot \mathbf{n}_i) \cdot \mathbf{n}_i \tag{7}$$

Using this equation stability of normal force computation depends only on the value of reference simplex angle $\tilde{\varphi}_i$.

Internal force of star-shaped simplex meshes does not act in the normal direction but in the direction of a deformational ray and is defined by

$$\mathbf{F}_{int} = \tilde{P}_i - P_i \tag{8}$$

where P_i is the vertex on which the force is acting and $\tilde{P}_i$ is the point, which lies on the deformational ray and its simplex angle with respect to the neighbours of P_i is equal to the reference simplex angle (see Fig. 4).

The point $\tilde{P}_i$ can be computed as a intersection of the deformational ray through P_i and the part of sphere on which all points has their simplex angles with respect to the neighbours of P_i equal to the reference simplex angle. The intersection is given by

$$\tilde{P}_i = O + \mathbf{v}_i \tilde{t} \tag{9}$$

where O is the center of deformation, $\mathbf{v}_i = \frac{P_i - O}{\|P_i - O\|}$ is the unit directional vector of the deformational ray through vertex P_i and $\tilde{t}$ is equal to

$$\tilde{t} = \mathbf{v}_i \cdot (O - \tilde{O}_i) + \delta\sqrt{\tilde{R}_i^2 + (\mathbf{v}_i \cdot (O - \tilde{O}_i))^2 - \|O - \tilde{O}_i\|^2} \tag{10}$$

where $\delta = 1$ if $\tilde{\varphi}_i < 0$ and $\delta = -1$ otherwise. $\tilde{R}_i = |\frac{r_i}{sin\tilde{\varphi}_i}|$ and $\tilde{O}_i = C_i + \mathbf{n}_i \tilde{R}_i cos\tilde{\varphi}_i$.

The reference simplex angle $\tilde{\varphi}_i$ can be computed in the following manners

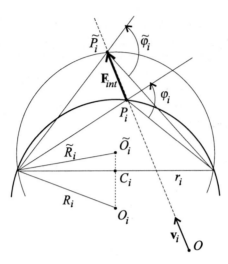

Fig. 4. Computation of internal force $\mathbf{F}_{int}$. The force is acting along the ray $O + \mathbf{v}_i t$ in order to move the vertex P_i with simplex angle φ_i to the new position $\tilde{P}_i$ where simplex angle is equal to the reference simplex angle $\tilde{\varphi}_i$.

- C^0 *constraint.* $\tilde{\varphi}_i$ is set to φ_i and therefore no internal force is acting. The surface can freely bend around vertex P_i.
- C^1 *constraint.* $\tilde{\varphi}_i$ is set to 0 and accordingly each vertex moves towards its center of curvature in the case of Delingette method or towards the center of deformation in the case of star-shaped meshes.
- *shape constraint.* $\tilde{\varphi}_i$ is set to constant value φ_i^0. This case is important for spherical shape reconstruction. The constants φ_i^0 are calculated according to initial surface (sphere or ellipsoid).
- *simplex shape continuity or* C^2 *constraint.* $\tilde{\varphi}_i$ is set to an average value of the simplex angles at neighbouring vertices.

External Force Computation. Problem of external force computation is broadly and deeply discussed in [5]. The expression of the external force depends on the nature of the input data. When star-shaped simplex meshes are being used, it is important to let the external force (as well as the other forces) act in the direction of deformational rays. The method which we used for external force computation is mentioned in the next section.

3   Application to Cell Nuclei Segmentation

Segmentation and reconstruction of the boundaries of cell nuclei is essential in many biological studies. Reliable 3-D model of nucleus is for example necessary for the measurement of some topographical parameters (e.g. distance between nucleus boundary and genes.). Measured topographical parameters are statistically evaluated and therefore a large number of nuclei must be processed in an

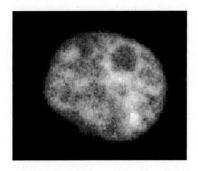 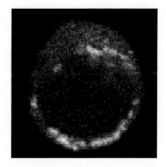

Fig. 5. (Left) A xy slice of the HL-60 input dataset. Volume of the nucleus is stained. (Right) A xy slice of the HT-29 input dataset. Nuclear envelope of the nucleus is stained. Some stain was washed away from the envelope and only its part is visible.

efficient and reliable manner. Visualisation of the reconstructed model of nucleus boundary is also important for understanding its shape.

We have performed nucleus reconstruction on two types of input images.

HL-60 – DAPI stained chromatin of 3-D fixed HL-60 cells, i.e the whole volume of nuclei is visualised. A typical xy slice of this input dataset is in Fig. 5 (left). Voxels with the highest gradient intensity determine the nucleus boundary.

HT-29 – nuclear envelope of 3-D fixed nuclei obtained from stabilised cell line of human colon adenocarcinoma HT-29. The nuclear envelope was visualised using Lamin B. A typical xy slice of the input dataset is in Fig. 5 (right). The voxels of the highest intensity values correspond to the nuclear envelope. Because the nuclear envelope is eroded during the process of specimen preparation, only parts of the nuclear envelope are clearly visible. Reconstruction algorithm have to deal with missing data. The voxels with the lower intensities corresponds to the places, from which the Lamin B was not properly washed away.

Two methods which were described in the previous section were applied on mentioned data:

SS – Star shaped simplex meshes (section 2).

GM – General method proposed by Delingette[5] with the change in normal force computation (stable formula 7 was used).

Shape constraint was used for determination of reference simplex angle in the both methods. The reference simplex angles of vertices were set to the values computed from the initial surface. Hence, the internal force was keeping the initial spherical (ellipsoidal) shape.

Input datasets were preprocessed before deformation process. Gaussian smoothing and intensity normalisation [13] was used. Input images were filtered by LoG (Laplacian of Gaussian) instead of Gaussian in experiment with HL-60 cells. A mKD-tree [14] was constructed for N voxels with the highest intensities

Table 1. Comparison of SS and GM methods (HL-60 input dataset). Testing was accomplished for fifteen differnt combinations of parametres α, β and γ for each method. Results for SS method are on the first line in each cell and results for GM method are on the second line. n is the number of iterations to achieve stable state, t is time of deformation and μ is mean distance between the input points and the final mesh. Symbol ∞ means that computation was oscillating.

α,β	Damping factor γ														
	0.1			0.25			0.5			0.75			1		
	n	t	μ	n	t	μ	n	t	μ	n	t	μ	n	t	μ
0.9, 0.1	66	12.54	4.68	63	11.97	4.67	69	13.11	4.8	32	6.08	5.1	25	4.75	6.23
	62	14.88	4.8	60	14.4	4.82	87	20.88	4.85	24	5.76	5.55	25	6.0	6.18
0.8, 0.2	68	12.92	4.11	43	8.17	4.15	56	10.64	4.22	74	14.06	4.26	83	15.77	4.3
	502	120.48	4.2	72	17.28	4.24	45	10.8	4.26	62	14.88	4.29	68	16.32	4.32
0.7, 0.3	75	14.25	3.79	44	8.36	3.88	58	11.02	3.88	72	13.68	3.89	94	17.86	3.9
	∞	∞	?	∞	∞	?	102	24.48	3.89	118	28.32	3.9	76	18.24	3.95

(hundreds on each slice was enough in our application). m-closest points to given point can be obtained efficiently using mKD-trees. An ellipsoid was taken as the initial surface. The ellipsoid generation was based on ellipse fitting [6] on each slice.

An external force $\mathbf{F}_{ext}$ was computed as a projection of the following force $\mathbf{F}$ onto the deformational ray trough given vertex P_i.

$$\mathbf{F} = \sum_{j=1}^{m} w_j X_j \tag{11}$$

where X_j are m closest points to given vertex P_i and w_j is defined by

$$w_j = \begin{cases} 0, & X_j - P_i > const \\ \frac{I(X_j)}{(X_j - P_i)^2}, & \text{otherwise} \end{cases} \tag{12}$$

where $I(X_j)$ is intensity of point X_j.

Deformation was computed until the change of mesh was insignificant. Each method was performed on each dataset for fifteen times and always with different parameters α, β and γ. Dumping factor γ has iterated over values 0.1, 0.25, 0.5, 0.75 and 1 and the couple (α, β) over $(0.9, 0.1)$, $(0.8, 0.2)$ and $(0.7, 0.3)$. Three values were logged for every execution of each method:

- The number of iterations n needed to achieve stable state,
- the time of deformation t and
- mean distance μ between the input points and the final mesh.

Times were measured on processor Pentium III 500MHz, RAM 128MB and OS Debian Linux. Results are summarized in tables 1 and 2.

Tables show that accuracy expressed by means of the mean distance between model and data is very similar for both methods. However, on the other side

Table 2. Comparison of SS and GM methods (HT-29 input dataset). This table is organized in the same manner as table 1.

α,β	Damping factor γ														
	0.1			0.25			0.5			0.75			1		
	n	t	μ	n	t	μ	n	t	μ	n	t	μ	n	t	μ
0.9, 0.1	75	16.5	12.59	47	10.38	12.38	71	15.62	12.24	57	12.54	11.25	74	16.28	11.24
	∞	∞	?	∞	∞	?	60	16.8	12.48	70	19.6	11.99	64	17.92	11.78
0.8, 0.2	79	17.38	10.36	41	9.02	10.37	81	17.82	9.95	90	19.8	9.81	88	19.36	9.72
	∞	∞	?	∞	∞	?	∞	∞	?	∞	∞	?	110	30.8	10.95
0.7, 0.3	94	20.68	9.14	62	13.64	8.98	57	12.54	8.57	82	18.04	8.61	89	19.58	8.59
	∞	∞	?	∞	∞	?	∞	∞	?	∞	∞	?	∞	∞	?

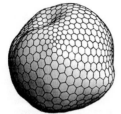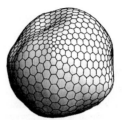

Fig. 6. Final meshes in HL-60 experiment, $\gamma = 0.5$, $\alpha = 0.9$, $\beta = 0.1$ (Left) SS method (Right) GM method.

it is impossible to decide exactly what result better approximates the border of real cell nucleus. An expert in biology have to make a selection what method and what parameters are most appropriate for a given application.

A lot of experiments with GM method have not converged. We have investigated this problem of oscillations and discovered that all oscillations were due to tangential forces. Therefore we believe that the reason why the star-shaped method have not ever oscillated is that there are no tangential forces. However this statment we are not able to proof at this moment.

Sum of α and β is intensionally equal to one. Changing the ratio of this two parameters influences on minimisation process. This ratio express balance between the internal and external forces. User can change the shape of spherical object by handling this ratio and drive model either more closer to input data or more closer to initial spherical model. An α, β ratio handling can be used for segmentation of noisy or pure data. General method is for α, β ratio handling less suitable than star-shaped method because it oscillate for some α and β.

Fig. 6 shows some final meshes of both methods for HL-60 dataset. A number of vertices of simplex meshes was 2700. In fig. 7 and 8 the projection of final mesh obtained by the application of SS method onto some xy and xz slices of input image is depicted .

Fig. 9 shows some final meshes of both methods for HT-29 dataset. In fig. 10 and 11 the projection of final mesh obtained by the application of SS method onto some xy and yz slices of input HT-29 image is depicted.

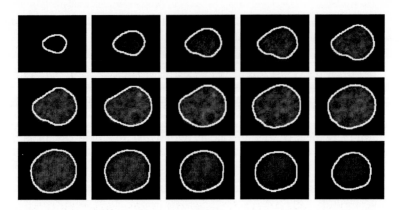

Fig. 7. Results in xy slices, HL-60 experiment, $\gamma = 0.5$, $\alpha = 0.9$, $\beta = 0.1$, SS method. The final surface was projected onto the input data.

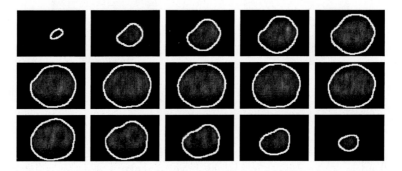

Fig. 8. Results in xz slices, HL-60 experiment, $\gamma = 0.5$, $\alpha = 0.9$, $\beta = 0.1$, SS method. The final surface was projected onto the input data.

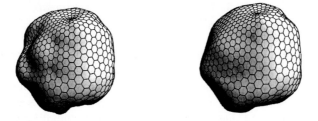

Fig. 9. Final meshes in HT-29 experiment, $\gamma = 0.5$, $\alpha = 0.9$, $\beta = 0.1$ (Left) SS method (Right) GM method.

4   Conclusion

A new method for spherical object reconstruction based on deformation of star-shaped simplex meshes was proposed. The new method provides similar results

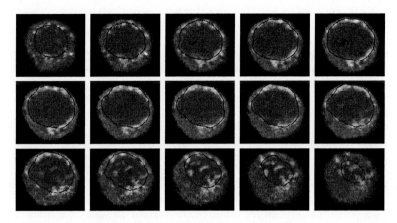

Fig. 10. Results in xy slices, HT-29 experiment, $\gamma = 0.75$, $\alpha = 0.9$, $\beta = 0.1$, SS method. The final surface was projected onto the input data.

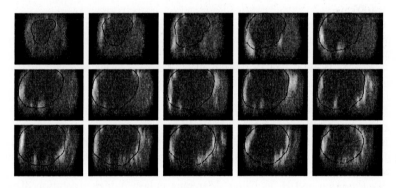

Fig. 11. Results in yz slices, HT-29 experiment, $\gamma = 0.75$, $\alpha = 0.9$, $\beta = 0.1$, SS method. The final surface was projected onto the input data.

as a Delingette general method [5], from which we drew inspiration. However, the new method is easier model and therefore it is faster. In adition, it has achieved a stable state more often then general method. We will study method further, because there are some not answered questions. The most important is, for which values of coefficients α and β is the minimisation stable. Answer to this question is important to further progress of the new method.

Acknowledgments

This work was supported by the Ministry of Education of the Czech Republic (Project No. MSM-143300002) and by the Academy of Sciences of the Czech Republic (Grants No. S5004010 and No. B5004102).

References

1. P. S. Umesh Adiga and B. B. Chaudhuri. Deformable models for segmentation of CLSM tissue images and its application in FISH signal analysis. *Analytical Cellular Pathology*, 18(4):211–225, 1999. ISSN 0921-8912.
2. P. Bamford and B. Lovell. Unsupervised cell nucleus segmentation with active contours. *Signal Processing Special Issue: Deformable Models and Techniques for Image and Signal Processing*, 71(2), 1998.
3. C. Ortiz de Solórzano, E. García Rodriguez, A. Jones, D. Pinkel, J. W. Gray, D. Sudar, and S. J. Lockett. Segmentation of confocal microscope images of cell nuclei in thick tissue sections. *Journal of Microscopy*, 193:212–226, 1999.
4. H. Delingette. Simplex meshes: a general representation for 3D shape reconstruction. Technical Report 2214, INRIA, France, 1994.
5. H. Delingette. General object reconstruction based on simplex meshes. *International Journal of Computer Vision*, 32(2):111–146, 1999.
6. A. Fitzgibbon, M. Pilu, and R. B. Fisher. Direct least square fitting of ellipses. *IEEE Transactions on Pattern Analysis and Machine Inteligence*, 21(5):476–480, May 1999.
7. F. Guilak. Volume and surface area measurement of viable chondrocytes in situ using geometric modelling of serial confocal sections. *Journal of Microscopy*, 173(3):245–256, 1993.
8. M. Kass, A. Witkin, and D. Terzopoulos. Active contour models. *International Journal of Computer Vision*, 1(4):133–144, 1987.
9. M. Kozubek, S. Kozubek, E. Lukášová, A. Marečková, E. Bártová, M. Skalníková, and A. Jergová. High-resolution cytometry of FISH dots in interphase cell nuclei. *Cytometry*, 36:279–293, 1999.
10. L. Kubínová, J. Janáček, F. Guilak, and Z. Opatrný. Comparison of several digital and stereological methods for estimating surface area and volume of cell studied by confocal microscopy. *Cytometry*, 36:85–95, 1999.
11. W. E. Lorensen and H. E. Cline. Marching cubes: A high resolution 3D surface construction algorithm. In *Computer Graphics (Proceedings of SIGGRAPH '87)*, volume 21, pages 163–169, 1987.
12. H. Netten, I. T. Young, L. J. Van Vliet, H. J. Tanke, H. Vrolijk, and W. C. R. Sloos. FISH and chips: automation of fluorescent dot counting in interphase cell nuclei. *Cytometry*, 28:1–10, 1997.
13. W. K. Pratt. *Digital Image Processing*. John Wiley & Sons, Inc., New York, second edition, 1991.
14. F. P. Preparata and M. I. Shamos. *Computational geometry : an introduction*. Springer-Verlag, 1985.

Gabor Feature Space Diffusion via the Minimal Weighted Area Method

Chen Sagiv[1], Nir A. Sochen[1], and Yehoshua Y. Zeevi[2]

[1] Department of Applied Mathematics
University of Tel Aviv
Ramat-Aviv, Tel-Aviv 69978, Israel
chensagi@post.tau.ac.il, sochen@math.tau.ac.il
[2] Department of Electrical engineering
Technion – Israel Institute of Technology
Technion City, Haifa 32000, Israel
zeevi@ee.technion.ac.il

Abstract. Gabor feature space is elaborated for representation, processing and segmentation of textured images. As a first step of preprocessing of images represented in this space, we introduce an algorithm for Gabor feature space denoising. It is a geometric-based algorithm that applies diffusion-like equation derived from a minimal weighted area functional, introduced previously and applied in the context of stereo reconstruction models [6, 12]. In a previous publication we have already demonstrated how to generalize the intensity-based geodesic active contours model to the Gabor spatial-feature space. This space is represented, via the Beltrami framework, as a $2D$ Riemannian manifold embedded in a $6D$ space. In this study we apply the minimal weighted area method to smooth the Gabor space features prior to the application of the geodesic active contour mechanism. We show that this "Weighted Beltrami" approach preserves edges better than the original Beltrami diffusion. Experimental results of this feature space denoising process and of the geodesic active contour mechanism applied to the denoised feature space are presented.

Keywords: Gabor analysis, Geometric-based algorithms, Geodesic active contours, Beltrami framework, Anisotropic diffusion, image manifolds, minimal weighted area method.

1 Introduction

Textured image segmentation is an important issue in image analysis. However, real world textures are difficult to model. Among the approaches to the analysis of textures are local geometric primitives [9], local statistical features [3], random field models [8, 4] and the FRAME theory [23] which combines filtering theory and Markov random field modeling through the maximum entropy principle. Another approach, based on the human visual system has emerged, in which texture features are extracted using Gabor filters [19].

The motivation for the use of Gabor filters in texture analysis is double fold. First, it is believed that simple cells in the visual cortex can be modeled by Gabor

M.A.T. Figueiredo, J. Zerubia, A.K. Jain (Eds.): EMMCVPR 2001, LNCS 2134, pp. 621–635, 2001.

functions [16, 5], and that the Gabor scheme provides a suitable representation for visual information in the combined frequency-position space [18]. Second, the Gabor representation has been shown to be optimal in the sense of minimizing the joint two-dimensional uncertainty in the combined spatial-frequency space [7]. The analysis of Gabor filters was generalized to multi-window Gabor filters [24] and to Gabor-Morlet wavelets [18, 24, 17, 15], and studied both analytically and experimentally on various classes of images [24].

A great deal of attention has been devoted in recent years to the "snakes", or active contour models, which were proposed by Kaas et al [10] for intensity based image segmentation. In this framework an initial contour is deformed towards the boundary of an object to be detected. The evolution equation is derived from minimization of an energy functional, which obtains a minimum for a curve located at the boundary of the object. A major drawback of the classical snakes algorithm is its dependence on the parameterization of the curve. This may actually lead to different results for different choices of parameterization.

The geodesic active contours model [2, 11] offers a different perspective for solving the boundary detection problem; It is based on the observation that the energy minimization problem is equivalent to finding a geodesic curve in a Riemannian space whose metric is derived from image contents. The geodesic curve can be found via a *parameterization invariant* geometric flow. Utilization of the Osher and Sethian level set numerical algorithm [20] allows automatic handling of changes of topology.

It was shown recently that the Gaborian spatial-feature space can be described, via the Beltrami framework [22], as a 4D Riemannian manifold [13] embedded in $\mathbb{R}^6$. Based on this approach, the intensity based geodesic active contours method was generalized to the Gabor-feature space of images [21]. It was shown that the geodesic snakes mechanism can be used for texture segmentation when applied to the Gabor spatial feature space of images rather than the intensity images themselves. The metric introduced in the Gabor space was used to derive the inverse edge indicator function E, which attracts in turn the evolving curve towards the boundary in the geodesic snakes schemes. Once the Gabor feature space of an image is derived, the scale and orientation for which the maximum amplitude of the transform was obtained are kept for each pixel. Thus, for each pixel, the maximum value of the Gabor transform coefficient and the orientation and scale that yield this maximum value are obtained. This approach results in a $2D$ manifold embedded in a $6D$ space. It was shown that using this approach the geodesic snakes yield good results when the textures are homogeneous and can be characterized by these maximum values.

However, the maximum values provide only partial information regarding image structure in the full Gabor feature space. This may, in turn, generate less than satisfactory results in case of more complex textures. One solution to this problem is to apply the geodesic snakes mechanism to the complete Gabor feature space and interpret the Gabor transform of an image as a function assigning for each pixel's coordinates, scale and orientation, a value. Thus, the Gabor transform of an image may be viewed as a $4D$ manifold embedded in $\mathbb{R}^6$.

An alternative solution is to improve the results obtained from the $2D$ manifold embedded in $6D$ space approach which we aim to achieve here.

We apply the weighted area minimization method to improve the results for the orientations which were determined by searching for the maximum value of the Gabor coefficients. We show that it better preserves edges than the Beltrami smoothing operator.

This paper is organized as follows: In section 2 we briefly review the Bayesian formulation in the context of image processing. In section 3 we describe the geodesic active contours method for intensity images. Next, in section 4 we describe the generation of the Gabor feature space. In section 5 we show how to apply the geodesic snakes mechanism in the Gabor feature space. In section 6 we describe the weighted area minimization method, and finally in section 7, we provide some preliminary results.

2 Bayesian Formulation

The Bayesian approach is useful in finding a compromise between the requirements of fidelity of a given image data, and our *a priori* knowledge or assumptions regarding the nature of "true" images. Accordingly, we consider an image to be made of an ensemble of interacting systems–i.e. pixels, wherein the gray level of each pixel is a realization of a random process. In other words, the gray level of each pixel is drown from a probability distribution that depends on the value of the given noisy image, as well as on a priori information reflecting assumptions about the structure and properties of natural images. For example, and in particular, the smoothness assumption can be interpreted as the "mean free path" of interactions among the above-mentioned pixel generating systems, resulting in some kind of a weighted averaging in a neighborhood of the pixel. The likelihood of an image, given the noisy data set of an image, is obtained by multiplication of the likelihood functions of all the pixels' gray levels. Given a pixel at the coordinates (x_i, y_i), according to Bayes rule

$$P_{x_i y_i}(I(x_i, y_i)|I_0(x_i, y_i)) = \frac{P_{x_i y_i}(I_0(x_i, y_i)|I(x_i, y_i))P_{x_i y_i}(I(x_i, y_i))}{P_{x_i y_i}(I_0(x_i, y_i))}, \quad (1)$$

and

$$P(I|I_0) = \prod_{i,j \in N \times N} P_{x_i y_i}(I(x_i, y_i)|I_0(x_i, y_i)), \quad (2)$$

where N is the size of the image, and in the left hand side of both (1) and (2) we have the posteriori probability distribution of either a pixel value (eq. 1) or of the entire image (eq. 2) that we wish to compute; Namely the probability of the gray value $I(x_i, y_i)$ (or of I), given the data $I_0(x_i, y_i)$ (or I_0). This distribution is calculated in the right hand side of both (1) and (2) as the probabilities of measuring $I_0(x_i, y_i)$ (or of I_0), given the "true" image, multiplied by the probability of $I(x_i, y_i)$ (I) being the true image. In other words, this second term reflects our prior assumption on the distribution of $I(x, y)$. The denominator depends only on $I_0(x_i, y_i)$ and therefore does not affect the optimization process of $I(x, y)$.

One often assumes a Gibbsian distribution, in which case the conditional probability becomes

$$P_{xy}(A|B) = \exp(-\alpha e(A, B)).$$

where $e(A, B)$ is an "energy density". Given this type of conditional probability equation (2) becomes

$$P(I|I_0) = \prod_{i,j \in N \times N} \frac{P_{x_i y_i}(I_0(x_i, y_i)|I(x_i, y_i))P_{x_i y_i}(I(x_i, y_i))}{P_{x_i y_i}(I_0(x_i, y_i))}$$

$$= \exp(-\alpha \int (e(I, I_0) - e(I_0))\, dx dy). \tag{3}$$

Determining which is the image that maximizes the posteriori probability, is equivalent to the selection of the image that minimizes the energy.

Our study generalizes this framework of the statistical approach to images, by considering the probability distribution of texture features and not only (and in the examples given herewith not at all) of the pixels' gray levels. We also choose somewhat non-standard fidelity term and smoothing term. A special form is assumed such that the two terms collapse into one. The technique is borrowed from recent results in stereo reconstruction models [6, 12] and our prior assumption is that textures (and/or other image features) are piecewise uniform.

3   Geodesic Active Contours

In this section we review the geodesic active contours method for non-textured images [2]. The generalization of the technique for texture segmentation is described in section 4.

Let $\mathbf{C}(q) : [0, 1] \to \mathbb{R}^2$ be a parametrized curve, and let $I : [0, a] \times [0, b] \to \mathbb{R}^+$ be the given image. Let $E(r) : [0, \infty[\to \mathbb{R}^+$ be an inverse edge detector, so that E approaches zero when r approaches infinity. Visually, E should represent the edges in the image. Minimizing the energy functional proposed in the classical snakes is generalized to finding a geodesic curve in a Riemannian space by minimizing:

$$L_R = \int E(|\nabla I(\mathbf{C}(q))|)\, |\mathbf{C}'(q)| dq. \tag{4}$$

We may see this term as a weighted length of a curve, where the Euclidean length element is weighted by $E(|\nabla I(C(q))|)$. The latter contains information regarding the boundaries within the image. The resultant evolution equation is the gradient descent flow:

$$\frac{\partial \mathbf{C}(t)}{\partial t} = E(|\nabla I|)k\mathbf{N} - (\nabla E \cdot \mathbf{N})\, \mathbf{N}, \tag{5}$$

where k denotes curvature.

If we now define a function U, so that $\mathbf{C} = ((x, y)|U(x, y) = 0)$, we may use the Osher-Sethian Level-Sets approach [20] and replace the evolution equation for the curve $\mathbf{C}$, with an evolution equation for the embedding function U:

$$\frac{\partial U(t)}{\partial t} = |\nabla U|\text{Div}\left(E(|\nabla I|)\frac{\nabla U}{|\nabla U|}\right). \tag{6}$$

A popular choice for the stopping function $E(|\nabla I|)$ is given by:

$$E(|\nabla I|) = \frac{1}{1 + |\nabla I|^2},$$

however, other image-specific functions may be used.

4   Feature Space and Gabor Transform

The Gabor scheme and Gabor filters have been studied by numerous researchers in the context of image representation, texture segmentation and image retrieval. A Gabor filter centered at the 2D frequency coordinates (U, V) has the general form of:

$$h(x, y) = g(x', y') \exp(2\pi i(Ux + Vy)) \tag{7}$$

where

$$(x', y') = (x\cos(\phi) + y\sin(\phi), -x\sin(\phi) + y\cos(\phi)), \tag{8}$$

$$g(x, y) = \frac{1}{2\pi\sigma^2}\exp\left(-\frac{x^2}{2\lambda^2\sigma^2} - \frac{y^2}{2\sigma^2}\right), \tag{9}$$

λ is the aspect ratio between x and y scales, σ is the scale parameter, and the major axis of the Gaussian is oriented at angle ϕ relative to the x-axis and to the modulating sinewave gratings.

Accordingly, the Fourier transform of the Gabor function is:

$$H(u, v) = \exp\left(-2\pi^2\sigma^2((u' - U')^2\lambda^2 + (v' - V')^2)\right) \tag{10}$$

where, (u', v') and (U', V') are rotated frequency coordinates. Thus, $H(u, v)$ is a bandpass Gaussian with its minor axis oriented at angle ϕ from the u-axis, and the radial center frequency F is defined by: $F = U^2 + V^2$, with orientation $\theta = \arctan(V/U)$. Since maximal resolution in orientation is desirable, the filters whose sinewave gratings are cooriented with the major axis of the modulating Gaussian are usually considered ($\phi = \theta$ and $\lambda > 1$), and the Gabor filter is reduced to: $h(x, y) = g(x', y')exp(2\pi iFx')$.

It is possible to generate Gabor-Morlet wavelets from a single mother-Gabor-wavelet by transformations such as: translations, rotations and dilations. We can generate, in this way, a set of filters for a known number of scales, S, and orientations K. We obtain the following filters for a discrete subset of transformations: $h_{mn}(x, y) = a^{-m}h(\frac{x'}{a^m}, \frac{y'}{a^m})$, where (x', y') are the spatial coordinates rotated by

$\frac{\pi n}{K}$ and $m = 0...S - 1$. Alternatively, one can obtain Gabor wavelets by loga-rithmically distorting the frequency axis [18] or by incorporating multiwindows [24]. In the latter case one obtains a more general scheme wherein subsets of the functions constitute either wavelet sets or Gaborian sets.

The feature space of an image is obtained by the inner product of this set of Gabor filters with the image:

$$W_{mn}(x,y) = R_{mn}(x,y) + iJ_{mn}(x,y) = I(x,y) * h_{mn}(x,y). \tag{11}$$

5   Application of Geodesic Snakes to the Gaborian Feature Space of Images

The proposed approach enables us to use the geodesic snakes mechanism in the Gabor spatial feature space of images by generalizing the inverse edge indicator function E, which attracts in turn the evolving curve towards the boundary in the classical and geodesic snakes schemes. A special feature of our approach is the metric introduced in the Gabor space, and used as the building block for the stopping function E in the geodesic active contours scheme.

Sochen et al [22] view images and image feature space as Riemannian man-ifolds embedded in a higher dimensional space. For example, a gray scale im-age is a $2D$ Riemannian surface (manifold), with (x,y) as local coordinates, embedded in $\mathbb{R}^3$ with (X,Y,Z) as local coordinates. The embedding map is $(X = x, Y = y, Z = I(x,y))$, and we write it, by abuse of notations, as (x,y,I). When we consider feature spaces of images, e.g. color space, statistical moments space, and the Gaborian space, we may view the image-feature information as a N-dimensional manifold embedded in a $N + M$ dimensional space, where N stands for the number of local parameters needed to index the space of interest and M is the number of feature coordinates. For example, we may view the Gabor transformed image as a 2D manifold with local coordinates (x,y) embedded in a 6D feature space. The embedding map is $(x,y,\theta(x,y),\sigma(x,y),R(x,y),J(x,y))$, where R and J are the real and imaginary parts of the Gabor transformed image, and θ and σ as the direction and scale for which a maximal response has been achieved. Alternatively, we can represent the Gabor transform space as a 4D manifold with coordinates (x,y,θ,σ) embedded in the same 6D feature space. The embedding map, in this case, is $(x,y,\theta,\sigma,R(x,y,\theta,\sigma),J(x,y,\theta,\sigma))$. The main difference between the two approaches is whether θ and σ are considered to be local coordinates or feature coordinates.

A basic concept in the context of Riemannian manifolds is distance. Con-sider, for example, we take a two-dimensional manifold Σ with local coordinates (σ_1,σ_2). Since the local coordinates are curvilinear, the distance is calculated using a positive definite symmetric bilinear form called the metric whose com-ponents are denoted by $g_{\mu\nu}(\sigma_1,\sigma_2)$:

$$ds^2 = g_{\mu\nu}d\sigma^\mu d\sigma^\nu, \tag{12}$$

where we used the Einstein summation convention: elements with identical su-perscripts and subscripts are summed over.

The metric on the image manifold is derived using a procedure known as pullback. The manifold's metric is then used for various geometrical flows. We shortly review the pullback mechanism. More detailed information can be found in [22].

Let $X : \Sigma \to M$ be an embedding of Σ in M, where M is a Riemannian manifold with a metric h_{ij} and Σ is another Riemannian manifold. We can use the knowledge of the metric on M and the map X to construct the metric on Σ. This pullback procedure is as follows:

$$(g_{\mu\nu})_{\Sigma}(\sigma^1, \sigma^2) = h_{ij}(X(\sigma^1, \sigma^2)) \frac{\partial X^i}{\partial \sigma^\mu} \frac{\partial X^j}{\partial \sigma^\nu}, \tag{13}$$

where we used the Einstein summation convention, $i, j = 1, \ldots, dim(M)$, and σ^1, σ^2 are the local coordinates on the manifold Σ.

If we pull back the metric of a 2D image manifold from the Euclidean embedding space (x,y,I) we get:

$$(g_{\mu\nu}(x,y)) = \begin{pmatrix} 1 + I_x^2 & I_x I_y \\ I_x I_y & 1 + I_y^2 \end{pmatrix}. \tag{14}$$

The determinant of $g_{\mu\nu}$ yields the expression: $1 + I_x{}^2 + I_y{}^2$. Thus, we can rewrite the expression for the stopping term E in the geodesic snakes mechanism as follows:

$$E(|\nabla I|) = \frac{1}{1 + |\nabla I|^2} = \frac{1}{\det(g_{\mu\nu})}.$$

We may interpret the Gabor transform of an image as a function assigning to each pixel's coordinates, scale and orientation, a value (W). Next, we get the scale and orientation for which we have received the maximum amplitude of the transform for each pixel. Thus, for each pixel, we obtain: W_{max}, the maximum value of the transform, θ_{max} and σ_{max} – the orientation and scale that yielded this maximum value. This approach results in a 2D manifold (with local coordinates (x, y)) embedded in a 6D space (with local coordinates $(x, y, R(x, y), J(x, y), \theta(x, y), \sigma(x, y))$. If we use the pullback mechanism described above we get the following metric:

$$(g_{\mu\nu}) = \begin{pmatrix} 1 + R_x^2 + J_x^2 + \sigma_x^2 + \theta_x^2 & R_x R_y + J_x J_y + \sigma_x \sigma_y + \theta_x \theta_y \\ R_x R_y + J_x J_y + \sigma_x \sigma_y + \theta_x \theta_y & 1 + R_y^2 + J_y^2 + \sigma_y^2 + \theta_y^2 \end{pmatrix} \tag{15}$$

We use the fact that the determinant of the metric is a positive definite edge indicator to determine E as the inverse of the determinant of $g_{\mu\nu}$. Here $g_{\mu\nu}$ is a function of the two spatial variables only x and y, therefore, we obtain an evolution of a 2D manifold in a 6D embedding space.

6 Smoothing of the Orientation Data by Application of the Weighted Area Minimization Method

In the previous section we have described how the Gabor feature space can be treated as a $2D$ manifold embedded in $6D$ space. We have used a maximum criterion to obtain a single orientation and scale for each pixel location. However, this information does not always well represent the textural information and is sensitive to local variations in the texture characteristics. Therefore, the resultant orientation data can be quite noisy. Also, some random noise can deteriorate the resultant data. Our aim is to reduce the amount of noise in the orientation data and obtain a smoother function to be used in the geodesic snakes mechanism.

We obtain the Gabor feature coefficients as a function of $x, y, \theta(x, y)$ and $\sigma(x, y)$. This discussion is devoted to the manipulation of θ, therefore we select a single scale σ and generate a set of Gabor filters for that scale, which differ in their orientation. Thus, the generated Gabor feature space is a function of $x, y, \theta(x, y)$. Our aim is to reduce the amount of noise in θ, whether its source is a heterogeneous texture or some random noise. We define an energy functional which minimizes the magnitude of the Gabor coefficients function weighted by an area element determined by $x, y, \theta(x, y)$.

$$\mathbf{S}(\theta) = \int D(x, y, \theta) \sqrt{g(\theta_x, \theta_y)} dx dy \tag{16}$$

where

$$D(x, y, \theta) = \frac{1}{(R^2 + J^2 + c)}$$

is a data fidelity term and g is the determinant of

$$(g_{\mu\nu}) = \begin{pmatrix} 1 + \theta_x^2 & \theta_x \theta_y \\ \theta_x \theta_y & 1 + \theta_y^2 \end{pmatrix}. \tag{17}$$

The combination $\sqrt{g}dxdy$, an area element of the orientation manifold $(x, y, \theta(x, y))$, is the term that forces smoothing as the orientation field reduces its overall area when it flows towards the optimal solution. For trivial data term the gradient descent process is the Beltrami flow that ignores any data edges that are not already very pronounced in the initial noisy guess. On the other hand a trivial metric for the orientation manifold results in decoupling of the different orientation values in different locations as the metric is the only place where derivatives of θ may appear. This decoupling leads to a simple solution: At each pixel the orientation for which maximum response is achieved is chosen. As we have noted above this leads to a noisy solution that may undermine the correctness of the segmentation process.

The constant c in the denominator has two roles: The first role is merely numeric, to avoid division in zero. The second role has a geometrical meaning since this constant determines the convergence properties of our scheme. If this constant is very small, the evolution depends more on the values of the Gabor transform, $(R^2 + J^2)$, and the smoothing of θ is less dominant. If the constant is very large compared with the values of the Gabor transform, then they are less dominant in the evolution, and the smoothing of θ is the same as in the Beltrami scheme.

Considering the Bayesian formulation we notice that we may rewrite the energy density as $e = (D - const)\sqrt{g} + const\sqrt{g}$. We note that the first term is a fidelity term that forces θ to align according to the orientation in the noisy original image while the second term pushes towards a minimal surface solution. Note that the $\sqrt{g}$ in the first term means that the fidelity term is to be thought of as a function *on the orientation manifold*. Choosing the same constant for both terms leads to the functional S written above. Note that we do indeed generalize the formalism by considering features, i.e. orientations in this specific implementation, rather than intensity. Our assumption is that images are piecewise continuous with respect to all the relevant image features/attributes. In the case of textureless images, i.e. gray level only, this continuity becomes identical to smoothness.

Thus, we process the manifold $\theta(x, y)$, while obtaining the maximum value for the Gabor coefficients, so that the contribution and impact of each component leads to satisfactory result.

Using the Euler-Lagrange method we obtain the following equation:

$$\frac{\delta S}{\delta \theta} = -div\left(\frac{\nabla \theta}{(R^2 + J^2)(x, y, \theta(x, y))\sqrt{g}}\right) - \frac{(R^2 + J^2)_\theta(x, y, \theta(x, y))\sqrt{g}}{(R^2 + J^2)^2(x, y, \theta(x, y))} \quad (18)$$

According to the steepest descent method the evolution equation for θ is:

$$\theta_t = -\frac{\delta S}{\delta \theta} \quad (19)$$

7   Results and Discussion

The Beltrami flow, being a nonlinear diffusion scheme, offers advantages in processing and analysis of images compared with linear diffusion. In the context of the present study it preserves edges more accurately. We use a similar approach to the Beltrami flow, where the Gaborian orientation data, θ, is treated as a $2D$ manifold embedded in $3D$ space, (x, y, θ). Our aim is to smooth the orientation information when accounting for the maximal Gabor coefficients obtained. Following the minimal weighted area diffusion, we can use θ as the input to the geodesic snakes algorithm. Geodesic snakes is an efficient geometric flow scheme for boundary detection, where the initial conditions include an arbitrary function U which implicitly represents the curve, and a stopping term E which contains the information regarding the boundaries in the image. We generalize the definition of gradients, usually considered in the context of intensity gradients over (x, y) to other possible gradients in scale and orientation. This gradient information is the input function E to the newly generalized geodesic snakes flow.

Next, we present the results of the minimal weighted area method compared to the Beltrami scheme. [For the complete set of full size images and a demo see the web-page: **http://www-visl.technion.ac.il/emmcvpr2001**].

In this study we have generated the Gabor wavelets for eight orientations, the scale being kept constant. In the geodesic snakes mechanism U was initiated to be a signed distance function [2].

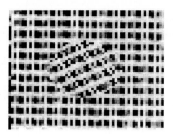

Fig. 1. An image of textures taken from the Brodatz album of textures [1]. The circular object is generated from the background texture after rotation by 30 degrees.

The first image (Fig. 1) is taken from the Brodatz album of textures [1]. The circular object is generated from the background texture by rotating it by 30 degrees. We apply the Gabor transform to this image and obtain the maximal values of the Gabor coefficients per pixel, and the orientation for which the maximal values were obtained. In figure (2(a)) we see that the orientation information is a piece-wise constant function and that it clearly captures the boundary between object and background. In figure (2(b)) we see the orientation information after random noise was added to it. When the Beltrami flow is applied to the noisy orientation image, if the edges are to be better preserved, we should compromise on the degree of smoothing of the background, as can be seen in figure (2(c)). If further smoothing is desired, the edges are smeared (Fig. 2(d)). When the Gabor coefficients are accounted for, we obtain a high degree of smoothing while preserving the sharpness of the edges (Fig. 2(e)).

The inter-relations between the Beltrami flow and the weight of the Gabor coefficients can be seen in the next example. By changing the constant value in the denominator from values larger than the mean value of $R^2 + J^2$ (equivalent to the Beltrami flow) to smaller than the mean value we control the impact of the Beltrami numerator to the Gabor denominator.

The second image is similar to the first one, however, here the rotation is done by 45 degrees (Fig. 3). In figure (4(a)) we see the relevant orientation data after application of the Gabor transform and obtaining the maximal values of the Gabor coefficients per pixel. As we did before, we add random noise to the orientation information (4(b)), and apply the smoothing procedures to remove it. Next, we evaluate the effect of changing the constant value. When the constant is big in comparison to the average value of $R^2 + J^2$, the weighted minimal area method is equivalent to the Beltrami flow (Fig. 4(c)). As we decrease this constant the impact of the Gabor coefficients is more evident and we obtain the same degree of smoothing without damaging the edges (Fig. 4(d,e)) . This is because the weighing of the Gabor coefficients in the Beltrami flow tends to keep the edges better than when applying the original Beltrami flow, where the only constraint is on the smoothing of the θ manifold. However, when the constant value is in the range of $R^2 + J^2$, the Gabor coefficients are very dominant comparing to the smoothing of the θ manifold, and the evolution of θ can be

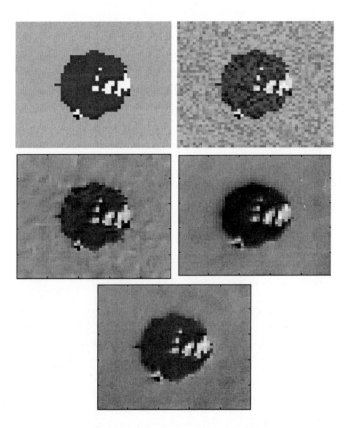

Fig. 2. a. The original orientation information following the application of the Gabor transform and using the maximum criteria (top left). b. The orientation information following addition of random noise (top right). c. Results of the Beltrami diffusion when the process is halted so that significant edges are still evident (middle left). d. If further smoothing is desired, the edges are smeared when the Beltrami diffusion is applied (middle right). e. The result obtained following application of the minimal weighted area method (bottom).

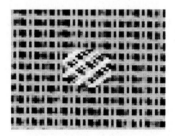

Fig. 3. This image is taken from the Brodatz album of textures [1]. The circular object is generated from the background texture by rotating it by 45 degrees.

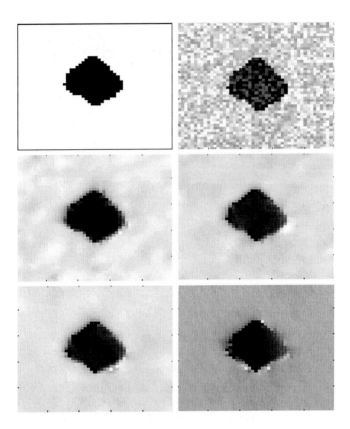

Fig. 4. a. The original orientation information following the application of the Gabor transform and using the maximum criteria (top left). b. The orientation information following addition of random noise (top right). The results of application of the weighted minimal area method are presented, where the mean value of $R^2 + J^2$ is about 200. The difference between the results is the value of the constant in the denominator. c. c =10,000 (middle left). d. c = 800 (middle right). e. c = 600 (bottom left). f. c = 200 (bottom right).

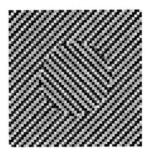

Fig. 5. This image is a synthesized texture composed of linear combination of spatial sinewave gratings of different orientations where some random noise was added to it.

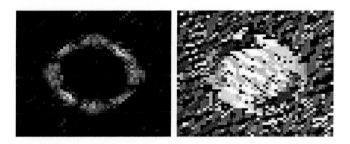

Fig. 6. The maximal values of the Gabor coefficients per pixel are obtained along with the relevant orientation information. a. The magnitude of the Gabor coefficients (left). b. The orientation information (right).

led to local minima. This is manifested in the white dots that appear when the constant is equal to 200 (Fig. 4(f)).

In the next example, we demonstrate how the different smoothing processes affect the results of the geodesic snakes mechanism. The original image is a synthesized texture composed of linear combination of spatial sinewave gratings of different orientations where some random noise was added to it (Fig. 5).

After application of the Gabor filters the maximal value of the Gabor coefficients per pixel is calculated (Fig. 6(a)) and the orientation image obtained is noisy (Fig. 6(b)). When the Beltrami flow is applied to the noisy orientation image we obtain a smooth result (Fig. 7(a)). However, the edges are more dominant when the Gabor coefficients are accounted for (Fig. 7(b)).

Next we use the smoothed θ obtained to calculate the stopping term E in the geodesic snakes mechanism. The stopping term obtained following the Beltrami diffusion is seen in figure (7(c)), and the one obtained following the minimal weighted area method can be seen in figure (7(d)). The resultant boundaries obtained can be seen in figure (7(e+f)). The most evident difference between the two results can be seen on the top right hand side of the boundaries. It is clear that using the minimal weighted area method the edges are better captured and detected.

Currently we expand this study to the other Gaborian features, such as the scale parameter σ and the sine grating frequency F. We explore the behavior of each parameter when considered separately, and also the coupling between these parameters. Another natural continuation of this work is to apply the results of Kimmel and Sochen [14] in order to obtain a more robust orientation diffusion where the orientations manifold is embedded in $R^2 \otimes S^1$. By properly choosing the local coordinate systems for both manifolds the problem arising from the cyclic nature of angles is addressed.

References

1. P. Brodatz, Textures: A photographic album for Artists and Designers, New York, NY, Dover, 1996.

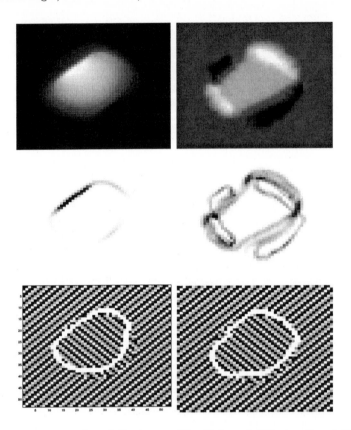

Fig. 7. The orientation data following: a. The Beltrami diffusion (top left), b. The minimal weighted area method (top right). The stopping term obtained when using: c. The Beltrami diffusion (middle left), d. The minimal weighted area method (middle right). The resultant boundary following the application of the geodesic snakes using: e. The Beltrami diffusion(bottom left). f. The minimal weighted area method (bottom right).

2. V. Caselles and R. Kimmel and G. Sapiro, "Geodesic Active Contours", *International Journal of Computer Vision*, 22(1), 1997, 61-97.
3. R. Conners and C. Harlow "A Theoretical Comparison of Texture Algorithms"*IEEE Transactions on PAMI*, 2, 1980, 204-222.
4. G.R. Cross and A.K. Jain, "Markov Random Field Texture Models" *IEEE Transactions on PAMI*, 5, 1983, 25-39.
5. J.G. Daugman, "Uncertainty relation for resolution in space, spatial frequency, and orientation optimized by two-dimensional visual cortical filters", *J. Opt. Soc. Amer.* 2(7), 1985, 1160-1169.
6. O. Faugeras and R. Keriven, "Variational Principles, surface evolution PDE's, level set methods, and the stereo problem ",*IEEE Trans. on Image Processing*, 7(3), (1998) 336-344.
7. D. Gabor "Theory of communication"*J. IEEE* , 93, 1946, 429-459.

8. S. Geman and D. Geman "Stochastic relaxation, Gibbs distribution and the Bayesian restoration of images", *IEEE Transactions on PAMI*, 6, 1984, 721-741.
9. B. Julesz "Texton Gradients: The Texton Theory Revisited", *Biol Cybern*, 54, (1986) 245-251.
10. M. Kaas, A. Witkin and D. Terzopoulos, "Snakes: Active Contour Models", *International Journal of Computer Vision*, 1, 1988, 321-331.
11. S. Kichenassamy, A. Kumar, P. Olver, A. Tannenbaum and A. Yezzi, "Gradient Flows and Geometric Active Contour Models",*Proceedings ICCV'95*, Boston, Massachusetts, 1995, 810-815.
12. R. Kimmel, "3D Shape Reconstruction from Autostereograms and Stereo", Special issue on PDEs in Image Processing, Computer Vision, and Computer Graphics, Journal of Visual Communication and Image Representation. In press..
13. R. Kimmel, N. Sochen and R. Malladi, "On the geometry of texture", Proceedings of the 4th International conference on Mathematical Methods for Curves and Surfaces, St. Malo, 1999.
14. R. Kimmel and N. Sochen. "Orientation Diffusion or How to Comb a Porcupine ? ", Special issue on PDEs in Image Processing, Computer Vision, and Computer Graphics, Journal of Visual Communication and Image Representation. In press.
15. T.S. Lee, "Image Representation using 2D Gabor-Wavelets", *IEEE Transactions on PAMI*, 18(10), 1996, 959-971.
16. S. Marcelja, "Mathematical description of the response of simple cortical cells", *J. Opt. Soc. Amer.*, 70, 1980, 1297-1300.
17. J. Morlet, G. Arens, E. Fourgeau and D. Giard, "Wave propagation and sampling theory - part 2: sampling theory and complex waves", *Geophysics*, 47(2), 1982, 222 - 236.
18. M. Porat and Y.Y. Zeevi, "The generalized Gabor scheme of image representation in biological and machine vision", *IEEE Transactions on PAMI*, 10(4), 1988, 452-468.
19. M. Porat and Y.Y. Zeevi, "Localized texture processing in vision: Analysis and synthesis in the gaborian space", *IEEE Transactions on Biomedical Engineering*, 36(1), 1989, 115-129.
20. S.J. Osher and J.A. Sethian, "Fronts propagating with curvature dependent speed: Algorithms based on Hamilton-Jacobi formulations", *J of Computational Physics*, 79, 1988, 12-49.
21. C. Sagiv, N. Sochen, and Y.Y. Zeevi , "Gabor Space Geodesic Active Contours", G. Sommer, Y.Y. Zeevi (Eds.), Algebraic Frames for the Perception-Action Cycle, *Lecture Notes in Computer Science* , Vol. 1888, Springer, Berlin, 2000.
22. N. Sochen, R. Kimmel and R. Malladi , "A general framework for low level vision", *IEEE Trans. on Image Processing*, 7, (1998) 310-318.
23. S.C. Zhu, Y.N. Wu and D.B. Mumford, "Equivalence of Julesz ensembles and FRAME models", *International Journal of Computer Vision*, 38(3), 2000, 247-265.
24. M. Zibulski and Y.Y. Zeevi, "Analysis of multiwindow Gabor-type schemes by frame methods", *Applied and Computational Harmonic Analysis*, 4, 1997, 188-221.

3D Flux Maximizing Flows

Kaleem Siddiqi and Alexander Vasilevskiy

McGill University
School of Computer Science &
Center for Intelligent Machines
3480 University Street
Montréal, QC H3A 2A7, Canada
{siddiqi,sasha}@cim.mcgill.ca

Abstract. A number of geometric active contour and surface models have been proposed for shape segmentation in the literature. The essential idea is to evolve a curve (in 2D) or a surface (in 3D) so that it clings to the features of interest in an intensity image. Several of these models have been derived, using a variational formulation, as gradient flows which minimize or maximize a particular energy functional. However, in practice these models often fail on images of low contrast or narrow structures. To address this problem we have recently proposed the idea of maximizing the rate of increase of flux of an auxiliary vector field through a curve. This has lead to an interpretation as a 2D gradient flow, which is essentially parameter free. In this paper we extend the analysis to 3D and prove that the form of the gradient flow does not change. We illustrate its potential with level-set based segmentations of blood vessels in a large 3D computed rotational angiography (CRA) data set.

1 Introduction

Level-set based numerical methods for hyperbolic conservation laws developed by Osher and Sethian [14] for curvature-dependent flame propagation were introduced to the computer vision community for shape analysis by Kimia et al. [8]. Such models were later adapted to the problem of shape segmentation independently by Caselles et al. [3] and Malladi et al. [13]. Here the essential idea was to halt an evolving curve in the presence of intensity edges by multiplying the evolution equation with an image-gradient based stopping potential. This led to new active contour models which, when implemented using level set methods, handled changes in topology due to the splitting and merging of multiple contours in a natural way. These geometric flows for shape segmentation were later given formal motivation as well as unified with the classical energy minimization formulations through several independent investigations [4, 7, 16, 17]. The main idea was to modify the Euclidean arc-length or the Euclidean area by a scalar function and to then derive the resulting gradient evolution equations. Mathematically this amounted to defining a new metric on the plane, tailored to the given image, and then deriving the corresponding gradient flows. The results

M.A.T. Figueiredo, J. Zerubia, A.K. Jain (Eds.): EMMCVPR 2001, LNCS 2134, pp. 636–650, 2001.
© Springer-Verlag Berlin Heidelberg 2001

generalized to the case of evolving surfaces in 3D by adding one more dimension to the variational formulation.

Recently there have been other advances in the use of geometric flows in computer vision, which have both theoretical and practical value. First, it has been recognized that a practical weakness of most geometric flows with stopping terms based purely on local image gradients is that they may "leak" in the presence of weak or low contrast boundaries, are not suitable for segmenting textures and typically require the initial curve or curves to lie entirely inside or outside the regions to be segmented. Thus, a number of researchers have sought to derive flows which take into account the statistics of the regions enclosed by the evolving curves [15, 21]. Further developments include multi-phase motions, which allow triple points to be captured [5], as well as the incorporation of an external force field based on a diffused gradient of an edge map [20]. Second, most geometric flows are not able to capture elongated low contrast structures well, such as blood vessels viewed in 2D and 3D angiography images. At places where such structures are narrow, edge gradients may be weak due to partial volume effects and it is also unclear how to robustly measure region statistics. Approaches to regularizing the flow in 3D by introducing a term proportional to mean curvature have the unfortunate effect of annihilating such structures. To address this issue, Lorigo et al. have proposed the use of active contours with co-dimension 2 (curves in 3D) [12]. The idea is to regularize the flow by a term proportional to the curvature of a 3D curve. The approach is grounded in the level set theory for mean curvature evolution of surfaces of arbitrary co-dimension [1] and has a variational formulation along with an energy minimizing interpretation. However, the derived flow is later modified with a (heuristic) multiplicative term to tailor it to blood vessel segmentation [12].

We have recently suggested an alternate approach to segmenting blood vessels in angiography images, which is motivated by the observation that blood flows in the direction of vessels. Brightness in angiography images is proportional to the magnitude of the blood flow velocity. This leads to the constraint that in the vicinity of blood vessel boundaries, the gradient vector field of the image should be locally orthogonal to them. Thus, a natural principle to use towards the recovery of these boundaries is to maximize the inward flux of the gradient vector field through an evolving curve (in 2D) or surface (in 3D). The derivation of the 2D flux maximizing flow was presented in [18] and lead to an elegant interpretation which is essentially parameter free. In the current paper we prove that the extension to 3D has the same form, a calculation which is more subtle. We also illustrate the potential of the 3D flux maximizing flow with several new simulations of blood vessels segmented from a large 3D computed rotational angiography (CRA) data set.

2   3D Flux Maximizing Flows

Let $\mathcal{S} : [0,1] \times [0,1] \to \mathcal{R}^3$ denote a compact embedded surface with (local) coordinates (u, v). Let $\mathcal{N}$ be the inward unit normal. We set

$$S_u := \frac{\partial S}{\partial u}, \quad S_v := \frac{\partial S}{\partial v}.$$

Then the infinitesimal area on S is given by

$$dS = (\|S_u\|^2\|S_v\|^2 - \langle S_u, S_v \rangle^2)^{1/2} du\, dv$$
$$= \|S_u \wedge S_v\| du\, dv.$$

Let $V = (V_1(x, y, z), V_2(x, y, z), V_3(x, y, z))$ be a vector field defined for each point (x, y, z) in $\mathcal{R}^3$. The total inward flux of the vector field through the surface is defined by the surface integral

$$Flux(t) = \int_0^{A(t)} \langle V, \mathcal{N} \rangle\, dS, \tag{1}$$

where $A(t)$ is the surface area of the evolving surface. The main contribution of the current paper is the proof of the following theorem

Theorem 1. *The direction in which the inward flux of the vector field V through the surface S is increasing most rapidly is given by $\frac{\partial S}{\partial t} = div(V)\mathcal{N}$.*

It turns out that the flux maximizing flow has the same form in 2D, a calculation which we presented in [18]. However, the proof is more subtle for the 3D case.

Proof: The essential idea is to calculate the first variation of the flux functional with respect to t:

$$Flux'(t) = \underbrace{\int_0^{A(t)} \langle V_t, \mathcal{N} \rangle\, dS}_{I_1} + \underbrace{\int_0^{A(t)} \langle V, \mathcal{N}_t \rangle\, dS}_{I_2}.$$

With $S = (x(u, v, t), y(u, v, t), z(u, v, t))$, the unit normal vector is given by the normalized cross product of two vectors in the tangent plane:

$$\mathcal{N} = \frac{S_u \wedge S_v}{\|S_u \wedge S_v\|} = \frac{(N_1, N_2, N_3)}{\|S_u \wedge S_v\|}$$
$$= \frac{(y_u z_v - y_v z_u), (x_v z_u - x_u z_v), (x_u y_v - x_v y_u)}{\|(y_u z_v - y_v z_u), (x_v z_u - x_u z_v), (x_u y_v - x_v y_u)\|}. \tag{2}$$

I_1 is then given by

$$\int_0^1 \int_0^1 \langle S_t, (N_1 \nabla V_1 + N_2 \nabla V_2 + N_3 \nabla V_3) \rangle\, du\, dv,$$

where the integrand is the inner product of S_t with another vector. We shall now simplify I_2 so that it takes on a similar form. It turns out to be advantageous to express the unit normal vector in Eq. (2) as $\frac{S_u \wedge S_v}{\|S_u \wedge S_v\|}$ and expand it in terms of the partial derivatives $x_u, x_v, y_u, y_v, z_u, z_v$ only later. With $dS = \|S_u \wedge S_v\| du\, dv$, I_2 can be rewritten as

$$\int_0^1 \int_0^1 \langle V, (S_u \wedge S_v)_t \rangle\, du\, dv.$$

The trick now is to eploit the fact that for any vectors A, B and C, the following properties of inner products and cross products hold:

$$A \wedge B = -B \wedge A$$
$$\langle A, (B \wedge C) \rangle = \langle (A \wedge B), C \rangle$$
$$(A \wedge B)_t = (A_t \wedge B) + (A \wedge B_t).$$

Hence, I_2 can be written as

$$I_2 = \int_0^1 \int_0^1 \langle \mathcal{V}, (\mathcal{S}_{ut} \wedge \mathcal{S}_v + \mathcal{S}_u \wedge \mathcal{S}_{vt}) \rangle \, du \, dv$$

$$= \int_0^1 \int_0^1 \langle \mathcal{V}, (\mathcal{S}_{ut} \wedge \mathcal{S}_v) \rangle \, du \, dv + \int_0^1 \int_0^1 \langle \mathcal{V}, (\mathcal{S}_u \wedge \mathcal{S}_{vt}) \rangle \, du \, dv$$

$$= \int_0^1 \int_0^1 -\langle \mathcal{V}, (\mathcal{S}_v \wedge \mathcal{S}_{ut}) \rangle \, du \, dv + \int_0^1 \int_0^1 \langle \mathcal{V}, (\mathcal{S}_u \wedge \mathcal{S}_{vt}) \rangle \, du \, dv$$

$$= \int_0^1 \underbrace{\left[\int_0^1 -\langle (\mathcal{V} \wedge \mathcal{S}_v), \mathcal{S}_{ut} \rangle \, du \right]}_{I_3} dv + \int_0^1 \underbrace{\left[\int_0^1 \langle (\mathcal{V} \wedge \mathcal{S}_u), \mathcal{S}_{vt} \rangle \, dv \right]}_{I_4} du$$

Using integration by parts, I_3 works out to be

$$\underbrace{-\langle (\mathcal{V} \wedge \mathcal{S}_v), \mathcal{S}_t \rangle]_0^1}_{\text{equals } 0} + \int_0^1 \langle \mathcal{S}_t, (\mathcal{V} \wedge \mathcal{S}_v)_u \rangle \, du$$

Similarly, using integration by parts, I_4 works out to be

$$\underbrace{\langle (\mathcal{V} \wedge \mathcal{S}_u), \mathcal{S}_t \rangle]_0^1}_{\text{equals } 0} - \int_0^1 \langle \mathcal{S}_t, (\mathcal{V} \wedge \mathcal{S}_u)_v \rangle \, dv$$

Combining I_3 and I_4, I_2 works out to be

$$\int_0^1 \int_0^1 \langle \mathcal{S}_t, (\mathcal{V} \wedge \mathcal{S}_v)_u - (\mathcal{V} \wedge \mathcal{S}_u)_v \rangle \, du \, dv.$$

It can now be seen that the integrand in I_2 has the desired form of the inner product of $\mathcal{S}_t$ with another vector. Hence, combining I_1 and I_2, the first variation of the flux is

$$\int_0^1 \int_0^1 \langle \mathcal{S}_t, N_1 \nabla V_1 + N_2 \nabla V_2 + N_3 \nabla V_3 + (\mathcal{V} \wedge \mathcal{S}_v)_u - (\mathcal{V} \wedge \mathcal{S}_u)_v \rangle \, du \, dv.$$

Note that

$$(\mathcal{V} \wedge \mathcal{S}_v)_u - (\mathcal{V} \wedge \mathcal{S}_u)_v = (\mathcal{V}_u \wedge \mathcal{S}_v) + (\mathcal{V} \wedge \mathcal{S}_{vu}) - (\mathcal{V} \wedge \mathcal{S}_{uv}) - (\mathcal{V}_v \wedge \mathcal{S}_u)$$
$$= (\mathcal{V}_u \wedge \mathcal{S}_v) - (\mathcal{V}_v \wedge \mathcal{S}_u).$$

Hence, the first variation of the flux can be written as the surface integral

$$\int_0^{A(t)} \left\langle \mathcal{S}_t, \frac{N_1 \nabla V_1 + N_2 \nabla V_2 + N_3 \nabla V_3 + (\mathcal{V}_u \wedge \mathcal{S}_v) - (\mathcal{V}_v \wedge \mathcal{S}_u)}{\|\mathcal{S}_u \wedge \mathcal{S}_v\|} \right\rangle dS.$$

Thus, for the inward flux to increase as fast as possible, the two vectors should be made parallel:

$$\mathcal{S}_t = \frac{N_1 \nabla V_1 + N_2 \nabla V_2 + N_3 \nabla V_3 + (\mathcal{V}_u \wedge \mathcal{S}_v) - (\mathcal{V}_v \wedge \mathcal{S}_u)}{\|\mathcal{S}_u \wedge \mathcal{S}_v\|}. \tag{3}$$

The above expression for the 3D flux maximizing gradient flow can be further simplified by noting that the components of the flow in the tangential plane to the surface $\mathcal{S}$ affect only the parametrization of the surface, but not its evolved shape. Hence, they can be dropped. The normal component of the flow can be calculated by taking the inner product of the right hand side of Eq. (3) with the unit normal vector in Eq. (2) to give

$$\mathcal{S}_t = \langle \frac{N_1 \nabla V_1 + N_2 \nabla V_2 + N_3 \nabla V_3 + (\mathcal{V}_u \wedge \mathcal{S}_v) - (\mathcal{V}_v \wedge \mathcal{S}_u)}{\|\mathcal{S}_u \wedge \mathcal{S}_v\|}, \frac{\mathcal{S}_u \wedge \mathcal{S}_v}{\|\mathcal{S}_u \wedge \mathcal{S}_v\|} \rangle \mathcal{N}$$

It is now a straightforward task to expand the terms in the expression by using Eq. (2):

$$\mathcal{S}_t = \frac{(y_u z_v - y_v z_u)}{\|\mathcal{S}_u \wedge \mathcal{S}_v\|^2} (V_{1x}(y_u z_v - y_v z_u) + V_{1y}(x_v z_u - x_u z_v) + V_{1z}(x_u y_v - x_v y_u))$$

$$+ \frac{(x_v z_u - x_u z_v)}{\|\mathcal{S}_u \wedge \mathcal{S}_v\|^2} (V_{2x}(y_u z_v - y_v z_u) + V_{2y}(x_v z_u - x_u z_v) + V_{2z}(x_u y_v - x_v y_u))$$

$$+ \frac{(x_u y_v - x_v y_u)}{\|\mathcal{S}_u \wedge \mathcal{S}_v\|^2} (V_{3x}(y_u z_v - y_v z_u) + V_{3y}(x_v z_u - x_u z_v) + V_{3z}(x_u y_v - x_v y_u))$$

$$+ \frac{1}{\|\mathcal{S}_u \wedge \mathcal{S}_v\|^2} \langle (\mathcal{V}_u \wedge \mathcal{S}_v), (y_u z_v - y_v z_u, x_v z_u - x_u z_v, x_u y_v - x_v y_u) \rangle$$

$$- \frac{1}{\|\mathcal{S}_u \wedge \mathcal{S}_v\|^2} \langle (\mathcal{V}_v \wedge \mathcal{S}_u), (y_u z_v - y_v z_u, x_v z_u - x_u z_v, x_u y_v - x_v y_u) \rangle.$$

With

$$\mathcal{V}_u \wedge \mathcal{S}_v = (z_v(V_{2x}x_u + V_{2y}y_u + V_{2z}z_u) - y_v(V_{3x}x_u + V_{3y}y_u + V_{3z}z_u),$$
$$x_v(V_{3x}x_u + V_{3y}y_u + V_{3z}z_u) - z_v(V_{1x}x_u + V_{1y}y_u + V_{1z}z_u),$$
$$y_v(V_{1x}x_u + V_{1y}y_u + V_{1z}z_u) - x_v(V_{2x}x_u + V_{2y}y_u + V_{2z}z_u)).$$

and

$$-\mathcal{V}_v \wedge \mathcal{S}_u = (-z_u(V_{2x}x_v + V_{2y}y_v + V_{2z}z_v) + y_u(V_{3x}x_v + V_{3y}y_v + V_{3z}z_v),$$
$$-x_u(V_{3x}x_v + V_{3y}y_v + V_{3z}z_v) + z_u(V_{1x}x_v + V_{1y}y_v + V_{1z}z_v),$$
$$-y_u(V_{1x}x_v + V_{1y}y_v + V_{1z}z_v) + x_u(V_{2x}x_v + V_{2y}y_v + V_{2z}z_v))$$

the terms can be grouped and simplified. The curious result is that most cancel, leaving the following simple and elegant form for the 3D flux maximizing flow:

$$\mathcal{S}_t = (V_{1x} + V_{2y} + V_{3z})\mathcal{N} = div(\mathcal{V})\mathcal{N} \qquad \square \tag{4}$$

Remark: The flux maximizing flow is a hyperbolic equation since it depends solely on the external vector field $\mathcal{V}$ and not on properties of the evolving surface. It is easy to see that the flow will drive towards and then converge to a zero level set of the divergence of $\mathcal{V}$. Thus, the existence and uniqueness of a solution to Eq. (4) is guaranteed, unless the vector field is everywhere non-conservative.

3   Blood Vessel Segmentation

3.1   Background

We shall now show how the 3D flux maximizing flow can be tailored to the problem of segmenting blood vessels in angiography images. We begin by reviewing some of the recent approaches which have been proposed in the literature. Wilson and Noble have introduced a Gaussian mixture model to characterize the physical properties of blood flow [19]. The parameters are estimated using the EM algorithm and structural criteria are then used to refine the initial segmentation. Krissian et al. propose a method which incorporates a Gaussian model for the intensity distribution as a function of distance from vessel centerlines, and exploits properties of the Hessian to obtain geometric estimates [11]. Koller et al. have also introduced a multi-scale method for the detection of curvilinear structures in 2D and 3D data [9] which combines the responses of steerable linear filters and also exploits the Hessian matrix to obtain geometric estimates. Bullitt et al. have introduced a method for obtaining 3D vascular trees which calculates vessel centerlines as intensity ridges in the data and estimates vessel width via medialness calculations [2]. It should be noted that several of the above approaches require second derivative computations, e.g., to compute the Hessian. Numerically accurate estimates of principal curvature magnitudes and directions are obtained only when the intensity images have been suitably smoothed. Approaches to smoothing the data while preserving and enhancing vessel-like structures include [10, 6].

Whereas the potential of several of the above approaches has been empirically demonstrated, their ability to recover low contrast thin vessels remains unclear. A recent framework which has been developed with this as one of its goals is the work of Lorigo et al. [12]. The main idea is to regularize a geometric flow in 3D using the curvature of a 3D curve, rather than the classical mean curvature based regularizations which tend to annihilate thin structures. The work is grounded in the recent level set theory developed for mean curvature flows in arbitrary co-dimension [1]. This flow is given by [12]:

$$\psi_t = \lambda(\nabla\psi, \nabla^2\psi) + \rho(\nabla\psi.\nabla\mathbf{I})\frac{g'}{g}\nabla\psi.\mathbf{H}\frac{\nabla\mathbf{I}}{\|\nabla\mathbf{I}\|}$$

Here ψ is an embedding surface whose zero level set is the evolving 3D curve, λ is the smaller nonzero eigen value of a particular matrix [1] g is an image-dependent weighting factor, $\mathbf{I}$ is the intensity image and $\mathbf{H}$ is its Hessian. For numerical simulations the evolution of the curve is depicted by the evolution of an ϵ-level set. It should be noted that without the multiplicative factor $\rho(\nabla\psi.\nabla\mathbf{I})$ the evolution equation is a gradient flow which minimizes a weighted curvature functional. The multiplicative factor is a heuristic which modifies the flow so that normals to the ϵ-level set align themselves (locally) to the direction of image intensity gradients (the inner product of $\nabla\psi$ and $\nabla\mathbf{I}$ is then maximized). However, with the introduction of this term the flow loses its pure energy minimizing interpretation.

3.2   The 3D Flux Maximizing Flow

The intuition behind using the 3D flux maximizing flow for blood vessel segmentation is illustrated in Figure 1. Here a cross section through an idealized blood vessel (a bright region in a uniform darker background) is depicted. It is clear that if one considers the gradient $\nabla\mathbf{I}$ of the original intensity image $\mathbf{I}$ to be the vector field $\mathcal{V}$ whose inward flux through the evolving surface is to be maximized, then the optimal configuration is for the evolving surface to align itself locally to the blood vessel boundaries. However, an important consideration in the implementation of Eq. (4) is that since the divergence of the vector field needs to be calculated, implicitly second derivatives of $\mathbf{I}$ are being used. The numerical computation can be made much more robust by exploiting a consequence of the divergence theorem. The divergence at a point is defined as the net *outward* flux per unit volume, as the volume about the point shrinks to zero. Via the divergence theorem,

$$\int_{\Delta v} \mathrm{div}(\mathcal{V})dv \equiv \int_s < \mathcal{V}, \mathcal{N} > dS. \qquad (5)$$

Here Δv is the volume, s is its bounding surface, $\mathcal{N}$ is the outward normal at each point on the surface, and dv and dS are volume and surface area elements.

   For our numerical implementations we use this outward flux formulation (which gives a measure proportional to the divergence) along the boundaries of spheres of varying radii, corresponding to a range of 3D blood vessel widths. The chosen flux value at a particular location is the maximum (magnitude) flux over the range of radii. In contrast to other multi-scale approaches where combining information across scales is non-trivial [11] normalization across scales is straightforward in our case. One simply has to divide by the number of entries in the discrete sum that approximates Eq. (5). Locations where the total outward flux is negative (or equivalently the total inward flux is positive) correspond to sinks; locations where the total outward flux is positive correspond to sources, as illustrated in Figure 1. Hence, the inward flux maximizing flow in Eq (4) has the desirable effect that, when seeds are placed within blood vessels, the sinks drive the seeds towards the vessel boundaries and the sources outside prevent the flow from leaking.

3.3   Level Set Implementation

In order to implement the flow, we use the level set representation for compact embedded surfaces, due to Osher and Sethian [14]. Let $\mathcal{S}(u, v, t) : [0, 1] \times [0, 1] \times$

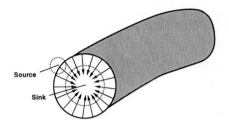

Fig. 1. An illustration of the gradient vector field of an angiography image along a cross-section of a 3D blood vessel. Assuming a uniform background intensity, at the scale of the vessel's width the total inward flux is positive (a sink). Outside the vessel, at a smaller scale, the total inward flux is negative (a source).

$[0, \tau) \to \mathbf{R}^3$ be a family of compact embedded surfaces evolving according to the surface evolution equation

$$\mathcal{S}_t = F\mathcal{N},$$

where F is an arbitrary (local) scalar speed function and $\mathcal{N}$ is inward unit normal to the surface. Then it can be shown that if $\mathcal{S}(u, v, t)$ is represented by the zero level set of a smooth and Lipschitz continuous function $\Psi : \mathbf{R}^3 \times [0, \tau) \to \mathbf{R}$, the evolving hypersurface Ψ satisfies

$$\Psi_t = F \, \|\nabla \Psi\| \, .$$

This last equation is solved using a combination of straightforward discretization and numerical techniques derived from hyperbolic conservation laws [14]. For hyperbolic terms, care must be taken to implement derivatives with upwinding in the proper direction. The evolving surface $\mathcal{S}$ is then obtained as the zero level set of Ψ.

4 Examples

In earlier work we have presented simulations of the flux maximizing flow on both 2D (retinal) and 3D (head) MRA data [18]. In this section we present new experiments on a $360 \times 330 \times 420$ computed rotational angiography (CRA) data set of the head, from which we have selected four distinct regions containing vascular networks of varying complexity. All examples were implemented in a level-set framework.

The evolution results are presented in Figures 2, 3, 4 and 5. For each region a maximal intensity projection of the data is shown on the top left, followed by the evolution of a few 3D spheres. These spheres were placed somewhat sparsely in regions of high flux. Notice how the spheres elongate in the direction of blood vessels. The main blood vessels, which have the higher inward flux, are the first to be captured. This is the expected evolution since it maximizes the rate of increase of inward flux through the evolving surface. Put another way, the evolution has the intuitive behaviour that it follows the direction of blood flow

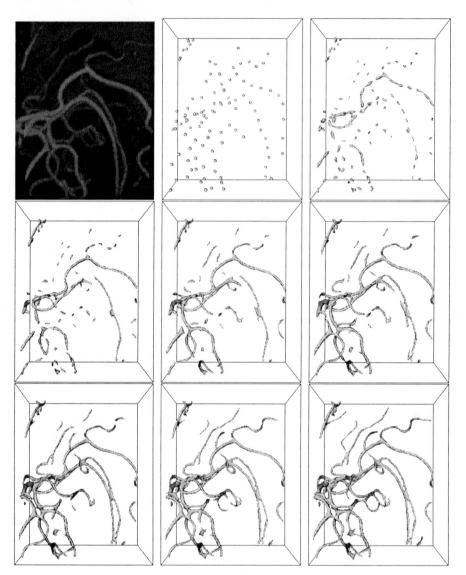

Fig. 2. An illustration of the flux maximizing flow for a portion of a $360 \times 330 \times 420$ 3D CRA image of blood vessels in the head. A maximum-intensity projection of the region being viewed is shown on the top left. The other images depict the evolution of a few isolated spheres. Notice how the evolution follows the direction of blood flow to reconstruct the blood vessel boundaries.

to reconstruct the blood vessel boundaries. Our own experience with developing and implementing some of the related geometric flows in the literature is that many would fail in low contrast regions or would not be able to capture the thinner vessels.

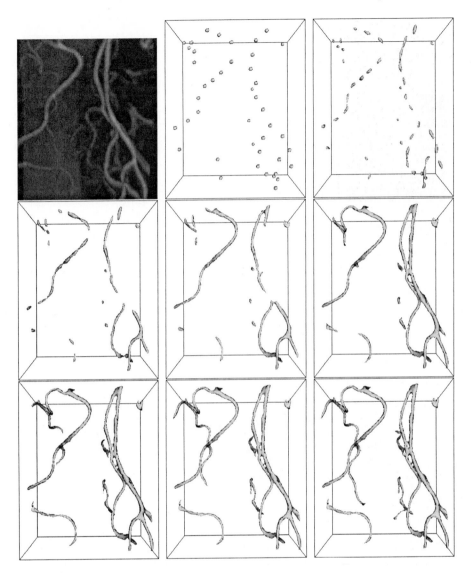

Fig. 3. An illustration of the flux maximizing flow for a portion of a $360 \times 330 \times 420$ 3D CRA image of blood vessels in the head. A maximum-intensity projection of the region being viewed is shown on the top left. The other images depict the evolution of a few isolated spheres. Notice how the evolution follows the direction of blood flow to reconstruct the blood vessel boundaries.

We should also point out that although CRA data is of higher resolution than MRA, the vessel structures exhibit a wider range of intensities and there are also a number of other structures whose intensities overlap with those of the thin vessels. Thus, simple thresholding of the intensity data generally gives poor

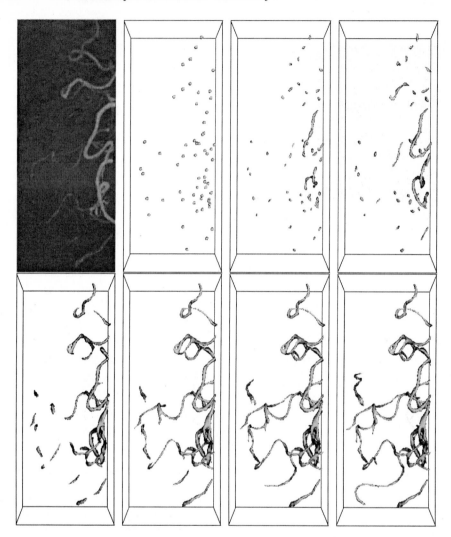

Fig. 4. An illustration of the flux maximizing flow for a portion of a 360 × 330 × 420 3D CRA image of blood vessels in the head. A maximum-intensity projection of the region being viewed is shown on the top left. The other images depict the evolution of a few isolated spheres. Notice how the evolution follows the direction of blood flow to reconstruct the blood vessel boundaries.

results, although this is a commonly used initialization step in many algorithms including the approach of [12]. This point is illustrated in Figure 6. The first row shows the results of a high threshold on the four regions, where as one would expect, many thin low contrast vessels are not captured. As the threshold is decreased, more thin vessels are captured, but also many voxels are incorrectly labeled as vessels (Figure 6, second row). The segmentation results obtained by

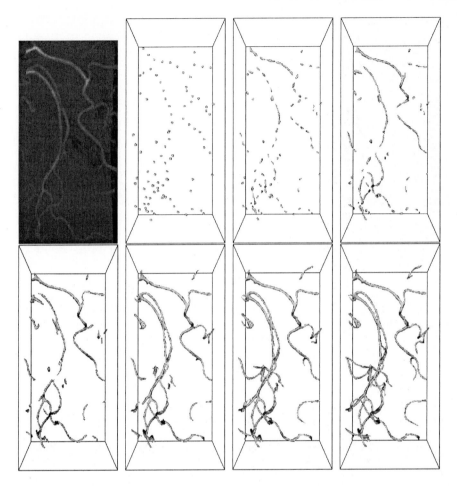

Fig. 5. An illustration of the flux maximizing flow for a portion of a $360 \times 330 \times 420$ 3D CRA image of blood vessels in the head. A maximum-intensity projection of the region being viewed is shown on the top left. The other images depict the evolution of a few isolated spheres. Notice how the evolution follows the direction of blood flow to reconstruct the blood vessel boundaries.

the flux maximizing flow are repeated in the last row. The arrows point to some of the thin low contrast vessels that are successively captured, but are not seen even in the low threshold case.

5   Conclusion

In recent work we proposed the flux maximizing flow and derived its form for the case of closed curves evolving in the plane [18]. We also suggested that its form remains the same in higher dimensions. The main contribution of the current paper is the formal derivation of the flux maximizing flow in 3D. We have also

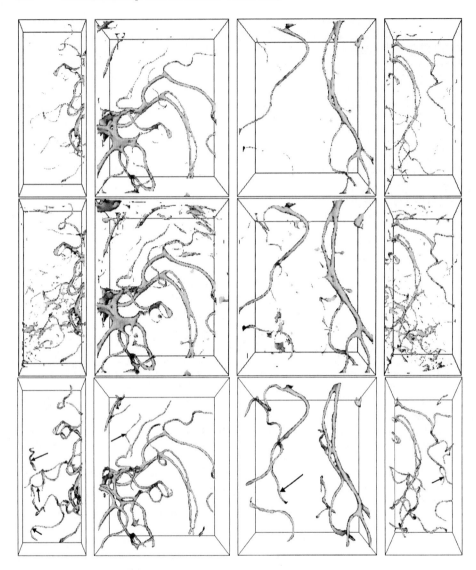

Fig. 6. A comparison of the segmentation results obtained by the flux maximizing flow with simple thresholding on the four different regions of the CRA image. FIRST ROW: A conservative high threshold fails to capture many thin low contrast vessels. SECOND ROW: A lower threshold captures some of the thinner vessels but also incorrectly labels many voxels. THIRD ROW: The segmentation results obtained by the flux maximizing flow. The arrows point to some of the thin low contrast vessels that are successively captured, but are not seen even in the low threshold case.

carried out a number of new simulations on a large CRA data set. These have the intuitive behaviour that the evolution follows the direction of blood flow to reconstruct blood vessel boundaries. The results suggest the potential of the approach to capture low contrast thin vessels, and also illustrate the advantages of the method over thresholding the original intensity image, which is a common initialization step in many vessel reconstruction algorithms.

More work remains to be done to validate this technique against ground truth or expert segmentations, and we are beginning to do this in collaboration with our colleagues in medical imaging. It would also be interesting to see whether a regularization term such as that used in [12] could be incorporated in the derivation of the flux maximizing flow from first principles.

Acknowledgements This work was supported by grants from the Canadian Foundation for Innovation, FCAR Quebec and the Natural Sciences and Engineering Research Council of Canada. We are grateful to Vincent Hayward, Terry Peters and David Holdsworth for giving us access to the vessel CRA data.

References

1. L. Ambrosio and H. M. Soner. Level set approach to mean curvature flow in arbitrary codimension. *Journal of Differential Geometry*, 43:693–737, 1996.
2. E. Bullitt, S. Aylward, A. Liu, J. Stone, S. K. Mukherjee, C. Coffey, G. Gerig, and S. M. Pizer. 3d graph description of the intracerebral vasculature from segmented mra and tests of accuracy by comparison with x-ray angiograms. In *IPMI'99*, pages 308–321, 1999.
3. V. Caselles, F. Catte, T. Coll, and F. Dibos. A geometric model for active contours in image processing. *Numerische Mathematik*, 66:1–31, 1993.
4. V. Caselles, R. Kimmel, and G. Sapiro. Geodesic active contours. In *ICCV'95*, pages 694–699, 1995.
5. T. Chan and L. Vese. An efficient variational multiphase motion for the mumford-shah segmentation model. In *Asilomar Conference on Signals and Systems*, October 2000.
6. A. Frangi, W. Niessen, K. L. Vincken, and M. A. Viergever. Multiscale vessel enhancement filtering. In *MICCAI'98*, pages 130–137, 1998.
7. S. Kichenassamy, A. Kumar, P. Olver, A. Tannenbaum, and A. Yezzi. Gradient flows and geometric active contour models. In *ICCV'95*, pages 810–815, 1995.
8. B. B. Kimia, A. Tannenbaum, and S. W. Zucker. Toward a computational theory of shape: An overview. *Lecture Notes in Computer Science*, 427:402–407, 1990.
9. T. M. Koller, G. Gerig, G. Székely, and D. Dettwiler. Multiscale detection of curvilinear structures in 2-d and 3-d image data. In *ICCV'95*, pages 864–869, 1995.
10. K. Krissian, G. Malandain, and N. Ayache. Directional anisotropic diffusion applied to segmentation of vessels in 3d images. In *International Conference On Scale Space Theories in Computer Vision*, pages 345–348, 1997.
11. K. Krissian, G. Malandain, N. Ayache, R. Vaillant, and Y. Trousset. Model-based multiscale detection of 3d vessels. In *CVPR'98*, pages 722–727, 1998.
12. L. M. Lorigo, O. Faugeras, E. L. Grimson, R. Keriven, R. Kikinis, A. Nabavi, and C.-F. Westin. Codimension-two geodesic active contours for the segmentation of tubular structures. In *CVPR'2000*, volume 1, pages 444–451, 2000.
13. R. Malladi, J. A. Sethian, and B. C. Vemuri. Shape modeling with front propagation: A level set approach. *IEEE Transactions on Pattern Analysis and Machine Intelligence*, 17(2):158–175, February 1995.

14. S. J. Osher and J. A. Sethian. Fronts propagating with curvature dependent speed: Algorithms based on hamilton-jacobi formulations. *Journal of Computational Physics*, 79:12–49, 1988.

15. N. Paragios and R. Deriche. Geodesic active regions for supervised texture segmentation. In *ICCV'99*, pages 926–932, September 1999.

16. J. Shah. Recovery of shapes by evolution of zero-crossings. Technical report, Dept. of Mathematics, Northeastern University, Boston, MA, 1995.

17. K. Siddiqi, Y. B. Lauzière, A. Tannenbaum, and S. W. Zucker. Area and length minimizing flows for shape segmentation. *IEEE Transactions on Image Processing*, 7(3):433–443, 1998.

18. A. Vasilevskiy and K. Siddiqi. Flux maximizing geometric flows. In *ICCV'2001*, July 2001.

19. D. L. Wilson and A. Noble. Segmentation of cerebral vessels and aneurysms from mr aniography data. In *IPMI'97*, pages 423–428, 1997.

20. C. Xu and J. Prince. Snakes, shapes and gradient vector flow. *IEEE Transactions on Image Processing*, 7(3):359–369, 1998.

21. A. Yezzi, A. Tsai, and A. Willsky. A statistical approach to snakes for bimodal and trimodal imagery. In *ICCV'99*, pages 898–903, September 1999.

Author Index

Lecture Notes in Computer Science

For information about Vols. 1–2091
please contact your bookseller or Springer-Verlag

Vol. 2136: J. Sgall, A. Pultr, P. Kolman (Eds.), Mathematical Foundations of Computer Science 2001. Proceedings, 2001. XII, 716 pages. 2001.

Vol. 2138: R. Freivalds (Ed.), Fundamentals of Computation Theory. Proceedings, 2001. XIII, 542 pages. 2001.

Vol. 2139: J. Kilian (Ed.), Advances in Cryptology – CRYPTO 2001. Proceedings, 2001. XI, 599 pages. 2001.

Vol. 2141: G.S. Brodal, D. Frigioni, A. Marchetti-Spaccamela (Eds.), Algorithm Engineering. Proceedings, 2001. X, 199 pages. 2001.

Vol. 2142: L. Fribourg (Ed.), Computer Science Logic. Proceedings, 2001. XII, 615 pages. 2001.

Vol. 2143: S. Benferhat, P. Besnard (Eds.), Symbolic and Quantitative Approaches to Reasoning with Uncertainty. Proceedings, 2001. XIV, 818 pages. 2001. (Subseries LNAI).

Vol. 2144: T. Margaria, T. Melham (Eds.), Correct Hardware Design and Verification Methods. Proceedings, 2001. XII, 482 pages. 2001.

Vol. 2146: J.H. Silverman (Eds.), Cryptography and Lattices. Proceedings, 2001. VII, 219 pages. 2001.

Vol. 2147: G. Brebner, R. Woods (Eds.), Field-Programmable Logic and Applications. Proceedings, 2001. XV, 665 pages. 2001.

Vol. 2149: O. Gascuel, B.M.E. Moret (Eds.), Algorithms in Bioinformatics. Proceedings, 2001. X, 307 pages. 2001.

Vol. 2150: R. Sakellariou, J. Keane, J. Gurd, L. Freeman (Eds.), Euro-Par 2001 Parallel Processing. Proceedings, 2001. XXX, 943 pages. 2001.

Vol. 2151: A. Caplinskas, J. Eder (Eds.), Advances in Databases and Information Systems. Proceedings, 2001. XIII, 381 pages. 2001.

Vol. 2152: R.J. Boulton, P.B. Jackson (Eds.), Theorem Proving in Higher Order Logics. Proceedings, 2001. X, 395 pages. 2001.

Vol. 2153: A.L. Buchsbaum, J. Snoeyink (Eds.), Algorithm Engineering and Experimentation. Proceedings, 2001. VIII, 231 pages. 2001.

Vol. 2154: K.G. Larsen, M. Nielsen (Eds.), CONCUR 2001 – Concurrency Theory. Proceedings, 2001. XI, 583 pages. 2001.

Vol. 2157: C. Rouveirol, M. Sebag (Eds.), Inductive Logic Programming. Proceedings, 2001. X, 261 pages. 2001. (Subseries LNAI).

Vol. 2158: D. Shepherd, J. Finney, L. Mathy, N. Race (Eds.), Interactive Distributed Multimedia Systems. Proceedings, 2001. XIII, 258 pages. 2001.

Vol. 2159: J. Kelemen, P. Sosík (Eds.), Advances in Artificial Life. Proceedings, 2001. XIX, 724 pages. 2001. (Subseries LNAI).

Vol. 2161: F. Meyer auf der Heide (Ed.), Algorithms – ESA 2001. Proceedings, 2001. XII, 538 pages. 2001.

Vol. 2162: Ç. K. Koç, D. Naccache, C. Paar (Eds.), Cryptographic Hardware and Embedded Systems – CHES 2001. Proceedings, 2001. XIV, 411 pages. 2001.

Vol. 2164: S. Pierre, R. Glitho (Eds.), Mobile Agents for Telecommunication Applications. Proceedings, 2001. XI, 292 pages. 2001.

Vol. 2165: L. de Alfaro, S. Gilmore (Eds.), Process Algebra and Probabilistic Methods. Proceedings, 2001. XII, 217 pages. 2001.

Vol. 2166: V. Matoušek, P. Mautner, R. Mouček, K. Taušer (Eds.), Text, Speech and Dialogue. Proceedings, 2001. XIII, 452 pages. 2001. (Subseries LNAI).

Vol. 2167: L. De Raedt, P. Flach (Eds.), Machine Learning: ECML 2001. Proceedings, 2001. XVII, 618 pages. 2001. (Subseries LNAI).

Vol. 2168: L. De Raedt, A. Siebes (Eds.), Principles of Data Mining and Knowledge Discovery. Proceedings, 2001. XVII, 510 pages. 2001. (Subseries LNAI).

Vol. 2170: S. Palazzo (Ed.), Evolutionary Trends of the Internet. Proceedings, 2001. XIII, 722 pages. 2001.

Vol. 2172: C. Batini, F. Giunchiglia, P. Giorgini, M. Mecella (Eds.), Cooperative Information Systems. Proceedings, 2001. XI, 450 pages. 2001.

Vol. 2174: F. Baader, G. Brewka, T. Eiter (Eds.), KI 2001: Advances in Artificial Intelligence. Proceedings, 2001. XIII, 471 pages. 2001. (Subseries LNAI).

Vol. 2175: F. Esposito (Ed.), AI*IA 2001: Advances in Artificial Intelligence. Proceedings, 2001. XII, 396 pages. 2001. (Subseries LNAI).

Vol. 2176: K.-D. Althoff, R.L. Feldmann, W. Müller (Eds.), Advances in Learning Software Organizations. Proceedings, 2001. XI, 241 pages. 2001.

Vol. 2177: G. Butler, S. Jarzabek (Eds.), Generative and Component-Based Software Engineering. Proceedings, 2001. X, 203 pages. 2001.

Vol. 2180: J. Welch (Ed.), Distributed Computing. Proceedings, 2001. X, 343 pages. 2001.

Vol. 2181: C. Y. Westort (Ed.), Digital Earth Moving. Proceedings, 2001. XII, 117 pages. 2001.

Vol. 2182: M. Klusch, F. Zambonelli (Eds.), Cooperative Information Agents V. Proceedings, 2001. XII, 288 pages. 2001. (Subseries LNAI).

Vol. 2184: M. Tucci (Ed.), Multimedia Databases and Image Communication. Proceedings, 2001. X, 225 pages. 2001.

Vol. 2186: J. Bosch (Ed.), Generative and Component-Based Software Engineering. Proceedings, 2001. VIII, 177 pages. 2001.

Vol. 2188: F. Bomarius, S. Komi-Sirviö (Eds.), Product Focused Software Process Improvement. Proceedings, 2001. XI, 382 pages. 2001.

Vol. 2189: F. Hoffmann, D.J. Hand, N. Adams, D. Fisher, G. Guimaraes (Eds.), Advances in Intelligent Data Analysis. Proceedings, 2001. XII, 384 pages. 2001.

Vol. 2190: A. de Antonio, R. Aylett, D. Ballin (Eds.), Intelligent Virtual Agents. Proceedings, 2001. VIII, 245 pages. 2001. (Subseries LNAI).

Vol. 2191: B. Radig, S. Florczyk (Eds.), Pattern Recognition. Proceedings, 2001. XVI, 452 pages. 2001.

Vol. 2193: F. Casati, D. Georgakopoulos, M.-C. Shan (Eds.), Technologies for E-Services. Proceedings, 2001. X, 213 pages. 2001.

Vol. 2196: W. Taha (Ed.), Semantics, Applications, and Implementation of Program Generation. Proceedings, 2001. X, 219 pages. 2001.